RB Acc № 1449

PERCUTANEOUS ABSORPTION

DERMATOLOGY

series editors

Charles D. Calnan
Consultant Dermatologist
University of London-British Postgraduate Medical Federation
St. John's Hospital for Diseases of the Skin
London, England

Howard I. Maibach
Department of Dermatology
University of California School of Medicine
San Francisco, California

Volume 1 Neonatal Skin: Structure and Function, *edited by Howard I. Maibach and Edward K. Boisits*
Volume 2 Allergic Contact Dermatitis to Simple Chemicals: A Molecular Approach, *edited by Gilles Dupuis and Claude Benezra*
Volume 3 Contact and Photocontact Allergens: A Manual of Predictive Test Methods, *by Thomas Maurer*
Volume 4 Cutaneous Infestations and Insect Bites, *edited by Milton Orkin and Howard I. Maibach*
Volume 5 Psoriasis, *edited by Henry H. Roenigk, Jr. and Howard I. Maibach*
Volume 6 Percutaneous Absorption: Mechanisms—Methodology—Drug Delivery, *edited by Robert L. Bronaugh and Howard I. Maibach*

Additional Volumes in Preparation

PERCUTANEOUS ABSORPTION

Mechanisms — Methodology — Drug Delivery

Edited by

ROBERT L. BRONAUGH
Division of Toxicology
Food and Drug Administration
Washington, D.C.

HOWARD I. MAIBACH
Department of Dermatology
University of California
School of Medicine
San Francisco, California

MARCEL DEKKER, INC.　　　　　New York and Basel

Library of Congress Cataloging-in-Publication Data
Main entry under title:

Percutaneous absorption.

(Dermatology ; v. 6)
Grew out of the Percutaneous Absorption Symposium held April 27, 1983 at the Food and Drug Administration in Washington, D.C.
Includes bibliographies and index.
1. Dermatopharmacology—Congresses. 2. Skin absorption—Congresses. I. Bronaugh, Robert L., [date]. II. Maibach, Howard I. III. Percutaneous Absorption Symposium (1983 : Washington, D.C.) IV. Series: Dermatology (Marcel Dekker, Inc.) ; v. 6
[DNLM: 1. Skin Absorption—congresses. W1 DE5084 v.6 / WR 102 P4285 1983]

RL801.P47 1985   615'.67   85-15970
ISBN 0-8247-7363-2

COPYRIGHT © 1985 by MARCEL DEKKER, INC. ALL RIGHTS RESERVED

Neither this book nor any part may be reproduced or transmitted in any form or by any means, electronic or mechanical, including photocopying, microfilming, and recording, or by any information storage and retrieval system, without permission in writing from the publisher.

MARCEL DEKKER, INC.
270 Madison Avenue, New York, New York 10016

Current printing (last digit):
10 9 8 7 6 5 4 3 2 1

PRINTED IN THE UNITED STATES OF AMERICA

Introduction to the Series

Many dermatologists along with other doctors and scientists were surprised by the views of an eminent medical Nobel Prize winner who said that all the major discoveries in biology have been made and little can be expected from now on. The scientific achievements of the past 40 years, even in relation to medicine alone, have been so phenomenal that one may wonder if there is anything of importance left for future generations. The same attitude may be taken with regard to medical books, and especially in relation to dermatology. So much has been written over the past 30 years that one may question whether there are any books of value left to be written. Nothing could be further from the truth.

The functions of medical journals and medical books are different. As the number, diversity, and output of journals expands, so does the need for medical books; this is as true for dermatology as for any other branch of medicine. And it is equally true for the subdivisions of dermatology. Some doctors may regret increasing subspecialization within a single branch such as dermatology, but it is a reflection of the steady and inevitable increase in knowledge within the subject. Specialized clinics and departments are now the norm rather than the exception within many university dermatological centers. Their outward manifestation is the growth of subspecialty journals in relation to such subjects as dermatological surgery and oncology, contact dermatitis and occupational dermatoses, microbiology, and pediatric dermatology.

The subdivision of subjects such as dermatology today is a reflection of the subdivision of internal medicine 40 years ago, and it produces similar opposing groups of antagonists. The dearth of the general dermatologist may come to be mourned in the same way as has the dearth of the general physician. But the practical clinical dermatologist and the physician who has responsibility for the care of patients with skin disease will usually depend more on books than on journals when he/she needs help. This is particularly true of dermatologists who work away from university centers, especially outside Western Europe and North America, and who constitute a "silent majority." Although there is still a place for the comprehensive textbook, the growth of specialist books has shown the need for such condensation of recent specialist information.

Marcel Dekker, Inc. has decided to meet this need with a selective series of books on particular branches of dermatology, especially in fields which have frontiers with more than one scientific discipline. The emphasis, however, will be on the information requirements of dermatologists whose responsibilities involve not only the clinical care of patients, but also extend to education and research.

Charles D. Calnan, M.D.
Howard I. Maibach, M.D.

Preface

The impetus for this book results from the 25 speakers at the "Percutaneous Absorption Symposium" held April 27, 1983 at the Food and Drug Administration in Washington, D.C. The overflow crowd of more than 500 persons at this meeting demonstrates the increasing interest in skin permeation, which is due primarily to the recognition of the skin as an important portal of entry of chemicals into the body. The penetration of substances is sometimes desirable and promoted, as in the case of drug delivery, for either a local or systemic effect. At other times, interest in percutaneous absorption stems from a concern about the dermal exposure to potentially toxic agents in topical drug and cosmetic products or agents encountered in the workplace or environment.

This book is our effort to provide a forum for a more complete exposition of the area than has previously been available. Its multiauthored approach supplements the recent excellent texts by Brian Barry (*Dermatological Formulations: Percutaneous Absorption*, Marcel Dekker) and Hans Schaefer, Achim Zesch and Gunter Stuttgen (*Skin Permeability*, Springer-Verlag).

The chapters are divided into three general areas: Mechanisms of Absorption, Methodology, and Drug Delivery. Of course, some chapters could have been placed in more than one of these areas, so the classification is somewhat arbitrary.

The Mechanisms of Absorption section contains chapters dealing with studies on the various factors that affect percutaneous absorption. Pathways of penetration, mathematical models, metabolism, binding, and pharmacokinetics are examples of topics discussed.

In the Methodology section, the various in vivo and in vitro techniques used to measure skin penetration are covered. Chapters include other factors influencing the methodology such as: animal models, volatility of test compound, multiple dosing, artificial membranes, and blood flow studies.

Procedures are discussed for use in the transdermal delivery of drugs. Topics include the effects of penetration enhancers on absorption, optimizing absorption, and the topical delivery of drugs to muscle tissue.

It is hoped that the book will be useful as a source of ideas and references to those engaged in percutaneous absorption studies. For those just planning to begin, the Methodology section, in particular, should be useful.

Robert L. Bronaugh
Howard I. Maibach

Contributors

John H. Anderson, D.V.M. Associate Veterinarian, California Primate Research Center, University of California, Davis, California

Dennis M. Anjo, Ph.D.* Staff Research Associate, Department of Dermatology, University of California School of Medicine, San Francisco, California

Michael B. Aufrere, Ph.D.† Standard Oil Company of California, Richmond, California

Brian W. Barry, Ph.D., D.Sc., F.P.S., C.Chem., F.R.S.C. Professor, Department of Pharmaceutical Technology, University of Bradford, Bradford, West Yorkshire, England

Charanjit R. Behl, M.S., Ph.D. Research Fellow, Pharmacy Research and Development, Hoffmann-LaRoche, Inc., Nutley, New Jersey

Nancy H. Bellantone, Ph.D. Research Scientist, Pharmaceutical Research and Development, Pfizer, Inc., Groton, Connecticut

Irvin H. Blank, Ch.E., Ph.D. Associate Biochemist, Department of Dermatology, Massachusetts General Hospital, Boston, Massachusetts

Robert L. Bronaugh, Ph.D. Research Pharmacologist, Division of Toxicology, Food and Drug Administration, Washington, D.C.

**Present affiliation*: Assistant Professor, Department of Chemistry, California State University, Long Beach, California
†Deceased

Contributors

Daniel A.W. Bucks, M.A. Staff Research Associate, Department of Dermatology, University of California School of Medicine, San Francisco, California

Eugene R. Cooper, Ph.D.* Section Head, Health and Personal Care Division, Miami Valley Laboratories, Proctor and Gamble Company, Cincinnati, Ohio

Neal Corbin, Ph.D.† Armour Research Center, Armour-Dial, Inc., Scottsdale, Arizona

Sandrine I. Courtheoux, Ph.D. Research Worker, Laboratoire de Pharmacologie, Universite de Paris-Sud, Chatenay Malabry, France

Janis L. Demetrulias Toxicologist, Product Safety and Regulatory Affairs, Armour-Dial, Inc., Scottsdale, Arizona

Louis B. Fisher, Ph.D. Manager, Department of Consultant and Medical Relations, Mary Kay Cosmetics, Inc., Dallas, Texas

Gordon L. Flynn, Ph.D. Professor of Pharmaceutics, University of Michigan College of Pharmacy, Ann Arbor, Michigan

Torsten Fredriksson, M.D., Ph.D. Department of Dermatology, Central Hospital, Västeras, Sweden

Christopher L. Gummer, Ph.D. Research Fellow, Department of Dermatology, University of California School of Medicine, San Francisco, California

Richard H. Guy, M.A., Ph.D., C.Chem., M.R.S.C. Assistant Professor, Departments of Pharmacy and Pharmaceutical Chemistry, University of California School of Pharmacy, San Francisco, California

Jonathan Hadgraft, M.A., D.Phil., C.Chem., F.R.S.C.§ Lecturer in Pharmacy, Department of Pharmacy, University of Nottingham, Nottingham, England

Barbara W. Kemppainen, Ph.D.** Research Pharmacologist, Toxicology and Biological Constituents, Research Unit, R.B. Russell Research Center, U.S. Department of Agriculture, Agricultural Research Service, Athens, Georgia

---

Present affiliations:
*Director, Drug Delivery, Alcon Laboratories, Inc., Fort Worth, Texas
†Deceased
‡Consultant, International Drug Development, Paris, France
§Professor of Pharmaceutical Chemistry, The Welsh School of Pharmacy, University of Wales Institute of Science and Technology, Cardiff, Wales
** Department of Pharmacal Sciences, Auburn University School of Pharmacy, Auburn, Alabama

Contributors

James McMaster Staff Research Associate, Department of Dermatology, University of California School of Medicine, San Francisco, California

Howard I. Maibach, M.D. Professor, Department of Dermatology, University of California School of Medicine, San Francisco, California

Jean-Paul Marty, Ph.D. Professor of Pharmaceutics, Laboratoire de Pharmacie Galenique, Faculté de Pharmacie, Université de Picardie, Amiens, France

Efraim Menczel, Ph.D. Director, Pharmaceutical Administration, Ministry of Health, State of Israel, Jerusalem, Israel

Sergio Nacht, Ph.D. Director, Biomedical Research, Richardson-Vicks, Inc., Shelton, Connecticut

Patrick K. Noonan, Ph.D. Manager Pharmacokinetics and Drug Metabolism, Research and Development Division, Key Pharmaceuticals, Inc., Miami, Florida

Helen North-Root, Ph.D. Manager, Department of Product Safety and Regulatory Affairs, Armour-Dial, Inc., Scottsdale, Arizona

Ervin Novak, M.D., Ph.D. Senior Research Physician, Department of Infectious Diseases Research, The Upjohn Company, Kalamazoo, Michigan

Judith G. Pace, Ph.D. Principal Investigator, Pathophysiology Division, U.S. Army Medical Research Institute of Infectious Diseases, Fort Detrick, Frederick, Maryland

Boyd J. Poulsen, Ph.D. Director and Vice President, Institute of Pharmaceutical Sciences, Syntex, Palo Alto, California

Joseph L. Rabinowitz, Ph.D. Veterans Administration Medical Center, University of Pennsylvania, Philadelphia, Pennsylvania

Martin D. Rabinowitz Veterans Administration Medical Center, University of Pennsylvania, Philadelphia, Pennsylvania

William G. Reifenrath, Ph.D. Research Chemist, Division of Cutaneous Hazards, Letterman Army Institute of Research, San Francisco, California

Ronald T. Riley, Ph.D. Research Pharmacologist, Toxicology and Biological Constituents Research Unit, R.B. Russell Research Center, U.S. Department of Agriculture, Agricultural Research Service, Athens, Georgia

Hans Schaefer, Ph.D. Professor and Director, Centre International de Recherches Dermatologiques, Valbonne, France

Wolfgang Schalla, M.D. Head, Department of Pharmacokinetics and Clinical Pharmacology, Centre International de Recherches Dermatologiques, Valbonne, France

Thomas S. Spencer, Ph.D. Manager, Department of Dermal Research, S.C. Johnson & Son, Inc., Racine, Wisconsin

John Surinchak, M.D., Ph.D. Department of Dermatology, University of California School of Medicine, San Francisco, California

Ethel Tur, M.D.[*] Visiting Assistant Professor, Department of Dermatology, University of California School of Medicine, San Francisco, California

Jacques L. Wepierre, M.Sc. Professor, Department of Pharmacology, Faculté de Pharmacie, Université de Paris-SUD, Chatenay Malabry, France

Ronald C. Wester, Ph.D. Assistant Research Dermatologist, Department of Dermatology and Assistant Adjunct Professor, Department of Pharmacy, University of California School of Medicine, San Francisco, California

Leszek J. Wolfram, Ph.D. Vice President of Research, Clairol, Inc., Stamford, Connecticut

Paul K. Wotton, Ph.D. Research Pharmacist, Department of Pharmacy, University of Nottingham, Nottingham, England

David Yeung, M.S. Senior Research Investigator, Department of Dermatological Research, Personal Care Division, Richardson-Vicks, Inc., Shelton, Connecticut

Joel L. Zatz, Ph.D. Professor of Pharmaceutics, Department of Pharmacy, Rutgers University College of Pharmacy, Piscataway, New Jersey

---

[*]*Present affiliation*: Senior Attending Physician, Department of Dermatology, Ichilov Medical Center, Tel Aviv, Israel

Contents

Introduction to the Series   iii
Preface   v
Contributors   vii

MECHANISMS OF ABSORPTION

1. **Mathematical Models of Percutaneous Absorption**   *Richard H. Guy and Jonathan Hadgraft*   3

   Models utilizing Fick's first law • Models utilizing Fick's second law • Pharmacokinetic models • References

2. **Mechanism of Percutaneous Absorption from Physicochemical Evidence**   *Gordon L. Flynn*   17

   General techniques of membrane characterization • Partitioning effects on percutaneous absorption • Influence of pH on permeability of weak electrolytes • Barrier properties as revealed by membrane sectioning • Chemical and thermal effects and barrier property • Integration of anatomy with the physicochemical evidence • References

3. **Skin Binding During Percutaneous Penetration**   *Efraim Menczel, Daniel A.W. Bucks, Ronald C. Wester, and Howard I. Maibach*   43

   Epidermal retention of chemicals in percutaneous penetration • Dermal association with chemicals in percutaneous penetration • Binding affinity versus partitioning of chemicals into skin • tissue • Sequential binding of chemicals in percutaneous absorption • Conclusions • References

4. Skin Metabolism: Theoretical   *Richard H. Guy and Jonathan Hadgraft*   57

Theoretical models • References

5. Cutaneous Metabolism of Xenobiotics   *Patrick K. Noonan and Ronald C. Wester*   65

Steroid metabolism • Cutaneous metabolism of polycyclic aromatic hydrocarbons • Miscellaneous cutaneous metabolic reactions • Enzyme induction and inhibition • Pharmacological and toxicological implications of skin metabolism • Skin metabolism and percutaneous absorption • Discussion • References

6. Facilitated Percutaneous Absorption of Anionic Drugs   *Jonathan Hadgraft and Paul K. Wotton*   87

Facilitated transport: The mechanism • In vitro modeling of skin absorption • In vitro permeation of salicylate across human skin • References

7. The Effect of Hydration on the Permeability of the Skin   *Irvin H. Blank*   97

References

8. Structure-Activity Correlations in Percutaneous Absorption   *Ronald C. Wester and Howard I. Maibach*   107

Partition coefficient • Chemical structure and percutaneous absorption • Molecular weight • Ionization • Vapor pressure • Colinearity • Discussion • References

9. Dermatopharmacokinetics in Clinical Dermatology   *Ronald C. Wester and Howard I. Maibach*   125

Dose and dosing regimen: Clinical and toxicological implications • Individual and site variations • Percutaneous absorption in diseased skin • Special consideration for the neonate • References

10. Skin Delipidization and Percutaneous Absorption   *Efraim Menczel*   133

Skin lipids • Skin delipidization • Percutaneous absorption after skin delipidization • Percutaneous hazards of organic solvents • Conclusions • References

11. Skin Deposition and Penetration of Triclocarban   *Helen North-Root, Neal Corbin, and Janis Demetrulias*   141

Deposition • Percutaneous penetration • Discussion • References

Contents

12. Topical Pharmacokinetics of [^{14}C] Butylated Hydroxytoluene in the Guinea Pig   *Sandrine I. Courtheoux, Jean-Paul Marty, and Jacques L. Wepierre* ... 153

    Experimental • Results • Discussion • Conclusion • References

13. Percutaneous Absorption: Computer Simulation Using Multicompartmented Membrane Models   *Joel L. Zatz* ... 165

    Description of the models • Simulation studies • Conclusions • References

14. Influence of Age on Percutaneous Absorption of Drug Substances ... 183
    Charanjit R. Behl, Nancy H. Bellantone, and Gordon L. Flynn

    In vivo percutaneous absorption studies • In vitro skin permeation studies • References

15. In Vitro Studies on the Permeability of Infant Skin   *Louis B. Fisher* ... 213

    Materials and methods • Calculations • Results • Discussion • References

16. Predictability of In Vitro Diffusion Systems: Effect of Skin Types and Ages on Percutaneous Absorption of Triclocarban   *Ronald C. Wester, Howard I. Maibach, John Surinchak, and Daniel A. W. Bucks* ... 223

    Introduction • Materials and methods • Results and discussion • References

17. In Vivo Percutaneous Absorption of Paraquat from Hands, Legs, and Forearm of Man   *Ronald C. Wester, Howard I. Maibach, Daniel A. W. Bucks, and Michael B. Aufrere* ... 227

    Introduction • Materials and methods • Results • Discussion • References

18. Influence of Hydration on Percutaneous Absorption   *Ronald C. Wester and Howard I. Maibach* ... 231

    Early studies • Recent work • Directions for future work • References

METHODOLOGY

19. In Vivo Methods for Percutaneous Absorption Measurements ... 245
    Ronald C. Wester and Howard I. Maibach

    Importance of in vivo percutaneous absorption • In vivo methods • Factors and steps in percutaneous absorption • References

Contents

20. In Vivo Animal Models for Percutaneous Absorption *Ronald C. Wester and Howard I. Maibach* — 251

    Comparative in vivo studies • Comparative in vitro studies • The in vitro model • Discussion • References

21. Determination of Percutaneous Absorption by In Vitro Techniques *Robert L. Bronaugh* — 267

    In vitro methodology • In vivo/in vitro comparisons • Hydrophobic compounds • Animal models for human skin • Solubility properties of penetrant • Conclusions • References

22. Localization of Compounds in Different Skin Layers and Its Use as an Indicator of Percutaneous Absorption *Wolfgang Schalla and Hans Schaefer* — 281

    Methods • Drug concentrations in the skin • Drug concentration in diseased skin • Influx into the skin and efflux into the body • Calculations of percutaneous resorption • Conclusions and summary • References

23. Evaporation and Penetration from Skin *William G. Reifenrath and Thomas S. Spencer* — 305

    Modes of loss from the skin surface • Methods • Comparison of skin penetration and evaporation in vitro and in vivo • Factors affecting the evaporation and penetration process • Pharmacological significance of evaporation of chemicals from the skin • Conclusion • References

24. Dermal Decontamination and Percutaneous Absorption *Ronald C. Wester and Howard I. Maibach* — 327

    Effects of occlusion and washing • Conclusion: Substantivity • References

25. Radial Transport in the Dermis *Richard H. Guy, Jonathan Hadgraft, and Howard I. Maibach* — 335

    Experimental observations • Interpretation • Conclusion • References

26. Interrelationships in the Dose Response of Percutaneous Absorption *Ronald C. Wester and Howard I. Maibach* — 347

    Effects of concentration on percutaneous absorption • Effect of application frequency • Application frequency and toxicity • Discussion • References

27. Does Rubbing Enhance In Vivo Dermal Absorption? *James McMaster, Howard I. Maibach, Ronald C. Wester, and Daniel A. W. Bucks* — 359

    Introduction • Methods • Results • Discussion • References

Contents

28. Polychlorinated Biphenyls: Dermal Absorption, Systemic Elimination, and Dermal Wash Efficiency *Ronald C. Wester, Daniel A. W. Bucks, Howard I. Maibach, and John H. Anderson* 363
    Introduction • Materials and methods • Results • Discussion • References

29. Artificial Membranes and Skin Permeability *Sergio Nacht and David Yeung* 373
    Materials and methods • Results • Discussion • References

30. Receptor Fluid Penetrant Interactions and the In Vitro Cutaneous Penetration of Chemicals *Ronald T. Riley and Barbara W. Kemppainen* 387
    Methods • Results and discussion • References

31. Blood Flow Studies and Percutaneous Absorption *Richard H. Guy, Ethel Tur, Ronald C. Wester, and Howard I. Maibach* 393
    Experimental techniques • Results • Conclusions • References

32. Hair Dye Penetration in Monkey and Man *Leszek J. Wolfram* 409
    Experimental • Results • References

33. Penetration of Mycotoxins Through Excised Human Skin *Barbara W. Kemppainen, Ronald T. Riley, and Judith G. Pace* 423
    Methods • Results and discussion • References

34. In Vitro Methods Used to Study Dermal Delivery and Percutaneous Absorption *Boyd J. Poulsen and Gordon L. Flynn* 431
    In vitro diffusion studies: No membrane • Studies involving membranes other than the skin • In vitro studies in which skin is the membrane • Summary • References

35. Calculations of Body Exposure from Percutaneous Absorption Data *Richard H. Guy and Howard I. Maibach* 461
    Calculations • Conclusions • References

DRUG DELIVERY

36. Percutaneous Penetration as a Method of Delivery to Muscle and Other Tissues *Jean-Paul Marty, Richard H. Guy, and Howard I. Maibach* 469
    Experimental results • Conclusions • References

37. Optimizing Percutaneous Absorption *Brian W. Barry* 489
    Cadaver skin experiments: In vitro methods • Vasoconstrictor assay: In vivo method • Correlation between optimization theory

and clinical efficacy • Protocol for optimizing a dermatological formulation • References

38. **Percutaneous Absorption of Corticosteroids: Systemic Effects**   513
    Torsten Fredriksson

    Approach to the study • Methods and amounts • Frequency of application • Measurement of adrenal suppression • Areas of uncertainty • Special cases • References

39. **Vehicle Effects on Skin Penetration**   *Eugene R. Cooper*   525

    Diffusion factors • Compositional and structural factors • Penetration enhancers • Summary • References

40. **Absorption of Triethanolamine 7-[^{14}C]Salicylate in Human and Animal Joints**   *Joseph L. Rabinowitz and Martin D. Rabinowitz*   531

    Historical development • Methodology • Results • Conclusions • Summary • References

41. **In Vivo Skin and Nitroglycerin Transdermal Delivery**   541
    Ronald C. Wester

    Factors influencing percutaneous absorption • Apparent transdermal absorption rates (humans) • Summary • References

42. **Pharmacodynamics and Percutaneous Absorption: Minoxidil Stimulates Cutaneous Blood Flow in Balding Human Scalps**   *Ronald C. Wester, Howard I. Maibach, Richard H. Guy, and Ervin Novak*   547

    Introduction • Methods • Results • Discussion • References

43. **Vehicles as Penetration Enhancers**   *Christopher L. Gummer*   561

    Cosmetic and therapeutic effects • Vehicles as penetration enhancers • Drug solubility • Drug concentration • Skin/vehicle interface • Skin hydration • Partition coefficient • Vehicle additives • Ideal vehicles • References

44. **Effect of a Water Vapor Permeable Film on the Percutaneous Penetration of Hydrocortisone**   *Dennis M. Anjo and Howard I. Maibach*   571

    Materials and methods • Results • Discussion • References

Index   575

PERCUTANEOUS ABSORPTION

MECHANISMS OF ABSORPTION

1
Mathematical Models of Percutaneous Absorption

Richard H. Guy
University of California School of Pharmacy, San Francisco, California

Jonathan Hadgraft*
University of Nottingham, Nottingham, England

The skin forms a complex barrier to the external environment, maintaining body fluids within our system and excluding harmful substances. It would be very useful to be able to predict the rate at which materials penetrate the skin, to assess potential toxicological hazards and also to improve the way in which drugs are administered topically. The ability to predict quantitatively the absorption of substances through the skin has implications in the pharmaceutical, chemical, and cosmetic industries and also in environmental health. An accurate model describing skin penetration will also be of benefit in determining the relative importance of such variables as loss of compound from the skin surface (volatility and substantivity) and metabolism as the substance diffuses. One of the major difficulties in generating a good model is the inherent biological variation of the skin; the disease or damage condition of the skin also presents obstacles. Regional variations in the permeability of the stratum corneum are important but are difficult to quantify.

In establishing a model it is necessary to consider the fundamental physiology of the epidermis and relate this to the possible rate-determining steps in the permeation process. Since all compounds are thought to transfer by a passive diffusion mechanism, it is then possible to apply Fick's laws of diffusion to obtain a solution to the problem. Further simplifications are possible in some circumstances, and the diffusive properties of the epidermis may be related to the first-order rate constants generated in a pharmacokinetic model. This approach is particularly valuable if the mathematical treatment is to be used in a clinical context.

The structure of the skin relevant to the production of a mathematical model is given in Figure 1. It would be impossible to solve the diffusion equations if the

---
*Present affiliation: University of Wales Institute of Science and Technology, Cardiff, Wales

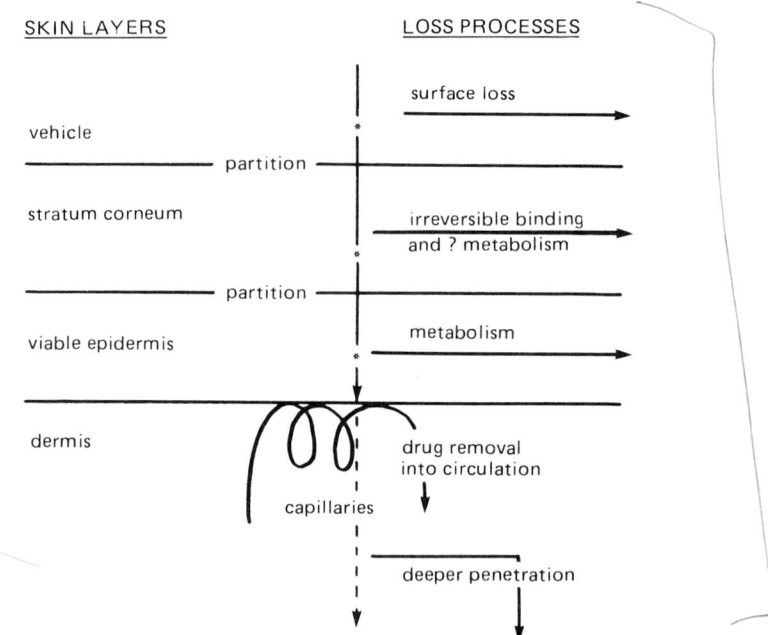

Figure 1 Schematic representation of the skin.

various layers of the skin were not considered to be homogeneous. Thus the layers themselves have different properties, but within a layer the barrier function is assumed constant. To a first approximation this is valid. It is thus possible to consider diffusion through the applied formulation, through the stratum corneum, and through the viable epidermis, and transport away from the site by the cutaneous vasculature. The models allow these diffusion steps to be examined and include partitioning between the various layers. It is also possible to include metabolic steps that occur as the molecule diffuses. Metabolism may be simulated by either first-order or Michaelis-Menten kinetics. With this type of approach it is possible to consider the following as potential rate-controlling factors.

1. *Diffusion through the delivery device/formulation.* Useful for assessing transdermal drug delivery systems.
2. *Diffusion through the stratum corneum.* The most common rate-limiting step.
3. *Diffusion through the viable epidermis.* A possible rate-controlling process for very lipophilic materials or for damaged skin.

MODELS UTILIZING FICK'S FIRST LAW

The most simple way of modeling the process of skin absorption is to assume that Fick's first law of diffusion is applicable. This may be a valid approximation in some in vitro experiments but is unlikely to be a true assumption in vivo. This stems from the fact that the stratum corneum is a very impermeable barrier, and therefore a long time is required to establish steady-state conditions. The length of time is unlikely to be attained in normal therapeutic or cosmetic applications. However it is important to study skin absorption in vitro, and several useful facts are exemplified by this type of analysis (Katz and Poulsen, 1971). The form of the equation often quoted is:

$$\frac{dQ}{dt} = \frac{D \cdot K_p c}{h}$$

where

dQ/dt = rate of skin penetration
D = effective diffusion coefficient of drug in stratum corneum
K_p = partition coefficient of drug between skin and vehicle
c = concentration of drug in vehicle (equation is valid only if it is assumed that the concentration of drug in receptor phase is zero)
h = effective thickness of skin barrier

Thus if we consider the interactions that exist between the drug, the vehicle, and the skin, we can see that the partition behavior is of paramount importance. The diffusion of the drug through the skin is also important, as is the driving force for diffusion, the concentration of the dissolved drug. It must be remembered however that this is a simplified equation; it will hold only for steady-state conditions and will not be valid if there are significant interactions, such as binding, between the drug and components of the skin.

The main characteristics of the permeant that influence the transfer rate are the partition coefficient and the diffusion coefficient in the stratum corneum. It is not easy to measure skin/vehicle partition coefficients, and these two constants are sometimes multiplied together to give a permeability constant. However by simple formulation changes it is possible to alter D, K_p, and c. In any formulation exercise designed to optimize delivery, it is these parameters that may be varied. The composition of the formulation should maximize the thermodynamic activity of the drug in the preparation (Higuchi, 1960). This is not always an easy task, since by increasing c we will decrease K_p. A balance has to be achieved between these two parameters (Ostrenga et al., 1971).

In the type of in vitro study where steady-state conditions prevail it is also possible to examine the component resistances of the different layers in the skin: the stratum corneum, the viable epidermis, and the dermis (Foreman and Kelly, 1976). When Fick's first law holds, the resistances may be summed:

$$R_{skin} = R_{stratum\ corneum} + R_{viable\ epidermis} + R_{dermis}$$

This type of evaluation of resistances is often useful in ascertaining the rate-limiting step to the overall transfer process.

In a heterogeneous structural model of the stratum corneum proposed by Michaels et al. (1975), the skin is represented in the form of "bricks and mortar," with the dead keratinized cells being the bricks and the intercellular channels the mortar. Using this simplified approach it is possible to develop Fick's first law to explain the different routes of penetration through the barrier layer. In this analysis it has been suggested that the interstitial lipid phase is the main barrier to penetration.

MODELS UTILIZING FICK'S SECOND LAW

We have already mentioned that in real situations steady-state conditions are unlikely to be established during the penetration of drugs across the skin. To analyze the fluxes and concentration profiles under these conditions, it is necessary to obtain solutions to Fick's second law of diffusion:

$$\frac{\partial c}{\partial t} = D \frac{\partial^2 c}{\partial x^2}$$

Solutions to this second-order differential equation are complex and depend on the boundary conditions for the experiment. To obtain simple analytical solutions to this differential equation, it is usually necessary to resort to approximations. However in some circumstances computer analyses have been used to obtain full solutions to the diffusion equation. Even so, some of these are valid only when the concentration gradient across the stratum corneum has attained steady state (Ando et al., 1977). Using this approach, the authors have examined the influence of metabolism in the skin with concurrent diffusion (see Chapter 4).

In vivo it is more pertinent to obtain solutions to Fick's second law of diffusion for non-steady-state conditions (Scheuplein, 1967). The solutions to this equation depend on the boundary conditions imposed by the experiment. In one case, the use of Franz-type diffusion cells with an infinite dose in the donor compartment, the following equation describes the amount of drug appearing in the receptor phase:

$$M = \frac{Dct}{h} - \frac{hc}{6} \frac{2hc}{\pi^2} \sum_{n=1}^{\infty} \frac{(-1)^n}{n^2} \exp\left(\frac{-Dn^2\pi^2 t}{h^2}\right)$$

where

    M = cumulative amount of drug in receptor phase
    D = diffusion coefficient of drug in skin
    h = thickness of skin
    c = concentration of drug in donor compartment
    t = elapsed time of experiment

The typical profile of M versus t is shown in Figure 2. At short time periods the equation above may be expressed (Hadgraft, 1979a; Rodgers et al., 1954; Short et al., 1970):

$$\log\left(\frac{M}{t^{3/2}}\right) = \log\left(\frac{8c}{h^2 \pi^{1/2}}\right) + \frac{3}{2} \log D - \frac{h^2}{9.2Dt}$$

This expression may be used to evaluate the diffusion coefficient of the drug and has also been used to analyze the in vivo penetration of esters of nicotinic acid

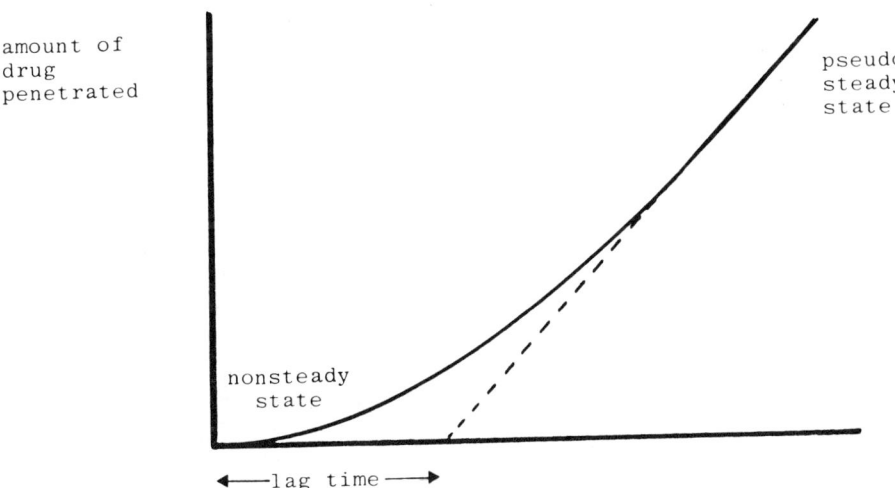

Figure 2 Typical profile of concentration versus time for diffusion through the epidermis.

(Albery and Hadgraft, 1979a,b). However the usual method of analyzing profiles such as those given in Figure 2 is to estimate the lag time (L) by extrapolation of the linear portion of the curve to the axis M = 0. The diffusion coefficient is then given by:

$$D = \frac{h^2}{6L}$$

Another complex series similar in form to that above describes the concentration profile of the drug in the stratum corneum. If u is the normalized concentration at distance x from the skin surface:

$$u = 1 - x + \frac{2}{\pi} \sum_{n=1}^{\infty} \left(\frac{-1}{n}\right)^n \exp\left(\frac{-n^2 \pi^2 Dt}{h^2}\right) \sin[n\pi(1-x)]$$

A typical profile and the results for the concentration distribution of glycerol in the stratum corneum of nude mice are given in Figure 3. This type of analysis is useful in predicting the concentration of drug throughout the skin and indicates targeting to specific regions of the epidermal barrier.

Theoretical papers using an idealized skin model have solved the diffusion equations for more than one layer (e.g., vehicle and stratum corneum, stratum corneum and viable epidermis). One example of the latter is the description of the reservoir effect of the stratum corneum as a function of the stratum corneum/viable epidermis partition coefficient (Hadgraft, 1979b). Even considering modest partition characteristics, it is possible for the drug to be held back in the stratum corneum. This is shown in Figure 4, which illustrates the fraction of the applied dose that arrives at the skin capillary network as a function of the time after application. Hydrocortisone, which has a skin/water partition coefficient of approximately 10 would still be present in the stratum corneum at a level of 10% of the original concentration 6 or 7 days postapplication. The fluorinated steroids have oil/water partition coefficients approximately 10 times that of hydrocortisone and would be expected to exhibit a more marked reservoir capacity.

This type of analysis has also been adopted to investigate the effect of the thickness of the applied base on the amount of drug reaching the systemic circulation (Guy and Hadgraft, 1980). Table 1 shows the ratios of drug released compared to the applied amount for the thickest application (1000 μm) at different time intervals. The data indicate that at short times after application, the vehicle thickness does not affect the amount penetrating but, as time progresses, significant deviations occur. An appreciation of this effect will be important in the rational design of transdermal drug delivery systems.

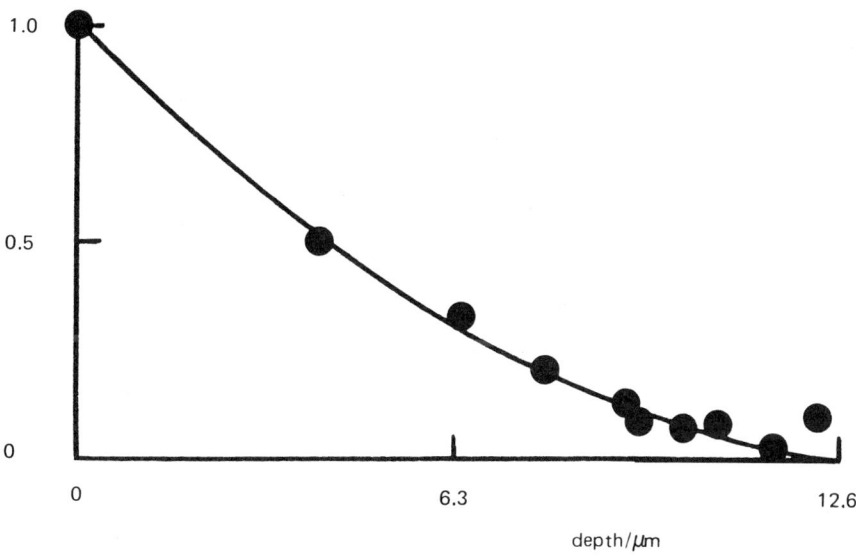

Figure 3 Profile of concentration versus distance of radiolabeled glycerol in the stratum corneum of nude mice. The concentration has been normalized with respect to the concentration in the outermost layer of the stratum corneum.

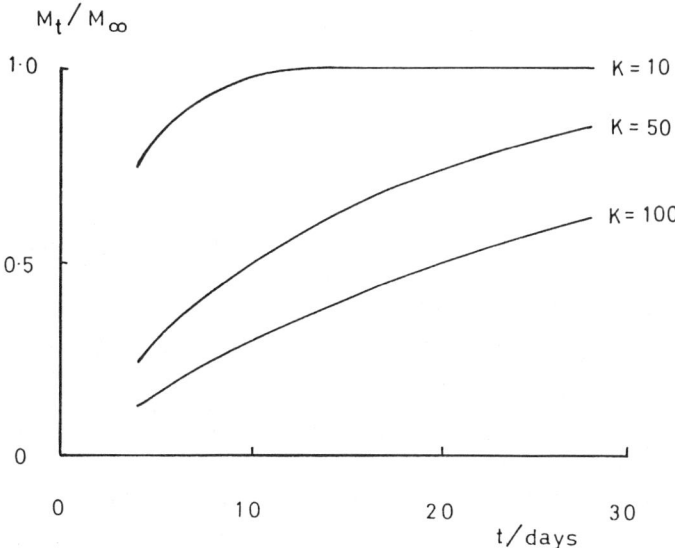

Figure 4 The dose fraction released into the dermal capillaries over a 28-day period following topical application of drugs with varying partition coefficients.

Table 1 Ratios of Drug Released Compared to the Applied Amount for the Thickest Application ($\ell_0 = 1000$ μm) at Different Time[a] Intervals

ℓ_0/μm	$\tau = 1$	$\tau = 2$	$\tau = 5$	$\tau = 10$	$\tau = 15$
100	0.022	0.039	0.071	0.092	0.098
250	0.024	0.045	0.098	0.158	0.194
500	0.024	0.048	0.111	0.197	0.269
750	0.024	0.048	0.114	0.211	0.294
1000	0.024	0.049	0.118	0.221	0.313

[a] $\tau = D_s t/\ell_s^2$ where t is time (sec) and D_s is the diffusion coefficient of the drug in the stratum corneum, the thickness of which is ℓ_s.

PHARMACOKINETIC MODELS

The ultimate aim of a mathematical model for percutaneous absorption is to provide a simple but effective means of estimating drug levels in the skin, blood, and urine following topical administration. In this context various attempts have been made at pharmacokinetic modeling. Such a model would be invaluable for assessing the merits of transdermal drug delivery. This approach has been adopted by Chandrasekaran et al. (1978), but the conclusions are specific to the drug scopolamine. For this compound the authors were able to obtain very good correlation between experimental and predicted urinary excretion data. Other individual drugs that have been subject to pharmacokinetic appraisal include norephedrine (Riegelman, 1974), methotrexate (Wallace and Barnett, 1978), and indomethacin (Naito and Tsai, 1981).

Ideally any model should have wide applicability, and for this reason the rate constants in the pharmacokinetic scheme should relate to the physicochemical properties of the diffusing drug. Guy et al. (1982) consider the relevance of these properties and the nature of the skin structure in their model, which is illustrated in Figure 5, where k_1 describes drug diffusion through the stratum corneum (this variable depends on the molecular weight and will be slow), k_2 relates to drug diffusion through the viable epidermis and may be estimated by consideration of characteristic diffusion rates in aqueous protein gels, and k_3 is a measure of the drug's affinity for the stratum corneum compared to the viable epidermis. The ratio k_3/k_2 may be regarded as the "partition coefficient" of the drug between the stratum corneum and the viable tissue. The larger the value of k_3, the higher the affinity for the stratum corneum and therefore the larger the reservoir effect. Finally, k_4 is the classic pharmacokinetic elimination rate constant following intravenous administration. This is a number that cannot be estimated but must be obtained experimentally. However, for most drugs this rate is routinely measured before marketing and is usually readily available.

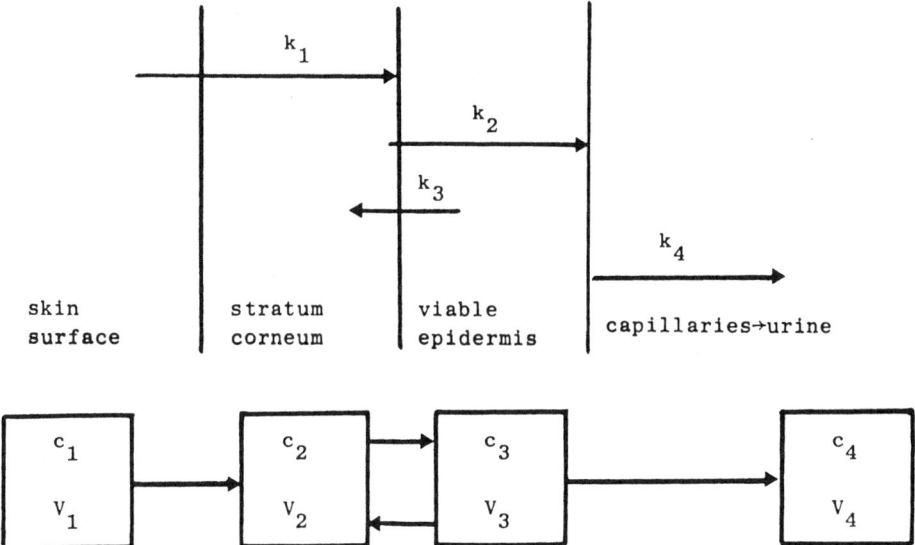

Figure 5 Schematic representation of the pharmacokinetic model.

An example of the pharmacokinetic approach is given in Figure 6. In this study the excretion pattern of testosterone was monitored and the results shown as the solid circles (Anjo et al., 1980). A theoretical analysis using the pharmacokinetic model described above is shown as a solid line (Guy et al., 1982). There is good agreement between the two showing the validity of this type of mathematical model.

The model has also been used to predict the disposition of the drug in the skin and plasma as a function of its physicochemical properties (Guy and Hadgraft, 1983, 1984). Another problem associated with topical delivery is consideration of multiple dosing to the same site. The pharmacokinetic model described above may be used to interpret this type of data, and Figure 7 shows the theoretical profile (Guy et al., 1983) and the experimental data for the multiple application of hydrocortisone (Wester et al., 1980). There is good agreement, and the difference in excretion pattern between labeled drug applied on day 0 and on day 7 may be attributed to the physicochemical properties of hydrocortisone. This steroid exhibits a reservoir or drug-binding effect and therefore takes several days to establish steady-state conditions. Hence greater elimination is exhibited after the second radioactive dose.

This modeling approach may also be used to assess vehicle effects by incorporating an input rate constant to the skin surface. The constant may be either first or zero order, but both will be assigned values dependent on the

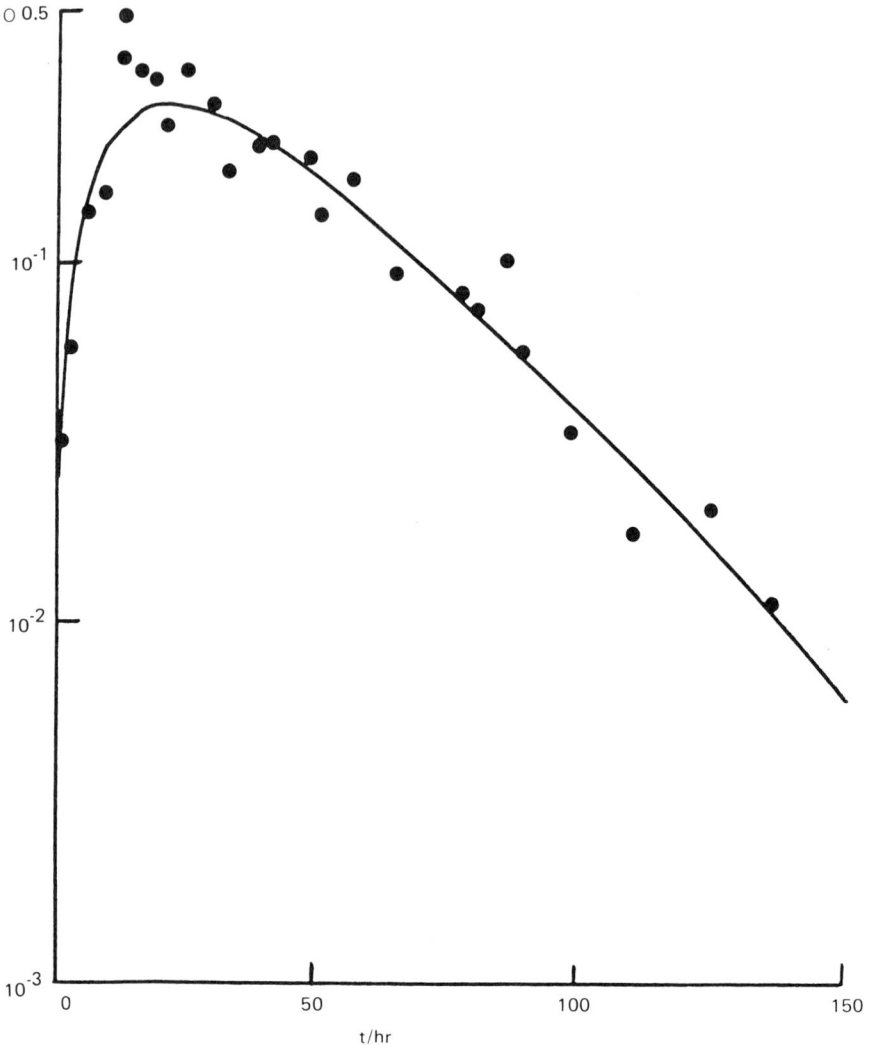

Figure 6 Urinary excretion data following topical administration of testosterone (●). Solid line is the theoretical model.

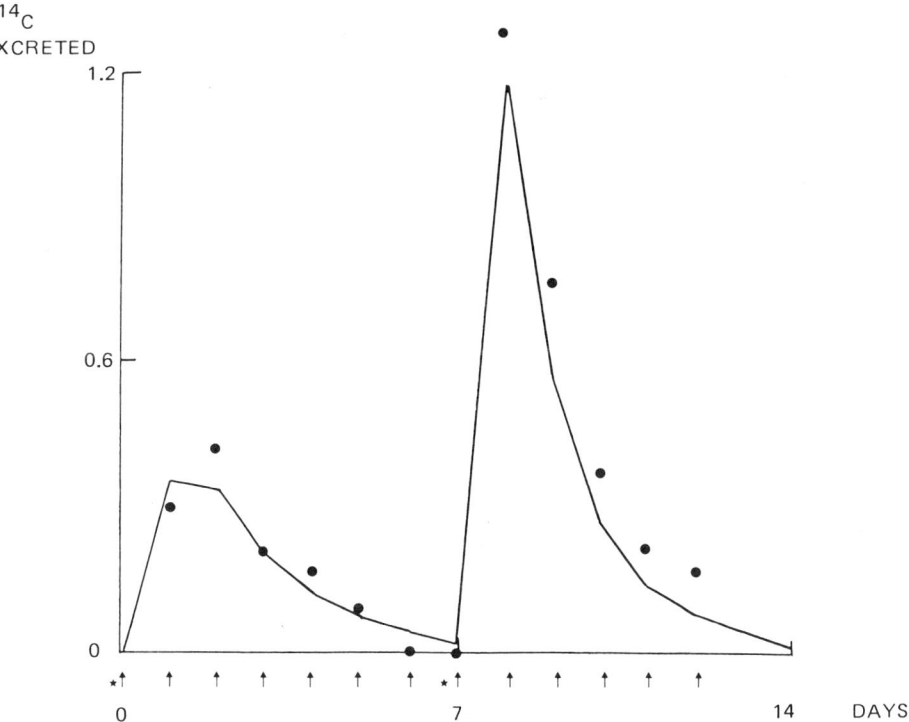

Figure 7 Percutaneous absorption of [^{14}C]hydrocortisone: ↑ represents hydrocortisone application and *↑ represents [^{14}C]hydrocortisone application. ● Represents experimental points, and the solid line is the theoretical curve predicted by the pharmacokinetic model.

nature of the vehicle or delivery system and the drug properties. In this way it will be possible to screen potential transdermal candidates, a topic of considerable current interest.

ACKNOWLEDGMENTS

We would like to thank Mrs. U. Lashmar for the data in Figure 3. We would also like to thank the following for financial assistance: the Burroughs Wellcome Fund, the Wellcome Trust, and Alza and Hoffmann La Roche.

REFERENCES

Albery, W. J. and Hadgraft, J. (1979a). Percutaneous absorption: Theoretical description. *J. Pharm. Pharmacol. 31*: 129-139.

Albery, W. J. and Hadgraft, J. (1979b). Percutaneous absorption: In vivo experiments. *J. Pharm. Pharmacol. 31*: 140-147.

Ando, H. Y., Ho, N. F. H., and Higuchi, W. I. (1977). Skin as an active metabolizing barrier. I: Theoretical analysis of topical bioavailability. *J. Pharm. Sci. 66*: 1525-1528.

Anjo, D. M., Feldman, R. J., and Maibach, H. I. (1980). Methods for predicting percutaneous penetration in man. In *Percutaneous Penetration of Steroids*. Edited by P. Mauvais-Jarvais, J. Wepierre, and C. F. H. Vickers. Academic, New York, pp. 31-51.

Chandrasekaran, S. K., Bayne, W., and Shaw, J. E. (1978). Pharmacokinetics of drug permeation through human skin. *J. Pharm. Sci. 67*: 1370-1374.

Foreman, M. and Kelly, I. (1976). The diffusion of nandrolone through hydrated human cadaver skin. *Br. J. Dermatol. 95*: 265-270.

Guy, R. H. and Hadgraft, J. (1980). A theoretical description relating skin penetration to the thickness of the applied medicament. *Int. J. Pharm. 6*: 321-332.

Guy, R. H. and Hadgraft, J. (1983). Physicochemical interpretation of the pharmacokinetics of percutaneous absorption. *J. Pharmacokinet. Biopharm. 11*: 189-203.

Guy, R. H. and Hadgraft, J. (1984). Prediction of drug disposition kinetics in skin and plasma following topical application. *J. Pharm. Sci. 73*: 883-887.

Guy, R. H., Hadgraft, J., and Maibach, H. I. (1982). A pharmacokinetic model for percutaneous absorption. *Int. J. Pharm. 11*: 119-129.

Guy, R. H., Hadgraft, J., and Maibach, H. I. (1983). Percutaneous absorption: Multidose pharmacokinetics. *Int. J. Pharm. 17*: 23-28.

Hadgraft, J. (1979a). Calculations of drug release rates from controlled release devices. The slab. *Int. J. Pharm. 2*: 177-194.

Hadgraft, J. (1979b). The epidermal reservoir: A theoretical approach. *Int. J. Pharm. 2*: 265-274.

Higuchi, T. (1960). Physical chemical analysis of percutaneous absorption process from creams and ointments. *J. Soc. Cosmet. Chem. 11*: 85-97.

Katz, M. and Poulsen, B. J. (1971). Absorption of drugs through the skin. In *Handbook of Experimental Pharmacology*, Vol. XXXVIII/1. Edited by B. B. Brodie and J. Gillette. Springer-Verlag, Berlin.

Michaels, A. S., Chandrasekaran, S. K., and Shaw, J. E. (1975). Drug permeation through human skin, theory and in vitro experimental measurement. *AIChEJ. 21*: 985-996.

Naito, S.-I. and Tsai, Y.-H. (1981). Percutaneous absorption of indomethacin from ointment bases in rabbits. *Int. J. Pharm. 8*: 263-276.

Ostrenga, J., Steinmetz, C., and Poulsen, B. (1971). Significance of vehicle composition. I. Relationship between topical vehicle composition, skin penetrability, and clinical efficacy. *J. Pharm. Sci. 60*: 1175-1179.

Riegelman, S. (1974). Pharmacokinetic factors affecting epidermal penetration and percutaneous absorption. *Clin. Pharmacol. Ther. 16*: 873-883.

Rodgers, W. A., Buritz, R. S., and Alpert, D. (1954). The diffusion coefficient, solubility and permeability of helium in glass. *J. Appl. Physiol. 25*: 868-875.

Scheuplein, R. J. (1967). Mechanism of percutaneous absorption. II. Transient diffusion and the relative importance of various routes of skin penetration. *J. Invest. Dermatol. 45*: 334-346.

Short, P. M., Abbs, E. T., and Rhodes, C. T. (1970). The effect of nonionic surfactants on the transport of testosterone across a cellulose acetate membrane. *J. Pharm. Sci. 59*: 995-998.

Wallace, S. M. and Barnett, G. (1978). Pharmacokinetic analysis of percutaneous absorption: Evidence of parallel penetration pathways for methotrexate. *J. Pharmacokinet. Biopharm. 6*: 315-325.

Wester, R. C., Noonan, P. K., and Maibach, H. I. (1980). Percutaneous absorption of hydrocortisone increases with long-term administration. *Arch. Dermatol. 116*: 186-188.

2
Mechanism of Percutaneous Absorption from Physicochemical Evidence

Gordon L. Flynn
University of Michigan College of Pharmacy, Ann Arbor, Michigan

GENERAL TECHNIQUES OF MEMBRANE CHARACTERIZATION

All living membranes are heterogeneous and composed of distinct macroscopic phases, and passive diffusion of molecules across the total barrier imposed by such membranes is necessarily dependent on the organization and sequencing of the phases encountered in the transport process. An inviolate rule of diffusion is that molecules follow the path of least diffusional resistance. The path of least resistance is determined by the physicochemical natures of the membrane's phases or by the densities, the viscosities and, where protein and other macromolecules are present, the extent of cross-linking and packing of such polymeric matter within the respective phases, all of which affect rates of diffusive movement. The path of least resistance is also affected by relative affinities of the phases for the permeant, the latter being responsible for the internal distribution of the permeant throughout the component physicochemical regimes of the membrane, and by the relative volumes of the phases.

The resistance of each distinct phase within a membrane can be characterized in specific terms that relate diffusion within a phase to all variables implicit in the generalizations above. Overall, a membrane may be regarded as a resistor of sorts in a circuit between two phases. The individual phases of the membrane determine the channeling of diffusive flows within the interior elements of the membrane based on their individual resistances and organization. The internal phase resistances are arranged either in series, in parallel, or as dispersed particulate resistors. When arranged in series the mass current or "diffusional flux" across the membrane is determined by the summed resistances of the laminae of the membrane. When in parallel the phases support separate currents that, in the simplest instance involving independency of the routes, are additive upon attainment of the steady state of diffusion. Dispersed phases act either as shunts, which hasten the diffusional process across the space they occupy when they are more permeable than the medium in which they are embedded, or they impede diffusion by blocking out volume otherwise available for diffusion when they are relatively impervious. The quantitative effects of dispersed phases on diffusion relate not only to the permeability of the particles but also to their numbers, sizes, shapes, and orientations in the diffusional field. Thus, while the principles of diffusion associated with dispersed phases are easy to generalize and understand, this particular complexity is difficult to deal with rigorously. The skin is so complex that all the foregoing have to be brought to bear in its barrier analysis.

Mathematically, the steady-state current J in a simple series barrier case can be represented by:

$$J = A \left(\frac{1}{R_1 + R_2 + \cdots + R_n} \right) (\Delta C) \tag{1}$$

where J has the units of mass per time. Here ΔC is the concentration drop across the membrane as measured in generally well-stirred, like phases external to but in contact with the membrane. When the external media are the same or even highly similar, ΔC accurately reflects the chemical potential difference existing across the membrane. In almost all skin permeation studies to date, the driving force for diffusion is the chemical potential gradient expressed across the tissue, no matter whether in vitro or in vivo methods have been used. The term

$$\frac{1}{R_1 + R_2 + \cdots + R_n} \tag{2}$$

is a mass transfer coefficient generally referred to as the permeability coefficient; $R_1, R_2, \ldots, R_n$ represent resistances of individual strata in the series, and it can be seen that the permeability coefficient is simply the reciprocal of the sum of these in the series barrier case. Thus the diffusional flux can be represented by:

$$J = A P (\Delta C) \tag{3}$$

where P is the permeability coefficient, a term that is analogous to conductivity in the electrical flux equation. Actually, Equation 3 is a general form of the mass transfer equation useful in describing steady-state mass transfer processes. Of course P itself takes different mathematical forms depending on the internal structural organization of a membrane. However P is always the reciprocal of the total diffusional resistance, no matter its source in the field of a membrane. In the simplest possible case of permeation, diffusion across an isotropic membrane, P takes a familiar form:

$$P = \frac{DK}{h} \tag{4}$$

where D is the membrane diffusion coefficient, K is the partition coefficient of the diffusant between the membrane and the medium external to the membrane, and h is the thickness of the membrane. Since this equation describes the situation where the resistance opposing the mass transfer process is derived from a single isotropic phase, the reciprocal of P yields the mathematical statement for the resistance of a singular resistor, that is, h/DK. It can be seen that in an isotropic phase, diffusional resistance is directly proportional to the thickness of the phase but inversely proportional to the mobility of the molecules (as reflected in the diffusion coefficient) and the partition coefficient.

It is intuitive that the resistance of the membrane should be smaller the thinner the membrane (smaller the value of h) and the greater the mobility of the molecules in the membrane (smaller the value of 1/D). The relationship of resistance to partition coefficient, however, needs some explaining. Fick's first law states that molecular flux per unit area across an isotropic field is proportional to the negative of the concentration gradient; that is,

$$\frac{J}{A} = -D\left(\frac{dC}{dx}\right) \tag{5}$$

In this equation D, which is the same diffusion coefficient as used above, is merely a proportionality coefficient which makes the relationship between the flux and concentration gradient exact. The concentration gradient is the rate of change of concentration with distance *within the membrane*. For a steady-state diffusional process operating across an isotropic membrane, and in the absence of complicating factors such as hydrodynamic layers, dC/dx can be represented by $(C_h - C_o)/h$, where the concentration terms are the concentrations actually in the membrane at its respective interfaces. Experimentally, concentrations are rarely if ever measured in the membrane proper. Rather, concentrations are measured in one or another of the media external to the membrane, and thus a partition coefficient is introduced to adjust external concentrations to the membrane's interfacial concentrations. The larger the partition coefficient into the membrane, the steeper the gradient within it, and therefore the greater the diffusional flux. Greater diffusional flux means less resistance to diffusion. In this manner the rate of diffusion is referenced to the medium in which the diffusant is applied through a partition coefficient, which becomes an explicit part of the diffusional resistance. The partition coefficient can be viewed as a capacity factor. Thus the diffusional resistance reflects elements of thickness, molecular mobility, and membrane capacity. This is as true for each pure phase of a complex membrane as it is for the single phase of the uncomplicated one-phase membrane.

When more than one phase of the membrane is continuous from one external surface to the other, the membrane is capable of supporting separate diffusional currents through each. In this instance the pathways are configured in parallel to one another, and the total flux of matter across the membrane is the sum of the fluxes of each route. In most instances independency of the routes is assumed, although this can be only approximately true. Where parallel currents contribute to the total current the total flux is expressed by:

$$J = A(f_1 P_1 + f_2 P_2 + \cdots + f_n P_n)(\Delta C) \tag{6}$$

where the term $f_1 P_1 + f_2 P_2 + \cdots + f_n P_n$ now defines the overall permeability coefficient P. It is notable that each path in parallel is described by its unique permeability coefficient P_i. Also, fractional areas of the routes, f_i's become important. A facile but very limited pathway may contribute less flux than a major pathway with higher internal resistance. Therefore relative area is also a factor in the resistance (or permeability coefficient) expression.

The presence of particles in the diffusional field also must be accounted for. For the purposes here, only the effects of inert and impervious particulates are considered. These block out area (or volume if considered in three dimensions) that otherwise could support a mass current. Diffusing matter must flow around the particulate obstacles, with a lengthening of the operative diffusional path. Terms are included in the rate equation to account both for the excluded area (or volume) and the increased tortuosity of the average molecule's diffusional course.

Series configuration of phases, parallel configuration of phases, and the presence of included phases all give membranes unique permeation behaviors; and with the right physicochemical probes such mechanistically important features can often be demonstrated, even for membranes as complex as the skin. Among the tools at one's disposal are (1) homolog and analog partitioning dependencies and the influences thereof on mass transfer across different types of membranes; (2) pH-partitioning relationships of weak electrolytes and their unique influences on mass transfer as a function of membrane type; (3) membrane sectioning techniques that isolate portions of a membrane for separate study; (4) stirring effects that help elucidate the role of hydrodynamic layers; (5) relationships between molecular size and the facility of diffusion through true pores and "pores" formed as the interstitial spaces between dense membrane components; (6) chemical and thermal effects that selectively alter the barrier properties of certain phases of a membrane to allow isolation and study of its other phases; and (7) enzyme inhibition techniques that allow factoring of enzyme influences from the gross mass transfer rate.

PARTITIONING EFFECTS ON PERCUTANEOUS ABSORPTION

General Observations

The permeability of biological tissues has long been thought to depend on the lipoidal character of the lipoprotein structure of its component cell membranes (Davson and Danielli, 1952; Overton, 1924). By inference drawn from membranes other than the skin and from very qualitative and mostly clinical observations on permeation of skin, early reviewers of the principles of percutaneous absorption imbued skin with lipidlike character (Blank, 1960; Calvery et al., 1946; Rothman, 1943, 1954; Tregear, 1964). However, it was not until Treherne (1956), Nogami and Hanano (1958), Loveday (1961), and Blank (1964) that unequivocal demonstrations of a relationship between oil/water (o/w) partitioning and skin penetration rate were provided.

Treherne's study was one of the first to employ excised skin (rabbit) in a diffusion cell for the purposes of defining its barrier characteristics, and he related obtained permeability coefficients to partition coefficients measured in vitro. Blank took an even more systematic approach by choosing the homologous alcohols as permeants. Partition coefficients of these increase systematically and exponentially, providing a wide range of partitioning values to test the fundamentally important idea that increasing lipophilicity enhances permeability. This general idea was greatly reinforced in a farsighted, theoretical article by T. Higuchi (1960), in which thermodynamic concepts of activity and activity coefficients were introduced into the percutaneous absorption picture. Activity coefficients of course determine the values of partition coefficients. These papers set the stage for the breakthrough conceptualizations of Scheuplein (1965, 1967) and Blank et al. (1967), which began anatomically accurate and physicochemically reasonable modeling of the skin membrane barrier.

Influence of Partitioning on Permeability

Studies with Alkyl Homologs

The partitioning of alkyl homologs between water-immiscible phases and water bears the following relationship to alkyl chain length:

$$\log K_n = \log K_0 + \Pi n \tag{7}$$

This is an especially useful relationship because it expresses a universal dependency, thereby allowing chain length n to be used in lieu of partition coefficients (log K_n) in theoretical analysis. Depending on the organic phase chosen, the value of Π, the slope of the log K_n versus n plot, can be as small or smaller than 0.3 and as large as 0.7. Values of 0.3 to 0.5 are typical for biological membranes (Yalkowsky and Flynn, 1973). At the lower end of the range it takes an addition of three methylene units to the alkyl chain to produce a 10-fold increase in partition coefficient. Two methylene units produce this effect when the Π value hovers around 0.5.

While partition coefficients are growing exponentially as the homologous series is ascended, there appears to be little concurrent effect on diffusion coefficients. This is because diffusivity in liquid media is sensitive only to the square root to cube root of volume. There is evidence the dependency is not much greater than this in noncrystalline polymers (Flynn et al., 1974).

The permeation of simple hydrophobic membranes by alkyl homologs applied to the membrane in aqueous solution often evidences a dominating influence of o/w partitioning on the permeability coefficient through the short to middle chain length members of the series. This is illustrated in Figure 1, where permeability coefficient profiles for three homologous series (Behl et al., 1984; Flynn and Yalkowsky, 1972; Hagen, 1979) permeating silicone rubber membranes are described. Silicone rubber is noncrystalline at room temperature and it has a solubility parameter not much greater than that of hexane, placing it on the extreme hydrophobic side of all materials. It is seen that log P for the short-chain members of each of these very different homologous series rises sharply and linearly with increased length of the alkyl chain. It will also be noticed that for each series the profile levels out at some long chain length.

This total pattern of permeability has the following basis. The resistance in these experiments comes from the membrane and watery boundary layers at the membrane's interfaces. These form a series barrier. The partition coefficients of the permeants between the bulk, well-mixed water in which the permeants are applied and the functionally unstirred water of the diffusion layers are all unity. Partitioning into the membrane follows the log K_n versus n homolog relationship expressed in Equation 7. At the shorter chain lengths the o/w partition coefficient is very small, and consequently the membrane resistance is high enough to totally control the rate of the permeation process (see discussion of Eq. 4). However, as the chain is lengthened, the resistance of the membrane is exponentially decreasing due to its reciprocal dependency on the o/w partition coefficient. The summed resistance of the boundary layers at the same time remains unchanged or even increases gradually due to the effect of increasing molecular size on diffusivity. Consequently, a point is reached where the low but unchanging resistance of the boundary layers assumes rate-controlling proportions. Such an overall pattern clearly marks a membrane as being "lipoidal." A mathematical treatment of this membrane/boundary layer situation has been given by Flynn and Yalkowsky (1972).

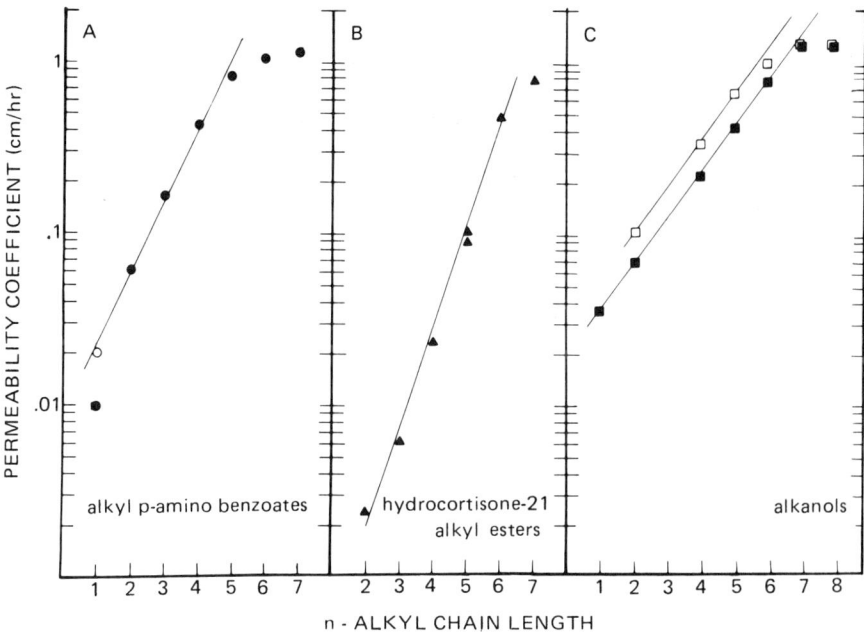

Figure 1 Series of plots of 37°C permeability coefficients as a function of alkyl chain length. All permeability coefficients are on the same scale. (A) Data for the alkyl-p-amino benzoates passing through 476-μm commercial silicone rubber films (Silastic 372, Dow Corning). An upper limit on the mass transfer coefficient of about 1.0 cm/hr is apparent. (B) The hydrocortisone-21-alkyl ester permeability coefficients obtained on a homemade 74-μm membrane at 25°C appear to be leveling off at a somewhat lower value. (C) Data for the homologous n-alkanols passing through 74-μm ($\square$) and 100-μm ($\blacksquare$) homemade silicone rubber membranes, respectively. These permeability coefficients level off at slightly above 1.0 cm/hr. A permeability of 1.0 cm/hr corresponds to a total diffusion layer thickness of several hundred micrometers.

Consider now the diffusion of homologs through a membrane by way of either molecularly sized interstices or macroscopic pores filled with the same solvent found outside the membrane. In this circumstance partition coefficients for all permeants between the conducting medium within the membrane and the applied medium will be near unity. Depending on the effective "pore" radius, diffusion coefficients can be relatively insensitive to the chain length or, if the "pores" are of molecular dimensions, they can even decrease sharply with chain length. "Pore" permeability coefficients through a homologous series thus either remain invariant or they decrease as the molecular size grows and the diffusivity decreases. When the external phase is water, such behavior, even if only over a two- or three-unit increase in chain length, is a certain sign of permeation by way of "aqueous pore pathways" across the membrane. A leveling out of the permeation profile does not indicate a "pore pathway" only when hydrodynamically generated boundary layers take away control of a permeation process from a lipid membrane as described above. A plateau also results when this occurs.

Scheuplein and co-workers (Blank et al., 1967; Scheuplein, 1965, 1967, 1976) systematically studied the permeation of homologous alkanols through membranes made of human epidermal sheets, proving unequivocally that the epidermal barrier has lipoidal qualities by way of the shape of the permeability pattern (Fig. 2A). They also isolated and studied skin strata from beneath the epi-

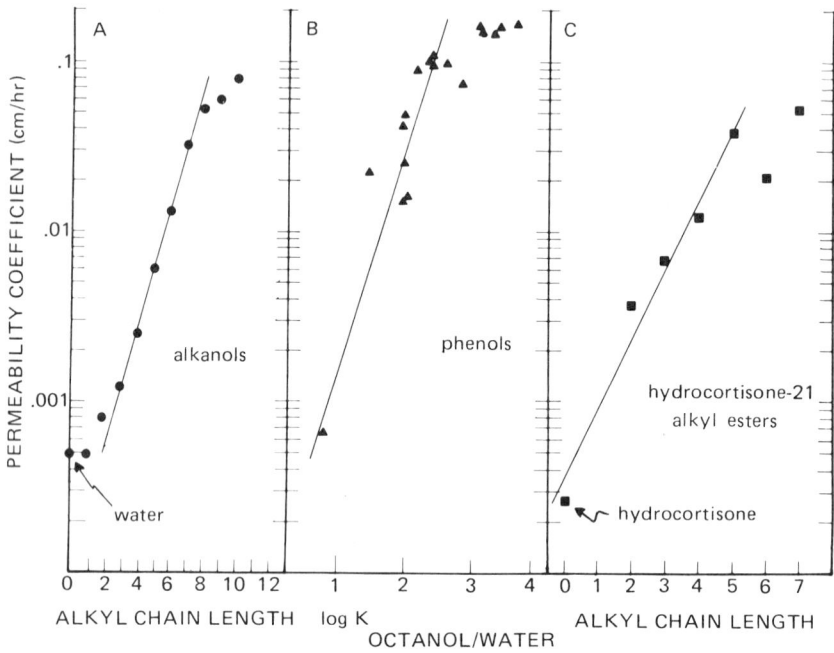

Figure 2 Plots of permeability coefficients of water and n-alkanols (A) and phenols (B) and hydrocortisone and its esters (C) as functions of increasing hydrophobicity. The latter property is measured in terms of increasing length of the alkyl chain for the two homologous series and in terms of octanol/water partition coefficients in the case of the phenols. A sigmoid character is evident with water and the alkanols. All three groups of homologs and analogs evidence leveling out of permeability coefficients as the members attain a high lipophilicity. The alkanol and phenol data were obtained with human epidermal sheets, while the steroid data were obtained using full thickness mouse skin membranes in which esterases were inhibited by p-nitrophenol. All permeability coefficients are on the same scale.

dermis, coming to the opposite conclusion that this diffusion zone of the skin behaves as a watery barrier to the alkanols.

While most of the alkanols exhibited partitioning-sensitive increases in P, the first two alkanol members (methanol and ethanol) had essentially the same permeability coefficient as water through the epidermis. Little was made of this at the time, but this observation now appears related to a different mechanism of permeation for these relatively small and quite polar substances. This trio of solutes appears to pass through intact skin by a pathway without an o/w partitioning dependency. Thus these workers also produced the first clear evidence of an alternative "aqueous pore pathway" through the skin's outer horny film. Earlier Treherne (1956) had also found the same permeability coefficient for methanol and ethanol, in this case through excised rabbit skin. And after the work from the Harvard laboratories other investigators demonstrated the same kind of permeability profile for alkanols permeating the skin of the hairless mouse (Behl et al., 1980a; Durrheim et al., 1980; Flynn et al., 1981c).

Most other published work with homologs is clearly supportive of a lipoidal pathway mechanism of permeation for whole skin or epidermis. For instance, using the ability of nicotinic acid esters to induce dilitation of superficial capillary beds, Stoughton et al. (1960) provided convincing evidence that the permeability of these homologs increases as their lipophilicity increases. In vitro permeation experiments with alkyl-substituted phenols (Roberts et al., 1977, 1978) shown in Figure 2B provides another unmistakable sign of some sort of o/w partitioning-dependent route. In Figure 2C some very recent data obtained for hydrocortisone and its homologous 21 esters are shown (Smith, 1982). These too pass through skin, in this instance hairless mouse skin, by way of a lipoidal route.

Data for one series, vidarabine and its homologous $5'$ esters (Gordon, 1981), do not fit well into the developing picture of a lipoidal skin membrane but rather are believed by this author to suggest another mechanism. Consider that, while vidarabine and its $5'$-octanoate ester differ in ether/water partition coefficient by roughly a factor of 10,000 (Flynn, 1971), the far more hydrophobic ester exhibits only a fourfold higher permeability coefficient. Permeability coefficients of the acetate and valerate esters fall on a line drawn between these two extremes. At first blush this observation seems totally inconsistent with all other research experience related here but, as will be seen momentarily, this observation is critical to the conclusion that drugs can diffusionally negotiate the stratum corneum in at least two different ways.

Studies Relating Skin Permeability to Partition Coefficients

Several studies have appeared in addition to those with homologs that illustrate much the same principles. Treherne's work has already been mentioned. It not only represented an early use of in vitro methods of permeation but was also one of the earliest works published involving the use of radioisotopes to follow the course of a permeation process. The permeability coefficients of small, polar nonelectrolytes were correlated with their ether/water partition coefficients. Curiously, while these data have been held up as demonstrating the lipophilicity of the skin membrane barrier, they actually lend credence to an opposing view, namely, that o/w partitioning is not exactingly related to the permeable coefficient. This is so because only a 100-fold change was found for the latter parameter, while partition coefficients ranged over four logarithmic orders. Even allowing for differences in the sensitivities of different partitioning systems to changing hydrophobicity of the partitioning molecules or, more specifically, for sensitivity differences between ether/water and skin lipoprotein/water partitioning systems, a much greater spread in the permeability coefficients must be exhibited to justify the conclusion that the skin (rabbit) functioned strictly as a lipoidal barrier.

Despite this criticism, Treherne's study still set important precedents for subsequent researchers in the area. In the above-mentioned studies by Scheuplein and co-workers, stratum corneum/water partition coefficients were assessed and correlated with the experimental permeability coefficients, with a good result, making the relation between the two factors totally obvious. These partition coefficients allowed the calculation of effective diffusion coefficients for the stratum corneum based on DK/h as the functional form of permeability coefficient, the first quantitative measures of their kind. The alkanol pattern of partitioning between water and the stratum corneum evidenced biphasic character. Such behavior is only consistent with a membrane having at least two solution domains, one watery and the other lipoidal. This essential partitioning pattern was also observed for mouse epidermis (Flynn et al., 1982). Here the reported partitioning values are about a factor of 5 too large as the dry weight and not the wet weight of the tissue was used in their estimation. When so corrected, they are exceedingly similar to the human stratum corneum/water values.

Later work from the Harvard laboratories (Scheuplein et al., 1969) correlated permeability coefficients of progestins, estrogens, and adrenal corticoids with stratum corneum/water as well as other partition coefficients. This steroid study added greatly to the evolving point of view that it is a hydrophobic horny layer that regulates the permeation rates of many chemicals. The study also established beyond doubt that some large as well as small nonelectrolytes "see" the stratum corneum as a nonpolar medium. Very small diffusion coefficients, on the order of 1×10^{-13} cm^2/sec, were estimated for the corticoids within the steroid group. These translate to breakthrough times (non-stationary-state periods) for permeation of the human epidermal membranes of a week's duration or more. Since the clinical response to topically applied corticosteroids is known to be prompt, the thought was introduced that another more facile but minor means of diffusion across or around the horny layer may exist to provide those few molecules that suppress inflammation.

Mechanism of Percutaneous Absorption

The permeability coefficients of a battery of organic compounds, large and small, polar and nonpolar, have been determined in the University of Michigan laboratories using a standardized diffusion cell procedure and excised hairless mouse skin as the membrane. They include most all the compounds studied by Treherne, the homologous alkanols, hydrocortisone and its esters, the vidarabine group of compounds, and some miscellaneous others. Additionally, the ether/water partition coefficients of all members of this diverse group of compounds either have been determined directly or have been calculated using reference experimental values along with known linear free energy relationships for the ether/water partitioning system (Flynn, 1972).

The values of the permeability coefficients determined experimentally are plotted against the respective ether/water partition coefficients on a log-log scale in Figure 3. This exposition of data provides a basis to unify the seemingly con-

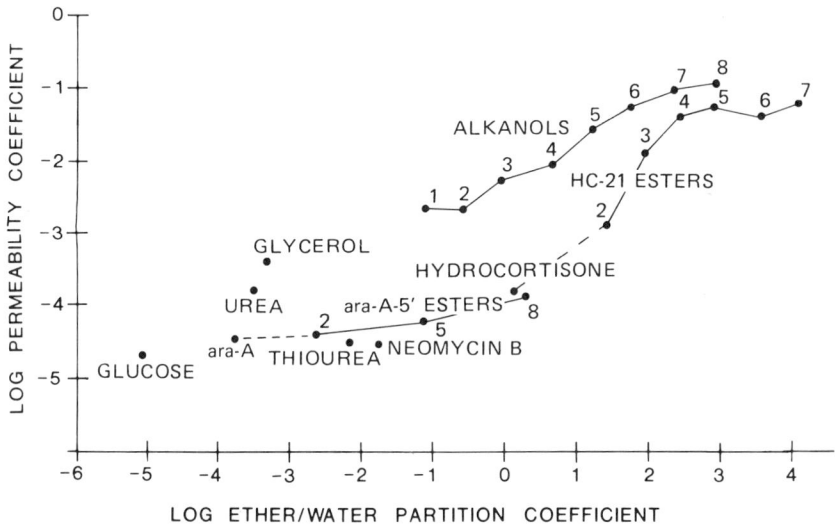

Figure 3 Collection of permeability coefficients (cm/hr) obtained with hairless mouse skin, specifically including data for the homologous n-alkanols, homologous hydrocortisone-21 (HC-21) esters, and homologous 5′-vidarabine (ara-A-5′) esters. These are plotted against the logs of their ether/water partition coefficients. The plot strongly suggests the existence of three distinguishable regimes of permeability in terms of polarity. Highly polar compounds of a given size pass through the tissue at about the same rate. The alkanol and steroid data are clearly confined to a regime exhibiting a distinct relation between permeability and o/w partitioning. At very high partition coefficients the data level off as tissue strata other than the stratum corneum assume rate control.

flicting literature observations mentioned previously. There appear to be well-demarcated zones of permeability behavior based on the degree of polarity of the permeants. Extremely nonpolar substances like the higher alcohols and the hexanoate and heptanoate esters of hydrocortisone permeate whole mouse skin as if significantly controlled by an aqueous diffusion barrier, and it has been reasoned that the cellular epidermis, the watery, fibrous dermis, and the true hydrodynamic layers are substantially rate controlling here. Compounds immediately to the left of these on the plot, namely, the rest of the hydrocortisone esters and the middle chain length alkanols, have the kind of pattern that is associated with passage across a lipid medium within the membrane. However, compounds much more polar that these, no matter whether large or small, seem to permeate as if o/w partitioning were not a factor. Many have order of magnitude higher permeabilities than could be anticipated on the basis of a lipoidal membrane. Vidarabine and its esters lie entirely in this polar zone, explaining their unexpected permeation insensitivity to partition coefficient. Glucose permeates on a par with these antiviral drugs, as does neomycin, a large molecule that carries multiple positive charges at neutral pH. Small nonelectrolytes seem to be uniformly more permeable than larger species of the same partition coefficient irrespective of polarity, which suggests significant molecular size effects. It was difficult to accurately assess the permeability coefficients of small polar nonelectrolytes because there were time dependencies to the rates of permeation. The values plotted here are those from the early few hours of the experiments. While there are no data as wide ranging in permeant polarity as these for membranes prepared from human skin, human tissue nevertheless seems to exhibit qualitative parallels to these behaviors. Proving this beyond doubt is worthy research, greatly in need of doing.

INFLUENCE OF pH ON PERMEABILITY OF WEAK ELECTROLYTES

The permeability behavior of weak electrolytes provides another general clue to the operational aspects of a given membrane. If the membrane is of the porous type, free and ionic species of weak electrolytes can diffuse with equal facility through the membrane, making the pH profile for permeation flat. On the other hand, if the membrane is lipoidal, ionic forms will be excluded from partitioning into the membrane because of thermodynamic constraints associated with the solution of ions in nonaqueous phases, with the important consequence that the membrane will preferentially support a current of the undissociated form, no matter its polarity. This does not mean that ionic species are totally forbidden from passing through the membrane, for ion pairing is possible and, in the form of ion pairs, a salt can be soluble to some extent within a lipid continuum and thereby can diffuse through it. All experience, however, suggests that a current associated with ion pairs is going to be exceedingly small, usually many log orders smaller than the flux of the free species at a comparable concentration differential (at or near where the pH is equal to the pK_a).

Few studies have been performed in which the permeation behavior of skin to weak electrolytes has been examined carefully. Loveday (1961) provides a complete pH profile for the permeation of salicylic acid through membranes made of the skin of a pig's ear. He states that "no significant variation of penetration was found above pH of 4." At lower pH the permeation rates increased dramatically, consistent with the expectation of facile diffusion of the functionally hydrophobic free salicylic acid species. The flux found above pH = 4 is attributable to the salicylate anion and, while smaller, it is nevertheless too large to be assigned to the diffusion of ion pairs, here undissociated sodium salicylate or some equivalent chemical form. Enough data are given to calculate the permeability coefficient of the anion, which is 2.3×10^{-2} cm/hr, a value about 10 times greater than observed for molecules like methanol and ethanol permeating human or hairless mouse skin membranes.

A plausible explanation for this large rate is that watery channels provide an alternative diffusional pathway through this skin. These could be in the horny structure itself, or they may arise as shunts through the stratum corneum provided by the skin's glands. In the absence of hard data supporting one or the other of these possibilities, it is impossible to make a definite assignment. However, since pig skin has a relatively nominal distribution of glands, and since it takes a plethora of such small glands to provide the observed flux, the suggestion is strong that the channels supporting the flux lie within the horny matrix itself. Arita et al. (1970) also studied salicylate permeation (guinea pig skin) and added a pH profile for a weak base, carbinoxamine, as well. By their index of permeation, the percentage of material absorbed after 6 hr of application of solutions of these substances in a cuplike cell inverted and placed on the living animal's abdomen, neither the anion of salicylic acid nor the cation of carbinoxamine seems to be absorbed. Thus, on the basis of these data it appears that this skin, which is furry and laced with appendageal shunts, does not allow the passage of ions.

We have recently studied the permeation of hairless mouse skin by phenolic compounds having significantly different pK_a's and also partitioning properties. Data for some of these are provided in Figure 4. The fluxes of the free species existing at low pH are favored, as is expected. At the same time there are measurable fluxes for all the phenols at high pH where essentially only the ionic forms are present. These data thus give added weight to the suggestion that, by some poorly defined means, ions are diffusionally negotiating the stratum corneum.

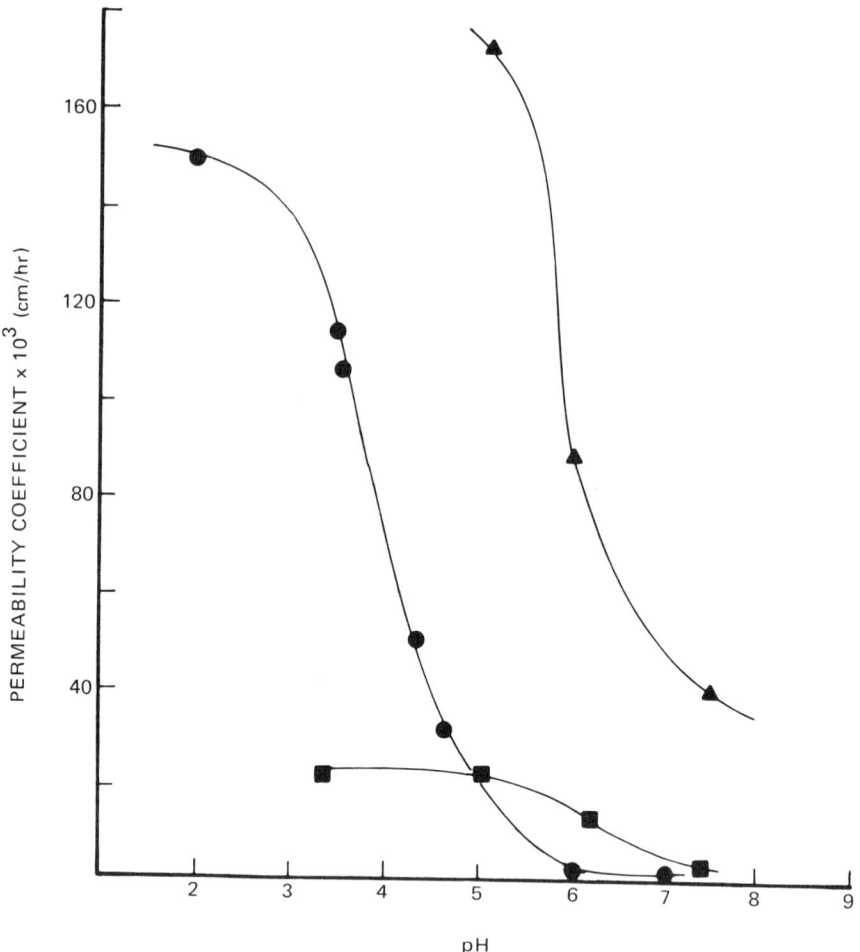

Figure 4 Permeability data for three phenols with different free species lipophilicities and different pK_a's. ●, 2,4-dinitrophenol, pK_a = 3.96; ■, 4-nitrophenol (pK_a = 7.15); ▲, 2,4,6-trichlorophenol (pK_a = 6.0).

BARRIER PROPERTIES AS REVEALED BY MEMBRANE SECTIONING

Wolf (1940) discovered that the stratum corneum of the skin can be systematically removed by repetitive application and removal of adhesive tape and touched off a series of experimental probes of the skin of enormous mechanistic importance. Blank (1953), for instance, in searching for the location of the barrier zone, measured the rate of water permeation of the skin as the skin is stripped.

This remained at near-normal levels until the lower reaches of the stratum corneum were attained, whereupon the increases were profound. These data were originally interpreted as meaning that the barrier was at the base of the horny structure. It has since been pointed out by Blank himself that the pattern is actually that expected for a stratum corneum of relatively uniform resistance (Blank, 1969). Monash (1957) systematically stripped human skin and related the time of onset of drug-induced local anesthesia to the number of strippings. It was concluded from the results of these pharmacological experiments that the whole stratum corneum constitutes the skin's major barrier element. Loveday (1961) also borrowed the stripping technique to show, with the aid of excised skin membranes in a diffusion cell, that the permeability of salicylic acid is markedly increased with increased numbers of strippings. He also favored the thought that the barrier qualities are more or less uniform throughout this tissue.

The studies above preceded systematic works of Scheuplein (1965, 1967) with human epidermis and of Flynn et al. (1981c) with mouse membranes. In these the resistance of each major layer of the skin to each of the homologous alcohols up to and including n-octanol was measured. As pointed out previously, the stratum corneum's lipoidally derived resistance varies with partitioning tendencies, and it systematically decreases as the alkyl chain is extended. On the other hand, the dermis—and, with few exceptions insofar as can be told by difference methods—the viable epidermis act as if they were a thickened, watery medium. Diffusion through these latter living strata is thought to be roughly one-tenth as facile as in bulk water. A decreasing stratum corneum involvement is noticed with the alkanols as the alkyl chain is increased in both human and mouse experiments. However, the stratum corneum is still in significant fractional control of the permeation rate for even the most hydrophobic alkanols of those studied. Behl et al. (1983) have reached essentially the same conclusion with phenol using stripping techniques as have Smith (1982) for hydrocortisone and its 21-alkyl esters and Linn (1982) for neomycin. A similar battery of techniques was used by Yu et al. (1979a,b) and a little later Gordon (1981) in their studies on the permeation of mouse skin membranes by vidarabine and some of its 5'-alkyl esters. Like all who preceded them, they also concluded that the principal barrier property of the skin resides in the stratum corneum and that it appears to be rather uniformly distributed throughout.

Some recent and as yet unpublished work by Govil at the University of Michigan adds confirming insight. Using better instrumentation than was available to Blank and other early investigators, the shape of the transepidermal water loss (TEWL) rate versus skin strippings profile has been carefully worked out on the living hairless mouse (Fig. 5). The profile has the shape expected when the horny layer is uniform in barrier quality. Total removal leads to a surface evaporation rate roughly that of an open surface of water. Of some importance, certain burns and chemical treatments leave the skin in the same condition without actual

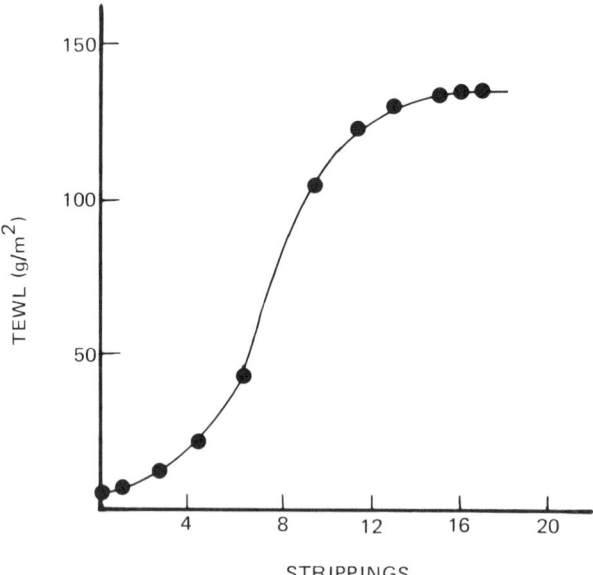

Figure 5 Relation of the water evaporation rate from the surface of the living mouse to the number of strippings of the mouse's skin. A maximum in the transepidermal water loss (TEWL) rate of 130 g/cm^2/hr is attained with about 15 strippings.

removal of the horny layer. Among other purposes, it is possible to show in this way that the barrier qualities of the skin are related in a direct way to the general integrity of the stratum corneum.

CHEMICAL AND THERMAL EFFECTS AND BARRIER PROPERTY

Some of the earliest experiments aimed at assessing the membrane properties of the skin have involved challenging it with solvents and measuring the effects of the treatments. Rothman (1943) characterized early experiments of Winternitz that dealt with absorption of strychnine from aqueous solutions as classical in this regard. This work showed that solvents such as ether, chloroform, and benzene enhance percutaneous absorption by altering the fundamental barrier-bearing properties of the skin. Starkenstein and Hendrych (1936) also demonstrated such effects. However, it was not until the advent of dimethyl sulfoxide (DMSO) and the recognition of the commercial possibilities of using such materials to promote the delivery of drugs through the skin that effort was concentrated on delineating these aspects. Stoughton and Fritsch (1964) assessed DMSO's ability to enhance the pharmacological activities of topically applied anticholinergic and vasoconstrictive agents and directly related the biological responses to increased drug penetration. Numerous studies with aprotic solvents (DMSO, DMA, and DMF) have followed. In most of these, observed enhancements of penetration have been large only when the organic solvents were applied in high concentration for relatively long periods of time. Several mechanisms have been advanced for the action, including elution of stratum corneum lipids (Allenby et al., 1969; Embery and Dugard, 1971), denaturation of stratum corneum structural keratin proteins (Montes et al., 1967; Scheuplein and Ross, 1970), and delamination of the horny layer by stress resulting from crosscurrents of highly water-reactive solvents and water itself (Chandrasekaran et al., 1977). Studies by Kurihara (1983) at the University of Michigan prove unequivocally that each of the mentioned causes is in fact partially responsible for the total observed behavior, with the dominant factor in a particular situation being the result of the concentration of DMSO and its method and duration of application to the skin. Generally, the effects here are so nonselective that few concrete inferences can be made about the barrier properties of the stratum corneum other than noting that the stratum corneum itself is the principal target of the chemical effects and also the main source of the skin's diffusional resistance.

Behl, Flynn, and co-workers (Behl et al., 1980b, 1981a; Flynn et al., 1981a, b), in an extensive series of experiments aimed at elucidating the degree of barrier compromise to skin as the result of thermal trauma, have added some important observations. Irrespective of the duration of burning, if the skin is burned at temperatures much lower than 75°C, it retains its essential barrier properties until such time that the devitalized tissue is digested and sloughed. This takes days (Flynn et al., 1981b). Thus, if this low burning temperature condition is met, it matters not whether the burn is first or fourth degree insofar as permeability of the wound immediately after receiving the wound is concerned. On the other hand, for burns inflicted at temperatures 85°C or higher, the permeability of the skin is immediately altered even if the depth of tissue damage is shallow. Some dramatic change must take place in the stratum corneum as the temperature approaches and exceeds 80°C. This change is clearly irreversible. Thermal analytical studies of Linn (1982) show that keratin denaturation explains the alteration in the tissue's properties. This is a form of a melting, and it takes place over the narrow temperature range specified. The thermal analysis data also suggest that despite measurable melting of lipids within the horny layer, these actually fuse at much lower temperatures. They also recrystallize quickly upon cooling of the stratum corneum samples. Therefore the melting of lipids does not appear to be responsible for the altered barrier integrity. While the densely packed keratin of the horny layer has long been presumed to tightly limit diffusion, these studies are among the first to experimentally implicate this molecular regime with the stratum corneum's unique membrane function. Considered together with certain solvent effects, it seems as if the removal of presumably intercellular lipids and the denaturation of intracellular protein produce the same end result—loss, to the point of totality in some instances—of the stratum corneum's diffusional resistance. There is no essential conflict here, in that any action that opens a facile route for diffusion through the stratum corneum will have this consequence.

One other group of experiments involving the unique chemical effects of phenol on the skin is revealing. It has long been known that phenol can be a lethal poison if applied to the skin as a saturated or near-saturated solution in water or, in a few troubling incidents, as the neat chemical (Deichmann, 1949). Several studies have related phenol contact with the skin to increased permeability of the skin. Particularly notable are the studies of Roberts et al. (1977) and of Behl et al. (1983) in that they provide the concentration dependency for phenol's effect. Whether the skin is of human or mouse origin, solutions of phenol in water less concentrated than 2% have little effect on the stratum corneum. However, when the concentration is 5% or more there is virtually instantaneous and complete destruction of the horny element. Though whole skin membranes treated in this fashion appear intact to the eye, permeability experiments show them to be no less permeable than skin membranes stripped free of stratum corneum.

It can be reasoned that aqueous phenolic solutions of 5-6% concentration hardly have the ability to elute the lipids of the horny layer as fat solvents do. While phenol may concentrate some in the intercellular space of the horny structure, it is equally hard to conceive of its presence there opening the floodgates. Rather, it seems that phenol is chemically denaturing keratin, as it is known to do with other proteins, opening the intracellular structure in a manner functionally equivalent to high-temperature denaturation. This provides a second important clue that the compactness and specific organization of the keratin matrix is critical to the high diffusional resistance of this tissue.

Such ideas give one pause, for they provide an easy and rational basis to explain many otherwise inexplicable mysteries associated with the skin barrier. Why, for instance, are premature infants with perfectly normal looking skins at high risk of absorbing every chemical they contact? Could it be that the final critical organization of the keratin is yet to be completed? Why do we see such profound differences in skin permeability across the animal kingdom? Different structural features, packing, and organization of keratin within the keratinocytes of different species provides a plausible explanation for the variability that exists here.

INTEGRATION OF ANATOMY WITH THE PHYSICOCHEMICAL EVIDENCE

The idea that the skin is first and foremost lipoidal is old, and this chapter adds very little that is new to this basic concept. Indeed, chemists have been designing drugs with this concept in mind for at least three decades. That the skin supports limited diffusion of highly polar permeants is also documented in the literature, but not nearly so convincingly. Most previous reviewers have ascribed the latter to appendageal shunts or have left the matter entirely open. The suggestion here of a heterogeneous stratum corneum with at least two distinct physicochemical regimes, each capable of separately conducting a stream of permeant, thus is relatively novel. One route, which may be through the intracellular keratin matrix, is considered "polar" and is seen as preferentially supporting the flux of polar substances. The other postulated route is thought to be through the intercellular lipid deposited in the final stages of cell specialization as described by Elias (1981). This regime is believed by many to be the "partitioning medium" that gives the skin its lipoidal membrane qualities. How possible is any of this? This question can be considered in the light of existing physicochemical and anatomical evidence.

Consider the presumed lipid route first. This could be through the keratin matrix by way of the lipid wrapping of the fibrils but, considering all evidence to date, it seems far more likely that the lipid of consequence is that lying in the seams of the cells. The total lipid of the stratum corneum has been variously estimated to be from about 10 to about 30% of the dry mass of the tissue. A reasonable estimate might be 15%. If the preponderance of this lipid material is intercellular and spread more or less uniformly between and around the edges of the platelet cells of the horny fabric, the intercellular lipid route viewed in the direction of inward diffusion would occupy about 1% of the diffusional area. This is so, for the bulk of the lipid lies in the lateral seams of the stratum corneum, given the flattened geometry of the horny cells. Essentially the same percentage is arrived at if one models the stratum corneum with a mortar and brick structure with cells of actual size, about 30 μm in diameter, and with spacings of 50 nm between cells as reported by Elias (1981).

When the cells are stacked directly over one another as they sometimes appear to be in histological section, a relatively straight route through the stratum corneum would exist. This route would have a great deal of lateral dead volume. Substance accumulating in this dead volume would do so at the expense of great lengthening of diffusion lag times. On the other hand, if the sheets of horny cells are more or less randomly overlayered, as they histologically appear to be over callused skin, this route around the horny cell platelets would be tortuous, with the steady-state diffusion course winding back and forth through a portion of the lipid material lying in the plane of the stratum corneum. More of the lipid mass would act as a conduit for diffusion in this instance, and there would be less dead space. The effective path would be longer. For horny platelets of 30 μm diameter and 0.5 μm width the upper limit on tortuosity might at first appear to be near 30, or half the diameter of the platelet divided by the width. This in fact overstates the tortuosity considerably, since when viewed as a three-dimensional array, there is no way to arrange the sheets of cells without some points of overlap of the vertical separations between the cell edges. These common "holes" through adjacent cell layers will act as funneling points for the diffusive current. Therefore a tortuosity of no more than 10 is actually indicated by the geometry.

How does the foregoing simplified and even schematic picture of the intercellular space square with experimental data on permeation of the stratum corneum? In the pioneering work on modeling of the skin mentioned previously, Scheuplein (1965, 1967, 1975) endowed all the skin's barrier phases with more or less uniform diffusional properties. Of specific interest here, the stratum corneum was, to a first approximation, considered to be a lipoprotein mosaic with a composite barrier quality. Based on careful permeation and partitioning studies with alkanols, an effective diffusion coefficient for most low molecular weight nonelectrolytes of 1×10^{-10} cm^2/sec was assigned to the horny material. We can consider the consistency of this value with a diffusion mechanism strictly through the intercellular route as described. To adjust it for steady-state diffusion, both the fractional area of the route and the effective tortuosity have to be explicitly considered. For exactly overlayered cells a factor of 100 in lost area must be accounted for in terms of increased diffusivity. In other words, to compensate for the blocking out of 99% of the area, the diffusion coefficient must be raised to 1×10^{-8} cm^2/sec. This value is not only highly reasonable for diffusion through a soft, lipoidal mass, it is even on the low side. A tortuosity factor of 10 for the highly disorganized stratum corneum cell packing is easily accommodated. That is, a diffusivity of 1×10^{-7} cm^2/sec is altogether reasonable, provided the intercellular space is aptly described here and is filled with a relatively noncrystalline lipid mixture. It is notable that partition coefficients would not have to be adjusted because all the model adjustment is tucked up in the diffusion coefficient.

This analysis of course does not prove the existence of the intercellular route any more than previous analyses prove the stratum corneum to be functionally isotropic. However, by not being able to rule out the possibility on physical grounds, it leaves open the question of whether intercellular diffusion is a viable part of the percutaneous absorption mechanism. It is profoundly interesting that upon consideration of relative fractional areas, the intercellular route as envisioned here would be roughly 10 times as important as the transfollicular route when the sebum of the latter pathway is, as a diffusion medium, comparable in physicochemical properties to the lipid lying in the thin seams between the stratum corneum cells.

The polar route, which is presumed to be directly through a limited, somewhat open portion of the hydrated protein mass of the keratinocytes, can now be considered. It will be remembered that the existence of such a watery path rests on several lines of evidence, most notably higher than expectable permeation rates of very polar species and comparable magnitudes of these rates, and the passage of ions through intact skin. Molecular species as these would be thermodynamically paralyzed by their unfavorable tendencies to partition into a purely lipid medium. Therefore they would not permeate lipid membranes at experimentally measurable rates. For the intact hairless mouse skin, measured permeability coefficients of molecular species as glucose and neomycin B are on the order of 1×10^{-5} cm/hr. Scheuplein (private communication, 1983) believes that human skin exhibits parallel behavior here but has suggested a somewhat lower limit of the permeability coefficient of 1×10^{-6} cm/hr for this tissue. These values are 1000 or more times smaller than those found on the upper side of the permeability coefficients of the parallel lipid route. Therefore, no doubt exists that the polar route as described is a highly restricted avenue of diffusive passage. The restrictive nature resides in factors other than gross fractional area, which is near unity.

There appear to be two reasons for the low permeability of the polar diffusional pathway. First, it is clear that the keratin of the fully differentiated cell is fibrous and is at least partially crystalline. It is woven into a compact structure. The density of packing and the crystallinity preclude a high degree of solubility of molecules in the intracellular matrix of the keratinocyte as well as facile diffusive mobility of the molecules that do dissolve. Based on partitioning sensitivities in the defined polar region of diffusion, the domain that does support diffusion appears to be water. This is almost certainly associated with the more open, hydratable parts of the intracellular matrix. The water sorption tendencies of keratin, which are enormous in callus but likely not as nearly so great with more typical stratum corneum, appear to be derived from the unusually high proportion in the protein structure of amino acids that have at their free ends ionic functionalities as carboxyl, sulfhydral, and amine groups. Counting mercapto end groups, about a third of the amino acid building blocks are ionic, a factor that sets keratin apart from all other proteins. The hydrated protein regime thus appears to be a highly ionic regime. Based on recent work of Walters et al. (1981, 1983) involving the human nail plate, the intracellular regime may have the ability to exclude hydrophobic molecules by something akin to a salting-out phenomenon. Be this as it may, the medium for diffusion is viewed here as water that is substantially bound up in the protein and is very limited in amount. When this protein structure is unraveled, as is done with heat and certain chemicals, at the least much more of it becomes available for diffusion, and it may even become more hydrated, rendering the stratum corneum useless as a membrane. While this description is speculative, it nevertheless accommodates all the diffusion observations set forth above.

Scheuplein (1975) has stated that "because of the great complexity of the skin barrier an exact mathematical solution of the diffusion problem is impractical." This author concurs fully. However, this should not deter us from considering the possibilities of various subtly different mechanisms and their worthiness for incorporation into barrier models. The foregoing discussions represent the synthesis of an idea of the barrier from facts selected from the literature. The general concept of at least two pathways, one lipoidal and the other watery, seems to be secured with hard data. What and exactly where these pathways lie within the stratum corneum or whether they are external to it by way of shunts is still subject to guess and argument. Such sifting of ideas as may result from speculative, hypothetical discussion can only improve our overall knowledge of the skin and its permeation behaviors. No matter the new twist in theory, it must be able to reasonably accommodate to known physicochemical facts developed experimentally for the skin barrier and also must fit into well-accepted concepts of the skin's anatomical design. This particular treatment is intended to show that within reasonable tolerances for known physical parameters, the concept of an intercellular lipid route is basically sound. All else set out above that relates to specific mechanisms must be considered to be food for thought and nothing more.

REFERENCES

Allenby, A. C., Creasey, N. H., Edginton, J. A. G., Fletcher, J. A., and Schock, C. (1969). Mechanism of action of accelerants on skin permeation. *Br. J. Dermatol. 81* (Suppl. 4): 47-55.

Arita, T., Hori, R., Anmo, T., Washitake, M., and Yajima, T. (1970). Studies on percutaneous absorption of drugs. I. *Chem. Pharm. Bull.* (Tokyo) *18*: 1045-1049.

Behl, C. R., Flynn, G. L., Kurihara, T., Harper, N., Smith, W., Higuchi, W. I., Ho, N. F. H., and Pierson, C. L. (1980a). Hydration and percutaneous absorption. I. Influence of hydration on alkanol permeation through hairless mouse skin. *J. Invest. Dermatol. 25*: 346-352.

Behl, C. R., Flynn, G. L., Kurihara, T., Smith, W., Gatmaitan, O., Higuchi, W. I., Ho, N. F. H., and Pierson, C. L. (1980b). Permeability of thermally damaged skin. I. Immediate influences of 60°C scalding on hairless mouse skin. *J. Invest. Dermatol. 25*: 340-345.

Behl, C. R., Flynn, G. L., Barrett, M., Linn, E. E., Higuchi, W. I., Ho, N. F. H., and Pierson, C. L. (1981a). Permeability of thermally damaged skin. IV. Influence of branding iron temperature on the mass transfer of water and *n*-alkanols acros hairless mouse skin. *Burns 8*: 86-98.

Behl, C. R., Flynn, G. L., Barrett, M., Walters, K. A., Linn, E. E., Mohamed, Z., Kurihara, T., Ho, N. F. H., Higuchi, W. I., and Pierson, C. L. (1981b). Permeability of thermally damaged skin. II. Immediate influences of branding at 60°C on hairless mouse skin permeability. *Burns 7*: 389-399.

Behl, C. R., Flynn, G. L., Fox, J. L., Smith, W. M., Durrheim, H. H., Hagen, T. A., Higuchi, W. I., and Ho, N. F. H. (1984). Permeability measurements on highly absorptive membranes. II. Permeation of silicone rubber membranes by the homologous *n*-alkanols. *J. Membrane Sci.* in press.

Behl, C. R., Linn, E. E., Flynn, G. L., Pierson, C. L., Higuchi, W. I., and Ho, N. F. H. (1983). Permeation of skin and eschar by antiseptics. I. Baseline studies with phenol. *J. Pharm. Sci. 72*: 391-397.

Blank, I. H. (1953). Further observations on factors which influence the water content of the stratum corneum. *J. Invest. Dermatol. 21*: 259-271.

Blank, I. H. (1969). Percutaneous absorption. Statement of problem and critical review of past methods. *J. Soc. Cosmet. Chem. 11*: 59-68.

Blank, I. H. (1964). Penetration of low-molecular-weight alcohols into skin. I. Effect of concentration of alcohol and type of vehicle. *J. Invest. Dermatol. 43*: 415-420.

Blank, I. H. (1969). Transport across the stratum corneum. *Toxicol. Appl. Pharmacol.* Suppl. 3: 23-29.

Blank, I. H., Scheuplein, R. J., and MacFarlane, D. J. (1967). Mechanism of percutaneous absorption. III. The effect of temperature on transport of nonelectrolytes across the skin. *J. Invest. Dermatol. 49*: 582-589.

Calvery, H. O., Draize, J. H., and Laug, E. P. (1946). The metabolism and permeability of normal skin. *Physiol. Rev. 26*: 495-540.

Chandrasekaran, S. K., Campbell, P. S., and Michaels, A. S. (1977). Effect of dimethyl sulfoxide on drug permeation through human skin. *AIChE J. 23*: 810-815.

Davson, H. and Danielli, J. F. (1952). *The Permeability of Natural Membranes*, 2nd ed. Cambridge University Press, London.

Deichmann, W. B. (1949). Local and systemic effects following skin contact with phenol—A review of the literature. *J. Indust. Hyg. Toxicol. 31*: 146-154.

Durrheim, H. H., Flynn, G. L., Higuchi, W. I., and Behl, C. R. (1980). Permeation of hairless mouse skin. I. Experimental methods and comparison with human epidermal permeation by alkanols. *J. Pharm. Sci. 69*: 781-786.

Elias, P. M. (1981). Lipids and the epidermal permeability barrier. *Arch. Dermatol. Res. 270*: 95-117.

Embery, G. and Dugard, P. H. (1971). The isolation of dimethyl sulfoxide soluble components from human epidermal preparations: A possible mechanism for dimethyl sulfoxide in effecting percutaneous migration phenomena. *J. Invest. Dermatol. 57*: 308-311.

Flynn, G. L. (1971). Structural approach to partitioning: Estimation of steroid partition coefficients based upon molecular constitution. *J. Pharm. Sci. 60*: 345-353.

Flynn, G. L. and Yalkowsky, S. H. (1972). Correlation and prediction of mass transport across membranes. I. Influence of alkyl chain length on flux-determining properties of barrier and diffusant. *J. Pharm. Sci. 61*: 838-852.

Flynn, G. L., Yalkowsky, S. H., and Roseman, T. J. (1974). Mass transport phenomena and models: Theoretical concepts. *J. Pharm. Sci. 63*: 479-510.

Flynn, G. L., Behl, C. R., Linn, E. E., Higuchi, W. I., Ho, N. F. H., and Pierson, C. L. (1981a). Permeability of thermally damaged skin. V. Permeability over the course of maturation of a deep partial thickness burn. *Burns 8*: 196-202.

Flynn, G. L., Behl, C. R., Walters, K., Gatmaitan, O., Wittkowsky, A., Kurihara, T., Ho, N. F. H., Higuchi, W. I., and Pierson, C. L. (1981b). Permeability of thermally damaged skin. III. Influence of scalding temperature on mass transfer of water and n-alkanols across hairless mouse skin. *Burns 8*: 47-58.

Flynn, G. L., Durrheim, H. H., and Higuchi, W. I. (1981c). Permeation of hairless mouse skin. II. Membrane sectioning techniques and influences on alkanol permeabilities. *J. Pharm. Sci. 70*: 52-56.

Gordon, N. A. (1981). A physical model approach to the simultaneous transport and bioconversion of prodrugs of vidarabine in the hairless mouse skin. Thesis, University of Michigan, Ann Arbor.

Hagen, T. A. (1979). Physicochemical study of hydrocortisone and hydrocortisone n-alkyl-21-esters. Thesis, University of Michigan, Ann Arbor.

Higuchi, T. (1960). Physical chemical analysis of percutaneous absorption process from creams and ointments. *J. Soc. Cosmet. Chem. 11*: 85-97.

Kurihara, T. (1983). Physicochemical study of the accelerant effects of DMSO on percutaneous absorption of an antiviral drug and other chemical prototypes. Thesis, University of Michigan, Ann Arbor.

Linn, E. E. (1982). Thermotropic effects on skin permeability. Thesis, University of Michigan, Ann Arbor.

Loveday, D. E. (1961). An in vitro method for studying percutaneous absorption. *J. Soc. Cosmet. Chem. 12*: 224-239.

Monash, S. (1957). Location of the superficial barrier to skin penetrability. *J. Invest. Dermatol. 29*: 367-376.

Montes, L. F., Day, J. L., Wand, C. J., and Kennedy, L. (1967). Ultrastructural changes in the horny layer following local application of dimethyl sulfoxide. *J. Invest. Dermatol. 48*: 184-196.

Nogami, H. and Hanano, M. (1958). Studies on percutaneous absorption. II. Effect of the incorporated substance. *Chem. Pharm. Bull.* (Tokyo) *6*: 249-255.

Overton, E. (1924). *Studien über die Narkose.* Fischer, Jena.

Roberts, M. S., Anderson, R. A., and Swarbrick, J. (1977). Permeability of human epidermis to phenolic compounds. *J. Pharm. Pharmacol. 29*: 677-683.

Roberts, M. S., Anderson, R. A., Swarbrick, J., and Moore, D. E. (1978). The percutaneous absorption of phenolic compounds: The mechanism of diffusion across the stratum corneum. *J. Pharm. Pharmacol. 30*: 486-490.

Rothman, S. (1943). The principles of percutaneous absorption. *J. Lab. Clin. Med. 28*: 1305-1321.

Rothman, S. (1954). In *Physiology and Biochemistry of Skin.* University of Chicago Press, Chicago, pp. 26-59.

Scheuplein, R. J. (1965). Mechanism of percutaneous adsorption. I. Routes of penetration and the influence of solubility. *J. Invest. Dermatol. 45*: 334-345.

Scheuplein, R. J. (1967). Mechanism of percutaneous absorption. II. Transient diffusion and the relative importance of various routes of skin penetration. *J. Invest. Dermatol. 48*: 79-88.

Scheuplein, R. (1975). Site variations in diffusion and permeability. In *The Physiology and Pathophysiology of the Skin*. Edited by A. Jarrett. Academic, New York, pp. 1731-1752.

Scheuplein, R. J. (1976). Percutaneous absorption after twenty-five years: Or "old wine in new wineskins." *J. Invest. Dermatol. 67*: 31-38.

Scheuplein, R. J. and Ross, L. (1970). Effects of surfactants and solvents on the permeability of epidermis. *J. Soc. Cosmet. Chem. 21*: 853-873.

Scheuplein, R. J., Blank, I. H., Brauner, G. J., and MacFarlane, D. J. (1969). Percutaneous absorption of steroids. *J. Invest. Dermatol. 52*: 63-70.

Smith, W. M. (1982). An inquiry into the mechanism of percutaneous absorption of hydrocortisone and its 21-*n*-alkyl esters. Thesis, University of Michigan, Ann Arbor.

Starkenstein, E. and Hendrych, F. (1936). Zur Physiologie und Pharmakologie der Sterine. II. Die Bedeutung des Cholesterins für Permeabilität und Resorption. *Arch. Exp. Pathol. Pharmakol. 182*: 664-687.

Stoughton, R. B. and Fritsch, W. (1964). Influence of dimethyl sulfoxide (DMSO) on human percutaneous absorption. *Arch. Dermatol. 90*: 512-517.

Stoughton, R. B., Clendenning, W. E., and Kruse, D. (1960). Percutaneous absorption of nicotinic acid and its derivatives. *J. Invest. Dermatol. 35*: 337-342.

Tregear, R. T. (1964). The permeability of skin to molecules of widely differing properties. In *Progress in Biological Sciences in Relationship to Dermatology*, vol. 2. Edited by A. Rook and R. H. Champion. Cambridge University Press, London, pp. 275-281.

Treherne, J. E. (1956). The permeability of skin to some nonelectrolytes. *J. Physiol. 133*: 171-180.

Walters, K. A., Flynn, G. L., and Marvel, J. R. (1981). Physicochemical characterization of the human nail. I. Pressure-sealed apparatus for measuring nail plate permeabilities. *J. Invest. Dermatol. 76*: 76-79.

Walters, K. A., Flynn, G. L., and Marvel, J. R. (1983). Physicochemical characterization of the human nail: Permeation pattern for water and the homologous alcohols and differences with respect to the stratum corneum. *J. Pharm. Pharmacol. 35*: 28-33.

Wolf, J. (1940). Das Oberflachenrelief der menschlichen Haut. *Z. Mikcosk-Anat. Forschung 47*: 351-355.

Yalkowsky, S. H. and Flynn, G. L. (1973). Transport of alkyl homologs across synthetic and biological membranes: A new model for chain length-activity relationships. *J. Pharm. Sci. 62*: 210-217.

Yu, C. D., Fox, J. L., Ho, N. F. H., and Higuchi, W. I. (1979a). Physical model evaluation of topical prodrug delivery—Simultaneous transport and bioconversion of vidarabine-5′-valerate. I. Physical model development. *J. Pharm. Sci. 68*: 1341-1346.

Yu, C. D., Fox, J. L., Ho, N. F. H., and Higuchi, W. I. (1979b). Physical model evaluation of topical prodrug delivery—Simultaneous transport and bioconversion of vidarabine-5'-valerate. II. Parameter definitions. *J. Pharm. Sci. 68*: 1347–1357.

3
Skin Binding During Percutaneous Penetration

Efraim Menczel
Ministry of Health, State of Israel, Jerusalem, Israel

Daniel A. W. Bucks, Ronald C. Wester, and Howard I. Maibach
University of California School of Medicine, San Francisco, California

Dr. Harvey M. Solomon stated: "It has long been recognized that the binding of various drugs to plasma proteins may profoundly influence the free concentration of such agents and, thus, markedly, alter the magnitude and duration of the pharmacologic response" (Solomon, 1973). The various aspects of protein binding studies were comprehensively reviewed with particular emphasis on drugs administered parenterally or orally (McElnay and D'Arcy, 1983; Meyer and Guttman, 1968; Vallner, 1977). Similar appreciation of these phenomena in skin research and therapy was limited (Artuc et al., 1980; Menczel and Maibach, 1972; Schaefer et al., 1981). Unequivocally, chemicals penetrating percutaneously are being withheld by various skin layers, foremost in the epidermis (Artuc et al., 1980; Baker et al., 1977; Blank and Gould, 1959; Epstein, 1977; Feldmann and Maibach, 1965; Fleischmajer and Witten, 1955; Lobitz and Daniels, 1961; Marzulli, 1962; Menczel and Maibach, 1970, 1972; Menczel et al., 1983, 1984; Samitz and Katz, 1976; Schaefer et al., 1981; Slaga et al., 1977; Vickers, 1963) but to a certain degree also in the dermis (Baker et al., 1977; Dikshith and Datta, 1972; Dikshith et al., 1973, 1974; Feldmann and Maibach, 1965; Fleischmajer and Witten, 1955; Fredriksson, 1961; Marzulli, 1962; Menczel and Goldberg, 1978; Menczel and Maibach, 1970, 1972; Menczel et al., 1983, 1984; Nagakawa et al., 1971; Schaefer et al., 1975; Wahlberg, 1965). Retention of a chemical by a cutaneous tissue does not necessarily mean that it is bound by that tissue. Some chemicals by virtue of their solubility parameters are partitioned into several skin strata or into sebum (Rutherford and Black, 1981). On the other hand, some chemicals retained by cutaneous layers possess a specific affinity of reversible binding nature (Artuc et al., 1980; Menczel and

Maibach, 1972; Menczel et al., 1983, 1984; Schaefer et al., 1981). Both processes may interact. The differentiation between binding and partitioning can be accomplished by using chemical techniques such as dialysis (Artuc et al., 1980; Menczel and Maibach, 1972; Slaga et al., 1977), charcoal adsorption (Epstein, 1977), gel filtration (Adachi, 1974), and ultracentrifugation (Adachi, 1974). Skin can therefore function as a reservoir for latent action of a drug (Vickers, 1963); it can also be a focus for allergic or detrimental manifestations (Blohm, 1957; Dikshith and Datta, 1972; Dikshith et al., 1973, 1974; Nagakawa et al., 1971; Samitz and Katz, 1976; Schaefer et al., 1981; Wahlberg, 1965). Isolation of specific binding cells for specific drugs is essential in the elaboration of activity mechanisms (Adachi, 1974; Baker et al., 1977; Dall'aqua et al., 1972; Epstein, 1977; Mitchell and Epstein, 1965; Schaefer et al., 1981; Slaga et al., 1977). The information gained leads to a better understanding of the percutaneous pathways of absorption (Schaefer et al., 1981; Wester and Maibach, 1983).

EPIDERMAL RETENTION OF CHEMICALS IN PERCUTANEOUS PENETRATION

The epidermis is the primary and most effective barrier to percutaneous penetration of chemicals. This function of the skin depends on the protective horny layer, the stratum corneum (Schaefer et al., 1981). The rate of diffusion of the penetrant through the stratum corneum is low for most chemicals. Moreover, some chemicals interact with the epidermal tissue in the course of percutaneous penetration. Vickers (1963) presented the epidermal reservoir concept exhibited by corticosteroidal reactivation 2 weeks after its topical application by a repeated occlusion with Saran wrap. The preferential accumulation in the epidermis of cortisol and corticosterone (Baker et al., 1977) was further elaborated into investigations on the receptor mechanisms involved (Epstein, 1977; Slaga et al., 1977). Testosterone has a fair rate of percutaneous penetration (Feldmann and Maibach, 1966; Menczel and Maibach, 1970). The epidermal affinity for this male hormone is high (Menczel and Maibach, 1972). The specific activity of bound dexamethasone—an anticarcinogenic agent—to skin fractions was two to five times as high in the epidermis as in the dermis (Slaga et al., 1977). Thyopyronine and 8-methoxypsoralen were found reversibly bound to epidermal tissue (Artuc et al., 1980). Benzene hexachloride and malathion, two pesticides of different chemical structures, were found bound to epidermal tissue to a greater extent than to dermal tissue (Menczel et al., 1983, 1984); these binding effects are not contradictory to the pesticides' high rates of percutaneous permeation (Feldmann and Maibach, 1974; Maibach and Feldmann, 1974). On the other hand, the percutaneous penetration of anionic surfactants is to a great extent inhibited by the immense binding affinity to the stratum corneum proteins (Blank and Gould, 1959; Lobitz and Daniels, 1961). Similar observations were recently reported for hair dyes (Bronaugh and Congdon, 1984). Epidermal binding phenomena are not limited to organic compounds. In a study of nickel sensitivity in allergic contact dermatitis, considerable amounts of nickel were detected bound to the epidermis. Also, in this case, the binding interfered with the total diffusion of nickel through the epidermal tissue (Samitz and Katz, 1976).

DERMAL ASSOCIATION WITH CHEMICALS IN PERCUTANEOUS PENETRATION

The barrier capacity of skin tissue beyond that of the stratum corneum has been considered to be minimal (Schaefer et al., 1981). However, accumulating reports indicate that the underlying skin layers, including the dermis, are far from being completely permeable to chemical penetrants. Using thorium X, Fleischmajer and Witten (1955) observed a double retention effect of this radioactive substance, one in the epidermis and the second in the dermis. From studies on percutaneous absorption of hydrocortisone, Feldmann and Maibach (1965) concluded that after removal of the stratum corneum, yet another significant barrier was present. In the course of an in vitro percutaneous penetration study of the male hormone testosterone, there was found an appreciable retention in the dermal layers (Menczel and Maibach, 1970). Figure 1 is a replica of this study. The binding association of this steroidal compound to skin was further elaborated (Menczel and Maibach, 1972). These results were confirmed in a permeation study where testosterone accumulated in the dermis subcutis boundary (Schaefer et al., 1975, 1981). Similarly, another steroidal glucocorticoid, triamcinolone acetonide, applied topically accumulates both in the epidermis and dermis (Baker et al., 1977). This is in contrast with other glucocorticoids investigated, namely, cortisol and corticosterone, which are preferentially associated with the epidermis. Fredriksson (1961) interpreted his results on the percutaneous penetration of parathion. This organophosphate pesticide is apparently retained in the corium. In experimental animals, cutaneous cytopathological and histopathological changes were induced by parathion (Dikshith and Datta, 1972). Malathion, a milder organophosphate pesticide, binds extensively to dermal tissue (Menczel et al., 1983) in vitro. The dermal binding association was assessed for benzene hexachloride (lindane), a commonly used insecticide and pesticide (Menczel et al., 1984). This chemical, particularly in combination with the pesticide diazinon, produces severe pathologic lesions in the epidermis and dermis of rats (Dikshith et al., 1973, 1974). The peculiar rate of percutaneous penetration of mercuric chloride was explained by its prolonged storage in the corium, from which it is further diffused (Wahlberg, 1965). Similarly, the in vitro percutaneous penetration of lidocaine hydrochloride was found to consist of two separate concomitant and different rates; one relates to the epidermal diffusion of the drug, the second to its dermal distribution, from which absorption takes place (Menczel and Goldberg, 1978). The high allergenic potency of

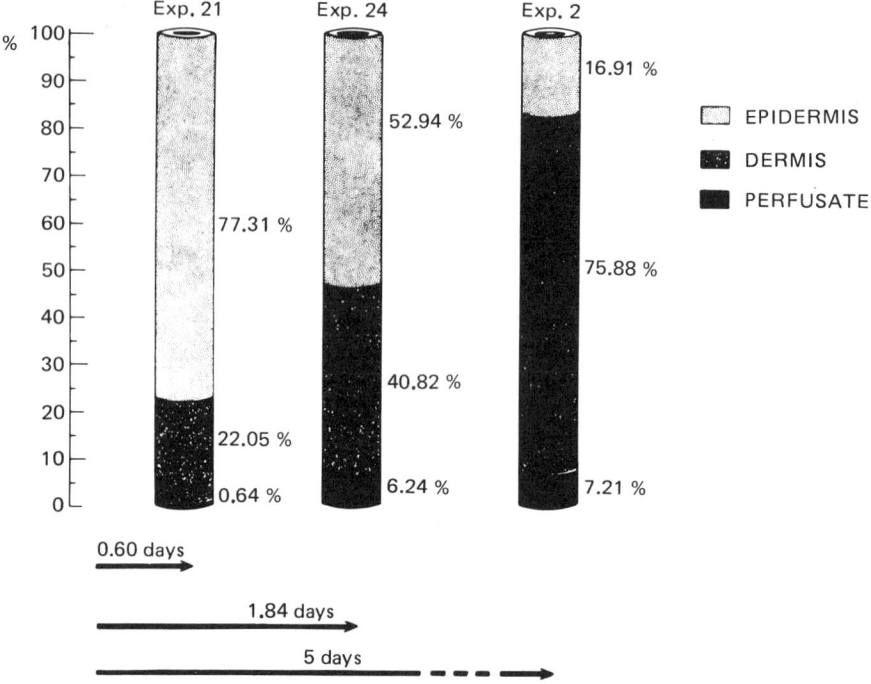

Figure 1 The relative distribution of [^{14}C] testosterone in the epidermis, dermis, and perfusate as function of the duration of percutaneous penetration experiments (autopsy human skin slices). (Courtesy of *Journal of Investigative Dermatology*.)

2,4-dinitrofluorobenzene and 2,4-dinitrochlorobenzene is related to the binding capacity of these compounds to proteins (Nagakawa et al., 1971; Schaefer et al., 1981). Marzulli (1962) distinctively outlined the varying capacities of the many skin barriers. As to a specific site, Adachi attempted to locate receptor proteins for androgens, such as dihydrotestosterone, through binding experiments with isolated sebaceous glands (Adachi, 1974). Accumulation of drugs in sebum has been demonstrated for germicides (Rutherford and Black, 1981). Binding studies were utilized to evaluate receptor mechanisms such as DNA to psoralen (Dall'aqua et al., 1972) or chloroquine to melanin (Mitchell and Epstein, 1965).

BINDING AFFINITY VERSUS PARTITIONING OF CHEMICALS INTO SKIN TISSUE

The retention of a chemical in any of the cutaneous tissue is a net outcome of either reversible affinity binding or partitioning of the substance between aqueous vehicle and tissue components (Artuc et al., 1980; Menczel and Maibach, 1972). This distinction can be ascertained by analyzing the data obtained from equilibration of the chemical dissolved in a suitable buffer with the specific skin tissue. In case of partitioning, the partition coefficient K can be derived from the concentration of the substance in the specific tissue D_T divided by its concentration D_B in an appropriate buffer (Artuc et al., 1980; Menczel and Maibach, 1972):

$$K = D_T/D_B \tag{1}$$

In its logarithmic form, a straight-line relationship is obtained with a slope equal to unity according to the following equation:

$$\log D_T = \log K + \log D_B \tag{2}$$

Reversible binding affinity can be described by the Freundlich adsorption isotherm, where the concentration of the tissue-bound substance D_{Tb} is related to that unbound D_F by an exponential term:

$$D_{Tb} = K \cdot D_F^a \tag{3}$$

where K and a are computed constants characteristic of the system involved. In its logarithmic form Equation 3 can be stated as follows:

$$\log D_{Tb} = \log K + a \log D_F \tag{4}$$

This is a straight-line relationship between $\log D_{Tb}$ and $\log D_F$, where $\log K$ is the intercept on the y axis and a is the slope that is less than unity.

The similarities of the relationships in Equations 2 and 4 are self-evident. When the value of a in Equation 4 approximates 1, it implicitly resembles Equation 2. Thus, the determination of slope *a* is the indicative of whether the chemical is partitioned or associatively bound (according to Freundlich adsorption isotherm) upon equilibration between its solution and the specific skin tissue (Artuc et al., 1980; Menczel and Maibach, 1972).

Except for the keratinous stratum corneum, the main binding constituent of tissues is albumin (Jusko and Gretch, 1976; McElnay and D'Arcy, 1983), a protein of high molecular weight that is also the chief drug-binding protein in plasma (McElnay and D'Arcy, 1983; Meyer and Guttman, 1968; Vallner, 1977). The dynamic equilibrium between the chemical bound to protein [PC] to the unbound chemical [C] is governed by K_a, the association constant, according to the law of mass action:

$$K_a = \frac{[PC]}{[P][C]} \tag{5}$$

where [P] is the free protein concentration. It follows that the ratio r of bound chemical to total protein [P_t] can be derived from Equation 5 as follows:

$$r = \frac{[PC]}{[P_t]} = \frac{[PC]}{[PC] + [P]} = \frac{n K_a [C]}{1 + K_a [C]} \tag{6}$$

where n is the number of binding sites. The Scatchard plot (Niazi, 1979; Scatchard, 1972) is a straight-line relationship obtained by rearrangement of Equation 6 and division by [C]:

$$\frac{r}{[C]} = n \cdot K_a - K_a \cdot r \tag{7}$$

where r/[C] is plotted on the y axis, r on the x axis, the slope obtained is K_a, and the intercept equals n · K_a. After substituting [P] in Equation 5 by n − [PC], which equals the concentration of the binding sites less that bound, the reciprocal of K_a is expressed as the dissociation constant K_d:

$$K_d = \frac{(n - [PC])[C]}{[PC]} = \frac{1}{K_a} \tag{8}$$

Rearrangement of Equation 8 will produce a straight-line, simplified Scatchard plot (Artuc et al., 1980):

$$[PC] = n - K_d \frac{[PC]}{[C]} \tag{9}$$

where [PC] is plotted on the y axis, [PC]/[C] on the x axis, n is the intercept, and the resulting slope will be K_d.

Figures 2a and 4b in Artuc et al. (1980) illustrate the estimation of epidermal binding parameters for thyopyronine by Freundlich adsorption isotherm (Eq. 4) and simplified Scatchard plot (Eq. 9), respectively.

SEQUENTIAL BINDING OF CHEMICALS IN PERCUTANEOUS ABSORPTION

Table 1 summarizes representative chemicals reported to be bound to one or more layers of the skin as well as those partitioned or retained therein.

Skin Binding During Percutaneous Penetration

The intense epidermal binding of chemicals is part of the skin's barrier mechanism, diminishing to a great extent cutaneous permeability (Marzulli, 1962; Samitz and Katz, 1976). The opposite effect is produced by dermal binding, which rather enhances percutaneous penetration by a dynamic uptake mechanism. The process is essentially similar to the absorption of plasma protein-bound drugs from the gastrointestinal tract. The more a drug is bound to plasma protein (= albumin), the better is its absorption following administration by the oral route (McElnay and D'Ary, 1983). Since passive diffusion is involved mainly in both these processes, Fick's law applies and accordingly an increase in the concentration gradient will augment the amount absorbed (McElnay and D'Arcy, 1983). The concentration gradient in percutaneous absorption is increased by binding the chemical in the absorbing side of the semipermeable membranes of the dermal layers.

In passive diffusion what indeed counts are the concentrations of the "free" (= unbound) chemical on both sides of membrane. Thus, the dermal protein-binding capacity for a chemical will determine the concentration gradient, which ultimately accelerates accordingly its dermal uptake. Provided plasma protein possesses binding affinity for the chemical, the same process repeats itself upon absorption; the chemical is subsequently carried away from the dermis through a drainage by the body fluids—in part as plasma protein bound. This in turn increases the concentration gradient, and percutaneous penetration is favored to the same degree as gastrointestinal absorption under similar circumstances. Diagrammatically these reactions can be presented as follows:

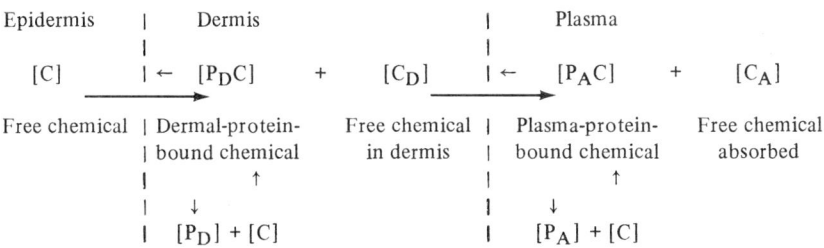

This sequence of events, first reported from one laboratory for the male hormone testosterone (Feldmann and Maibach, 1966; Menczel and Maibach, 1970, 1972), was further substantiated in another independent laboratory where penetration kinetics of sexual hormones were investigated (Schaefer et al., 1975). The magnitude of epidermal binding of testosterone exceeds by severalfold that of the dermis; but, because of the manyfold thicknesses of the dermis in comparison to the epidermis, far larger amounts are associatively bound in the dermis (Menczel and Maibach, 1970, 1972) (see also Fig. 1), from which it is further eluted by the body fluids. Testosterone is plasma protein bound (Doughday, 1959; Eiknes et al., 1954); its percutaneous absorption is enhanced.

Table 1 Epidermal and Dermal Retention Effects of Chemicals

Chemical	Reference	
	Epidermis	Dermis
2 Amino-4-nitrophenol	Bronaugh and Congdon, 1984	
4 Amino-2-nitrophenol	Bronaugh and Congdon, 1984	
Anionic surfactants	Blank and Gould, 1959; Blohm, 1957; Lobitz and Daniels, 1961	
Benzene hexachloride (lindane)	Dikshith et al., 1973, 1974[a]; Menczel et al., 1984	Dikshith et al., 1973, 1974[a]; Menczel et al., 1984
Benzyl alcohol	Menczel and Maibach, 1972; Slaga et al., 1977	Menczel and Maibach, 1972; Slaga et al., 1977
4 Chloro-m-phenylenediamine	Bronaugh and Congdon, 1984	
Corticosterone	Baker et al., 1977	
Cortisol	Baker et al., 1977	
Dexamethasone	Epstein, 1977; Slaga et al., 1977	
Dihydrotestosterone		Adachi, 1974[b]
2,4-Dinitrochlorobenzene	Nagakawa et al., 1971; Schaefer et al., 1981	Nagakawa et al., 1971; Schaefer et al., 1981
α-Estradiol	Artuc et al., 1980	
Fluocinolone acetonide	Vickers, 1963	

Germicides		Rutherford and Black, 1981[c]
Hydrocortisone	Feldmann and Maibach, 1965	Feldmann and Maibach, 1965
Lidocaine hydrochloride	Menczel and Goldberg, 1978	Menczel and Goldberg, 1978
Malathion	Menczel et al., 1983	Menczel et al., 1983
Mercuric chloride	Wahlberg, 1965	
5-Methoxypsoralen	Artuc et al., 1980	
8-Methoxypsoralen	Artuc et al., 1980	
Nickel sulfate	Samitz and Katz, 1976	
σ Phenylenediamine	Bronaugh and Congdon, 1984	
ρ Phenylenediamine	Bronaugh and Congdon, 1984	
Parathion	Dikshith and Datta, 1972; Fredriksson, 1961	Dikshith and Datta, 1972
Testosterone	Menczel and Maibach, 1970, 1972	Menczel and Maibach, 1970, 1972; Schaefer et al., 1975, 1981
Thiopyronine	Artuc et al., 1980	
Thorium X (THXCP)	Fleischmajer and Witten, 1955	Fleischmajer and Witten, 1955
Triamcinolone acetonide	Baker et al., 1977; Vickers, 1963	Baker et al., 1977

[a]With diazinon.
[b]Sebaceous glands.
[c]Sebum.

Three additional examples illustrate this principle:

1. 2,4-Dinitrochlorobenzene (DNCB) is an allergenic compound that rapidly binds to proteins, cutaneous included (Nagakawa et al., 1971; Schaefer et al., 1981); its percutaneous absorption is outstanding (Feldmann and Maibach, 1970a; Schaefer et al., 1981).

2. Benzene hexachloride (lindane), was found recently to be epidermal-dermal bound as well as being bound to plasma protein (Menczel et al., 1984). These findings are reproduced in Figures 2 and 3. Lindane is fairly well absorbed percutaneously (Feldmann and Maibach, 1970b).

3. The organophosphate pesticide malathion, proved to be bound both to epidermis and to dermis (Menczel et al., 1983); it ranks among the higher

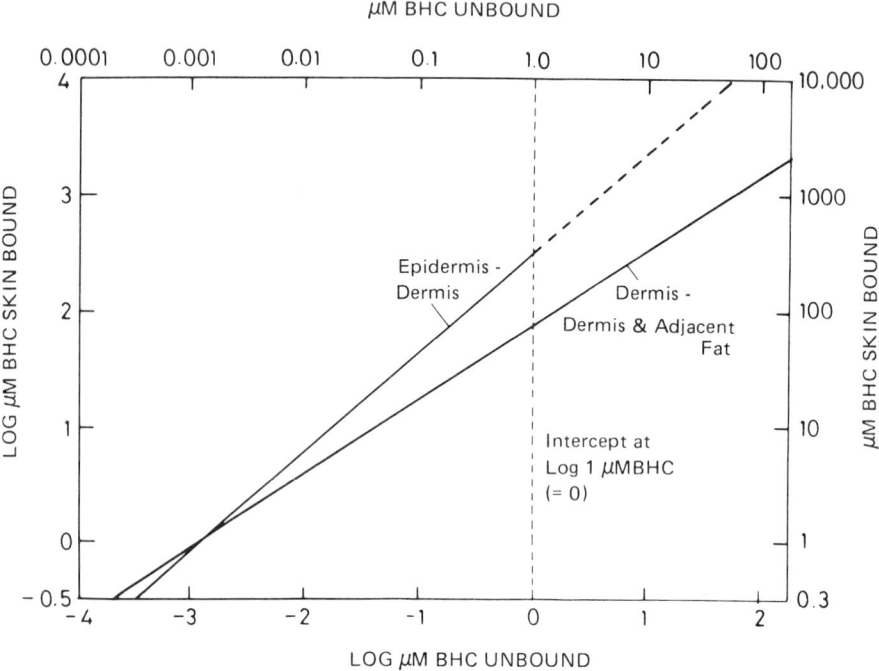

Figure 2 Isotherm binding capacity determinations of benzene hexachloride (BHC) (lindane) in autopsy human skin sections. Skin-bound BHC versus unbound BHC in aqueous buffer (pH 7.4) plotted according to the Freundlich adsorption isotherm. The binding slope is denoted by solid lines in the range of the concentrations tested and by a dashed line in the range of the extrapolated values. Slope (a of Eq. 4) values: 0.86 for the outer and middle and 0.66 for the inner sections of the skin. Bound per totum BHC at 75 μmole/liter = 99.8% for the outer and middle and 98.7% for the inner sections. (Courtesy of *Archives of Dermatology Research*.)

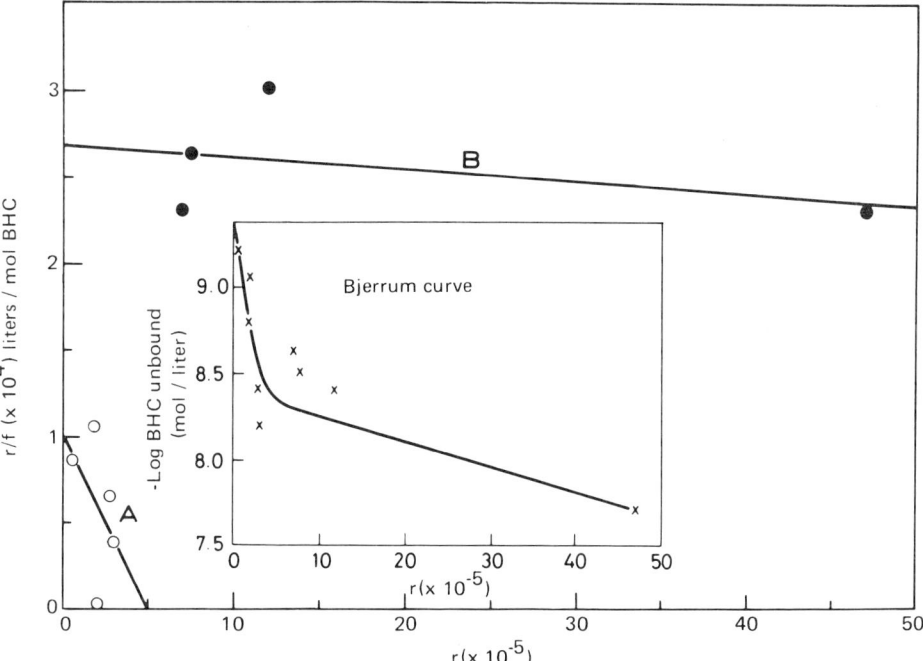

Figure 3 Scatchard plots for the binding of benzene hexachloride (BHC) (lindane) to plasma protein fraction (human 5%, USP): r = moles per liter of BHC bound per mole per liter of albumin in plasma protein fraction, f = moles per liter of BHC unbound (free—denoted [C] in Eq. 7). Insert: Bjerrum curve of $-\log$ BHC unbound versus r. Experimental values: ○, Scatchard plot A; ●, Scatchard plot B; ×, Bjerrum curve. The Bjerrum curve signifies two binding slopes: A and B. Slope values (K_a of Eq. 7): 2.00×10^8 and 7.27×10^6 liters per mole of BHC unbound for plots A and B, respectively. (Courtesy of *Archives of Dermatology Research*.)

percutaneously penetrating chemicals (Feldmann and Maibach, 1970a,b; Wester et al., 1983). The interaction of malathion with plasma proteins indicates a pattern of solubilization within the protein micelles (Mulley, 1964). For a wide range of concentrations, malathion's partitioning in plasma is characterized by about double concentration of that in aqueous buffer (Menczel et al., 1983) (see Fig. 4). Plasma solubilization of malathion produces a strong binding linkage (Eiknes et al., 1954; Goldstein et al., 1969) that affects the concentration gradient to a great extent, which sequentially promotes percutaneous penetration. On the other hand, the dissociation of malathion from the protein micelles is slow, and this might interfere with the rate of its urinary excretion (Eiknes et

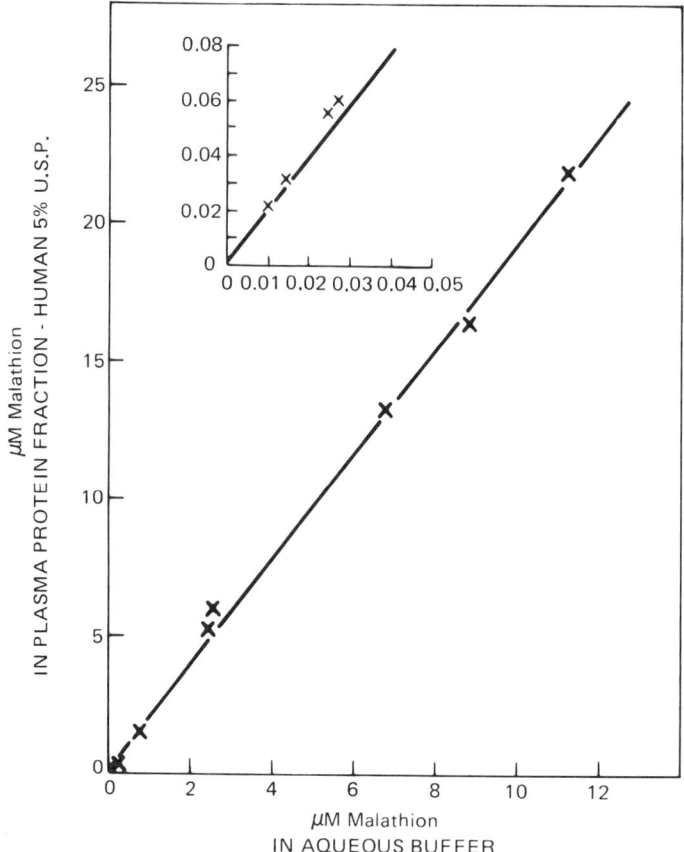

Figure 4 Solubilization of malathion in plasma. Equilibrium partitioning of malathion between aqueous buffer and plasma protein fraction (human 5%, USP) in micromolar concentrations. Ranges: 0.01-0.08 (insert) and 0.1-22 (main figure). For both plots ($n = 11$), by linear regression analysis the solubilization partitioning slope is 1.93 (r = correlation coefficient = .9988); experimental values denoted by X. (Courtesy of *Archives of Dermatology Research*.)

al., 1954; Goldstein et al., 1969). This could be a prime factor governing the toxicity of this pesticide, which also has medical applications (British National Formulary, 1981; Menczel et al., 1983).

CONCLUSIONS

The binding interactions of chemicals with various layers of skin have manifold consequences. They contribute primarily to the barrier function of the skin—

mostly of the epidermis. Through retention, according to the binding capacity of a chemical to skin proteins—or its partitioning—a reservoir depot is produced either in the epidermis or in the dermis, or in both these skin layers.

In addition, chemical binding to skin proteins affects the dynamic pathways of epidermal-dermal uptake and ultimate absorption by the body fluids. The sequential binding association with plasma proteins is a contributing factor in the kinetics of percutaneous penetration.

Moreover, the information on binding of chemicals to various strata of the skin is of utmost importance in the investigation of the pharmacologic activities and therapeutic responses, as well as to studies of allergic or deleterious toxic manifestations, both in healthy and diseased skin.

REFERENCES

Adachi, K. (1974). *J. Invest. Dermatol. 62*: 217.
Artuc, M., Reinhold, C., Stüttgen, G., and Gazith, J. (1980). *Arch. Dermatol. Res. 268*: 129.
Baker, J. R. J., Christian, R. A., Simpson, P., and White, A. M. (1977). *Br. J. Dermatol. 96*: 171.
Blank, J. H. and Gould, E. (1959). *J. Invest. Dermatol. 33*: 327.
Blohm, S. G. (1957). *Acta Dermatovenereol.* (Stockholm) *37*: 269.
Bronaugh, D. L. and Congdon, E. R. (1984). *J. Invest. Dermatol. 83*: 124.
British National Formulary, No. 2 (1981). British Medical Association, Pharmaceutical Press, London.
Dall'aqua, F., Marciani, S., Vedaldi, D., and Rodighiero, G. (1972). *FEBS Lett. 27*: 192.
Davson, H. and Danielli, J. F. (1943). *The Permeability of Natural Membranes*. Cambridge University Press, London.
Dikshith, T. S. S. and Datta, K. K. (1972). *Experientia 28*: 169.
Dikshith, T. S. S., Chandra, P., and Datta, K. K. (1973). *Experientia 29*: 684.
Dikshith, T. S. S., Datta, K. K., and Chandra, P. (1974). *Exp. Pathol. 9*: 219.
Doughday, W. H. (1959). *Physiol. Rev. 39*: 885.
Eiknes, K., Schellman, J. A., Lumry, R., and Samuels, L. T. (1954). *J. Biol. Chem. 206*: 411.
Epstein, E. (1977). *Clin. Res. 25*: 281A.
Feldmann, R. J. and Maibach, H. I. (1965). *Arch. Dermatol. 91*: 661.
Feldmann, R. J. and Maibach, H. I. (1966). *Arch. Dermatol. 94*: 649.
Feldmann, R. J. and Maibach, H. I. (1970a). *J. Invest. Dermatol. 54*: 399.
Feldmann, R. J. and Maibach, H. I. (1970b). *J. Invest. Dermatol. 54*: 435.
Feldmann, R. J. and Maibach, H. I. (1974). *Toxicol. Appl. Pharmacol. 28*: 126.
Fleischmajer, R. and Witten, V. H. (1955). *J. Invest. Dermatol. 25*: 223.
Fredriksson, T. (1961). *Acta Dermatovenereol.* (Stockholm) *41*: 353.
Goldstein, A., Aronow, L., and Kalman, S. M. (1969). *Principles of Drug Action*, Harper & Row, New York.
Jusko, W. J. and Gretch, M. (1976). *Drug Metab. Rev. 5*: 43.
Lobitz, W. C. and Daniels, F. D. (1961). *Annu. Rev. Physiol. 23*: 207.

McElnay, J. C. and D'Arcy, P. F. (1983). *Drugs 25*: 495.
Maibach, H. I. and Feldmann, R. J. (1974). *Systemic Absorption of Pesticides.* Report to the Federal Working Group on Pest Management from the Task Group, pp. 120–127.
Marzulli, F. N. (1962). *J. Invest. Dermatol. 39*: 387.
Menczel, E and Goldberg, S. (1978). *Dermatologica 156*: 8.
Menczel, E. and Maibach, H. I. (1970). *J. Invest. Dermatol. 54*: 386.
Menczel, E. and Maibach, H. I. (1972). *Acta Dermatovenereol.* (Stockholm) *52*: 38.
Menczel, E., Bucks, D., Maibach, H., and Wester, R. (1983). *Arch. Dermatol. Res. 275*: 403.
Menczel, E., Bucks, D., Maibach, H., and Wester, R. (1984). *Arch. Dermatol. Res. 276*: 326.
Meyer, M. C. and Guttman, D. E. (1968). *J. Pharm. Sci. 57*: 895.
Mitchell, W. and Epstein, J. H. (1965). *J. Invest. Dermatol. 45*: 482.
Mulley, B. A. (1964). In *Advances in Pharmaceutical Sciences*, Vol. 1. Edited by H. S. Bean, A. H. Beckett, and J. E. Charles. Academic, New York.
Nagakawa, S., Ueki, H., and Tanioky, K. (1971). *J. Invest. Dermatol. 57*: 269.
Niazi, S. (1979). *Textbook of Pharmaceutics and Clinical Pharmacokinetics.* Appleton-Century-Crofts, New York.
Rutherford, T. and Black, J. G. (1981). *Br. J. Dermatol. 81* (Suppl. 4): 75.
Samitz, M. H. and Katz, S. A. (1976). *Environ. Res. 11*: 34.
Scatchard, G. (1972). *Ann. N.Y. Acad. Sci. 51*: 660.
Schaefer, H., Zesch, A., Giera, M., Wendtker, N., and Bauer, E. (1975). *Arch. Dermatol. Forsch. 252*: 74.
Schaefer, H., Zesch, A., and Stüttgen, G. (1981). In *Handbuch der Haut und Geschlechtskrankheiten, Erganzungswerk 1/4B, Normal and Pathologic Physiology of the Skin*, Vol. III. Edited by G. Stüttgen, H. W. Spier, and E. Schwarz, Springer-Verlag, Berlin.
Slaga, T. J., Thompson, S., and Schwarz, J. A. (1977). *J. Inv. Dermatol. 68*: 307.
Solomon, H. M. (1973). *Ann. N.Y. Acad. Sci. 226*: 5.
Vallner, J. J. (1977). *J. Pharm. Sci. 66*: 447.
Vickers, C. F. H. (1963). *Arch. Dermatol. 88*: 72.
Wahlberg, J. E. (1965). *Acta Dermatovenereol.* (Stockholm) *45*: 415.
Wester, R. C. and Maibach, H. I. (1983). *Drug Metab. Rev. 14*: 169.
Wester, R. C., Maibach, H. I., Bucks, D. A. W., and Guy, R. H. (1983). *Toxicol. Appl. Pharmacol. 68*: 116.

4
Skin Metabolism
Theoretical

Richard H. Guy
University of California School of Pharmacy, San Francisco, California

Jonathan Hadgraft*
University of Nottingham, Nottingham, England

To what extent does cutaneous metabolism affect the topical or transdermal delivery of drugs? This question has not been adequately considered in the literature. The answer, however, is important for its own sake and has much relevance both to the selection of candidates for transdermal drug delivery and to the design and feasibility of topical prodrugs. Experimental study of skin metabolism is difficult, and it is probably fair to say that until somewhat recently, biotransformation of penetrating molecules has been assumed to be rather unimportant or unlikely. More substantial evidence, though, is now becoming available, (see Chap. 5) and it seems clear that cutaneous metabolism represents an area in which much further investigation will be conducted.

In this chapter, we shall discuss attempts to model mathematically the ramifications of concurrent metabolism on the percutaneous penetration process. The objective of this work has been to demonstrate the conditions under which skin biotransformation is important and to illustrate the consequent effects on the concentration versus time profiles of parent and metabolite in skin and plasma.

THEORETICAL MODELS

Mathematical treatments of skin metabolism and percutaneous absorption can be classified into three categories:

   Steady state
   Non-steady state
   Pharmacokinetic

**Present affiliation*: University of Wales Institute of Science and Technology, Cardiff, Wales

The approach and deductions of these different descriptions are now considered in turn.

Steady-State Model

In normal practice, steady-state conditions are not encountered. However, it may be instructive to ascertain the effect of cutaneous metabolism by assuming that a linear concentration gradient of the parent drug exists across the stratum corneum. This simplifies the mathematical analysis and enables one to assess the influence of simple physicochemical parameters on the resulting parent drug/metabolite disposition profiles. This approach has been adopted in some recent publications (Ando et al., 1977; Fox et al., 1979; Yu et al., 1979a,b) to consider, in a fundamental way, the effect of cutaneous biotransformation and to evaluate rationally topical prodrug delivery.

The authors solve the following diffusion equation:

$$\frac{\partial^2 c}{\partial x^2} - \frac{V_{max} c}{K_m + c} = 0 \tag{1}$$

The first term describes transcutaneous transport according to Fick's second law of diffusion; the second term represents the skin metabolic process in a conventional Michaelis-Menten fashion. Ando et al. (1977) made the initial attempt to use the equation and sought to demonstrate the manner in which topical bioavailability could be affected by skin metabolism. Fox et al. (1979) used a computational method and identified three factors that were important when simultaneous percutaneous absorption and biotransformation were considered: prodrug solubility, rate of prodrug to drug conversion, and ability of the prodrug to inhibit the metabolism of the drug. If this system can be developed to a sufficient extent, it should be possible to use the analysis to optimize the choice of the chemical structure of the prodrug.

In a series of publications, Yu et al. (1979a,b) describe the application of the model above to the evaluation of the skin metabolism of the prodrug vidarabine-5'-valerate. Enzyme distribution in the skin was shown to be significant, and the results from hairless mouse skin were assessed using the mathematical model. The results may be used predictively to estimate the therapeutic effect of the prodrug when it is applied topically.

Non-Steady-State Model

If a linear concentration gradient does not exist across the skin, the transport/bioconversion equation that applies is as follows:

$$\frac{\partial c}{\partial t} = \frac{\partial^2 c}{\partial x^2} - \frac{V_{max} c}{K_m + c} \tag{2}$$

Skin Metabolism: Theoretical

Complete analytical solutions to this expression have not been derived for skin, but there have been attempts to consider certain limiting cases that have proved instructive (Guy and Hadgraft, 1982; Hadgraft, 1980). The mathematical treatment in this type of approach establishes a simple physical model of the type illustrated in Figure 1. Hadgraft (1980) addressed the theoretical aspects of metabolism and assumed that linear biotransformation kinetics pertained. Metabolism was considered in both the stratum corneum and the viable epidermis. The mathematical deductions allow evaluation of the amount of unchanged penetrant reaching the dermal vasculature as a function of time. It was shown that this amount not only is dependent on the metabolism kinetics but also is a sensitive function of the effective partition coefficient of the molecule between the stratum corneum and the viable epidermis. This sensitivity is illustrated in Figure 2.

While linear enzyme kinetics may be adequate to describe cutaneous metabolism, it is of course conceivable that saturation of these systems may occur. Guy and Hadgraft (1982) have considered this possibility and have solved Equation 2 under conditions of saturable enzyme kinetics. Also considered as a variable in this work was the rate at which the absorbing species enters the skin from the applied phase. Clearly, in a saturable system, the input rate to the region in which biotransformation occurs will be a major determinant of the final "percentage of drug penetrating unchanged versus time" profile.

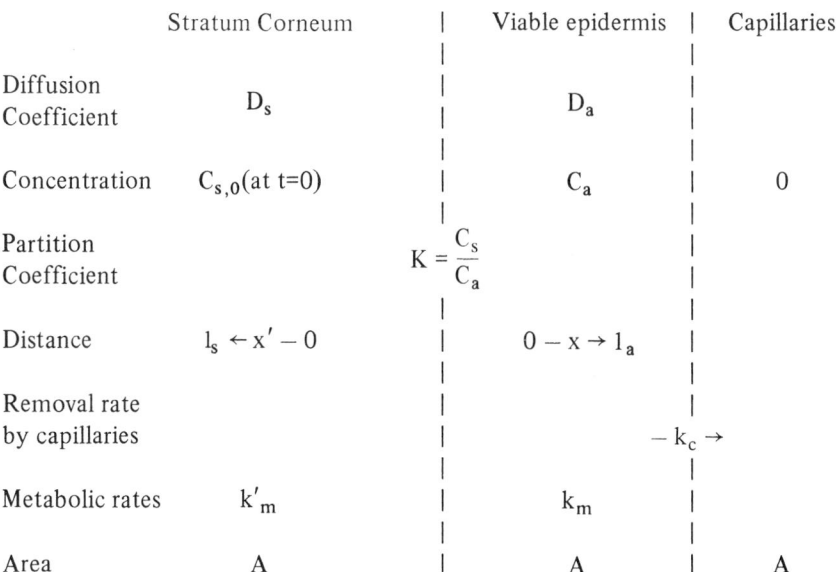

	Stratum Corneum	Viable epidermis	Capillaries
Diffusion Coefficient	D_s	D_a	
Concentration	$C_{s,0}$ (at t=0)	C_a	0
Partition Coefficient		$K = \dfrac{C_s}{C_a}$	
Distance	$l_s \leftarrow x' - 0$	$0 - x \rightarrow l_a$	
Removal rate by capillaries			$-k_c \rightarrow$
Metabolic rates	k'_m	k_m	
Area	A	A	A

Figure 1 Schematic representation of the skin structure.

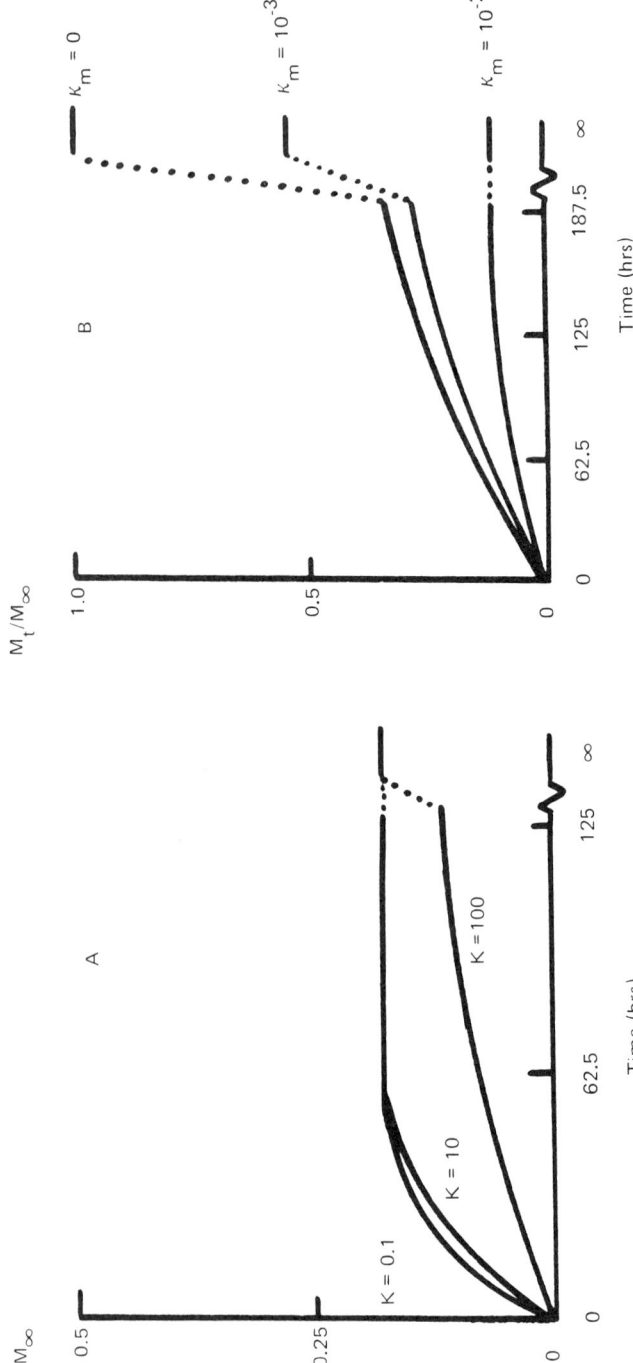

Figure 2 Release profiles showing the effect of metabolism kinetics and partition coefficient on the fraction of the applied parent compound that eventually reaches the capillaries (M_t/M_∞). (A) Effect of varying the stratum corneum/viable epidermis partition coefficient with a fixed first-order metabolic rate in the viable tissue ($k_m = 4.4 \times 10^{-5}$ sec^{-1}). (B) Effect of varying metabolic rate constant ($k_m = 0.1$ corresponds to $k_m = 4.4 \times 10^{-5}$ sec^{-1}) with a fixed partition coefficient of 100.

Skin Metabolism: Theoretical

At present, many of the results indicated by the non-steady-state treatments remain difficult to test because sufficiently precise information concerning enzyme levels and activities in skin does not exist. However, when these data become available, it may be expected that the results of this mathematical work, in which a realistic non-steady-state case has been considered, will be of much value in predicting the significance of the cutaneous metabolism of drugs.

Pharmacokinetic Model

Most recently, a more conventional pharmacokinetic approach has been adopted to tackle the question of concurrent skin transport and metabolism (Guy and Hadgraft, 1984). The approach is based on a simpler linear model, which has been established to describe the process of percutaneous absorption (Guy et al., 1982). The pharmacokinetic scheme is shown in Figure 3. First-order rate constants are assumed as in Chapter 1: k_1 describes stratum corneum transport of parent drug, k_2 relates to its movement further into the tissue across the viable epidermis, k_3 reflects the competition for the penetrant between the stratum corneum and the viable epidermis, and k_4 is the elimination rate constant of the parent drug from the dermal vasculature to the urine. Skin metabolism is represented in the model by the transformation rate constant k_5 of parent to metabolite in the viable epidermis; subsequent elimination of metabolite is described by k_6. Thus we assume that only one metabolite is formed in the skin and that the substrate concentration is low, so that the linear approximation to Michaelis-Menten kinetics can be used.

We have chosen to illustrate the utility of the simulation by calculating the plasma concentrations of parent drug and metabolite under a variety of situations. Such an approach is useful in assessing the potential of transdermal delivery candidates that may be susceptible to cutaneous metabolic deactivation. Equally, the model can be employed to determine the effectiveness of topical prodrugs for local therapy, since it is also straightforward to calculate skin levels of penetrant and metabolite.

The differential equations that describe the kinetics shown in Figure 3 are solved by standard procedures. The resulting expressions are sums of exponential functions (Guy and Hadgraft, 1984; Guy et al., 1982). To show how the plasma profiles can be influenced by alteration of the rate parameters in the model, two examples are given in Figures 4 and 5. In the situations considered, elimination and biotransformation rate constants are held invariant ($k_4 = k_5 = k_6 = 10^{-4}$ sec^{-1}). Transport across the viable epidermis also proceeds at the same rate in both cases ($k_2 = 10^{-3}$ sec^{-1}) and corresponds to an expected diffusional velocity for typical drug molecules in this region (Guy and Hadgraft, 1982; Scheuplein, 1967), that is, 10^{-7} cm^2/sec. The rate constants that are altered are k_1 and k_3: $k_1 = k_3 = 10^{-6}$ sec^{-1} in Figure 4; $k_1 = 10^{-5}$ sec^{-1} and $k_3 = 10^{-3}$ sec^{-1} in Figure

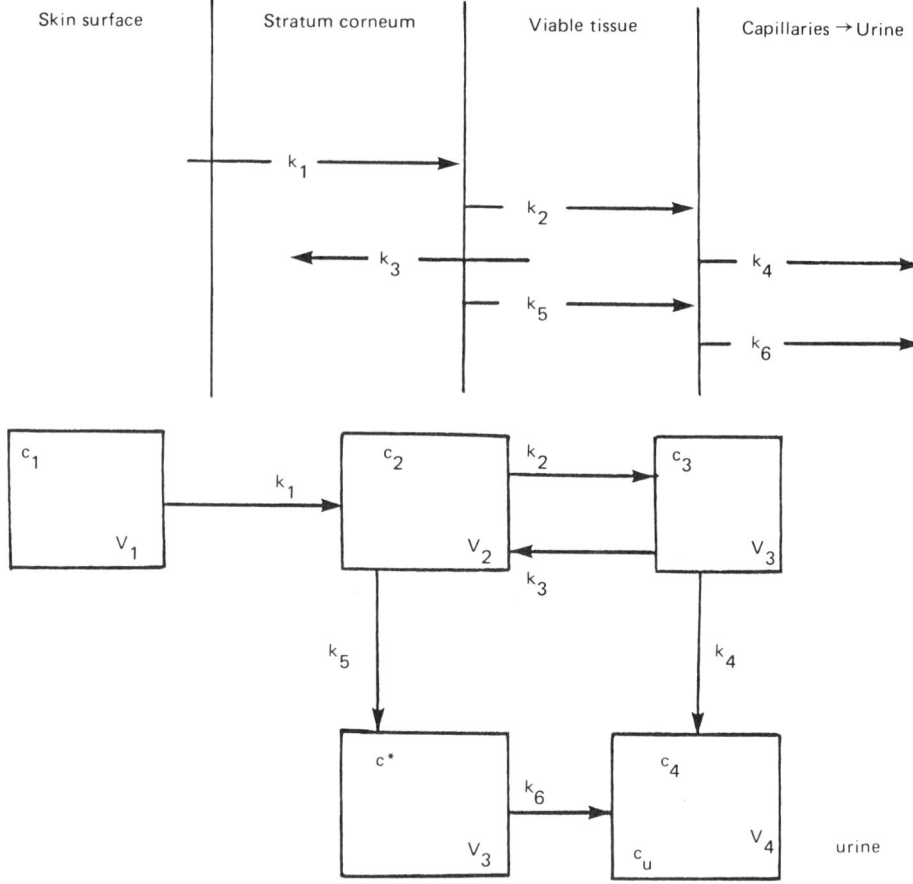

Figure 3 Schematic representation of the pharmacokinetics of skin absorption with concurrent metabolism.

5. Hence, the two examples illustrate (1) the effect of different trans-stratum corneum diffusion coefficients, and (2) the effect of changing the relative stratum corneum/viable epidermis partition coefficient. In Figure 4, the low k_3 value means that the drug molecule shows little affinity for the stratum corneum and moves relatively rapidly through the skin. Given the magnitude of k_5, little bioconversion is able to take place under these circumstances. In Figure 5, which corresponds to a much more lipophilic parent molecule, slower transcutaneous movement occurs and the metabolic process has a greater opportunity to act. The outcome of these differences is clearly indicated in the figures.

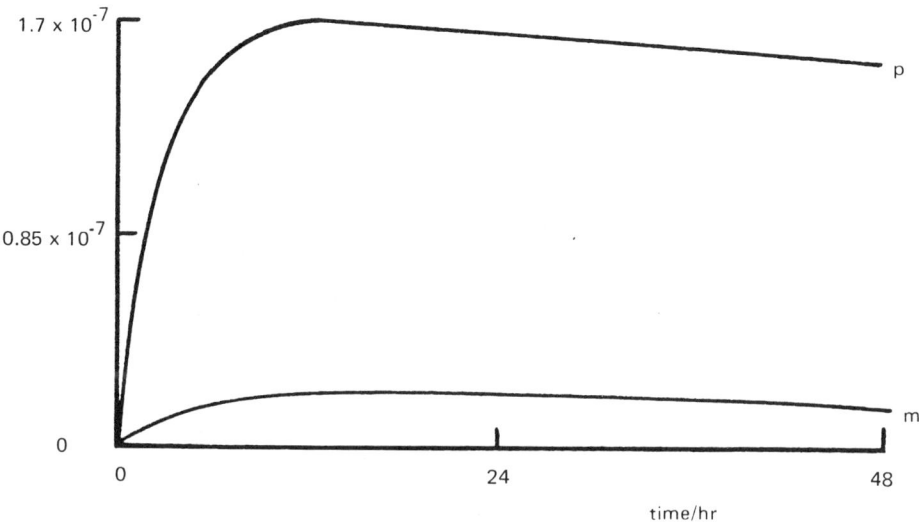

Figure 4 The fraction of the applied topical dose appearing in the plasma as parent compound (p) and metabolite (m) as a function of time for the following first-order rate constants (sec^{-1}): $k_1 = k_3 = 10^{-6}$; $k_2 = 10^{-3}$; $k_4 = k_5 = k_6 = 10^{-4}$.

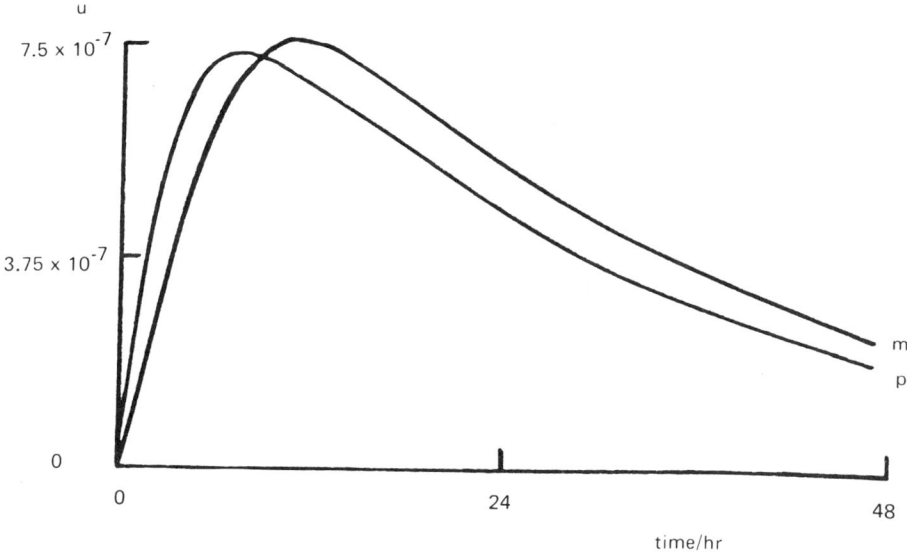

Figure 5 The fraction of the applied topical dose appearing in the plasma as parent compound (p) and metabolite (m) as a function of time for the following first-order rate constants (sec^{-1}): $k_1 = 10^{-5}$; $k_2 = k_3 = 10^{-3}$; $k_4 = k_5 = k_6 = 10^{-4}$.

It is believed that this type of analysis will facilitate assessment of the cutaneous metabolic process and will enable the importance of biotransformation on transdermal drug delivery to be determined. One may also expect that the approach will be useful in the rational design of topical prodrugs. Future application awaits the acquisition of more extensive and precise experimental in vivo data.

ACKNOWLEDGMENTS

We would like to thank the following for financial assistance: the Burroughs Wellcome Fund, the Wellcome Trust, and Alza and Hoffmann La Roche.

REFERENCES

Ando, H. Y., Ho, N. F. H., and Higuchi, W. I. (1977). Skin as an active metabolizing barrier. I. Theoretical analysis of topical bioavailability. *J. Pharm. Sci.* 66: 1525-1528.

Fox, J. L., Yu, C. D., Higuchi, W. I., and Ho, N. F. H. (1979). General physical model for simultaneous diffusion and metabolism in biological membranes. The computational approach for the steady state case. *Int. J. Pharm.* 2: 41-57.

Guy, R. H. and Hadgraft, J. (1982). Percutaneous metabolism with saturable enzyme kinetics. *Int. J. Pharm.* 11: 187-197.

Guy, R. H. and Hadgraft, J. (1984). Pharmacokinetics of percutaneous absorption with concurrent metabolism. *Int. J. Pharm.* 20: 43-51.

Guy, R. H., Hadgraft, J., and Maibach, H. I. (1982). A pharmacokinetic model for percutaneous absorption. *Int. J. Pharm.* 11: 119-129.

Hadgraft, J. (1980). Theoretical aspects of metabolism in the epidermis. *Int. J. Pharm.* 4: 229-239.

Scheuplein, R. J. (1967). Mechanism of percutaneous absorption. II. Transient diffusion and the relative importance of various routes of skin penetration. *J. Invest. Dermatol.* 45: 334-346.

Yu, C. D., Fox, J. L., Ho, N. F. H., and Higuchi, W. I. (1979a). Physical model evaluation of topical prodrug delivery–simultaneous transport and bioconversion of vidarabine-5'-valerate. I. Physical model development. *J. Pharm. Sci.* 68: 1341-1346.

Yu, C. D., Fox, J. L., Ho, N. F. H., and Higuchi, W. I. (1979b). Physical model evaluation of topical prodrug delivery–simultaneous transport and bioconversion of vidarabine-5'-valerate. II. Parameter determinations. *J. Pharm. Sci.* 68: 1347-1357.

5
Cutaneous Metabolism of Xenobiotics

Patrick K. Noonan
Research and Development Division, Key Pharmaceuticals, Inc., Miami, Florida

Ronald C. Wester
University of California School of Medicine, San Francisco, California

The skin is viewed as a passive membrane with a primary function of restricting the diffusion of substances into and out of the body. The skin, in its most simple form, can be described in terms of three basic layers: the epidermal and dermal layers, and subcutaneous fat. The outermost layer of the epidermis is the stratum corneum, often the major barrier to percutaneous absorption. Below the stratum corneum is the viable epidermal layer, the most metabolically active layer in skin (Laerum, 1969). This is a unique biological situation because any substance that penetrates the stratum corneum then is subjected to the drug-metabolizing properties of the viable epidermis. Lack of metabolism by the viable epidermis will allow free passage of the unchanged chemical into the systemic circulation. Metabolism of the chemical may reduce the pharmacologic and/or toxicologic activity of the chemical. However, the reverse can also occur. Skin-metabolizing enzymes can convert nonactive chemical moieties into active pharmacologic and toxicologic agents.

This chapter reviews the chemical-metabolizing potential of skin, relates this potential to enzyme induction and first-pass metabolism, and discusses some of the potential toxicologic implications.

Parts of this review have been published in *Dermatoxicology & Pharmacology* and are reproduced here with permission of the publisher.

STEROID METABOLISM

Topical administration of steroids (e.g., hydrocortisone) is commonly utilized for some dermatologic disorders. The skin plays an important role in the formation and catabolism of endogenous steroids and thus may regulate these endogenous hormones (Hsia, 1971). The following is a discussion of steroid metabolism by cutaneous enzymes.

Oxidation

There are several examples of the cutaneous metabolism of alcohol groups present in many steroids: Hsia et al. (1965) observed that hydrocortisone (Fig. 1) can be metabolized by human skin to cortisone. Wotiz et al. (1956) found that testosterone is metabolized to at least seven metabolites in human skin. The major metabolite is Δ4-androstene-3,17-dione (Fig. 2). Another example of alcohol oxidation involves the estrogen estradiol. Skin contains the metabolic enzymes necessary for the oxidation of estradiol to estrone (Weinstein et al., 1968). The reaction is shown in Figure 1. All these oxidations are catalyzed in skin by the enzyme 17β-hydroxysteroid dehydrogenase.

Faredin and co-workers (1969) incubated dehydroepiandrosterone (DHA) with abdominal slices of human skin and isolated several metabolites. The major metabolite (60%) was 7α-hydroxydehydroepiandrosterone (Fig. 2). A significant amount (16%) of the 7β-hydroxy metabolite was generated, along with an equal amount of the 7-keto metabolite.

This example demonstrates a well-known hepatic metabolite route (selective hydroxylation) in skin. In contrast with the cutaneous metabolic route, human hepatic enzymes produced only the 7α-hydroxylated metabolite of DHA. A mechanistic interpretation of this metabolic route was difficult, since two mechanisms were possible. One mechanism involves the presence of both a 7α- and a 7β-hydroxylase. In this case, either or both of these epimers could be oxidized to the ketone. The alternate mechanism would involve only a 7α-hydroxylase. In this case, the 7α-hydroxy-DHA would be oxidized to the 7-keto-DHA. Reduction of the 7-keto-DHA would then form a mixture of the two 7-hydroxy epimers. The mechanism has not been determined.

Reduction

The carbonyl groups of various steroids can be reduced by metabolic reactions in the skin. An example of this type of reaction was just mentioned regarding the possible reduction of 7-keto-DHA. Two more definitive examples involve the cutaneous reduction of the 20-oxo group of hydrocortisone (Hsia et al., 1965) and progesterone (Frost et al., 1969). In both cases, the 20-oxo group (carbonyl) is reduced to a secondary alcohol and yields two epimers. Figure 1 shows the reduction of progesterone by enzymes found in both human skin and vaginal mucosa.

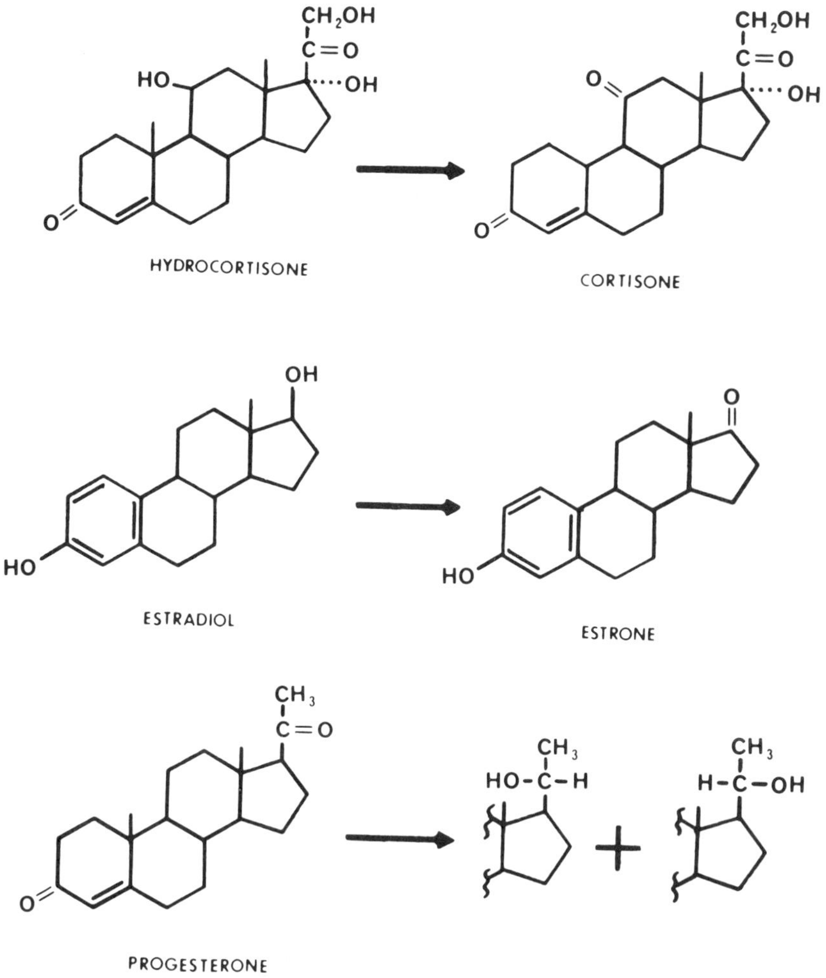

Figure 1 Cutaneous metabolism of several steroids. Top: hydrocortisone to cortisone; middle: estradiol to estrone; bottom: reduction of progesterone.

The hepatic metabolism of many steroids proceeds via the route of carbon-carbon double-bond reduction. The same reductase activity is present in skin. While hepatic microsomal systems often yield both α and β epimers, cutaneous metabolism exhibits more stereospecificity in that only the α epimers are produced. Some examples of cutaneous reductase activity have been shown for hydrocortisone, testosterone, and progesterone. Hydrocortisone was reduced to allodihydrocortisol by human skin (Hsia et al., 1965), testosterone via a 5α-

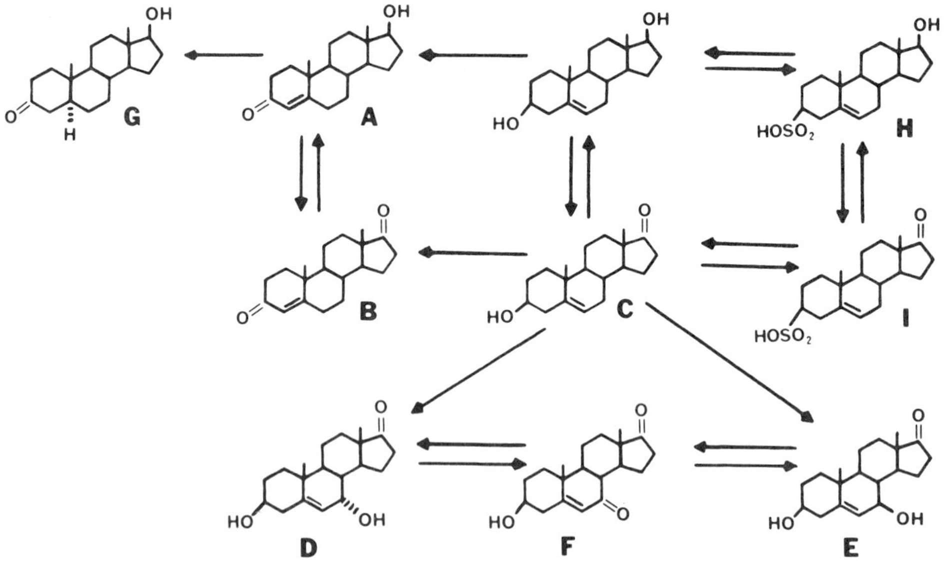

Figure 2 Metabolism of testosterone (A) and related steroids in human skin. (B) Δ4-Androstene-3,17-dione. (C) Dehydroepiandrosterone (DHA). (D) 7α-Hydroxy-DHA. (E) 7β-Hydroxy-DHA. (F) 7-keto-DHA. (G) 5α-Dihydrotestosterone. (H and I) Sulfate conjugates. (From Pannatier et al., 1978.)

reductase to 5α-dihydrotestosterone (Fig. 2). Progesterone has been shown to be reduced to 5α-pregnane derivatives by human skin (Frost et al., 1969).

Hydrolytic Reactions

Tauber and Toda (1976) investigated the biotransformation of diflucortolone valerate (DFV) in rat, guinea pig, and human skin. Guinea pig and rat skin hydrolyze DFV rapidly (half-life = 30-60 min) to diflucortolone (DF) and valeric acid. In vitro hydrolysis of DFV in human skin occurred much more slowly: only 5-15% DF was formed after 7 hr. In this case, absorption of the drug into the skin was the rate-limiting step, since it was found that the reaction proceeded more rapidly with injured skin.

Conjugation Reactions

The predominant conjugation reaction with steroids involves sulfate conjugation (Fig. 2). Berliner et al. (1968) isolated two water-soluble metabolites of [^{14}C]-DHA after incubation of [^{14}C]DHA with human abdominal skin (dermis and epidermis) for 5 days. These metabolites were identified as the sulfate conjugates.

In a similar study, Faredin et al. (1968) incubated [^{14}C]DHA with small pieces of normal human female abdominal skin. They also found the DHA-sulfate conjugate, from which they concluded that human skin contains sulfokinase activity. From these studies, skin may participate not only in phase I steroid biotransformation reactions but also in sulfate conjugation (phase II) reactions.

CUTANEOUS METABOLISM OF POLYCYCLIC AROMATIC HYDROCARBONS

Much interest has been devoted to the effects of polycyclic aromatic hydrocarbons (PAH) on the skin. As a group, various PAHs induce skin carcinomas. Metabolic activation is usually the first step toward the induction of skin cancers by these compounds. The study of the cutaneous metabolism of PAHs can yield important data regarding the structure of the ultimate carcinogenic responsible for tumor induction.

Benzo(a)pyrene

When benzo(a)pyrene (BP) is applied to human skin, it may be metabolized to several distinct metabolites. Figure 3 shows some of the metabolic products of BP formed during in vitro incubations with cultures of human epithelial cells. These metabolic reactions not only serve to detoxify BP, they also convert active BP to more reactive species, which may in turn react with cell macromolecules.

Basically these metabolites fall into three classes: phenols, quinones, and dihydrodiols (Fox et al., 1975). Two phenols were formed (3- and 9-hydroxy-BP) and were products of aromatic hydrocarbon hydroxylase (AHH), a nonspecific enzyme containing cytochrome P-450. Two dihydrodiols were formed, the 7,8- and 9,10-dihydrodiols (Fig. 3). Three quinones of BP were isolated from the incubation media, namely, the 1,6- and 3,6- and 6,12-quinones. These quinones could be formed spontaneously in culture media alone. However, the amounts formed by skin enzymes were significantly greater than that formed in control incubations.

Cutaneous metabolism of BP in the "K region" was not detectable, although it had been detected in hepatic incubations. Neither the 4,5-dihydrodiol nor the 4,5-epoxide of BP was detected. It may be possible that the 4,5-epoxide is unstable and covalently binds to cellular macromolecules before it can be converted to the dihydrodiol. However, Fox et al. (1975) were unable to show any significant binding to cells and were able to account for the remaining tritium label [^{3}H]BP, which was not metabolized. Selkirk et al. (1975) isolated the 4,5-dihydrodiol as a metabolite of BP by human hepatic microsomes. Therefore, because this metabolite was stable in a hepatic enzyme system, it should also have been stable in a cutaneous enzyme system. Thus, it seems highly unlikely that the 4,5-epoxide is formed by the cutaneous system.

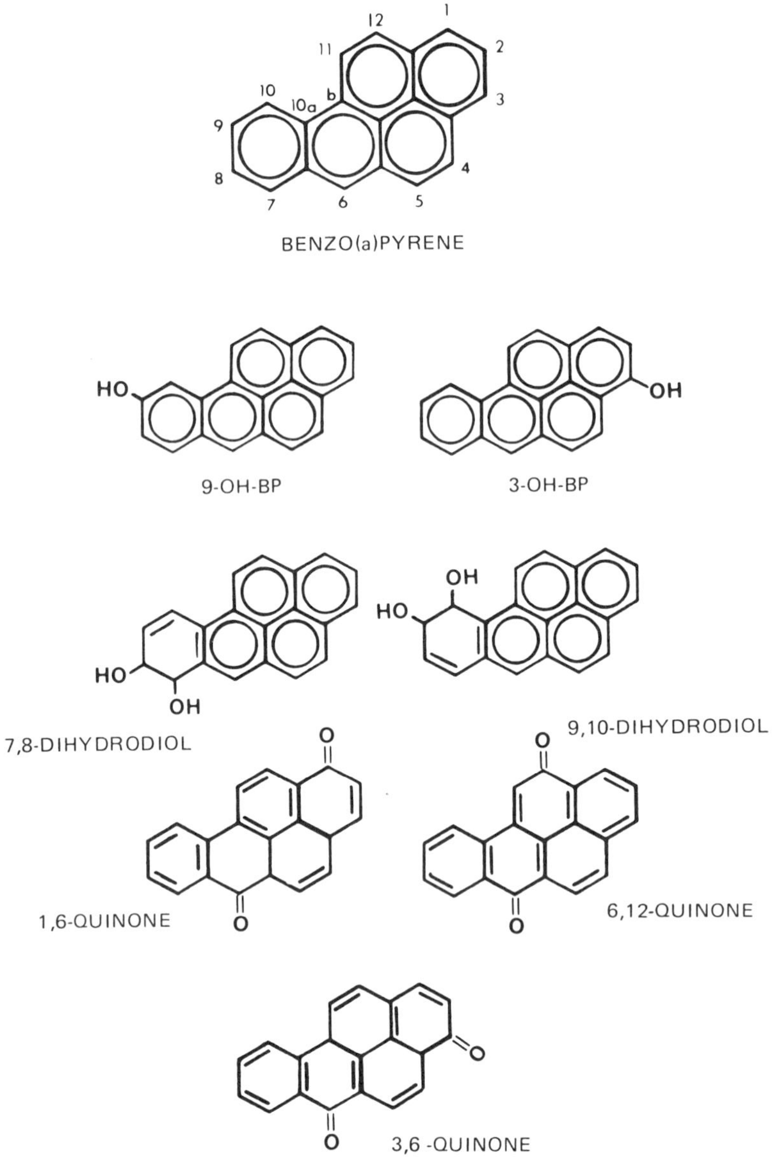

Figure 3 Metabolic products of benzo(*a*)pyrene formed in vitro during incubations with cultures of human epithelial cells. (From Fox et al., 1975.)

The enzyme epoxide hydrase, an important component necessary for the detoxification of the benzpyrene epoxides, has been demonstrated in skin (Bentley et al., 1976). These epoxides are thought to be responsible for the alkylation of macromolecules and ultimately for carcinogenicity. The presence of dihydrodiol metabolites has often been taken as evidence that an epoxide was formed, but was deactivated by the epoxide hydrase. The activity of this enzyme toward K-region epoxides has been measured in rat skin and compared to that activity from liver (Bentley et al., 1976). The activity of rat skin microsomal preparations toward BP-4,5-oxide was 60-fold lower than that of rat liver preparations. Similarly, cutaneous AHH activity has been found to be low. Pohl et al. (1976) found the AHH activity in skin toward BP to be 2% of that in liver. Although these activities are low, the presence of these minute amounts of enzyme may still offer a significant physiological protection mechanism.

Studies involving the metabolic activation of BP have been focusing on the "bay region" of the molecule and not the "K region." The bay region of BP would be identified by carbons 10, 10a, 10b, and 11 (Fig. 3). The tumorigenic activity of a material has often been correlated with the ability to covalently bind to DNA. Studies have shown that metabolites of benzpyrene-7,8-dihydrodiol were bound to DNA to a greater extent than any other BP metabolite (Borgen et al., 1973). These studies suggested that BP was metabolized to BP-7,8-dihydrodiol-9,10-epoxide, which was the ultimate carcinogen. Carcinogenicity studies of BP and its metabolites have been performed in mouse skin (Levin et al., 1977). BP-7,8-dihydrodiol was more carcinogenic than BP; BP-7,8-dihydrodiol was not carcinogenic if the 9,10 double bond was reduced. Note that if the 9,10 double bond was reduced, formation of the epoxide-diol is no longer possible in the bay region. BP-7,8-dihydrodiol-9,10-epoxide was a more potent carcinogen than BP (Kapitulunik et al., 1977).

The stereoselective binding of BP metabolites to macromolecules has been detected. The binding of BP-dihydrodiol-epoxides occurred with high stereoselectivity (Koreeda et al., 1978). These investigators isolated the macromolecular adducts that were formed when [^{3}H] BP was applied to the skin of mice. There are two stereochemical configurations for the BP-7,8-dihydrodiols; each may be metabolized to the respective 9,10-epoxide. The epoxide may then react with cellular nucleophiles such as DNA, RNA, or proteins. The in vivo binding to nucleic acids occurs preferentially to guanine at the 2-amino group (in both DNA and RNA). Both stereoisomers bind cellular components.

In the liver, once an aromatic compound has been oxidized to a phenol, it can be conjugated via a phase II reaction and eliminated. Skin tissues oxidize BP via AHH to hydroxylated metabolites, which would be available to conjugating enzyme systems if present. BP is metabolized both in vivo and in vitro by mouse skin to a mixture of glucuronide-conjugated benzpyrenols (Harper and Calcutt,

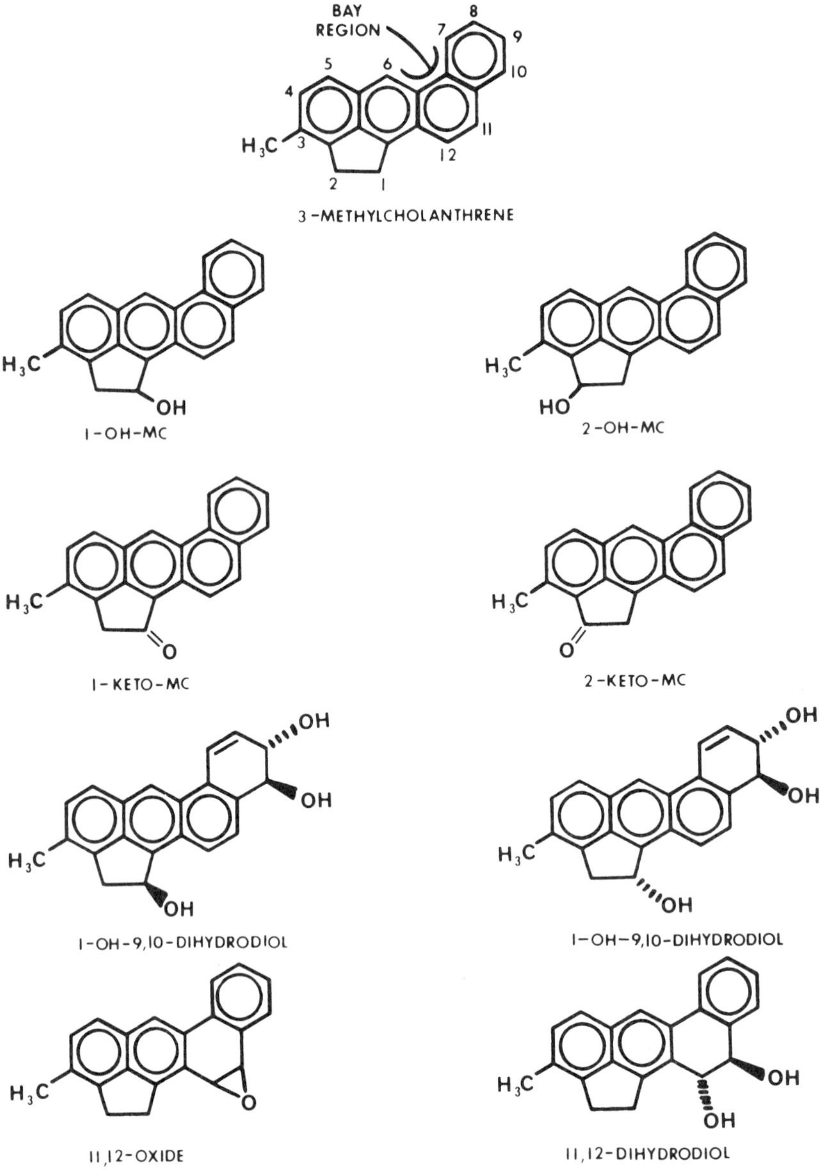

Figure 4 Structure of 3-methylcholanthrene (3-MC) and several hepatic metabolites of 3-MC. (From Levin et al., 1979.)

1960). In a separate study, these authors applied the same amount of either BP or 8-benzpyrenol to mouse skin and assayed the skin for metabolites. They found the same amount of glucuronide conjugate for both. They concluded that the hydroxylation of BP in this system was not the rate-limiting step, but, instead, glucuronidation of the metabolites was rate limiting. These authors also attempted to detect the corresponding sulfate conjugates. Sulfate conjugation had been identified as a metabolic route of elimination for steroids. They were unable to detect these in ATP-supplemented in vitro studies. Thus, they concluded that skin does not seem to have the capability of eliminating benzpyrenols as sulfate conjugates.

3-Methylcholanthrene

3-Methylcholanthrene (3-MC) is a polycyclic aromatic hydrocarbon and is a potent carcinogen. Experiments with BP have indicated that diol-epoxides in which the epoxide is located in the bay region are the ultimate carcinogenic metabolites. A similar mechanism (i.e., metabolic activation) may be applicable to 3-MC. Several metabolites of 3-MC (Fig. 4) have been identified (Levin et al., 1979). The structures shown are rat liver metabolites, but as discussed in the preceding section, skin also possesses the AHH activity necessary for such oxidations.

The metabolites in Fig. 4 were tested for tumor-initiating activity in mouse skin after single-dose applications (Levin et al., 1979) of 3–30 nmol. If it is assumed that metabolic activation was required before initiation, and that absorption of these is similar, then the compounds structurally most similar to the ultimate carcinogen would have been most active in this in vivo test. At the lowest (3-nmol) dose, 2-hydroxy-3MC was more tumorigenic than 3-MC; 1-hydroxy-9,10-dihydrodiol had very little activity. At the 10-nmol dose, 1-hydroxy-9,10-dihydrodiol was as active as both 3-MC and 2-hydroxy-3MC. The dihydrodiol metabolite was two to three times more active than 3-MC in producing pulmonary tumors and up to 10 times more active in producing hepatic tumors. These results indicated that 2-keto-3MC, 2-hydroxy-3MC, and 1-hydroxy-9,10-dihydriol-3MC were equipotent with 3-MC in tumor induction. Also, each of these were more active than the other metabolites (Fig. 4).

Wood et al. (1978) found 1-hydroxy-9,10-dihydrodiol-3MC was consistently the most active (in vitro) of the 3-MC metabolites, indicating that this metabolite may be a proximate carcinogen. Other recent studies in mouse skin have indicated that the 9,10-dihydrodiol-7,8-epoxide of 3-MC may be the ultimate carcinogen (Vigny et al., 1977a). DNA-bound adducts were isolated and found to be saturated in the 7, 8, 9, and 10 positions. This was consistent with the formation of the 7,8-epoxide-9,10-dihydrodiol of 3-MC.

As in the case of benzo(*a*)pyrene, metabolic activation of 3-MC is necessary for tumorigenic activity. Skin contains the necessary oxidative enzymes for this activation and deactivation. Epoxide hydrase was present (Bentley et al., 1976) and metabolized the 11,12-oxide of 3-MC to the corresponding dihydrodiol. Although these cutaneous enzymes are responsible for detoxifying most of the 3-MC, ironically, they are also responsible for the formation of reactive (toxic) metabolites.

Benzanthracene Derivatives

Members of the benzo(*a*)anthracene group of PAHs are among some of the most potent of PAH carcinogens. One of the most important members of this group is 7,12-dimethylbenz(*a*)anthracene (DMBA). DMBA undergoes aromatic and aliphatic oxidation by skin enzymes. DiGiovanni et al. (1977) showed that DMBA can be metabolized to at least three metabolites: 7-hydroxymethyl-12-methylbenzanthracene, 12-hydroxymethyl-7-methylbenzanthracene, and 7,12-di(hydroxymethyl)benzanthracene.

Since DMBA induces tumors in mouse skin, a reactive metabolite (e.g., an epoxide) is most likely produced. Slaga et al. (1979) found that the K-region epoxide (5,6-oxide) was a poor tumor initiator and probably not involved in tumorigenesis. As with other PAHs, metabolism at the bay region was most likely responsible for activity.

Vigney et al. (1977a) applied DMBA to mouse skin and isolated DNA adducts. They found that the 3,4-dihydrodiol-1,2-oxide of DMBA was involved in adduct formation. Additional evidence toward the bay-region theory was provided by Huberman and Slaga (1979). They tested the activity of several fluoro-DMBA derivatives on mouse skin. Fluorination at the 1, 2, or 5 position of DMBA decreased the activity by about 85%. On the other hand, the 11-fluoro-DMBA was as active as DMBA alone. These results showed that the bay region was involved in the metabolic activation of DMBA. Their results also suggested that substituents in the K region may also be able to affect the activation of DMBA.

The cutaneous metabolism of a DMBA derivative, 7-methylbenz(*a*)anthracene (7-MBA) has been investigated. Mouse skin metabolized 7-MBA to several dihydrodiol metabolites (1,2-, 3,4-, 5,6-, and 10,11-dihydrodiols). Additionally, adducts of 7-MBA have been isolated and were derived from 3,4-dihydrodiol-1,2-oxide of 7-MBA (Vigney et al., 1977b). Chouroulinkov et al. (1977) applied 7-MBA and each of the dihydrodiols above separately to mouse skin and found that the 3,4-dihydrodiol was the most active (tumor promoter) in this series. These data are in good agreement with those obtained from DMBA and the bay theory, that is, the dihydrodiol located next to the bay region (vicinal) yet leaving the region available for epoxide formation.

Bentley et al. (1976) found that microsome-bound epoxide hydrase was present in rat skin and capable of hydrating several different K-region epoxides from this PAH series. Epoxide hydrase activity was present but decreased in the

Cutaneous Metabolism of Xenobiotics

following order: phenanthracene-9,10-oxide > 7-MBA-5,6-oxide > benz(a)-anthracene-5,6-oxide > dibenz(a,h)anthracene-5,6-oxide. The K_m values of this enzyme ranged from 2.0 to 4.6 μM. They concluded that these "low K_m values indicate that epoxide hydrase could be efficient at removing active epoxides at the low concentrations at which they would be produced metabolically from low levels of ubiquitous hydrocarbons."

MISCELLANEOUS CUTANEOUS METABOLIC REACTIONS

Oxidations

The ability of skin to deaminate organic amines was documented by Hakanson and Möller (1963a). They incubated norepinephrine with rat, rabbit, mouse, and human skin; it was metabolized to dehydroxymandelic acid (DHMA). Thus, they were able to demonstrate the presence of monoamine oxidase (MAO) in skin.

These investigators also demonstrated (1963b) both DOPA (3,4-dihydroxyphenylalanine) decarboxylase and dopamine-β-oxidase activity in skin (rabbit, mouse, rat, and human). Dopamine-β-oxidase is an enzyme catalyzing the last reaction in the biosynthesis of norepinephrine. Mouse skin (which gave the highest yields) metabolized [^{14}C]DOPA and [^{14}C]dopamine to epinephrine. Thus, they established that all the enzymes involved in the biosynthesis of norepinephrine were present in skin.

Other dealkylations in skin were demonstrated by Pohl et al. (1976). They detected the presence of a mixed-function oxidase (MFO) that dealkylated 7-ethoxycoumarin (7-EC). The activity of this enzyme in skin was 2% of that in liver. Although deethylation of 7-EC was shown in skin, dealkylation of d-benzphetamine (N-demethylase activity) could not be detected.

Deaminase activity in skin was further demonstrated by Ando et al. (1977). They detected the enzyme adenosine deaminase in viable epidermis. This enzyme metabolized the drug vidarabine (9-α-d-arabinofuranosyladenine) to 9-α-d-arabinofuranosylhypoxanthine.

Pohl et al. (1976) showed that a mouse skin microsomal preparation contained aniline hydroxylase. This enzyme was able to metabolize aniline to p-aminophenol. Thus, they were able to show that the cutaneous oxidation of aromatic rings is not restricted to polycyclic aromatic hydrocarbons.

Reductive Reactions

Cutaneous reductive metabolism is not restricted to the steroids. An example of a nonsteroidal compound metabolized by the skin is croton oil, a tumor promoter in mouse skin. One of the most potent components of this oil is phorbol myristate acetate (PMA). When 25 μg of [^{3}H]PMA was painted on mouse skin (for 5 hr), about 2% of the dose was metabolized to the hydroxylated metabolite

(PHMA) via reduction of the carbonyl at the 5 position to yield the 5-β-hydroxy metabolite (Segal et al., 1975). This metabolite is a potent inflammatory agent on mouse skin. When [^{3}H]PHMA was painted on mouse skin, no PMA was formed, indicating that the reaction is not reversible. This study showed that cutaneous tissue contains the enzymes for reducing substances other than steroids. It is not known whether PHMA is actually the active tumor-producing agent (proximate carcinogen) in croton oil.

Conjugation Reactions

As mentioned for the hydroxylated metabolites of BP, the skin contains the enzymes necessary for glucuronidation (i.e., UDP-glucuronyl transferase). Other than BP metabolites, only a few other substrates have been shown to be glucuronidated by the skin. Stevenson and Dutton (1960) showed glucuronide synthesis in the skin. They demonstrated that the conjugation of o-aminophenol in skin was similar to that in liver. Rugstad and Dybing (1975) investigated glucuronidation in cultures of whole human skin and homogenates of these same cells. The homogenates were supplemented with UDPGA (UDP-glucuronic acid) to eliminate the possibility of any permeability barrier (through cell membranes). When p-nitrophenol (PNP), p-aminophenol (PAP), and bilirubin were used as substrates, only PNP and PAP were glucuronidated. Even though bilirubin was actively taken up by skin cells, it was not glucuronidated.

Hakanson and Möller (1963a) found that catechol-o-methyltransferase (COMT) was present in cutaneous tissues. They incubated norepinephrine (anaerobically) with skin from four species (rat, rabbit, mouse, and man) and were able to identify normetanephrine as a metabolite. This metabolic reaction was inhibited by pyrogallol, which is a specific COMT inhibitor. Bamshad (1969) observed that COMT was present in normal skin. He investigated the distribution of COMT between the dermis and epidermis versus the whole skin. He concluded that the activity of COMT was "much greater" in the epidermis than either the dermis or whole skin.

ENZYME INDUCTION AND INHIBITION

Cytochrome P-450, present in skin at low concentrations, is inducible by topical application of some of the same agents that induce hepatic metabolism (Alvares et al., 1973). Although phenobarbital is a known inducer of P-450 in hepatic systems, no induction of P-450 could be shown after topical administration to skin (Pohl et al., 1976). These authors applied phenobarbital for only 24 hr, during which time they monitored P-450 induction. Conney (1971) observed that maximum phenobarbital induction of zoxazolamine hydroxylase in rat liver microsomes occurred after 3-4 days of phenobarbital injections. It may be that phenobarbital induction of P-450 in skin takes much longer than 24 hr. Perhaps these investigators (Pohl et al., 1976) should have followed the induction for 3-7 days.

Pohl et al. (1976) also investigated the induction of P-450 in skin after topical application of 3-MC and 2,3,7,8-tetrachlorodibenzo-p-dioxin (TCDD) in skin. 3-MC caused a slight increase in cutaneous P-450 levels, but these levels returned to control levels within 72 hr. Percutaneous administration of TCDD not only caused cutaneous P-450 levels to increase, but doubled the hepatic levels of P-450. These studies show that cutaneous tissues do contain cytochrome P-450 and this cytochrome can be induced by at least two polycyclic aromatic hydrocarbons.

Many investigators have been unable to detect cytochrome P-450 in normal skin. Often these inconclusive results were caused by one or a combination of the following factors. First, the levels of P-450 in noninduced skin were low, often approaching the limits of the analytical methods available. Second, cytochrome oxidase is present in skin. This cytochrome causes a distorted difference spectrum, often masking the presence of low concentrations of P-450. Finally, cytochrome P-420 was often found in skin when P-450 could not be detected (Pohl et al., 1976). Cytochrome P-420 is an artifact of the solubilization process. P-450 is unstable; it is entirely possible that the small amount of P-450 present in skin degraded to P-420 during the isolation procedure. Since these studies were performed, various investigators have learned how to solubilize P-450 with minimal degradation. Using these new techniques, it should be possible to more carefully quantitate the levels of P-450 in induced and noninduced skin.

In addition to the cytochrome P-450s, many other enzymes can be either induced or inhibited after topical administration of various agents. The PAHs are known hepatic enzyme inducers, and evidence indicates that they are also cutaneous enzyme inducers. Dutton and Stevenson (1962) found that the topical application of BP increases the UDP-glucuronyl transferase activity in the skin. On the other hand, Rugstad and Dybing (1975) found that the glucuronidation rate of human skin epithelial cells (in culture) was not increased by either BP or benzanthracene. They suggested, though, that the conditions used in their cell cultures may have caused the cells to already be maximally induced.

Pohl et al. (1976) measured the enzyme induction of several cutaneous enzymes after topical applications of 3-MC (3 mg) or TCDD (0.3 μg). Application of 3-MC caused a temporary twofold increase in AHH activity, but this activity returned to noninduced levels 72 hr after dosing. Twenty-four hours after dosing with TCDD, the cutaneous AHH activity had increased eightfold, while at 72 hr the activity had increased to a value 30-fold greater than control levels. They noted that 3-MC was unable to induce the activities of either 7-EC or aniline hydroxylase in skin. TCDD, on the other hand, increased the deethylase activity fourfold after 24 hr and sevenfold after 72 hr.

As previously discussed, Fox et al. (1975) observed that the cutaneous metabolism of BP was significant even without prior induction. However, BP metabolism was increased even more upon induction. Interestingly, when hydrocortisone was applied simultaneously with the inducer, the metabolism of BP decreased significantly. The metabolic products that were decreased were the quinone and dihydrodiol metabolites. Thus, they showed that the cutaneous metabolism of BP could be either induced or inhibited under the proper conditions.

The effects of various topically applied MFO modifiers on the induction of AHH activity in skin were studied by Bowden et al. (1974). The modifiers used were phenobarbital, 1,2,5,6-dibenzanthracene (DBA), 7,12-dimethylbenz(a)-anthracene (DMBA), 5,6-benzoflavone (5,6-BF), and 7,8-benzoflavone (7,8-BF). Although phenobarbital significantly induces hepatic enzyme activity, no effect on cutaneous AHH activity was detected. Both AHH activity and induction were inhibited by 7,8-BF. Interestingly, DiGiovanni et al. (1977) later noted that 7,8-BF inhibited AHH activity in vitro. The activity of AHH in cutaneous tissues was increased by 5,6-BF, DMBA, and DBA. The levels of induction were 350, 600, and 1200%, respectively.

Bowden et al. (1974) and DiGiovanni et al. (1977) investigated the effects of these modifiers on the initiating potential (tumorigenic) of DMBA and DBA. Both 5,6-BF and 7,8-BF inhibited DMBA skin tumorigenesis in mice. DMBA binding to DNA, RNA, and proteins was inhibited by 7,8-BF, while only binding to DNA by DMBA was shown to be inhibited by 5,6-BF. The effects of 7,8-BF on DBA were opposite to those of DMBA; that is, 7,8-BF increased the carcinogenicity of DBA. DiGiovanni et al. (1977) also studied the modifying effects of 17β-estradiol on DMBA activity. The formation of all (detectable) metabolites of DMBA was inhibited by 17β-estradiol, yet it had no effect of the tumor initiation of DMBA.

From these data, it may be observed that inhibitors and inducers may affect both the activation and detoxification of drugs in the skin. For example, 7,8-BF inhibited the activation of DMBA to a greater extent than it inhibited detoxification of DMBA. Therefore, the carcinogenicity of DMBA was decreased. On the other hand, 7,8-BF inhibited the detoxification of DBA to a greater extent, which resulted in increased carcinogenicity (Bowden et al., 1974). Therefore, a given modifier may have different effects on various carcinogens, that is, either more or less carcinogenicity. This effect is dependent on the delicate balance between the activation and detoxification pathways.

PHARMACOLOGICAL AND TOXICOLOGICAL IMPLICATIONS OF SKIN METABOLISM

The chemical that is introduced into the systemic circulation is the final chemical species that penetrates the skin barrier. Some chemicals may be more toxic via a dermal route of administration than when administered orally. Topically applied hexachlorophene does not appear to be metabolized. It is absorbed into the bloodstream unchanged. In contrast, orally ingested hexachlorophene is metabolized extensively by the liver (Marzulli and Maibach, 1975). The metabolic detoxification potential seen with oral absorption is not present with dermal administration. Thus, the only barrier to hexachlorophene toxicity is the barrier to percutaneous absorption.

There is information that the routes of metabolism can differ with dermal and with oral administration (Greaves, 1971). With oral administration of [^{3}H]-cortisol, the urinary metabolites were mainly corticosteroids. With dermal administration the urinary metabolites were mainly oxosteroids. However, cortisol (hydrocortisone) is clinically effective; therefore, this metabolic difference would have no relevance unless one of the metabolites were an active moiety.

It can probably be assumed that most skin metabolism deactivates or detoxifies the applied chemical agent. Most skin metabolism that has been studied seems to indicate this. The most notable exception is found in connection with the activation by skin aryl hydrocarbon hydroxylase enzymes of chemical agents into potent carcinogens. Here, there is no doubt about the toxicological implications.

A study suggests that there may be a difference in the drug-metabolizing potential of normal and diseased skin. Aryl hydrocarbon hydroxylase activity was the same in both psoriatic lesions and noninvolved skin, but lower than the activity observed in normal volunteers. Preincubation of tissue with benzanthracene increased activity in both normal and noninvolved epidermis. However, no stimulation at all was observed in psoriatic lesions (Chapman et al., 1977b). It is unfortunate that more information like this is not available. Other than the possibility of skin metabolism being different in diseased skin, there are no other data on which to base speculation.

An unfortunate area of percutaneous toxicity occurs among infants, especially with preterm infants whose skin (and subsequent barrier function) is not completely developed (Singer et al., 1971). It is not known what role skin metabolism might play in the developing or full-term infant.

Quantitatively, it is difficult to assess the amount of skin metabolism that occurs in vivo because most skin metabolism studies are done in vitro. However, there are some in vivo studies that may quantitate skin metabolism. The lack of clinical effectiveness of cortisone suggests that there is not sufficient metabolism to hydrocortisone. With the topical application of [^{14}C]benzoyl peroxide, all the compound was metabolized to benzoic acid during in vitro absorption using human skin. All the radioactive material in the urine was benzoic acid following in vivo topical application to rhesus monkey. Renal clearance of the metabolite was sufficiently rapid to preclude hepatic conjugation with glycine to form hippuric acid (Nacht et al., 1981). The percutaneous first-pass metabolism of nitroglycerin has been estimated to be 20% during transdermal delivery (Wester et al., 1983).

SKIN METABOLISM AND PERCUTANEOUS ABSORPTION

In spite of the intensive study of percutaneous absorption, there is a persistent belief that skin viability has little importance in the movement of a chemical from the skin surface to the capillaries of the dermis. This concept of skin as a passive membrane has led to skin penetration theories dominated by laws of mass action and physical diffusion. It has led investigators to use skin excised from cadavers and stored frozen, or to use chemically isolated skin sheets. However, Smith and Holland (1981) showed that in vitro penetration of skin by benzo(*a*)pyrene is determined primarily by epidermal viability. Holland et al. (1984) then showed that benzo(*a*)pyrene penetration is directly related to the metabolically induced state of the skin, and can be destroyed by freezing the skin. Thus, the rate-limiting step of benzo(*a*)pyrene percutaneous absorption is that of metabolism in its transit through living skin.

Accepting that metabolism is an important factor in skin and percutaneous absorption, we can visualize a different concept for percutaneous absorption. For a great many compounds, especially low molecular weight alcohols, the stratum corneum appears to be a barrier of primary importance. For less polar molecules, such as benzo(*a*)pyrene and steroids, the lipid-saturated stratum corneum can be a sink for topically applied lipotropic materials; its function is more that of a sponge capable of absorbing a quantity of material, limited only by the solubility of the substance in sebaceous and epidermal lipids. The viability and metabolic activity of the epidermis will then determine the disposition of the substance in other parts of the skin and delivery to the capillaries in the dermis.

DISCUSSION

It is obvious that skin is not a passive barrier that merely restricts the diffusion of chemical agents into the body. The skin is viable, metabolizing membrane that can metabolize an assortment of topically applied substances before they become systemically available.

Enzyme systems in skin are highly inducible. For example, after TCDD exposure, the activity of aromatic hydrocarbon hydroxylase increases up to 30-fold and that of 7-ethoxycoumarin deethylase increases sixfold. Such changes in cutaneous metabolizing ability may potentially alter the availability of topically applied drugs.

Since the skin possesses many of the same enzymes that the liver does, it would be interesting to compare their relative activites. The activities of several cutaneous enzymes have been measured and compared to hepatic activities (Pohl et al., 1976). The activities of these enzymes in skin are low compared to

Table 1 Enzyme Activity Ratios Found in Skin, as Compared to Liver

Enzyme	Activity ratio (skin/liver)	
	Whole skin[a]	Epidermis[b]
Aromatic hydrocarbon hydroxylase	0.02	0.80
7-Ethoxycoumarin deethylase	0.02	0.80
Aniline hydroxylase	0.06	2.40
NADP-cytochrome C reductase	0.06	2.40

[a] Data calculated from Pohl et al. (1976)
[b] Assuming that epidermis is 2.5% of whole skin.

liver, typically 2-6% of the hepatic values (Table 1). Although these data indicate that cutaneous metabolism is low, this may not be representative of the in vivo situation.

The distribution of skin-metabolizing enzymes in skin is an important consideration. Laerum (1969) found that oxygen consumption was 5.4-fold greater in the epidermis than the dermis. Bamshad (1969) noted that the amount of enzyme catechol-o-methyltransferase was 8.3-fold greater in the epidermis. Weinstein et al. (1968) found that the epidermal metabolism of estradiol to estrone was greater than metabolism by the dermis. Finally, Chapman et al. (1977a) showed that 96.5% of AHH activity in skin was present in the epidermis. These data indicate that most of the enzyme activity of skin may be localized in the epidermal layer.

The epidermal thickness ranges from 0.06 to 0.1 mm. The dermis may be 2-4 mm thick. Therefore, the epidermis makes up only 2.5-3% of the total skin. This percentage may be even smaller if the subcutaneous layers are included in this calculation. The cutaneous enzyme activities reported in the literature were based on enzyme activities in whole skin homogenates. Assuming that these enzymes are constrained in to the epidermal layer, the real activities range from 80 to 240% of those in the liver (Table 1). Therefore, cutaneous enzymes are active and, in the epidermis, may equal or even exceed the activity of hepatic drug metabolizing enzymes.

Since the cutaneous metabolic activity has been shown to be high, it may be possible for these enzymes to exert a first-pass metabolic effect toward topically applied drugs. If a drug diffuses slowly through the epidermis, the skin may serve as a site of first-pass metabolism. Such metabolism may decrease both the amount of drug at the site of action (often the dermis) and the amount systemically available. On the other hand, if absorption is fast, the cutaneous enzymes may become saturated. In this case, a significant amount of drug may be absorbed into the systemic circulation without being metabolized.

The skin is a highly active metabolic organ. It contains a multitude of different drug-metabolizing enzymes, including a cytochrome P-450 system. These enzymes may be highly inducible in much the same way as the liver. Some information available suggests that there are pharmacological and toxicological implications in the cutaneous biotransformation of chemical agents that come in contact with the skin. When studying the availability of topically administered drugs or environmental contaminants, one must consider the metabolizing ability of the skin, which may affect bioavailability during the first passage through the skin.

REFERENCES

Alvares, A., Bickers, D., and Kappas, A. (1973). Alteration of hepatic microsomal hemoprotein by polychlorinated biphenyls. *Fed. Proc. 32*: 235.

Ando, H., Ho, H., and Higuchi, W. (1977). Skin as an active metabolizing barrier. I. Theoretical analysis of topical bioavailability. *J. Pharm. Sci. 66*: 1525-1528.

Bamshad, J. (1969). Catechol-*o*-methyltransferase in epidermis and whole skin. *J. Invest. Dermatol. 52*: 351-352.

Bentley, P., Schuassmann, H., Sims, P., and Oesch, F. (1976). Epoxides derived from various polycyclic hydrocarbons as substrates of homogeneous and microsome bound epoxide hydratase. *Eur. J. Biochem. 69*: 97-103.

Berliner, D., Pasqualini, J., and Gallegos, A. (1968). The formation of water soluble steroids by human skin. *J. Invest. Dermatol. 50*: 220-224.

Borgen, A., Davey, H., Castagnoli, N., Crocker, T., Rasmusse, R., and Wang, I. (1973). Metabolic conversion of benzo(*a*)pyrene by Syrian hamster liver microsomes and binding of metabolites to deoxyribonucleic acid. *J. Med. Chem. 16*: 502-506.

Bowden, G., Slaga, T., Shapas, B., and Boutwell, R. (1974). The role of aryl hydrocarbon hydroxylase in skin tumor initiation by 7,12-dimethylbenz(*a*)-anthracene and 1,2,5,6-dibenzanthracene using DNA binding and thymidine-^{3}H incorporation into DNA as criteria. *Cancer Res. 34*: 2634-2642.

Chapman, P. H., Rawlins, M. D., and Shuster, S. (1977a). Activity of aryl hydroxylase in adult human skin. *Br. J. Clin. Pharmacol. 4*: 393P.

Chapman, P. H., Rawlins, M. D., Rogers, S., and Shuster, S. (1977b). Aryl hydroxylase activity in psoriatic skin. *Br. J. Clin. Pharmacol. 4*: 644P.

Chouroulinkov, I., Gentil, A., Tierney, B., Grover, P., and Sims, P. (1977). The metabolic activation of 7-methylbenz(*a*)anthracene in mouse skin: High tumor initiating activity of the 3,4-dihydrodiol. *Cancer Lett. 3*: 247-253.

Conney, A. H. (1971). Environmental factors influencing drug metabolism. In *Fundamentals of Drug Metabolism and Disposition.* Edited by B. LaDu, H. Mandel, and E. Way. Williams & Wilkins, Baltimore, pp. 253-278.

DiGiovanni, J., Slaga, T., Berry, D., and Juchau, M. (1977). Metabolism of 7,12-dimethylbenz(*a*)anthracene in mouse skin with high pressure liquid chromatography. *Drug Metab. Disposition 5*: 295-301.

Dutton, G. and Stevenson, I. (1962). The stimulation by 3,4-benzpyrene of glucuronide synthesis in skin. *Biochim. Biophys. Acta 58*: 633-634.

Faredin, I., Toth, I., Fazekas, A., Kokai, K., and Julesz, M. (1968). Conjugation in vitro of (4-14C) dehydroepiandrosterone to (4-14C) dehydroepiandroserone sulfate by normal human female skin slices. *J. Endocrinol. 41*: 295-296.

Faredin, I., Fazekas, A., Toth, I., Kokai, K., and Julesz, M. (1969). Transformation in vitro of (4-14C)-dehydroepiandrosterone into 7-oxygenated derivatives by normal human male and female skin slices. *J. Invest. Dermatol. 52*: 357-361.

Fox, C., Selkirk, J., Price, F., Croy, R., Sanford, K., and Fox, M. (1975). Metabolism of benzo(*a*)pyrene by human epithelial cells in vitro. *Cancer Res. 35*: 3551-3557.

Frost, P., Gomez, E., Weinstein, G., Lamas, J., and Hsia, S. (1969). Metabolism of progesterone-4-^{14}C in vitro in human skin and vaginal mucosa. *Biochemistry 8*: 948-952.

Gelboin, H., Kinoshita, N., and Weibel, F. (1972). Microsomal hydroxylases: Induction and role in polycyclic hydrocarbon carcinogenesis and toxicity. *Fed. Proc. 31*: 1298-1309.

Greaves, M. S. (1971). The in vivo catabolism of cortisol by human skin. *J. Invest. Dermatol. 57*: 100-107.

Hakanson, R. and Möller, H. (1963a). On metabolism of noradrenaline in the skin: Activity of catechol-*o*-methyltransferase and monoamine oxidase. *Acta Dermatovenereol.* (Stockholm) *43*: 552-555.

Hakanson, R. and Möller, H. (1963b). On formation of noradrenaline in the skin: Activity of dopamine-β-oxidase. *Acta Dermatovenereol.* (Stockholm) *43*: 548-551.

Harper, K. and Calcutt, G. (1960). Conjugation of 3:4-benzpyrenols in mouse skin. *Nature 186*: 80-81.

Holland, J. M., Kao, J. Y., and Whitaker, M. J. (1984). A multisample apparatus for kinetic evaluation of skin penetration in vitro: The influence of viability and metabolic status of the skin. *Toxicol. Appl. Pharmacol. 72*: 272-280.

Hsia, S. L. (1971). Steroid metabolism in human skin. In *Modern Trends in Dermatology*, Vol. 4. Edited by P. Borrie, Butterworth, London, pp. 69-88.

Hsia, S., Mussallem, J., and Witten, V. (1965). Further metabolic studies of hydrocortisone-4-^{14}C in human skin. *J. Invest. Dermatol. 45*: 384-390.

Huberman, E. and Slaga, T. J. (1979). Mutagenicity and tumor-initiating activity of fluorinated derivatives of 7,12-dimethylbenz(*a*)anthracene. *Cancer Res. 39*: 411-414.

Kapitulunik, J., Levin, W., Conney, A. H., Yagi, H., and Jerina, D. M. (1977). Benzo(*a*)pyrene 7,8-dihydrodiol is more carcinogenic than benzo(*a*)pyrene in newborn mice. *Nature 266*: 378-380.

Koreeda, M., Moore, P., Wislocki, P., Levin, W., Conney, A., Yagi, H., and Jerina, D. (1978). Binding of benzo(*a*)pyrene 7,8-diol-9,10-epoxides to DNA, RNA and protein of mouse skin occurs with high stereoselectivity. *Science 199*: 778-781.

Laerum, O. D. (1969). Oxygen consumption of basal and differentiating cells from hairless mouse epidermis. *J. Invest. Dermatol. 52*: 204–211.

Levin, W., Wood, A., Wislocki, P., Kapitulunik, J., Yaki, H., Jerina, D., and Conney, A. (1977). Carcinogenicity of benzo-ring derivatives of benzo(*a*)-pyrene on mouse skin. *Cancer Res. 37*: 3356–3361.

Levin, W., Buening, M. K., Wood, A., Chang, R., Thakker, D., Jerina, D., and Conney, A. (1979). Tumorigenic activity of 3-methylcholanthrene metabolites on mouse skin and in newborn mice. *Cancer Res. 39*: 3549–3553.

Marzulli, F. N. and Maibach, H. I. (1975). Relevance of animal models: The hexachlorophene story. In *Animal Models in Dermatology*. Edited by H. I. Maibach. Churchill Livingstone, New York, pp. 156–167.

Nacht, S., Yeung, D., Beasley, J. N., Jr., Anjo, M. D., and Maibach, H. I. (1981). Benzoyl peroxide: Percutaneous penetration and metabolic disposition. *J. Am. Acad. Dermatol. 4*: 31–37.

Pannatier, A., Jenner, P., Testa, B., and Etter, J. (1978). The skin as a drug-metabolizing organ. *Drug Metab. Rev. 8*: 319–343.

Pohl, R., Philpot, R., and Fouts, J. (1976). Cytochrome P-450 content and mixed function oxidase activity in microsomes isolated from mouse skin. *Drug Metab. Disposition 4*: 442–450.

Rugstad, H. and Dybing, E. (1975). Glucuronidation in cultures of human skin epithelial cells. *Eur. J. Clin. Invest. 5*: 133–137.

Segal, A., Van Durren, B., and Maté, U. (1975). The identification of phorbolol myristate acetate as a new metabolite of phorbol myristate acetate in mouse skin. *Cancer Res. 35*: 2154–2159.

Selkirk, J., Croy, R., and Gelboin, H. (1975). Isolation and characterization of benzo(*a*)pyrene-4,5-epoxide as a metabolite of benzo(*a*)pyrene. *Arch. Biochem. Biophys. 168*: 322–326.

Singer, E. J., Wegmann, P. C., Lehman, M. D., Christensen, M. S., and Vinson, L. J. (1971). Barrier development, ultrastructure, and sulfhydryl content of the fetal epidermis. *J. Soc. Cosmet. Chem. 22*: 119–137.

Shaw, J. and Chandrasekaran, S. (1978). Controlled topical delivery of drugs for systemic action. *Drug Metab. Rev. 8*: 223–233.

Slaga, T., Gleason, G., DiGiovanni, J., Sukumaran, K., and Harvey, R. (1979). Potent tumor-initiating activity of the 3,4-dihydrodiol of 7,12-dimethylbenz(*a*)anthracene in mouse skin. *Cancer Res. 39*: 1934–1936.

Smith, L. H. and Holland, J. M. (1981). Interaction between benzo(*a*)pyrene and mouse skin in organ culture. *Toxicology 21*: 47–57.

Stevenson, I. and Dutton, G. (1960). Mechanism of glucuronide synthesis in skin. *Biochem. J. 77*: 19P.

Tauber, V. and Toda, T. (1976). Biotransformation of diflucortolone valerate in the skin of rat, guinea pig and man. *Arzneim.-Forsch. (Drug Res.) 26*: 1484–1487.

Vigny, P., Duquesne, M., Coulomb, H., Tierney, B., Grover, P., and Sims, P. (1977a). Fluorescence spectral studies on the metabolic activation of 3-methylcholanthrene and 7,12-dimethylbenz(*a*)anthracene in mouse skin. *FEBS Lett. 82*: 278–282.

Vigny, P., Duquesne, M., Coulomb, H., Labombe, C., Tierney, B., Grover, P., and Sims, P. (1977b). Metabolic activation of polycyclic hydrocarbons. *FEBS Lett. 75*: 9-12.

Weinstein, G., Frost, P., and Hsia, S. (1968). In vitro conversion of estrone and 17β-estradiol in human skin and vaginal mucosa. *J. Invest. Dermatol. 51*: 4-10.

Wester, R. C., Noonan, P. K., Smeach, S., and Kosobud, L. (1983). Pharmacokinetics and bioavailability of intravenous and topical nitroglycerin in the rhesus monkey. Estimate of percutaneous first-pass metabolism. *J. Pharm. Sci. 72*: 745-748.

Wood, A., Chang, R., Levin, W., Thomas, P., Ryan, D., Stoming, T., Thakker, D., Jerina, D., and Conney, A. (1978). Metabolic activation of 3-methylcholanthrene on its metabolites to products mutagenic to bacterial and mammalian cells. *Cancer Res. 38*: 3398-3404.

Wotiz, H., Mescon, H., Doppel, H., and Lemon, H. (1956). The in vitro metabolism of testosterone by human skin. *J. Invest. Dermatol. 26*: 113.

6
Facilitated Percutaneous Absorption of Anionic Drugs

Jonathan Hadgraft* and Paul K. Wotton
University of Nottingham, Nottingham, England

The ability of any drug to exert its pharmacological action depends not only on that drug's potency, but also on its ability to reach the desired site of action, that is, its bioavailability. In the case of topically applied drugs, the word "bioavailability" refers to the difference between the amount of drug applied to the skin and the amount reaching the site of action itself (Idson, 1983). The ease with which a drug can penetrate the skin from a topical formulation depends primarily on two factors. First the drug must be able to diffuse from the vehicle to the skin surface, and second the drug must be able to overcome the skin barrier. Both these processes depend on the physical properties of the drug, the vehicle, and the barrier itself (Ostrenga et al., 1971).

The main barrier to percutaneous absorption is accepted to be the stratum corneum, a heterogeneous tissue composed of 8-16 layers of flat keratinized cells. The cell membranes also contain lipids that provide stability, insolubility, and resistance. Besides this the cells act as the graveyard for all the by-products of the death of epidermal cells, such as water-soluble proteins and amino acids (Katz and Poulsen, 1971). The cells are arranged in a highly organized structure. The major route of penetration through this barrier is thought to be by intracellular diffusion (even though the diffusional resistance is high), although there is some evidence to suggest penetration occurs via intercellular (Albery and Hadgraft, 1979), and transappendageal routes (Katz and Poulsen, 1971).

It is the physicochemical nature of the drug itself that is the important factor in determining whether it will cross what is essentially a lipoidal membrane. In general, lipid-soluble drugs penetrate the skin better than water-soluble drugs. Thus inorganic and organic acid salts normally penetrate the skin very poorly, on account of their high polarity. Bodor et al. (1980) utilized the prodrug approach

---

**Present affiliation*: University of Wales Institute of Science and Technology, Cardiff, Wales

to the problem to improve the percutaneous delivery of disodium cromoglycate. This was achieved with some success by producing a series of esters more lipid soluble than the parent compound. There are many other such compounds, that except for their highly polar nature would be useful as topically applied drugs. One novel method of accelerating the transport of anionic drugs across the skin is that of facilitated transport, a process developed by the chemical engineering industry.

FACILITATED TRANSPORT: THE MECHANISM

Biological carrier facilitated transport mechanisms have been known for many years, the uptake of glucose into red blood cells being an example (Levin, 1969). Such polar molecules would otherwise be insoluble within the membrane, but their passage is facilitated by a carrier macromolecule with which they temporarily combine, within the membrane itself. Such a combination is reversible and resembles that between an enzyme and its substrate.

Babcock et al. (1980) used a tertiary amine to transport uranium anions from an aqueous donor compartment, through an organic membrane, to an aqueous receptor phase. A pH gradient was used as the driving force to concentrate the anion against its own concentration gradient. The amine picks up the anion on one side of the membrane and carries it across by diffusion as a neutral complex. Ions of opposite charge may be carried in the same direction, or ions of like charge may be carried in the opposite direction. These modes of transport are referred to as cotransport and countertransport, respectively.

This mechanism may be utilized to attempt to facilitate the transport of anions across the stratum corneum. Since the pH of the surface of the skin is between 4.2 and 5.6 (Katz and Poulsen, 1971) and the dermal pH is 7.3-7.4 (i.e., the physiological pH), a ready-made pH gradient already exists to provide the driving force for facilitated transport, in the presence of a suitable carrier molecule. A vehicle of pH 5 would be well tolerated by the skin.

A well-defined model system, based on the rotating diffusion cell (Albery et al., 1976), has been used to assess the potential of this technique (Barker and Hadgraft, 1981). The epidermal barrier is simulated by using a suitable membrane filter, impregnated with isopropyl myristate (IPM), a liquid representative of skin lipids (Poulsen et al., 1968). To facilitate the transport of anionic drug molecules across this membrane, a carrier molecule is introduced into the IPM. The use of various tertiary amines as proposed carrier molecules has been investigated.

At the lower pH of the donor compartment/membrane interface, (representative of the skin surface), the carrier molecule protonates, and combines with the drug anion to produce an electrically neutral ion pair. This ion pair is now able to partition into the lipid phase and diffuse down its concentration gradient, toward the opposite interface. When it reaches this interfacial region, it encounters the higher pH of the receptor compartment (pH 7.4) and is encouraged to deprotonate, with the subsequent release of the anion. The carrier is free to shuttle back to the original interface and pick up another drug molecule, and the process is repeated. This is illustrated schematically in Figure 1.

Since the skin is the target membrane, rather than a synthetic polymer, we are severely limited not only in terms of the small pH gradient available, but also in the choice of carrier molecules. For efficient transport to take place, the carrier should possess a pK_a between 5 and 7.4 so that it will protonate at pH 5 to enable ion pairing at the skin surface, but will deprotonate at pH 7.4 to release the anion. The ideal carrier should also possess the following properties: First it must be nontoxic and nonsensitizing. It should also be nonvolatile and lipophilic, so that it will remain in the stratum corneum, where it is required to function. The carrier should also be inert to the various skin constituents. It should have some surfactant properties so that it may readily be adsorbed and desorbed at the relevant interface. Finally it should be cosmetically and pharmaceutically acceptable and preferably readily available.

In previous studies it has been shown that there are some bis(2-hydroxypropyl) amines that might satisfy the criteria above (Barker and Hadgraft, 1981). More recently, the Ethomeens, a group of ethoxylated tertiary amines derived from natural fats and oils, have been investigated. These compounds have been employed in the cosmetics industry as conditioning agents in hair product formulations (Ciba, 1965; Société Monsavon-l'Oréal, 1959). Godfrey (1966) gives an

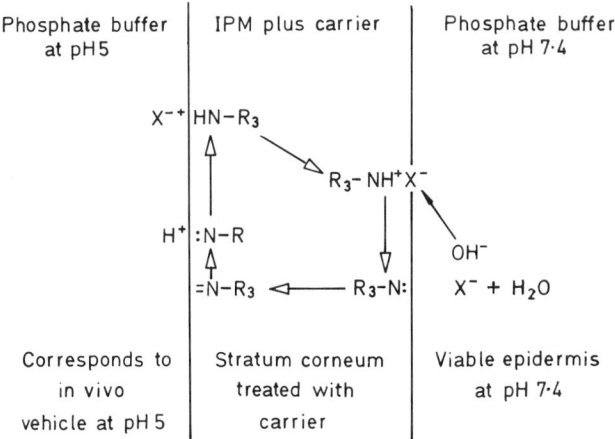

Figure 1 Schematic diagram of the facilitated transport of X^-.

account of their uses in cosmetics. They are therefore considered to be good candidates for potential carrier molecules.

IN VITRO MODELING OF SKIN ABSORPTION

The rotating diffusion cell has been used as an in vitro model to study the transport of anionic solutes across a lipoidal membrane. This cell uses the hydrodynamics of the rotating disk system to impose a known pattern of convective flow in aqueous phases on both sides of the membrane (Albery et al., 1976).

The membrane consists of a mixed cellulose ester membrane filter, impregnated with IPM containing dissolved carrier. This is achieved by saturating the filter with IPM and carefully removing any excess with a soft tissue. The method has been shown to be reproducible.

Earlier experiments utilized methyl orange as the model anion, but recently ionized salicylate has been used as the model drug, since its use in this system has been documented (Guy and Hadgraft, 1981). Resorcin brown R (RBR) has been used as a model for a dianionic drug because it bears some structural resemblance to disodium cromoglycate (Fig. 2), a potential topical drug (Barker et al., 1984). The rate of appearance of the anionic solutes is monitored continuously using a flow-through cell in a spectrophotometer.

Barker and Hadgraft (1981) showed that a series of bis(2-hydroxypropyl)-amines were capable of facilitating the transport of methyl orange across an IPM-supported membrane, against its own concentration gradient, by utilizing a pH gradient of 5-7.4 to provide the driving force. Moreover the efficiency of the car-

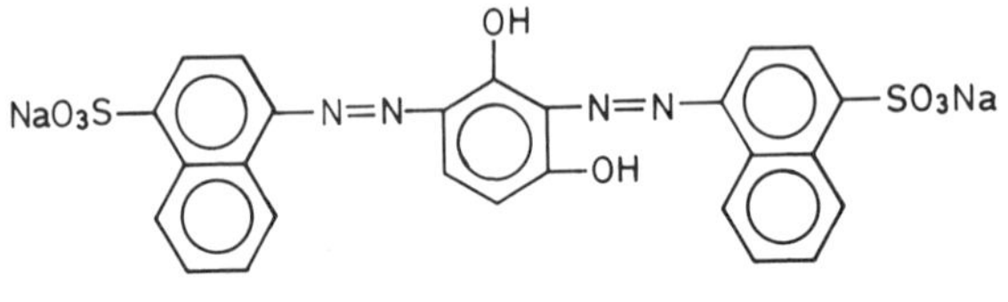

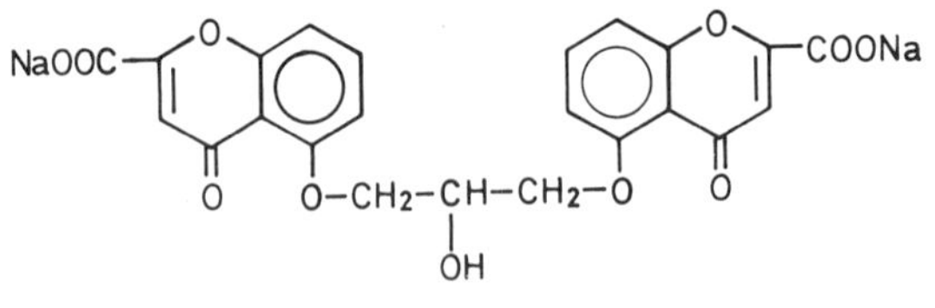

Figure 2 Structures of resorcin brown R (I) and disodium cromoglycate (II).

riers in this particular system was found to be related to their alkyl chain length. Of a series of carriers ranging from C12 to C18 the longer the alkyl chain, the more efficient the carrier. This is to be expected, since as the carbon chain length increases, so too does the lipophilicity of the amine, and a more soluble ion pair will result. Of the amines synthesized, a C18 carbon chain was found to be the optimum length for an efficient carrier in this model. Two bis(2-hydroxybutyl) amines, N-octadecyl and N-hexadecyl were also synthesized and tested for their ability to act as carriers. They were found to transport RBR more efficiently than N-octadecyldiisopropanolamine (C18 prop), a result that is difficult to explain, since there are unlikely to be any significant differences between the two series of compounds, either in terms of their pK_a's, or of their lipophilicities. They were also found to transport salicylate against a concentration gradient, although to a lesser extent than RBR. C18 prop transported salicylate and RBR equally. These findings are difficult to rationalize, since on a stoichiometric basis, one would expect salicylate to be transported more readily than RBR, but the results might be due to the difference in the hydrophobicities of the two anions, and the stabilization of the ion pair at the interfacial region.

The influence of RBR concentration on transport rates is shown in Figure 3. The shape of the curves indicates that the coupled transport flux tends toward a limiting value, suggesting that some form of saturated carrier kinetics is occurring.

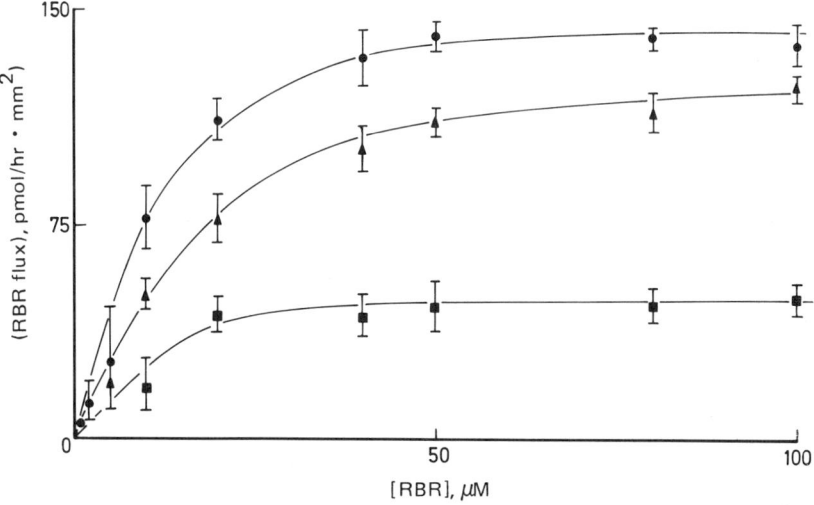

Figure 3 Relationship between RBR flux and RBR concentration: ●, 0.01M N-octadecyldiisobutanolamine; ▲, 0.01M N-hexadecyldiisobutanolamine; ■, 0.1M N-octadecyldiisopropanolamine.

To develop a facilitated transport scheme for commercial use, it is desirable to use compounds that are readily available and pharmaceutically acceptable. The Armeens and Ethomeens have been investigated with these criteria in mind. Their ability to transport salicylate across an IPM-impregnated filter was tested. To produce a system more relevant to the in vivo situation, these experiments were conducted with a concentration gradient of salicylate in the direction of transport. Some potent carriers were found, notably Ethomeens S12, T12, and HT12. Of the Armeens, DM16D was found to be a good carrier, however its bad smell does not make it a good candidate for use in topical formulations. Other Ethomeens were found to be unsuitable for use in the rotating diffusion cell, causing interfacial instability in some cases, but this does not necessarily exclude them from use in possible future formulations.

The method of analyzing data from the rotating diffusion cell is to plot the inverse forward rate constant against the inverse square root of the rotation speed of the cell. Figure 4 is a typical graph. The forward rate constant relates to the flux of anion across the membrane, the interfaces, and the stagnant diffusion layers. From this type of analysis one can determine the k forward at infinite rotation speed (i.e., with no stagnant diffusion layers on either side of the membrane). It is seen that Ethomeen S12 increased the forward rate constant approximately three times for salicylate, going from a 0.1M solution in pH 5 buffer, to a pH 7.4 buffer solution. Ethomeen S12 is also capable of transporting salicylate against

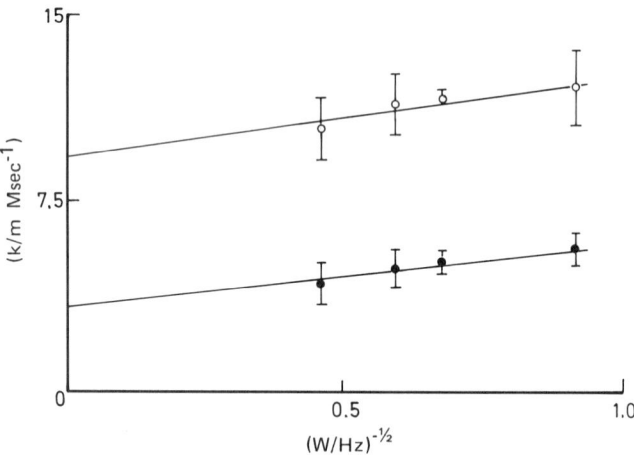

Figure 4 Relationship between the inverse forward rate constant and the square root of the rotation speed as measured in a rotating diffusion cell: ○, salicylate (0.1M in donor compartment) transporting across IPM from pH 5 to pH 7.4; ●, the same, but the IPM contains 0.1M Ethomeen S12.

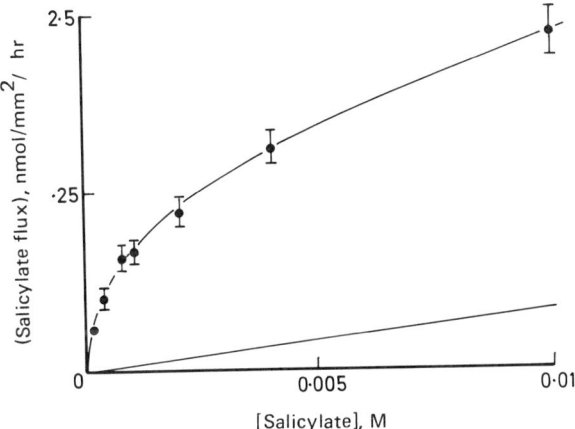

Figure 5 Relationship between salicylate flux and salicylate concentration for 0.1M Ethomeen S12. The lower linear relationship is diffusion without carrier transport; upper curve is a combination of diffusion plus carrier transport.

its own concentration gradient, utilizing a pH gradient of 5-7.4. Similar results were obtained for the related Ethomeens, T12 and HT12, and Armeen DM16D.

To study the effect of solute concentration on transfer, a pH gradient of 6.0-7.4 was employed. A pH stat was used to maintain the pH at 6, to minimize the unwanted transfer of buffer anions and un-ionized salicylate across the membrane. The results of this experiment are shown in Figure 5. Diffusion in a system without the carrier present occurred to the small extent shown; however, in the presence of carrier the flux was improved markedly. The shape of the curve indicates that again, as expected, some form of saturated carrier kinetics is occurring. The shape of the curve has been reported previously in systems where diffusion and carrier transport occur simultaneously (Neame and Richards, 1971).

These results indicate that carrier molecules provide a useful mechanism whereby negatively charged drug molecules may be transferred across an artificial lipid membrane in a well-defined model system. Using the information obtained in this type of experiment, one can now apply this concept in an attempt to enhance the percutaneous absorption of anionic drugs in vivo.

IN VITRO PERMEATION OF SALICYLATE ACROSS HUMAN SKIN

In vitro studies using excised human skin have shown that the long-chain alkanolamines are capable of enhancing the delivery of ionized salicylate across such membranes, from a number of vehicles. For example, salicylate absorption from long-chain alkanolamine salicylate white soft paraffin ointments was found to be significantly greater than that from a diethylamine salicylate formulation. However the production of a coupled transport membrane within the epidermis has yet to be evaluated thoroughly, although these results show that an ion pair consisting of a long-chain alkanolamine and an anion is capable of traversing the epidermal barrier. Impregnation of the epidermal barrier with carrier molecules that would remain there to act in a coupled transport system will provide a more appropriate model.

The ointment formulations were also tested on a previously evaluated rabbit model (Davis et al., 1981). The results showed an increased bioavailability from alkanolamine salicylates compared to diethylamine salicylate. An encouraging observation was a lack of skin irritation after application of the ointment.

These preliminary investigations indicate that carrier-facilitated transport may provide a useful method of drug delivery, although it is evident that much more work is needed to evaluate its potential in biological systems.

REFERENCES

Albery, W. J. and Hadgraft, J. (1979). Percutaneous absorption: In vivo experiments. *J. Pharm. Pharmacol. 31*: 140-147.

Albery, W. J., Burke, J. F., Leffler, E. B., and Hadgraft, J. (1976). Interfacial transfer studied with a rotating diffusion cell. *J. C. S. Faraday 1*: 72, 1618-1626.

Babcock, W. C., Baker, R. W., Lachapelle, E. D., and Smith, K. L. (1980). Coupled transport membranes. II. The mechanism of uranium transport with a tertiary amine. *J. Membrane Sci. 7*: 71-87.

Barker, N. and Hadgraft, J. (1981). Facilitated percutaneous absorption: A model system. *Int. J. Pharm. 8*: 193-202.

Barker, N., Hadgraft, J., and Wotton, P. K. (1984). Facilitated transport across liquid-liquid interfaces and its relevance to drug diffusion across biological membranes. *J. C. S. Faraday Disc. 77*: 97-104.

Bodor, N., Zupan, J., and Selk, S. (1980). Improved delivery through biological membranes. VII. Dermal delivery of cromoglycic acid (cromolyn) via its prodrugs. *Int. J. Pharm. 7*: 63-75.

Ciba Limited (1965). Shampoos. U.K. Patent 1,014,887, Dec. 31.

Davis, S. S., Hadgraft, J., and Al-Khamis, K. (1981). Percutaneous absorption of methyl salicylate from polyethylene glycol vehicles. *J. Pharm. Pharmacol. 33*: 97P.

Godfrey, K. M. (1966). Cationic emulsifiers in cosmetics. *J. Soc. Cosmet. Chem. 17*: 17-27.

Guy, R. H. and Hadgraft, J. (1981). Interfacial transport of salicylic acid. *J. Colloid Interfacial Sci. 81*: 69-74.

Idson, B. (1983). Vehicle effects in percutaneous absorption. *Drug Metab. Rev.* *14*: 2, 207-222.
Katz, M. and Poulsen, B. J. (1971). In *Handbook of Experimental Pharmacology*, Vol. 28. Edited by B. B. Brodie and J. Gillette. Springer-Verlag, Berlin.
Levin, R. J. (1969). *The Living Barrier. A Primer on Transfer Across Biological Membranes.* Heinemann, London, p. 95.
Neame, K. D. and Richards, T. G. (1972). *Elementary Kinetics of Membrane Carrier Transport.* Blackwell, Oxford, p. 54.
Ostrenga, J., Steinmetz, C., and Poulsen, B. J. (1971). Significance of vehicle composition. I. Relationship between topical vehicle composition, skin permeability, and clinical efficacy. *J. Pharm. Sci. 60*: 1175-1179.
Poulsen, B. J., Young, E., Coquilla, V., and Katz, M. (1968). Effect of topical vehicle composition on the in vitro release of flucinolone acetonide and its acetate ester. *J. Pharm. Sci. 57*: 928-933.
Société Monsavon-l'Oréal (1959). Improvements in or relating to materials for cleansing the hair. U.K. Patent 823,303, Nov. 11, 1959.

7
The Effect of Hydration on the Permeability of the Skin

Irvin H. Blank
Massachusetts General Hospital, Boston, Massachusetts

The stratum corneum is the rate-limiting barrier in human skin. There are several factors that affect the permeability of nondiseased stratum corneum. They include: (1) thickness, (2) integrity, (3) previous contact with organic solvents or surfactants, (4) temperature, and (5) hydration.

Permeability is inversely proportional to the thickness of the stratum corneum. Thickness varies from site to site on the same individual and for the same site will vary from individual to individual. The thickness of this tissue at one site may vary from time to time depending on its exposure to ultraviolet radiation and to physical stress (friction, trauma). Some types of physical stress may affect its structural integrity. Chemical alterations may also affect its permeability. Organic solvents or surfactant solutions will remove lipids and will increase its permeability to most substances. The temperature of the skin is relatively constant but may vary somewhat in low- and high-temperature environments. Diffusion is a process quite sensitive to small changes in temperature. Increased hydration of keratinized tissue increases its permeability to most substances. It is this relationship that this chapter discusses.

Hydration of the stratum corneum may be increased by soaking the skin in water, by subjecting it to environments of high relative humidity, and by covering it with a membrane that is relatively impervious to water (occlusion) so that the endogenous water that normally escapes into the environment will be trapped and will hydrate the stratum corneum. The increased efficacy of a topical therapeutic agent as a result of occlusion may result from increased penetration through the endogenously hydrated tissue. Wurster and Kramer (1961) showed that hydrating the stratum corneum increased the penetration of methyl, ethyl, and glycol salicylates. Polano (1976) and Scheuplein and Ross (1974) showed an increase in the penetration of steroids as the stratum corneum became hydrated. Behl et al. (1980) have examined, in detail, the effect of hydration on the penetration of water and the alkanols. Hydration of hairless mouse skin for up to 30 hr had very little effect on the permeability constants for water, methanol, and ethanol. The permeability constants for butanol and hexanol were doubled by such hydration and were increased for heptanol and octanol but not doubled. The authors state that their results "indicate that there are complex molecular structure-permeability relationships operating in skin."

Penetration through hydrated stratum corneum will be increased if the partition coefficient, that is, solubility in stratum corneum/solubility in vehicle, increases or if the diffusion constant increases as the stratum corneum hydrates. With hydration the stratum corneum gets somewhat thicker, which decreases the penetration.

The partition coefficient can be measured experimentally, as can thickness. Under some conditions, thickness can be calculated. Diffusion constant cannot be determined directly but can be calculated when flux has been determined and the concentration of the penetrant in the presenting solution is known.

Of considerable interest is the effect of hydration of the stratum corneum on the penetration of water itself through this tissue. Forty years ago King (1945) studied the effect of hydration on the penetration of water through keratin membranes (cow's horn). The diffusion constant increased as the tissue became hydrated. Scheuplein (1965) observed increasing diffusion of water through human stratum corneum as it became increasingly hydrated. In diffusing through the stratum corneum, the water molecule encounters many restraining forces and its activation energy is 15 kcal/mol, three times greater than the activation energy for the self-diffusion of water. As the stratum corneum hydrates over a period of hours to days, pathways develop in the stratum corneum through which water molecules diffuse more easily.

In vivo, there is a continuous diffusion of water from within the body through the stratum corneum and into the environment, the transepidermal water loss (TEWL). This is passive diffusion, and it occurs because of the water concentration gradient in the stratum corneum; the part of this tissue adjacent to the granular layer is strongly hydrated and the part in equilibrium with the environment is drier. The water content of the inside layer remains relatively constant, but that of the outside layer increases if the relative humidity increases.

Thus it is seen that in vivo the concentration gradient decreases as the environmental humidity increases, which will cause a decrease in TEWL. However, as the drier part of the stratum corneum hydrates, the diffusion constant increases, which will increase the TEWL. It is not easy to predict which of these factors will predominate and whether, therefore, TEWL will decrease or increase as the relative humidity increases.

TEWL can be measured, but the techniques are not entirely satisfactory, especially when an attempt is being made to determine the effect on environmental relative humidity on TEWL. Newer techniques are being developed that may result in more accurate measurements. If diffusion constants for water diffusing through pieces of stratum corneum of different degrees of hydration are known, TEWL can be calculated.

We developed an in vitro method for measuring the flux of tritiated water (HTO) across pieces of stratum corneum of a uniform and known water content (Blank et al., 1984). Figure 1 shows the type of diffusion chamber used. When salt solutions of known concentration are held in the chamber reservoirs for 2-3 days, the stratum corneum will have uniform water content, which will be determined by the relative humidity of its environment. Figure 2 shows the relation between environmental relative humidity and water content of the tissue (Spencer et al., 1975).

After equilibrium has been attained, HTO is introduced into the donor side, and the rate at which it diffuses through the stratum corneum and accumulates in the receptor is determined by counting small aliquots of the receptor fluid. A representative curve of the rate at which HTO accumulates in the receptor is seen in Figure 3. Once flux has been determined, the donor and receptor solutions are discarded and a salt solution of a different salt concentration is introduced into the chamber. A new equilibrium is established and new flux determined. The process is repeated for a total of four different relative humidities.

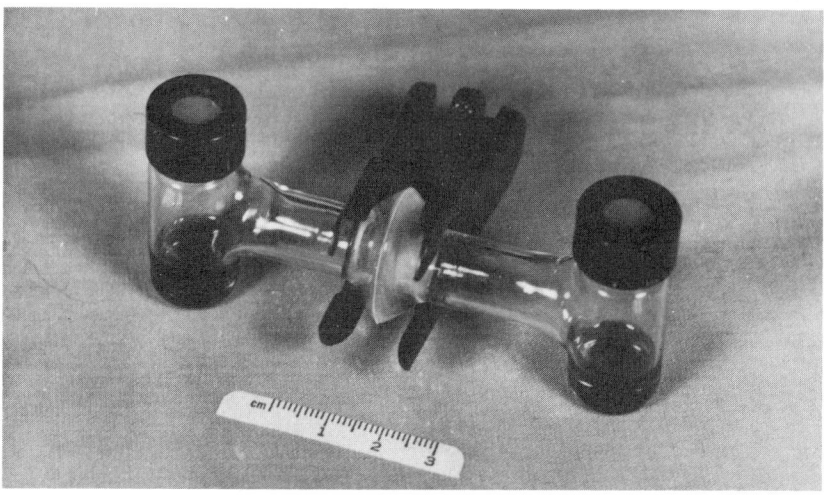

Figure 1 Diffusion chamber.

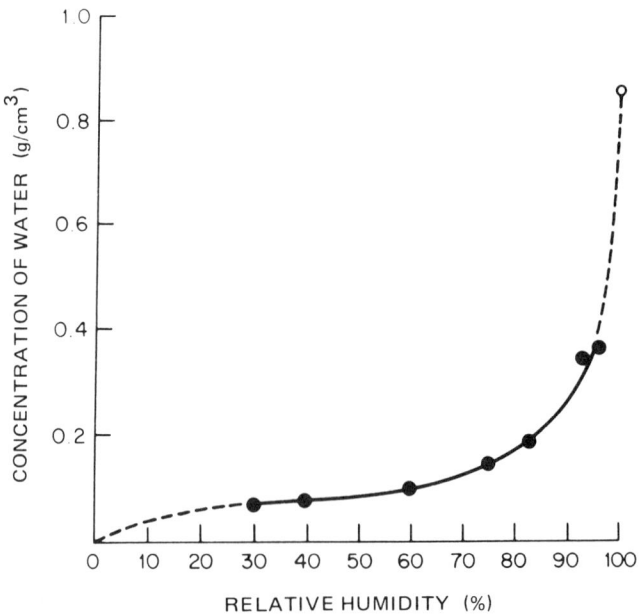

Figure 2 Concentration of water in stratum corneum in equilibrium with air at 30°C as a function of relative humidity. (Adapted from Spencer et al., 1975.)

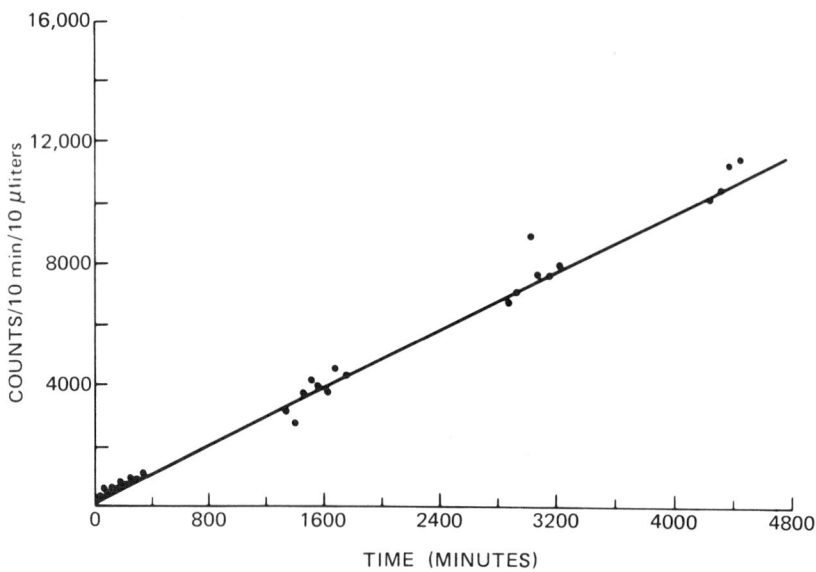

Figure 3 Diffusion of HTO through the stratum corneum, showing the amount of HTO in the receptor as a function of time.

From such flux measurements, diffusion constant can be calculated using the following form of Fick's equation:

$$J_s = \frac{K_m D_m}{\delta}(C_d - C_r)$$

where

J_s = flux
K_m = partition coefficient
D_m = diffusion constant
δ = thickness
C_d = concentration of the penetrant in the donor
C_r = concentration of the penetrant in the receptor

The value of C_d is known; C_r is so low compared to C_d that it may be considered to be zero. Blank et al. (1984) indicate how K_m and δ were calculated from a knowledge of the water content of the tissue and the salt solutions and also show the calculations for the diffusion constants. Table 1 shows the diffusion constants for the skin of three subjects at four levels of hydration. It is not clear why the diffusion constant appears to decrease as the relative humidity increases from 81 to 93%, a range over which flux increases, as is to be expected.

From a knowledge of these diffusion constants and the water content of the innermost and outermost layers of the stratum corneum, the thickness of the stratum corneum in vivo, the TEWL, and the water concentration profile at the different environmental humidities can be calculated (see appendix, Blank et al., 1984, for these calculations). Figures 4-6 give these data. Wu (1983) has also de-

Table 1 Diffusivity of Water in Stratum Corneum as a Function of Its Water Content

Relative humidity (%)	Water content, c_m (g/cm³)	Diffusivity, D ($\times 10^{10}$ cm²/sec)		
		Subject A	Subject B	Subject C
46	0.096	3.19	3.19	2.50
62	0.127	4.30	3.52	2.93
81	0.194	9.26	9.57	4.01
93	0.358	8.11	8.34	3.77

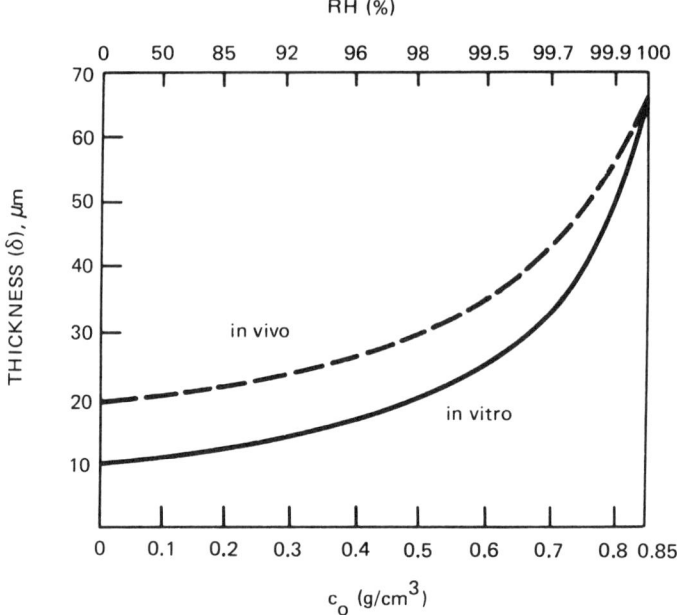

Figure 4 Calculated thickness (δ) of stratum corneum versus surface water concentration (c_0) for in vivo and in vitro conditions. Corresponding relative humidities (RH) are shown. These curves assume an in vitro dry thickness of 10 μm.

termined the water concentration profile of the stratum corneum from water diffusivity data.

It is seen that over a wide range of environmental humidity (0-80%) the transepidermal water loss remains relatively constant; there is a slow decrease. At higher humidities there is a precipitous decrease. Over the years, various investigators (Goodman and Wolf, 1969; Grice et al., 1972; Lamke and Wedin, 1971; Spruit and Malten, 1969) have shown somewhat larger drops in TEWL as humidity increases up to 80%; but as methods for the experimental measurement of TEWL improve, it is predicted that measured TEWL will be nearly that shown in Figure 5.

The work presented here also indicates that the water concentration profile remains nearly constant over the 0-80% relative humidity range. It is, of course, possible that the small increase in water concentration in the surface layers of the stratum corneum, as the humidity approaches 80%, will cause significant differences in the mechanical characteristics of this tissue (stiffness, tensile strength, viscoelasticity, etc.). Much larger changes in water concentration

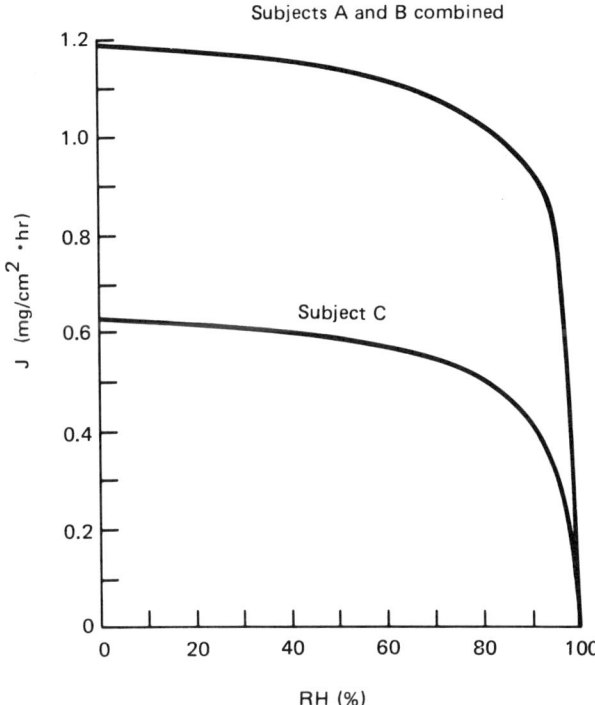

Figure 5 Calculated in vivo water flux (J) versus relative humidity (RH). (The curves for Subjects A and B in Table 1 are so similar they have been combined.)

throughout the thickness of the tissue are seen at relative humidities in excess of 80%.

Transepidermal water loss is a somewhat unique example of skin permeability. The in vivo water concentration gradient is such that water is continually lost from within the body into the environment. When we are looking at the effect of hydration on TEWL, water is, of course, responsible for hydration, but also it is the water molecule, the movement of which is being monitored. At any one relative humidity, a water concentration gradient is established in vivo such that the concentrations of water in the various layers of the stratum corneum differ but each remains relatively constant, and because of the gradient water will still move through the tissue.

Most of the time when percutaneous absorption is being studied, the movement of various molecules into the body is observed. For such movement, the gradient is the reverse of that for water diffusing out of the skin; rarely is the penetration of water into the skin observed. As a rule, hydration (exogenous or

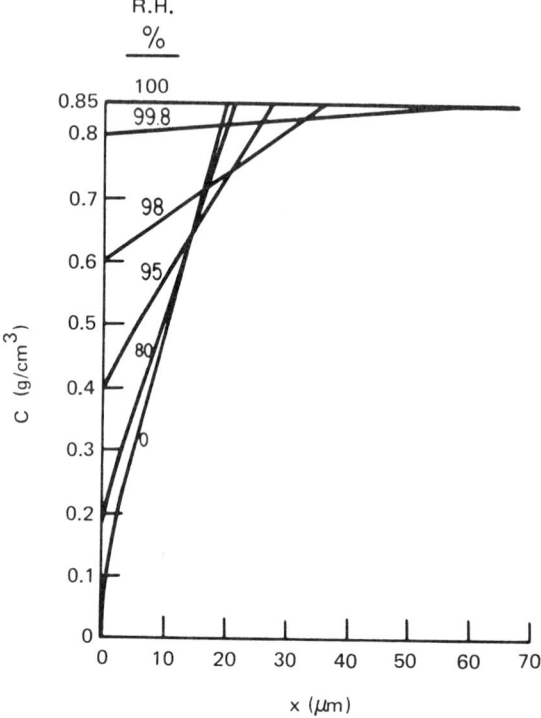

Figure 6 Calculated in vivo water concentration profiles at various relative humidities for subject A; c is the concentration of water at depth x, within the stratum corneum.

endogenous) increases the penetration of substances into the skin in contrast to the decrease in TEWL as the stratum corneum hydrates with increasing relative humidity. This decrease apparently results from the decrease in concentration gradient, which is a larger factor than any increase that would accompany increased diffusivity. The increase in penetration of most substances into the skin that accompanies hydration apparently results from an increase in diffusivity. It is theoretically possible that for strongly lipid-soluble penetrants, hydration would cause a decrease in partition coefficient large enough to result in decreased penetration. Since hydration can influence diffusivity, partition coefficient, thickness, and concentration gradient (for water only), the effect of hydration on penetration cannot always be predicted.

REFERENCES

Behl, C. R., Flynn, G. L., Kurihara, T., Harper, N., Smith, W., Higuchi, W. M., Ho, N. F. H., and Pierson, C. L. (1980). *J. Invest. Dermatol. 75*: 346.

Blank, I. H., Maloney, J., III, Emslie, A. G., Simon, I., and Apt, C. (1984). *J. Invest. Dermatol. 82*: 188.

Goodman, A. B. and Wolf, A. V. (1969). *J. Appl. Physiol. 26*: 203.

Grice, K. A., Sattar, H., and Baker, H. (1972). *J. Invest. Dermatol. 58*: 343.

King, G. (1945). *Trans. Faraday Soc. 41*: 479.

Lamke, L. O. and Wedin, B. (1971). *Acta Dermatovenereol.* (Stockholm) *51*: 111.

Polano, M. K. (1976). *Arch. Dermatol. 112*: 675.

Scheuplein, R. J. (1965). *J. Invest. Dermatol. 45*: 334.

Scheuplein, R. J. and Ross, L. (1974). *J. Invest. Dermatol. 62*: 353.

Spencer, T. S., Linamen, C. E., Akers, W. A., and Jones, H. E. (1975). *Br. J. Dermatol. 93*: 159.

Spruit, D. and Malten, K. E. (1969). *Dermatologica 138*: 418.

Wu, M. (1983). *J. Soc. Cosmet. Chem. 34*: 191.

Wurster, D. E. and Kramer, S. F. (1961). *J. Pharm. Soc. 50*: 288.

8
Structure-Activity Correlations in Percutaneous Absorption

Ronald C. Wester and Howard I. Maibach
University of California School of Medicine, San Francisco, California

The skin has both hydrophilic and hydrophobic regions. The theory of skin absorption postulates that lipid-soluble substances pass through the cell membranes because of their lipid content, whereas water-soluble substances pass through cell membranes because of their hydrated proteinaceous content. While this is a simplification, the water/lipid solubility characteristics of the skin structure are important. This chapter discusses the chemical composition and physical characteristics of compounds that allow them to penetrate the water/lipid system of skin.

PARTITION COEFFICIENT

The partition coefficient is a measure of the ability of a chemical to separate between two immiscible phases. The phases consist of an organic solvent such as octanol or heptane, and water, either distilled or a buffered solution. The lipid solubility and the water solubility characteristics of the chemical will allow it to proportionately partition between the organic phase and the water phase. It is this chemical characteristic that is likened to the partition of a chemical between lipid and water phases of skin. Therefore, the partition coefficients of varied chemicals have been compared to their ability to penetrate skin. Bartek and LaBudde (1975) determined the percutaneous absorption of a series of chemicals in various animal species, comparing the percutaneous absorption of these chemicals in animals to those values obtained by Feldmann and Maibach (1969, 1970, 1974) in man. Bartek and LaBudde also determined the partition coefficients of the chemicals in a heptane/buffer system. Table 1 shows the partition

Table 1 Partition Coefficient (heptane/buffer)[a] and Percutaneous Absorption

Chemical	Partition coefficient	Dose absorbed in man (%)
N-Acetylcysteine	0.0004	2.43
Cortisone	0.002	3.38
Caffeine	0.005	47.6
Testosterone	1.81	13.2
Parathion	14.4	9.7
DDT	28.5	10.4
Lindane	32.9	9.3
Malathion	33.2	8.2
Haloprogin	45.4	11.0
Butter yellow	100.8	21.6

[a] Buffer = 0.1 M phosphate buffer, pH 7.4.
Source: Bartek and LaBudde (1975).

coefficient and percutaneous absorption data for the chemicals. The chemicals are arranged by increasing partition coefficient and show the related percentage dose absorbed of that chemical in man. The lower the partition coefficient, the more water soluble the chemical. N-Acetylcysteine has the lowest partition coefficient of this series with a value of 0.0004, and its percentage dose absorbed in man is also the lowest, 2.43%. The compound with the highest percutaneous absorption in this series (aside from caffeine) is butter yellow. It has a percentage dose absorbed of 21.6% in man. It also has the highest partition coefficient: it is 100% soluble in the organic phase of heptane. The other compounds (cortisone, testosterone, parathion, DDT, lindane, malathion, and haloprogin) all show an increase in partition coefficient, that is, an increase in lipid solubility. Correspondingly, percentage dose absorbed in man also tended to increase, the lone exception being caffeine. Although partition coefficients are not predictive of percutaneous absorption in man, this series of compounds shows some correlation between increased partition coefficient and increased percentage dose absorbed. For testosterone, parathion, DDT, lindane, malathion, and haloprogin, the partition coefficient increased from 1.8 for testosterone to 45.4 for haloprogin. However, the percutaneous absorption is essentially the same—13.2% for testosterone and 11% for haloprogin. Therefore, it appears that a partition coefficient by itself will give only a limited indication as to whether a compound will be absorbed in man.

Table 2 In Vitro Permeability Coefficients, Threshold Concentrations for Damage, Solubility, and Partition Data for Various Phenol Compounds

Solute	Permeability coefficient (cm/min × 10^4)	Damage threshold concentration (% w/v)[a]	Solubility (% w/v)	$\log_{10} P$[b]
Resorcinol	0.04	n*		0.8
p-Nitrophenol	0.93	0.9	1.4	1.96
n-Nitrophenol	0.94	0.8	1.3	2.00
Phenol	1.37	1.5	7.8	1.46
Methyl hydroxybenzoate	1.52	n	0.2	1.96
n-Cresol	2.54	1.0	2.5	1.96
o-Cresol	2.62	0.9	2.5	1.95
p-Cresol	2.92	8.85	2.1	1.95
β-Naphthol	4.65	n	0.1	2.84
o-Chlorophenol	5.51	0.8	2.2	2.15
p-Ethylphenol	5.81	n	0.5	2.40
3,4-Xylenol	6.00	n	0.5	2.35
p-Bromophenol	6.02	0.95	1.5	2.59
p-Chlorophenol	6.05	0.75	2.4	2.39
Thymol	8.80	n	0.1	3.34
Chlorocresol	9.16	n	0.5	3.10
Chloroxylenol	9.84	n	0.03	3.39
2,4,6-Trichlorophenol	9.90	n	0.09	3.69
2,4-Dichlorophenol	10.01	n	0.5	3.01

[a]Key: n = no damage observed for any concentration of solute up to saturation; n* = no damage up to 40% w/v.
[b]Octanol/water partition coefficient of solute = P.
Source: Roberts et al. (1977).

Table 2 gives the in vitro permeability coefficients and partition data for various phenolic compounds. The partition coefficient P is the octanol/water partition coefficient. Resorcinol had the lowest permeability coefficient (0.04) and the lowest partition coefficient (0.8). Conversely, 2,4-dichlorophenol had a permeability coefficient of 10.01 and a partition coefficient in octanol/water of 3.08. Generally, as the permeability coefficient for these phenol compounds increased, the partition coefficient between octanol and water increased. Figure 1

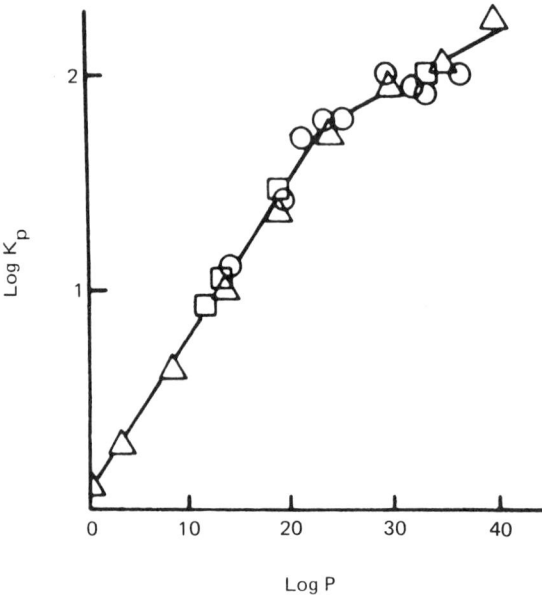

Figure 1 Relation between the in vitro determined permeability coefficients (k_p) of solutions through human epidermis from aqueous solutions and the solutes' octanol/water partition coefficients (P). O, phenolic compounds; □, aromatic alcohols; △, aliphatic alcohols. Ordinate: log ($k_p \times 10^6$ cm/min). (From Roberts et al., 1975.)

shows the relationship between the permeability coefficient of solutions through human epidermis from aqueous solutions and the solutes' octanol/water partition coefficient. The linear portion of the plot of log K_p against P value has a slope of about 0.6. A similar slope was found when stratum corneum/water partition coefficients were plotted against octanol in water (Roberts et al., 1975). Thus, the partition coefficient appears to be a factor in the penetration of these phenol compounds through skin.

Table 3 shows the in vitro determined permeability constants and partition coefficients for a series of steroids. The partition coefficients shown are K_m, which is the stratum corneum/water partition coefficient; K_{ac}, which is the amyl caproate/water partition coefficient; and K_{hex}, the hexadecane/water partition coefficient. The steroids are arranged by decreasing permeability constant. Progesterone had the highest permeability constant of 1500 cm/hr $\times$ 10^{-6}. It also had the highest partition coefficient between amyl caproate and water and highest partition coefficient between hexadecane and water. Generally, as the permeability constant of the steroids decreased, the partition coefficient between

Table 3 In Vitro Permeability Constants and Partition Coefficients for Steroids[a]

Steroid	K_p (cm/h × 10⁻⁶)	K_m	K_{ac}	K_{hex}
Progesterone	1500	104	56	17.0
Prognenolone	1500	50	52	4.2
Hydroxypregnenolone	600	43	49	1.6
Hydroxyprogesterone	600	40	46	2.5
Cortexone	450	37	30	3.0
Testosterone	400	23	16	2.6
Cortexolone	75	23	11.2	0.1
Corticosterone	60	17	6.8	0.02
Cortisone	10	8.5	1.5	0.28
Hydrocortisone	3	7	1.3	0.0009
Aldosterone	3	6.8	–	–
Estrone	3600	46	80	3.0
Estradiol	300	46	66	0.6
Estriol	40	23	1.6	0.2

[a]Key: K_p = permeability constant; K_m = stratum corneum/water partition coefficient; K_{ac} = amyl caproate/water partition coefficient; K_{hex} = hexadecane/water partition coefficient.
Source: Scheuplein et al. (1969).

the stratum corneum and water also decreased. The correlation was good. Similarly, the partition coefficient of both amyl caproate and hexadecane with water also decreased as the permeability constant decreased. Therefore, a good correlation exists for steroids between in vitro determined permeability constants and partition coefficients, especially between the stratum corneum and water.

The three estrogen steroids are presented separately in Table 3. The permeability coefficients of the three similarly structured chemicals vary widely, estrone having a high and estriol a low permeability coefficient. The corresponding partition coefficient between stratum corneum and water does not correlate with the permeability constants of these estrogens. The partition coefficient of amyl caproate and water tended to correlate with the estrogens, but not in a 1 = 1 relationship. Similarly, the partition coefficients for hexadecane and water do not correlate well with the permeability of the estrogens. In summary, there is a general relationship between in vitro determined permeability constants and partition coefficients; however, exceptions, as shown with the estrogens, exist. Therefore, partition coefficients for steroids suggest both high and low permea-

Table 4 Alcohol In Vitro Permeability

Molecule (aqueous solutions)	Permeability constant for solute, K_p (cm/hr)
H_2O	0.5
Methanol	0.5
Ethanol	0.8
Propanol	1.4
Butanol	2.5
Pentanol	6.0
Hexanol	13.0
Heptanol	32.0
Octanol	52.0
Nonanol	60.0

Source: Blank et al. (1967).

bility constants, but not by linear relationships. This suggests, at least in part, a parabolic (or bilinear) dependence of penetration on $\log P$.

Table 4 gives the permeability constants for a series of alcohols. Blank and coworkers (1967) obtained these results for a series of normal primary alcohols applied to dilute aqueous solutions. They found that the in vitro determined permeability constants were directly proportional to the water partition coefficients. However, they noted that before solubility factors can be related to flux, the stratum corneum/vehicle partition coefficient, rather than the ether-water partition coefficient, must be known. Table 4 illustrates the influence of lipid solubility and molecular structure on permeability. As the alcohols add on one carbon in series, the permeability constant increases at a 1:1 ratio. Adding carbon atoms increases the lipid solubility end of the molecule. Therefore, as this series of alcohols decreased from water solubility toward more lipid solubility, permeability constants increased proportionately.

Feldmann and Maibach determined steroid penetration in vivo in man. Anjo et al. (1980) took the penetration data and/or half-life data for these compounds and correlated it with the compounds' solubility in benzene or olive oil. The best correlations were obtained from a plot of benzene solubility and half-life of penetration (Fig. 2). The most common method of correlating physical properties of a group of related compounds with penetration of biomembranes is by using linear free energy relationships. This has been done for gastrointestinal contractility, barbiturate binding, and skin penetration. Table 5 shows the linear free energy correlations of steroid solubility with skin penetration. The best

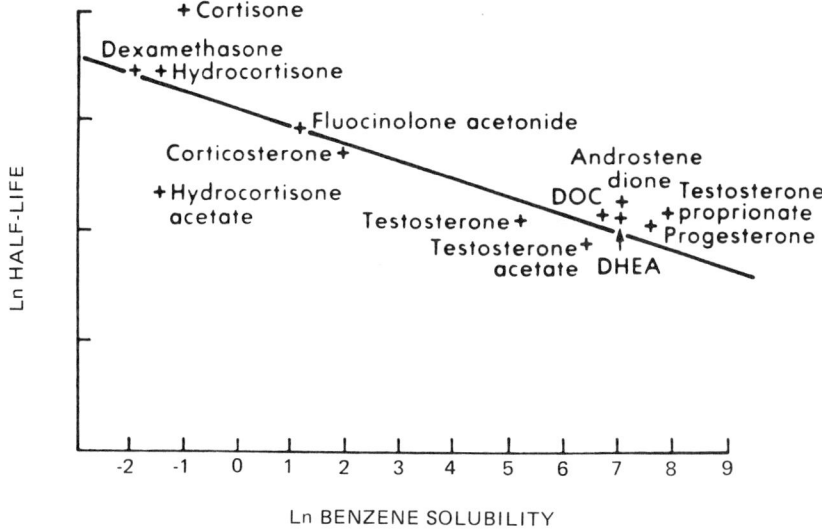

Figure 2 A correlation of benzene solubility with penetration half-life in man with steroids (DHEA = dihydroepiandrosterone, DOC = deoxycholic acid). (From Anjo et al., 1980.)

correlation was between benzene solubility and the half-life of the compounds as the bioresponse.

Thus, as seen from the examples above, a correlation between some parameter of bioresponse in terms of percutaneous absorption and lipid solubility exists. The bioresponse is percutaneous absorption, whether it is an in vitro permeability constant or an in vivo percentage dose absorbed. Also shown was

Table 5 Linear Free Energy Correlation of Steroid Solubility with Skin Penetration[a]

Solute	Bioresponse	Slope, m	Intercept, b	Linear correlation, P
Olive oil	5-day excretion	0.238	1.16	0.01
Benzene	5-day excretion	0.217	0.861	0.005
Olive oil	Half-life	0.163	3.86	0.0008
Benzene	Half-life	0.151	4.13	0.0006

[a]The slope, intercept, and linear correlation were determined using a least squares log-log regression calculation on a desktop microcomputer.
Source: Anjo et al. (1980).

the correlation of half-life of a compound with benzene solubility. It is apparent that there is a correlation between partition coefficient and the penetration of a compound into skin. However, the partition coefficient is not predictive of percutaneous absorption, but can distinguish between probable high and probable low absorption. Both the ratio of partition coefficient and the amount of solubility may be important in future study designs. Since concentration affects absorption and solubility/saturation is important for the ratio of partition, perhaps better control of these parameters would give better experimental results.

CHEMICAL STRUCTURE AND PERCUTANEOUS ABSORPTION

Figure 3 shows the steroid structures of closely related androgens and the percentage dose absorbed through skin in vitro. Absorption of testosterone was

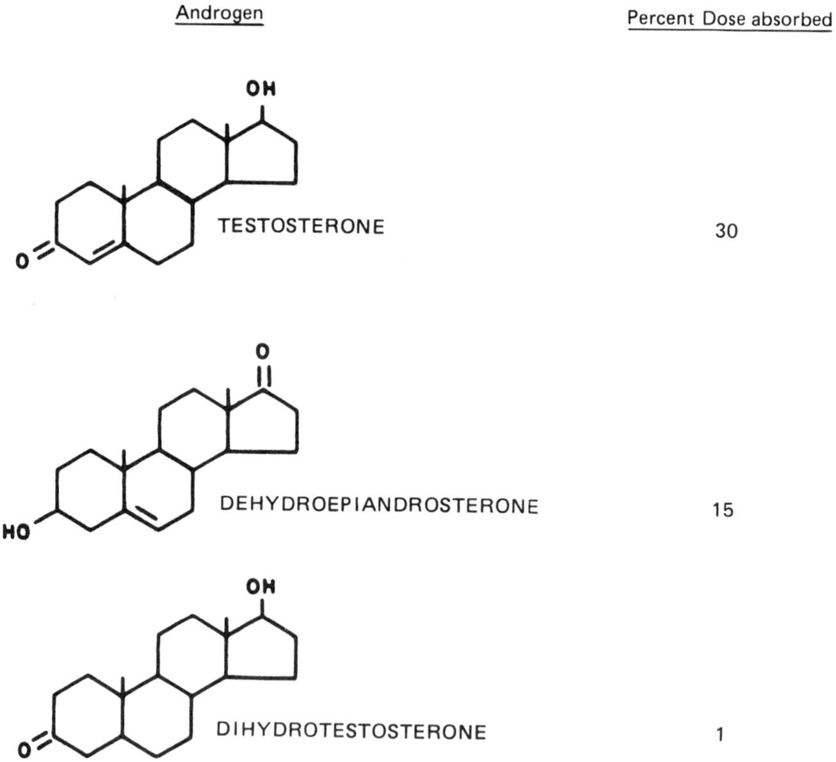

Androgen	Percent Dose absorbed
TESTOSTERONE	30
DEHYDROEPIANDROSTERONE	15
DIHYDROTESTOSTERONE	1

Figure 3 Steroid structures and in vitro absorption. (From Schaefer et al., 1981.)

30% of applied dose. The percutaneous absorption of dihydrotestosterone was only 1%, a decrease by a factor of over 30. Yet in this case, the chemical modification was just the addition of two hydrogen molecules to a double bond in the A ring of the steroid. A slightly more drastic chemical modification, that of dehydroepiandrosterone, restored skin permeability to the chemical. For these closely related androgens, the percutaneous absorption can vary greatly.

Figure 4 shows the steroid structures of closely related estrogens and their in vitro permeability constants. Estrone had the highest permeability constant. The permeability of estriol decreased by a factor of 12, with the chemical modification of reducing the ketone on the sixteenth position of the molecule. The addition of a second hydroxyl group to estriol further decreased the permeability constant by a factor of 7.56. Thus, for this series of compounds, chemical modifications greatly change the in vitro permeability constant of the chemical.

Figure 5 shows the chemical structures of two closely related progestins and their in vitro permeability constants. The addition of a hydroxy group to progesterone decreased the permeability constant from 1500 to 600; again a chemical modification on a large molecule having a large effect on its permeability constant.

Figure 6 shows the steroid structures of a series of corticoids and their corresponding permeability constants. The permeability constant of cortexone was

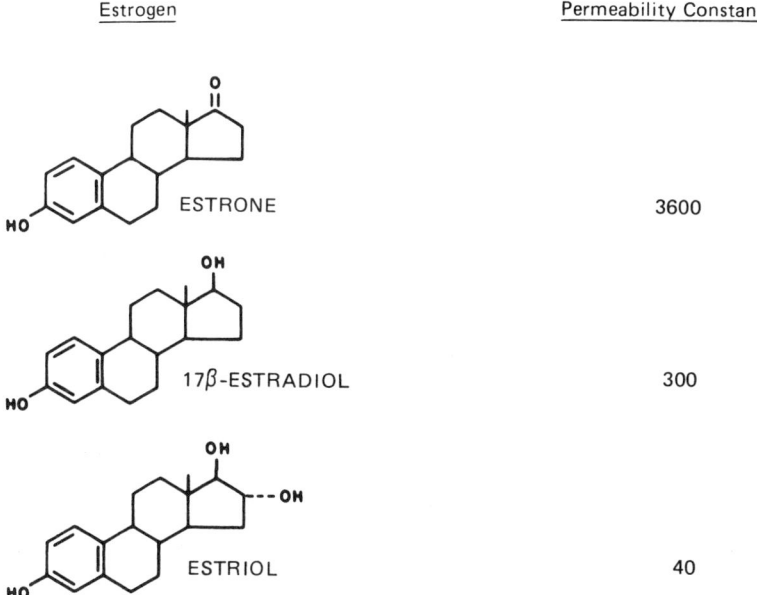

Figure 4 Steroid structures and in vitro absorption. (From Schaefer et al., 1981.)

Progestin	Permeability Constant
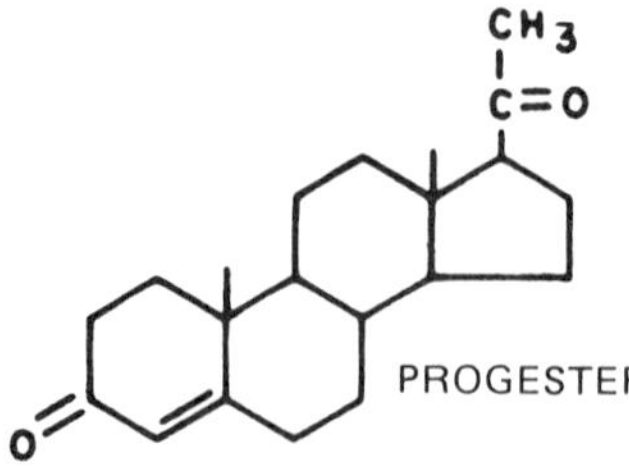 PROGESTERONE	1500
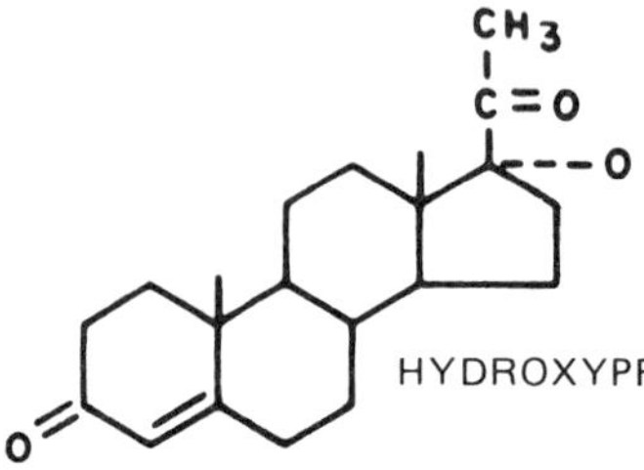 HYDROXYPROGESTERONE	600

Figure 5 Steroid structures and in vitro absorption. (From Schaefer et al., 1981.)

450. The addition of a hydroxyl group to form cortexolone decreased the permeability constant by a factor of 3.

The foregoing examples illustrate that chemical modifications can cause large changes in the ability of a chemical to permeate the skin. Scheuplein (1980) stated that the decrease in steroid permeability with the addition of polar groups was primarily due to a decrease in the diffusion constant, not the partition coefficient. It arises from the increased degree of chemical interaction between the increasingly polar steroids and the lipid-protein-water matrix within the stratum corneum. However, it is noteworthy that these chemical modifications are expected when examining the compounds above. This brings into question the role of metabolism and the designs of the studies from which permeability data are obtained. For most in vitro and in vivo studies, radiolabeled material is used. The dose is applied to the skin and radioactivity is measured, either in the cup apparatus for the in vitro studies, or in urine for in vivo studies. Radioactivity measurements do not distinguish between applied chemical and metabolites. Thus, if the radioactive material is metabolized within the skin, the permeability constant may be for the metabolite or, more likely, a mixture of an applied compound and its metabolite. Moreover, when any permeability constant data or

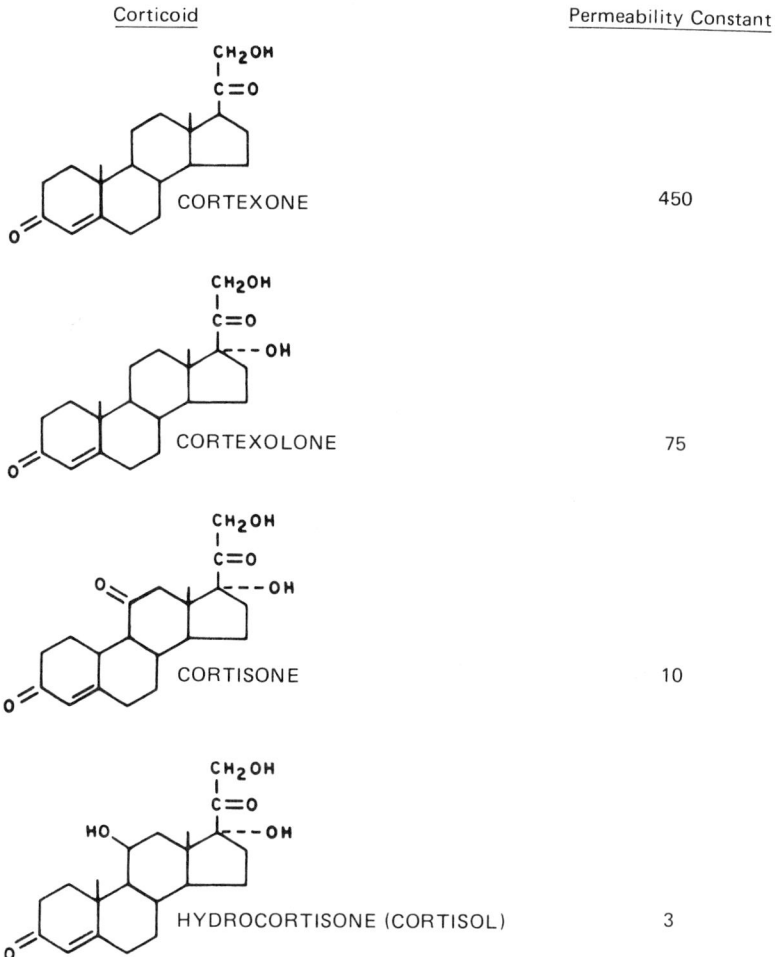

Figure 6 Steroid structures and in vitro absorption. (From Schaefer et al., 1981.)

skin absorption data are correlated with partition coefficients or chemical structure or the like, the study design that was used to determine these data should be examined. For instance, the partition coefficient of hydrocortisone would be determined and the compound applied to skin. The compound that actually penetrates the skin and from which the permeability data are obtained may be a mixture of hydrocortisone and its metabolites (one of which is cortisone). Therefore, the inability of partition coefficients and other physical parameters to directly predict chemical penetration may be due to the limitations of the study

Table 6 Structure and in Vitro Permeability

Solute	Formula	Permeability constant, K_p (cm/hr)
Ethyl ether	C–C–O–CC	15-17
2-Butanone	$\overset{\overset{\displaystyle O}{\|\|}}{\text{C–C–CC}}$	4-5
1-Butanol	C–C–C–C–OH	2-4
2-Ethoxy ethanol	C–C–O–C–C–OH	0.2-0.3
2-3 Butanediol	$\overset{\text{OH OH}}{\underset{\text{C–C–C–C}}{\|\quad\|}}$	0.05

Source: Scheuplein and Blank (1971).

design, namely, the use of radioactivity and the inability to distinguish between applied chemical and metabolites.

Table 6 shows the structure of a series of solutes, their molecular formulation, and their permeability constants. These chemicals all have the same number of carbon atoms, namely, four. What differs is the position of an introduced oxygen atom and corresponding addition of hydroxyl groups. As discussed above, for the modifications listed, the permeability constants change drastically. Ethyl ether has a permeability constant in the range of 15-17, and 2,3-butanediol has a permeability constant of 0.05.

MOLECULAR WEIGHT

The data on alcohol permeability in Table 4 show an increase in permeability constant with an increase in molecular weight (Blank et al., 1967). However, the addition of carbon atoms to the molecule and, therefore, the increased molecular weight, did not cause the increase in permeability constant by itself. The increase in carbon length increased the lipid solubility of the chemical and thus increased the permeability constant. For example, steroids exhibit large permeability constant differences with minor molecular weight modifications. The addition of a hydrogen atom, with the molecular weight of 1, to a steroid with a molecular weight of 300 or more greatly changes the permeability constant. Obviously, a molecular weight increase of 1 for molecules with a molecular weight of 300 or more suggests that molecular weight per se does not influence percutaneous absorption. Thus, the lower limit for both molecular weight and size for which percutaneous absorption becomes a limiting factor needs to be determined. High molecular weight polymers such as plastics probably cannot surmount the skin barrier.

Many observers assume a molecular weight of 5000 to be the lower limit, but the lack of validity of this generalization is demonstrated by the example of heparin. The data seem to indicate that heparin (molecular weight 17,000) could penetrate through skin (Schaeffer et al., 1981). Thus, the actual molecular weight limit has not yet been shown. There must be some limit; one could generalize that movement through the skin, including the stratum corneum, probably can be predicted to decrease with increasing molecular weight due to the concomitant reduction and diffusion coefficient in water. Since the mass of individual molecules increases sharply with increasing molecular weight, correspondingly fewer molecules per square centimeter of skin can be applied. Thus, the quantities of compounds in the skin expressed as moles would exhibit a disproportionate decrease with increasing molecular weight.

IONIZATION

The ionization of a weak electrolyte in aqueous solution decreases penetrability (Loomis, 1980). Small ions penetrate slowly: sodium, potassium, bromine, and aluminum penetrate with permeability constants of 10^{-6} cm^{-1}/hr. The pH of the applied solution influences not only the degree of ionization but also the percutaneous absorption of the applied chemical. Figure 7 shows the mean relative absorption of 0.239M unbuffered chromium solutions and initial pH values applied to guinea pig skin in vivo. The mean relative absorption between pH 3 and 5 was low. However, between pH 5 and 7 the relative absorption greatly increased and stayed increased above pH 7. Thus, the pH of the applied material is extremely important in the penetration of an ionized material.

Dipole Moment

8-Methoxypsoralen resembles dithranol in terms of electron charge distribution and ability to penetrate the skin, although the kinetics in distribution in the original skin layers are completely different. The structure of 8-methoxypsoralen exhibits considerable charge separation, which supports a working hypothesis that high dipole moment could bestow good absorption properties (Schaeffer et al., 1981). The difference in electron charge may assist molecules to distribute themselves between the different components or layers of skin and, thus, readily penetrate skin.

Amphiphilic Molecules

Amphiphilic molecules are typified by a high affinity to the fatty lipophilic phases as well as the aqueous phase of the multilayer structure of the skin's stratum corneum. In some instances, they are completely miscible with both phases: acetone, dimethyl sulfoxide, and similar substances are unlimitedly

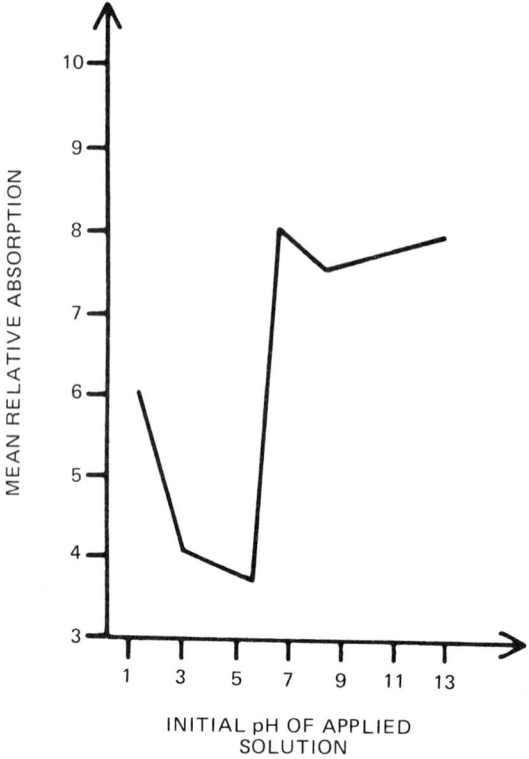

Figure 7 Mean relative absorption from 0.239M unbuffered chromium solutions of different initial pH; guinea pig skin, in vivo. (From Wahlberg, 1973.)

miscible in most lipids and in water. Thus, the barrier function of the multilayer skin system to these compounds is reduced or even eliminated, since it is based on the poor solubility of a substance in one of these two skin layers. An example of the relationship between chemical structure and absorption is provided by dithranol and its corresponding triester, 1,8,9-triacetoxyanthracene, in which the three hydroxy groups are sterified with acetic acid. The high penetration, permeation, and percutaneous absorption of dithranol is not only reduced by esterification but also so fundamentally altered that completely different kinetics pertain (Schaeffer et al., 1981).

VAPOR PRESSURE

Human skin repeatedly comes in contact with chemicals in the vapor state. This occurs as a result of exposure to laboratory procedures, industrial processes, and

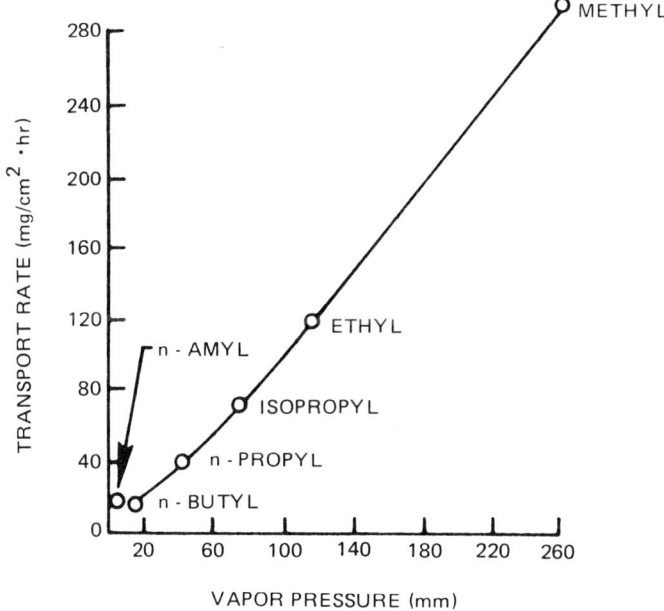

Figure 8 Average transport rates of various acetates through stratum corneum conjunction membrane versus vapor pressure at 30°C (vapor state diffusion experiment). (From Wurster, 1978.)

environmental processes, and environmental pollution by gases and chemical vapor. The transfer of chemicals in a vapor state across human skin is of interest from a standpoint of evaluating potential health hazards as well as the application of therapeutic procedure. Wurster (1978) has predicted a linear relationship between the transport rate and the vapor pressure. The relationship applies to an ideal system where a gas at different pressures is in contact with a membrane and the solubility of the gas in the membrane is directly proportional to the vapor pressure. Figure 8 shows the transport rates of a homologous series of acetate esters in a stratum corneum conjunction membrane plotted as a function of the vapor pressure of the penetrant. Although departure from linearity is apparent, the dependence of the transport rate on the vapor pressure is evident.

COLINEARITY

This chapter has attempted to deal with individual parameters of chemical structure and physicochemical properties, and how these parameters affect percutaneous absorption. However, it is obvious that a single chemical modification invokes multiple changes in the properties of that chemical. Since only a tiny fraction of the almost infinite number of possibilities can be studied in drug modification, redundancy must be minimized. Testing two congeners that have the same physiochemical properties (colinearity) is most likely to be less valuable than testing two with different properties (Hansch and Leo, 1979).

DISCUSSION

The data base that allows the prediction of percutaneous absorption from a chemical structure (and properties) consists mainly of two types of experiment. In the first, several investigations examined chemical structure and compared them to the extent of percutaneous absorption observed in in vivo studies of human forearm skin by Feldmann and Maibach. These data are most relevant to man even though they represent a simplified biological situation. Since there are now 10 steps identified in skin penetration (Wester and Maibach, 1983), it is likely that predictions about compounds and their percutaneous absorption may become more accurate when additional quantitative data are applied. Furthermore, we now realize that permeability characteristics of compounds have many other specialized aspects, such as metabolism and binding, that influence flux. Inclusion of these data as part of a predictive scheme should add reliability to future experimental results.

The second type of experimental data relates in vitro flux to the physical properties of a chemical. The extrapolation of these data to the in vivo situation in man presents even additional complexity. Relevance of in vitro data to in vivo situations cannot be assumed.

REFERENCES

Anjo, D. M., Feldmann, R. J., and Maibach, H. I. (1980). Methods for predicting percutaneous penetration in man. In *Percutaneous Absorption of Steroids*. Edited by P. Mauvais-Jarvis, C. F. H. Vickers, and J. Wepierre. Academic, New York, pp. 31-51.

Bartek, M. J. and LaBudde, J. A. (1975). Percutaneous absorption, in vivo. In *Animal Models in Dermatology*. Edited by H. I. Maibach. Churchill Livingstone, New York, pp. 103-120.

Blank, I. H., Scheuplein, R. J., and MacFarlane, D. J. (1967). Mechanism of percutaneous absorption. III. The effect of temperature on the transport of non-electrolytes across the skin. *J. Invest. Dermatol. 49*(6): 582-589.

Feldmann, R. J. and Maibach, H. I. (1969). Percutaneous penetration of steroids in man. *J. Invest. Dermatol. 52*(1): 89-94.

Feldmann, R. J. and Maibach, H. I. (1970). Absorption of some organic compounds through the skin in man. *J. Invest. Dermatol. 54*(5): 399-404.

Feldmann, R. J. and Maibach, H. I. (1974). Percutaneous penetration of some pesticides and hervicides in man. *Toxicol. Appl. Pharmacol. 28*: 126-132.

Hansch, C. and Leo, A. (1979). Substituent constants for correlation analysis in chemistry and biology. In *Cluster Analysis and the Design of Congener Sets.* Edited by Wiley, New York, pp. 48-63.

Loomis, T. A. (1980). Skin as a portal of entry for systemic effects. In *Current Concepts in Cutaneous Toxicity.* Edited by Drill and Lazar. Academic, New York, pp. 153-169.

Roberts, M. S., Triggs, E. J., and Anderson, R. A. (1975). Permeability of solutes through biological membranes measured by a desorption technique. *Nature* 257: 225-227.

Roberts, M. S., Anderson, R. A., and Swarbrick, J. (1977). Permeability of human epidermis to phenolic compounds. *J. Pharm. Pharmacol.* 29: 677-683.

Schaeffer, H., Zesch, A., and Stüttgen, G. (1981). Skin permeability. In *Handbuch der Haut und geschlechtskrankheiten Erganzungswerk*, Band I/48 (*Normal and Pathologic Physiology of the Skin,* Vol. III). Edited by G. Stüttgen, H. Spier, and E. Schwarz. Springer-Verlag, Berlin.

Scheuplein, R. J. and Blank, I. H. (1971). Permeability of the skin. *Physiol. Rev.* 51(4): 702-474.

Scheuplein, R. J., Blank, I. H., Brauner, G. J., and MacFarlane, D. J. (1969). Percutaneous absorption of steroids. *J. Invest. Dermatol.* 52(1): 63-70.

Wahlberg, J. E. (1973). Percutaneous absorption. *Curr. Probl. Dermatol.* 5: 1-36.

Wester, R. C. and Maibach, H. I. (1983). Cutaneous pharmacokinetics: 10 Steps to percutaneous absorption. *Drug Metab. Rev.* 14: 169-205.

Wurster, D. E. (1978). Some physical-chemical factors influencing percutaneous absorption from dermatologicals. *Curr. Probl. Dermatol.* 7: 156-171.

9
Dermatopharmacokinetics in Clinical Dermatology

Ronald C. Wester and Howard I. Maibach
University of California School of Medicine, San Francisco, California

Percutaneous absorption is the process or processes by which a topically administered drug or chemical enters the skin and the systemic circulation of the body. The skin is recognized both as a barrier to absorption and as a primary route to the systemic circulation. The skin's barrier properties are often, but not uniformly, impressive. Fluids and precious chemicals are retained reasonably well within the body, while at the same time hundreds of foreign chemicals are partially restricted from entering the systemic circulation. Many physicians have been frustrated in their attempts to deliver drugs into the skin. Concurrently, the skin is a primary body contact with the environment, as well as the route by which many chemicals enter the skin and systemic circulation. The physician here must face the ever-growing list of occupational diseases.

The process of percutaneous absorption starts with vehicle release of the chemical to the skin, then proceeds into the various kinetics and factors affecting it. This chapter discusses some factors that may guide physicians in their understanding of percutaneous absorption.

DOSE AND DOSING REGIMEN: CLINICAL AND TOXICOLOGICAL IMPLICATIONS

Foremost among the parameters affecting percutaneous absorption are concentration of applied dose, surface area, and time of exposure. As the concentration

---
*Reprinted from *Seminars in Dermatology* 2: 81-84, 1983, with permission of the editor and publisher.

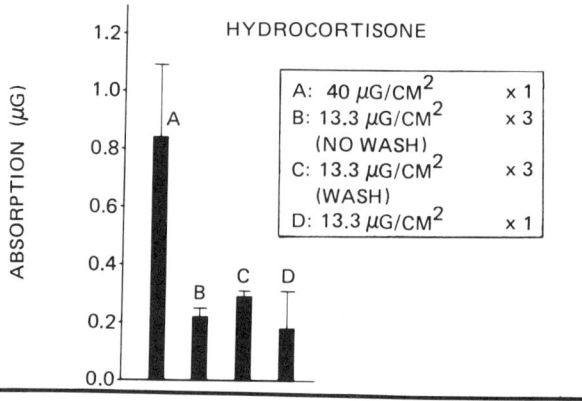

Figure 1 Percutaneous absorption of hydrocortisone following single and multiple daily applications. (From Wester and Maibach, 1977.)

of applied dose is increased, the total amount absorbed into the skin and body increases. Increasing the surface area of the applied dose also increases the total amount absorbed into the body. Moreover, the longer a chemical remains on the skin, the greater its chance to penetrate skin. Therefore, the greatest therapeutic and toxocological potential for percutaneous absorption can occur when a high concentration of chemical is spread over a large part of the body and remains in situ for an extended period of time. However, it also follows that for a drug to penetrate skin and reach its therapeutic threshold, drug concentration and time of exposure may be relevant. This is illustrated in Figure 1 for hydrocortisone, where the total amounts absorbed per 24-hr application were different for single and divided doses. Absorption from one application of a high hydrocortisone concentration was greater than absorption of the same concentration applied in equally divided doses. The single dose was of higher concentration and remained on the skin longer than the divided doses. Therefore, more drug penetrated the skin. A practical ramification is that in clinical practice, one daily application of a topical drug may be all that is needed in some disease entities.

The dosing regimen may also have toxicological implications for the occupational dermatologist. Table 1 gives the incidence of epidermal tumors for various doses and frequency of applications for shale oil components. The total dose per week was the same (40 mg). When the 40 mg was divided into more frequent applications, the number of animals with epidermal cancer decreased. The 40-mg dose applied once had the highest concentration per unit of skin surface area; it was on the skin for the longest time, and it produced the highest incidence of epidermal cancer.

Table 1 Incidence of Epidermal Tumors

Shale oil component	Skin application dose and frequency (mg/times)	Total dose (mg)	Number of animals with epidermal cancer
OSCO No. 6	10/1X	40	2
	20/2X	40	4
	40/1X	40	13
PCSO II	10/4X	40	11
	20/2X	40	17
	40/1X	40	19

Source: Wilson and Holland (1982).

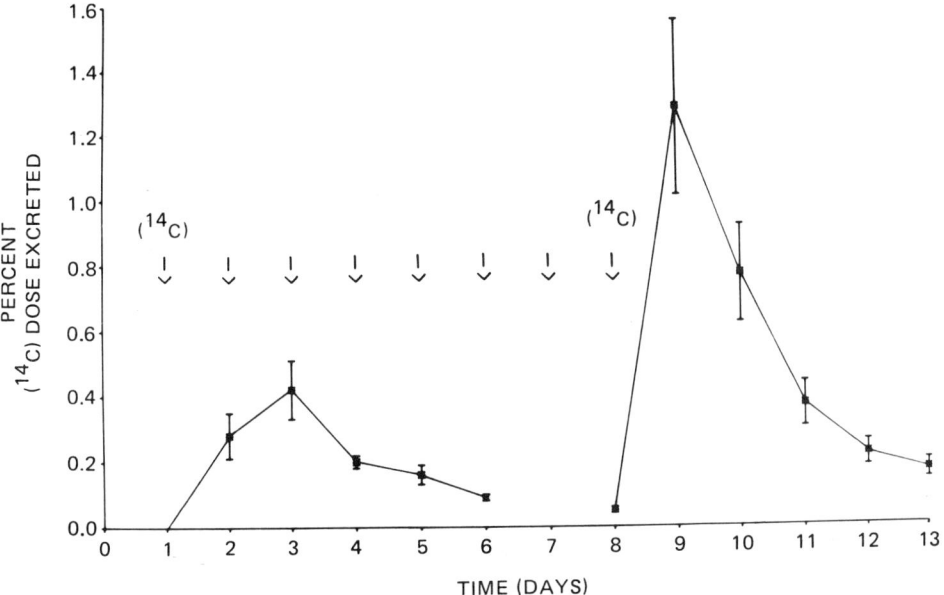

Figure 2 Percutaneous absorption of hydrocortisone following single and long-term application.

Another relevant deviation from acute administration studies is that of chronic administration studies (Wester and Maibach, 1980). Drugs that alter the condition of the skin (hydrocortisone, salicylic acid) also alter the barrier function of skin, resulting in different absorption for subsequent chronic application (Fig. 2). The relevance to in vivo percutaneous absorption is that the skin is a viable tissue, able to change and respond to topical administration.

INDIVIDUAL AND SITE VARIATIONS

The percutaneous absorption of hydrocortisone was studied in 18 healthy adult males. The median absorption was 0.9% of applied dose. However, the absorption for several individuals was one-third as much, whereas one subject absorbed three times more than the median (Fig. 3). The variation was as might be expected in almost any biological system. Physicians should consider individual variation when evaluating the response or nonresponse to topical therapy (Maibach, 1976).

The extent of absorption also depends on the anatomical site to which the chemical is applied (Feldmann and Maibach, 1967). There is obvious practical significance in that high total absorption is found for head, neck, and axilla, where both cosmetic and environmental exposure are greater. The female genitalia show greater absorption than forearm skin surface, but not so great as scrotal skin. The general pattern of regional variation holds for different types of chemicals.

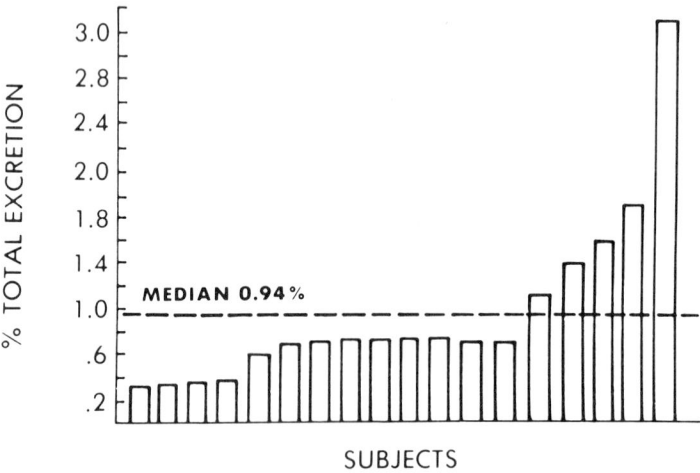

Figure 3 Individual variation in the percutaneous absorption of hydrocortisone.

Dermatopharmacokinetics

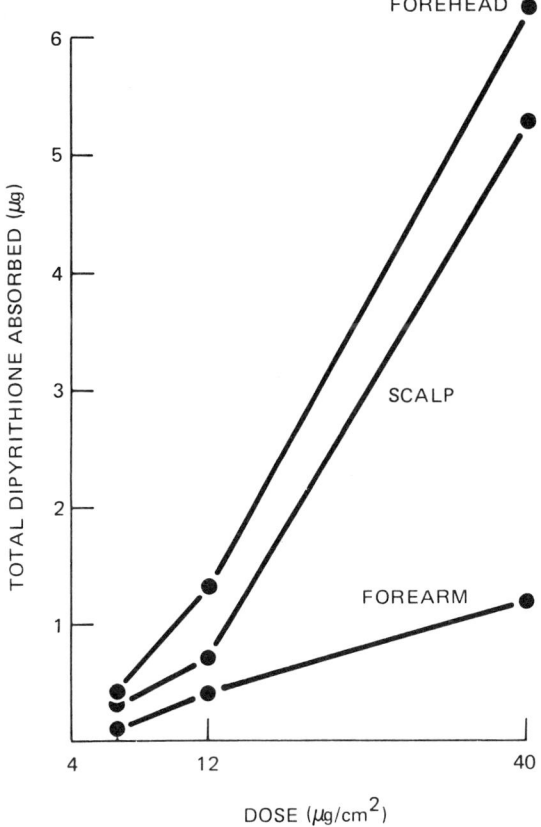

Figure 4 Interrelationships of applied concentration and skin site in percutaneous absorption of dipyrithione. (From Wedig et al., 1977.)

Percutaneous absorption is an interrelationship of many factors (Wester and Maibach, 1983a,b). Figure 4 illustrates this for dose and site variation for dipyrithione topical absorption (Wedig et al., 1977). As the dose increased, the total amount absorbed always increased, and the absorption for some skin sites was greater than for others.

PERCUTANEOUS ABSORPTION IN DISEASED SKIN

Percutaneous absorption of hydrocortisone and certain other dermatological drugs usually is determined in normal subjects; however, usually drugs are clinically applied to diseased skin. It has been assumed that diseased skin has

Table 2 Hydrocortisone Percutaneous Absorption in Psoriasis

Parameter	Absorption (%, ±SD)	
	Psoriatic patients	Control subjects
Percentage of dose absorbed	2.45 ±1.2	2.32 ±1.4
Literature (Maibach, 1976)		1.87 ±1.6
Elimination half-life (hr)	32.0 ±4.6	40.4 ±10.1

Source: Wester et al. (1983).

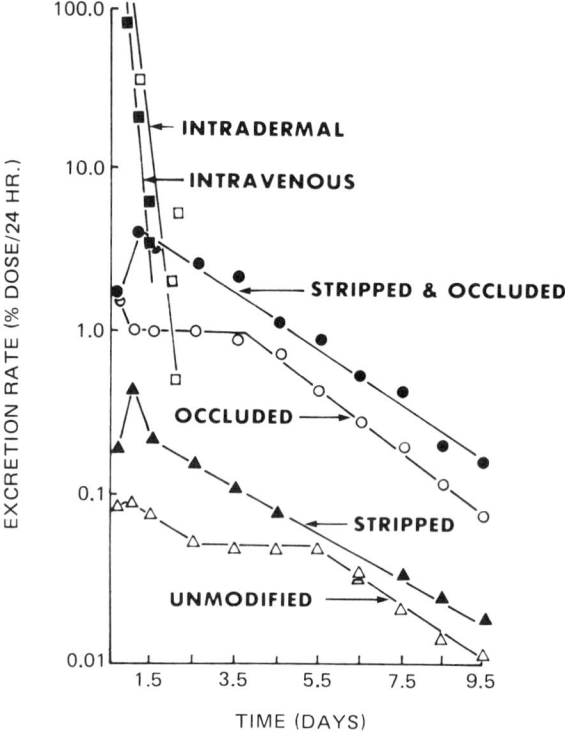

Figure 5 Excretion time curve for hydrocortisone: intravenous and intradermal administration compared with topical application to unmodified, stripped, and occluded skin.

Table 3 Aqueous Partition Coefficients of Hydrocortisone with Normal and Psoriatic Stratum Corneum

Stratum corneum type	Aqueous partition coefficient (mean ± standard error)
Normal sheet (abdominal)	1.04 ± 0.88
Normal powdered (plantar)	1.70 ± 0.47
Psoriatic	1.94 ± 0.42

damaged barier properties and that this will result in enhanced penetration. The skin in acute exfoliative erythroderma is far more permeable than normal skin (unpublished observations). The percutaneous absorption of 1,3-bis(2-chloroethyl)-1-nitrosourea (BCNU) carmustine in mycosis fungoides was 7.2% for uninvolved skin and 20.6% for diseased skin (Zackheim et al., 1977). These studies tend to indicate that the hypothesis of damaged barrier properties may be true. However, this is not the case for stable psoriasis plaques and hydrocortisone absorption.

Hydrocortisone was applied to sharply defined erythematous plaques with silvery scales of four hospitalized psoriatic patients. The absorption was 2.4%. The absorption of the same dose for six normal subjects was 2.3% (Table 2). Thus, for presumably stable psoriatic plaques, the percutaneous absorption of hydrocortisone is the same as for normal skin (Wester et al., 1983). Therefore, other diseased skin and other drugs may show different absorption. From a practical clinical perspective, drugs such as hydrocortisone probably do not readily penetrate psoriatic plaques. Therefore, continued use of penetrating vehicles and treatment such as occlusion (Fig. 5) to enhance penetration (and clinical effectiveness) probably is warranted.

Table 3 gives the aqueous partition coefficients of hydrocortisone with normal and psoriatic stratum corneum. The binding of hydrocortisone was the same for normal and diseased skin. Therefore, the initial contact (binding) of the drug and diseased skin is the same as for normal skin.

SPECIAL CONSIDERATION FOR THE NEONATE

Little is known about percutaneous absorption in children and infants; yet the greatest toxicological response has been seen following topical administration in the infant. Preterm infants probably are most susceptible to topical poisoning because they have increased skin permeability. The skin barrier properties are probably intact at the time of normal birth; however, susceptibility to topical poisoning continues. There seems to be a tendency to smear drugs over large areas of the infant and then cover with diaper, rubber pants, and other clothing. This combination of large surface area, clothing occlusion, and natural wetness (sweat, urine) can tend to drive drug into the infant. Other kinetic considerations, such as the infant's different ratio of surface area to body weight, add to the toxicological potential (Wester and Maibach, 1982). These factors, combining with the inherent toxicity of a chemical such as hexachlorophene, can result in infantile poisoning following topical application.

REFERENCES

Feldmann, R. J. and Maibach, H. I. (1967). Regional variation in percutaneous penetration of [^{14}C] cortisol in man. *J. Invest. Dermatol. 48*: 181.

Maibach, H. I. (1976). In vivo percutaneous penetration of corticoids and unresolved problems in their efficacy. *Dermatologica 152* (Suppl.): 11.

Wedig, J. H., Feldmann, R. J., and Maibach, H. I. (1977). Percutaneous penetration of the magnesium sulfate adduct of dipyrithione in man. *Toxicol. Appl. Pharmacol. 41*: 1.

Wester, R. C. and Maibach, H. I. (1977). Frequency of application on percutaneous absorption of hydrocortisone. *Arch. Dermatol. 113*: 620.

Wester, R. C. and Maibach, H. I. (1980). Percutaneous absorption of hydrocortisone increases with long-term administration. *Arch. Dermatol. 116*: 186.

Wester, R. C. and Maibach, H. I. (1982). Comparative percutaneous absorption. In *Neonatal Skin: Structure and Function.* Edited by H. I. Maibach and E. K. Boisits, Dekker, New York, pp. 137-147.

Wester, R. C. and Maibach, H. I. (1983a). Cutaneous pharmacokinetics: 10 steps to percutaneous absorption. *Drug Metab. Rev. 14*: 169-205.

Wester, R. C. and Maibach, H. I. (1983b). In vivo percutaneous absorption. In *Dermatotoxicology,* 2nd ed. Edited by F. N. Marzulli and H. I. Maibach. Hemisphere, Washington, D.C., p. 131.

Wester, R. C., Bucks, D. A. W., and Maibach, H. I. (1983). In vivo percutaneous absorption of hydrocortisone in psoriatic patients and normal volunteers. *J. Am. Acad. Dermatol. 8*: 645-647.

Wilson, J. S. and Holland, L. M. (1982). The effect of application frequency on epidermal carcinogenesis assays. *Toxicology 24*: 45.

Zackheim, H. S., Feldmann, R. J., Lindsay, C., and Maibach, H. I. (1977). Percutaneous absorption of 1,3-bis(2-chloroethyl)-1-nitrosourea (BCNU, carmustine) in mycosis fungoides. *Br. J. Dermatol. 97*: 65.

10
Skin Delipidization and Percutaneous Absorption

Efraim Menczel
Ministry of Health, State of Israel, Jerusalem, Israel

Skin lipids are a major constituent of the epidermal barrier, impermeable to a great extent to many chemicals. The barrier capacity of the skin ought to be diminished by its delipidization through extraction of the fatty materials. Several reports indicated that defatting excised skins by organic solvents increased the skin permeability to penetrants. This effect was not reproduced in humans in a clinical trial of percutaneous penetration of hydrocortisone cream following skin delipidization by 1:1:1 trichlorethane. Various implications of these results were considered in relation to the hazards of common industrial solvents as far as percutaneous penetration is concerned.

SKIN LIPIDS

The nature of the fatty, glossy appearance of human skin was investigated both physically and chemically. Complete wetting of human skin could be obtained only by organic solvents or with mineral oil, indicating the hydrophobicity of skin surface (Rosenberg et al., 1973). The barrier function of the outer layer of the skin, the stratum corneum, depends on its mosaic of lipid and protein content (Fukuyama et al., 1976). Lamellar bodies synthesized in the deeper layer, the stratum spinosum, are involved in the deposition of lipid-rich constituents in the intercellular spaces of the stratum corneum. Skin lipogenesis is a continuous dynamic process. The polar glycolipids and free sterols are metabolized into sphingolipids and neutral, nonpolar free fatty acids and cholesterol esters. These persist to form the bilayers of the stratum corneum (Elias, 1981; Elias and Friend, 1975; Elias et al., 1977, 1979; Grayson and Elias, 1982; Olah and

Rohlich, 1970). Whereas whole stratum corneum contains approximately 10% lipids, its membrane complex consist of about 50% lipid materials (Grayson and Elias, 1982). Total lipids in acetone extracts from skin in humans varied between 32.7 and 40% (Wilkinson, 1969). Moreover, cholesterol from the epidermis is diluted with products from the sebaceous glands as they increase with maturity (Ramasatry et al., 1969). The lipid areas of the stratum corneum were considered as the major pathway of fatty soluble skin penetrants, whereas the aqueous soluble ingredients diffuse through the proteinaceous constituents (Rasmussen, 1979).

SKIN DELIPIDIZATION

Organic solvents are commonly used in the extraction of fats, in the removal of grease, and in degreasing. The solvents used for skin delipidization can be classified as water miscible or water immiscible. The water-miscible solvents used were methanol (Blank et al., 1967), ethanol (Berenson and Burch, 1951; Blank et al., 1967; Fredriksson, 1969; Matoltsy et al., 1968; Scheuplein and Ross, 1970), and acetone (Berenson and Burch, 1951; Blank et al., 1967; Fredriksson, 1969; Mali, 1956; Matoltsy et al., 1968; Onken and Moyer, 1963; Scheuplein and Ross, 1970). The water-immiscible solvents employed in the skin defatting procedures range from the aliphatic hydrocarbon hexane (Onken and Moyer, 1963) to various chlorhydrocarbons such as chloroform (Blank et al., 1967; Fredriksson, 1969; Matoltsy et al., 1968; Sweeney and Downing, 1970), carbon tetrachloride (Blank et al., 1967); and 1:1:1 trichlorethane (Bucks et al., 1983). Diethyl ether solvent properties of lipids were extensively utilized (Berenson and Burch, 1951; Blank et al., 1967; Fredriksson, 1969; Mali, 1956; Matoltsy et al., 1968; Onken and Moyer, 1963; Scheuplein and Ross, 1970; Sweeny and Downing, 1979). Octanol pretreatment of excised skin was also attempted (Scheuplein and Ross, 1970). Mixtures of water-miscible and water-immiscible solvents efficiently extracted skin lipids. These were 92:8 diethyl ether-ethanol (Berenson and Burch, 1951; Blank et al., 1967), 2:1 chloroform-methanol (Blank et al., 1967; Scheuplein and Ross, 1970), and 1:1 acetone-diethyl ether (Berenson and Burch, 1951).

PERCUTANEOUS ABSORPTION AFTER SKIN DELIPIDIZATION

The changes in the barrier capacity of the skin following its delipidization were investigated by measuring either the rate of water permeation or the percutaneous penetration of chemicals. Table 1 summarizes the skin delipidization studies as related to the organic solvents used for skin defatting.

The in vitro water permeation experiments with excised skins have shown increased rates following delipidization (Berenson and Burch, 1951; Mali, 1956;

Table 1 Organic Solvents Employed in Investigations of Cutaneous Delipidization

Solvent	References	
	Water permeation	Percutaneous penetration
Acetone	Berenson and Burch, 1951; Mali, 1956; Matoltsy et al., 1968; Onken and Moyer, 1963; Scheuplein and Ross, 1970; Sweeney and Downing, 1970	Blank et al., 1967; Fredriksson, 1969
Carbon tetrachloride		Blank et al., 1967
Chloroform	Matoltsy et al., 1968; Sweeney and Downing, 1970	Blank et al., 1967; Fredriksson, 1969
Diethyl ether	Berenson and Burch, 1951; Mali, 1956; Matoltsy et al., 1968; Onken and Moyer, 1967; Scheuplein and Ross, 1970; Sweeney and Downing, 1970	Blank et al., 1967; Fredriksson, 1969
Ethanol	Berenson and Burch, 1951; Matoltsy et al., 1968; Scheuplein and Ross, 1970	Blank et al., 1967; Fredriksson, 1969
Hexane	Onken and Moyer, 1963	
Methanol		Blank et al., 1967
Octanol		Scheuplein and Ross, 1970
1:1:1 Trichlorethane		Bucks et al., 1983
Mixtures of solvents		
1:1 Acetone-diethyl ether	Berenson and Burch, 1951	
2:1 Chloroform-methanol	Scheuplein and Ross, 1970	Blank et al., 1967
92:8 Diethyl ether-ethanol		Blank et al., 1967

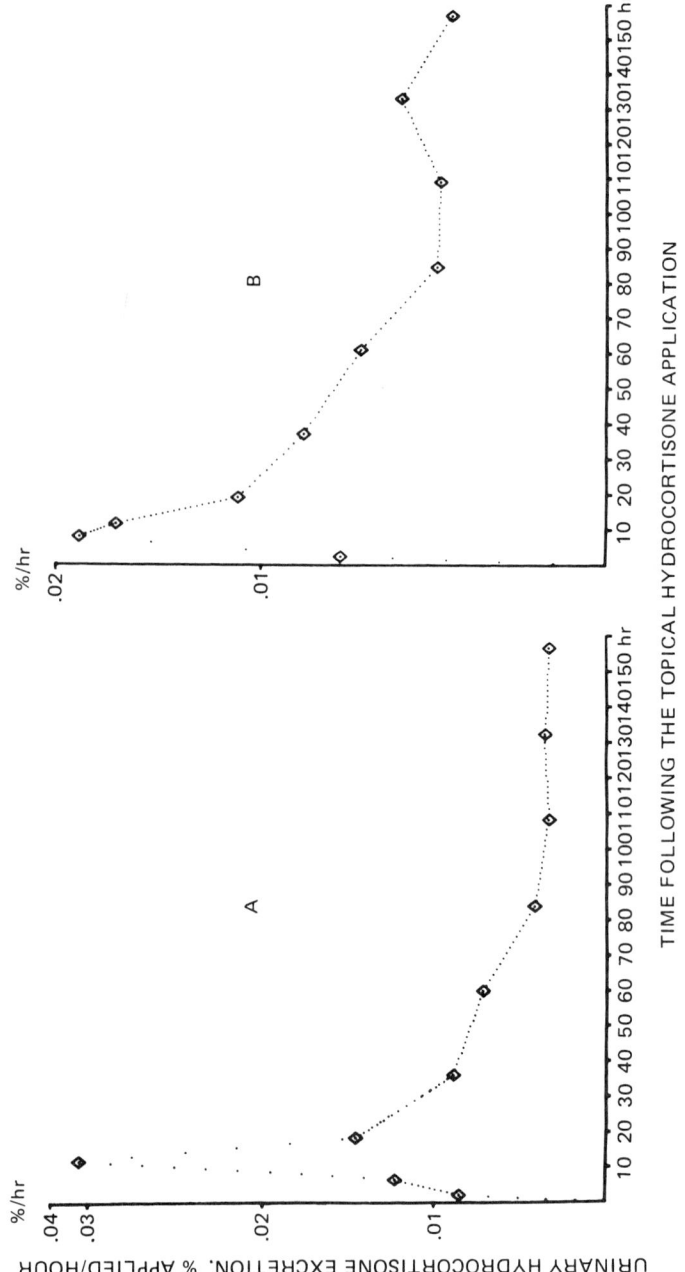

Figure 1 Computerized diagrams of average urinary excretion of hydrocortisone at preset time intervals in five subjects for 7 days. (A) Without delipidization, area under the curve (AUC) = 1.119 (rate × hr). (B) With delipidization of the skin by 1:1:1 trichlorethane: AUC = 1.112 (rate × hr) (The scaling of the y axis in the two curves is different). (From Bucks et al., 1983.)

Matoltsy et al., 1968; Onken and Moyer, 1963; Scheuplein and Ross, 1970; Sweeney and Downing, 1970). However, with different solvents these effects are quantitatively dissimilar. Acetone was found to be the least effective in reducing the cutaneous barrier to water permeation (Berenson and Burch, 1951; Mali, 1956). Mixtures of acetone and diethyl ether as well as of ethanol and diethyl ether were more effective. The maximum effects were attained with boiling 95% ethanol (Berenson and Burch, 1951; Mali, 1956) or diethyl ether (Berenson and Burch, 1951; Mali, 1956; Onken and Moyer, 1963). Extraction by acetone followed by hexane removed almost the entire water vapor barrier properties of the skin (Onken and Moyer, 1963); these were restored when the acetone-hexane extracts were replaced on the extracted skin section. In two independent investigations, the effectiveness of delipidizing solvents on water permeation was graded as follows: ethanol < acetone < diethyl ether < chloroform < chloroform-methanol mixture (Matoltsy et al., 1968; Scheuplein and Ross, 1970). The more lipids extracted by chloroform during delipidization, the higher the ratio of the postdelipidization water diffusion rate versus that of the initial (predelipidization) rate of the skin slices (Sweeney and Downing, 1970). For other solvents such as diethyl ether or acetone, there is no direct correlation between the amount of lipid extracted and the degree of alteration of the skin/water diffusion rate (Sweeney and Downing, 1970). It should be noted that even sorption of small amounts of octanol to skin slices resulted in doubling the diffusion rate of water (Scheuplein and Ross, 1970).

Percutaneous penetration following skin delipidization was assessed both by in vitro and in vivo methods. With excised skins thoroughly delipidized by the chloroform-methanol mixture, the permeability of the slowly penetrating propanol increased and was nearly equal to that of rapidly penetrating heptanol (Blank et al., 1967). Octanol sorption on excised skin slices nearly quadrupled the percutaneous penetration of butanol and butyric acid (Scheuplein and Ross, 1970). In guinea pigs the percutaneous penetration of an organophosphorus cholinesterase inhibitor (sarin) was evaluated with and without delipidization. The penetration was most rapid with diethyl ether or chloroform skin pretreatment; ethanol was slower, and the least effective pretreatment, namely, acetone, was far better than the control, whose skin was pretreated with distilled water (Fredriksson, 1969). In a crossover trial in humans, skin delipidization by 1:1:1 trichlorethane did not alter the pattern of hydrocortisone topical absorption as depicted in Figure 1 (Bucks et al., 1983).

PERCUTANEOUS HAZARDS OF ORGANIC SOLVENTS

Overexposure to organic solvents commonly used in industry may lead to toxic effects involving depression of the central nervous system and the respiratory center. Large amounts ingested or inhaled result in unconsciousness and peripheral vascular collapse, and deleteriously affect the liver and kidneys (Browning, 1965; Hamilton and Hardy, 1974; Stewart, 1971). Percutaneously, some solvents are more toxic than others. None of the guinea pigs survived topical application of either 2-chlorethanol or 1:1:2 trichloroethane; the same treatment with either benzene or toluene produced only minor toxic effects (Wahlberg, 1976; Wahlberg and Boman, 1978).

In spite of the lipid solubility, except for diethyl ether, the percutaneous penetration of organic solvents is limited (Blank et al., 1967; Stewart, 1971). [*Note*: Dimethyl sulfoxide (DMSO) is excluded because its destructive effect on the stratum corneum is not related to its lipid solubility.] Some solvents influence the vascularity of skin, which facilitates absorption of solutes (Brown and Box, 1971). The hazards of organic solvents may be aggravated if they are allowed to affect the natural skin barrier and promote percutaneous penetration of environmental intoxicants and allergens.

The findings of an in vitro study with excised skins indicate that following delipidization even with solvents most destructive to skin impermeability, barrier capacity is later restored, provided the contact is for relatively short periods (Blank et al., 1967). These results were confirmed in a clinical crossover trial where human skin was delipidized with 1:1:1 trichlorethane and the percutaneous penetration of hydrocortisone in a cream base was neither increased nor decreased (Bucks et al., 1983). It has been postulated that two factors probably combined to counteract the delipidization of healthy human skin. The dynamic lipid biogenesis (Elias, 1981; Elias and Friend, 1975; Elias et al., 1977, 1979; Grayson and Elias, 1982; Olah and Rohlich, 1970) and the lipids contained in the cream base substitute for the lipids removed from the skin through the defatting treatment by the organic industrial solvent (Bucks et al., 1983).

CONCLUSIONS

The application of organic solvents to the surface of the skin rich in lipids has been utilized as a research tool for more than a decade to detect the fine structures of the skin strata and their interactions.

Some generalizations presented in the earlier studies hold true. Many of the in vitro studies have not been substantiated in humans. It may be concluded:

1. The skin barrier cannot completely exclude both water-soluble and water-insoluble penetrants (Rasmussen, 1979).

2. The intercellular spaces of the skin, filled with hydrophobic and hydrophilic substances, appear to be the main pathway of percutaneous penetrants of both types (Elias, 1981).

3. The lipids extracted from the skin by its delipidization with organic solvents might affect the barrier capacity of the skin for rather short periods, since this capacity is restored through the dynamic intrinsic skin lipogenesis (Bucks et al., 1983; Elias, 1981).

4. Lipid ingredients of cream bases have a protective value for industrial workers overexposed to organic solvents. The fatty constituents of the creams prevent any loss of skin lipids or replace them extrinsically (Bucks et al., 1983).

ACKNOWLEDGMENT

The technical assistance of Mildred A. Cohen in preparing this presentation is gratefully acknowledged.

REFERENCES

Berenson, G. S. and Burch, G. E. (1951). *Am. J. Trop. Med. Hyg. 31*: 842.
Blank, I. H., Scheuplein, R. J., and MacFarlane, D. J. (1967). *J. Invest. Dermatol. 49*: 582.
Brown, V. K. H. and Box, V. L. (1971). In *Toxicological Problems of Drug Combinations. Proceedings of the Thirteenth Meeting of the European Society for the Study of Drug Toxicity.* Excerpta Medica Series, No. 254.
Browning, E. (1965). *Toxicity and Metabolism of Industrial Solvents.* Elsevier, Amsterdam.
Bucks, D. A. W., Maibach, H. I., Menczel, E., and Wester, R. C. (1983). *Arch. Dermatol. Res. 275*: 242.
Elias, P. M. (1981). *Int. J. Dermatol. 20*: 1.
Elias, P. M. and Friend, D. S. (1975). *J. Cell. Biol. 65*: 185.
Elias, P. M., Brown, B. E., Fritsch, P., Goerke, J., Gray, G. M., and White, R. J. (1979). *J. Invest. Dermatol. 73*: 339.
Elias, P. M., Goerke, J., and Friend, D. S. (1977). *J. Invest. Dermatol. 69*: 535.
Fredriksson, T. (1969). *Arch. Derm. Venereol. 49*: 55.
Fukuyama, K., Inoue, N., Suzuki, H., and Epstein, W. L. (1976). *Int. J. Dermatol. 15*: 473.
Grayson, S. and Elias, P. M. (1982). *J. Invest. Dermatol. 78*: 128.
Hamilton, A. and Hardy, H. L. (1974). *Industrial Toxicology.* Publishing Sciences Group, Acton, Mass.
Mali, J. W. H. (1956). *J. Invest. Dermatol. 27*: 451.
Matoltsy, A. G., Downes, A. M., and Sweeney, T. M. (1968). *J. Invest. Dermatol. 50*: 19.
Olah, J. and Rohlich, P. (1970). *Z. Zellforsch. Mikrosk. Anat. 73*: 205.
Onken, H. D. and Moyer, C. A. (1963). *Arch. Dermatol. 87*: 584.
Ramasatry, P., Downing, D. T., Pocht, P. E., and Strauss, J. S. (1969). *J. Invest. Dermatol. 52*: 383.
Rasmussen, J. E. (1979). In *Yearbook of Dermatology,* edited by R. L. Dobson. Yearbook, Chicago, pp. 15-38.
Rosenberg, A., Williams, R., and Cohen, G. (1973). *J. Pharm. Sci. 62*: 920.
Scheuplein, R. and Ross, L. (1970). *J. Soc. Cosmet. Chem. 21*: 853.
Stewart, R. D. (1971). *JAMA 215*: 1789.
Sweeney, T. M. and Downing, D. T. (1970). *J. Invest. Dermatol. 55*: 135.
Wahlberg, J. E. (1976). *Ann. Occup. Hyg. 19*: 115.
Wahlberg, J. E. and Boman, A. (1978). *Dermatologica 156*: 299.
Wilkinson, D. I. (1969). *J. Invest. Dermatol. 52*: 339.

11
Skin Deposition and Penetration of Triclocarban

Helen North-Root, Neal Corbin,† and Janis L. Demetrulias
Armour-Dial, Inc., Scottsdale, Arizona

The two principal factors to consider in the estimation of systemic exposure to ingredients in products used on the skin are the quantity applied and the quantity absorbed. In the case of bar soaps, exposure to the soap ingredients applied during showering or bathing is usually brief and difficult to quantitate. Consequently, the amount of material remaining on the skin after washing and rinsing (i.e., the amount deposited) comprises the major portion of material available for percutaneous absorption. Even though one may correctly assume that the amount of material remaining on the skin after washing and rinsing will be small, one cannot assume that this quantity is negligible, particularly where biologically active ingredients (e.g., perfumes and germicides) are involved.

3,4,4'-Trichlorocarbanilide (TCC, triclocarban) is a widely used germicide in deodorant bar soaps. Several investigators have attempted to quantitate the amount of TCC absorbed or deposited following application of soap suspensions or showering (Black et al., 1975; Howes and Black, 1976; Rutherford and Black, 1969; Scharpf et al., 1975). Under these conditions, little TCC was absorbed. Several factors appeared to influence the amount of TCC that was deposited on the skin. These factors included the vehicle, the concentration of TCC in the vehicle, the number of times the TCC-soap was applied, and the time lapse between soap application and determination of the amount of TCC deposited. For example, Black et al. (1975) encountered variable TCC deposition depending on whether the soap suspensions were freshly made or allowed to "equilibrate" for a week.

---
†Deceased

The studies described here were designed to identify a more representative animal model and a noninvasive procedure for quantitating the deposition of TCC on skin. Furthermore, the studies were designed with the idea that the procedure would be representative of the human use situation and could be adapted to human subjects.

The amount of TCC residue left on the skin after washing is only one factor to consider in the safety substantiation of this germicide. The extent to which the deposited TCC penetrates the skin could alter the margin of safety for this material. For this reason, the percutaneous penetration of the TCC residue left on the skin as the result of a simulated wash with TCC-soap was evaluated and compared to the results obtained from the more traditional approach, namely, to apply the material, leave it on the skin (no rinsing), and measure the amount excreted.

DEPOSITION

Development of a Method to Quantitate the Skin Deposition of Triclocarban in Bar Soap

The hairless mouse and the albino Sprague-Dawley rat were evaluated as models for studying TCC deposition because they are easily obtained, housed, and handled. The hairless mouse possesses a further advantage as a model because it does not require shaving before application of test material.

Materials and Methods

Materials. [^{14}C] 3,4,4'-Trichlorocarbanilide (uniformly labeled in the 3,4-dichlorophenyl ring) and unlabeled TCC were supplied by Monsanto Chemical Co., St. Louis. The specific activity of the [^{14}C] TCC was 4.54 mCi/mM. The radiopurity was determined by thin-layer chromatography (two developments in toluene-diethyl ether-glacial acetic acid, 80:20:1.5) to be 94% with no impurity containing greater than 0.05% of the total applied radioactivity. The purity of the unlabeled TCC was determined to be 95.2% by UV absorbance and melting point measurements.

[^{14}C] TCC was dissolved in acetone and diluted with unlabeled TCC in acetone (1 part labeled TCC to 2 parts unlabeled TCC). The mixture was dried by rotoevaporation and ground by mortar and pestle to a fine powder. A soap formulation was prepared by mixing sodium tallowate and cocoate, [^{14}C] TCC, glycerin, water, and perfume. Miniature soap bars or "pellets" were prepared by mixing the [^{14}C] TCC-soap with distilled water to yield a mixture with enough tackiness to press into pellets. A Parr pellet press (Parr Instrument Co., Moline Ill.) was used to press pellets of 3/8 in. diameter weighing approximately 0.2 g. The final concentration of [^{14}C] TCC in the soap pellet was determined to be 1.48%, versus the targeted concentration of 1.5%.

Soap previously prepared without TCC (placebo) was shaved and pressed into pellets of the size described above.

Animals. Ten-week old female hairless mice (HRS/J) were obtained from Jackson Laboratory, Bar Harbour, Maine. Each mouse was fitted with a plastic, flexible Elizabethan-type collar to keep the animal from ingesting the applied soap during the exposure period. A 1 cm × 3 cm treatment site was marked on the midline of each mouse's back.

Female Sprague-Dawley rats weighing 200–300 g were supplied by Charles River Breeding Laboratories, Wilmington, Mass. The hair on the back of each rat was clipped short using an Oster small animal clipper 24 hr before soap application. On the day of the study, each rat was anesthetized by an intraperitoneal injection of sodium pentobarbital and a 1 × 3 cm treatment site marked on the skin in the midscapular area. In a preliminary experiment to determine the effect the amount of hair might have on TCC deposition, the hair was clipped, or clipped and then shaved with a Gillette double-edge razor, or left unclipped.

Methods. Identical washing and rinsing procedures were followed for the rats and hairless mice. Each soap pellet, whether placebo or [^{14}C] TCC-soap, was moistened by briefly dipping it in distilled water. The moistened soap was gently applied using a side-to-side motion to the 3-cm^2 treatment site for 30 sec. The applied soap was left on the skin of the animal for an additional 9.5 min before it was rinsed from the site. The 10-min period was selected as an exaggerated simulated use regimen with the expectation that it would maximize TCC deposition. To assure thorough rinsing, the site was gently massaged while being rinsed with 50 ml of tap water slowly delivered from a syringe. The treatment site was blotted dry with a paper towel.

The rinse water was collected via a glass funnel into a glass bottle containing 20 ml of acetone. The acetone functioned to maintain the solubility of TCC in the rinse water, thereby providing homogeneity. The funnel and, in the case of the hairless mice, the plastic collar, were rinsed with additional 10-ml aliquots of acetone, which were subsequently added to the rinse water solution.

Determining the Residual Radioactivity in the Skin

Skin Excision Method. Following rinsing and drying, the rats and mice were immediately sacrificed by cervical dislocation and the treatment sites excised. The excised sites were solubilized in 4 cc of NCS tissue solubilizer (Amersham, Chicago) at 50°C overnight. The pH of the solubilized samples was adjusted to 6.5 by the addition of glacial acetic acid. Each sample was counted in 10 cc of OCS scintillation cocktail (Amersham). Considerable chemiluminescence was seen; therefore, the vials were counted several times to verify the stability of the counts per minute before further calculations (e.g., correcting for counting efficiency) were performed. The counting efficiency of the skin samples was greater than 50%.

Three mice and three rats were washed with placebo soap and subjected to the same procedures as the test animals to correct for background radioactivity.

Tape Strip/Skin Excision Method. Hairless mice were sacrificed by cervical dislocation immediately following the washing procedures. The treated sites were stripped 20 times with cellophane tape (Scotch 810-Magic Transparent Tape), and each tape was placed immediately in a scintillation vial and 10 ml of PCS (Amersham) was added. Tape stripping has been used successfully to remove chemicals deposited on the skin (Pinkus, 1951). The residual radioactivity remaining in the skin was determined by skin excision.

Three mice were washed with placebo soap and subjected to the same procedures described above to correct for background radioactivity.

Determining the Total Applied Radioactivity
Triplicate 0.5-ml aliquots of each rinse water solution were counted directly in PCS scintillation cocktail. The counting efficiency of the rinse solutions was greater than 80%.

Aliquots of rinse solution from placebo-treated sites were counted, and the resulting counts per minute used in determining the background radioactivity for these solutions.

Direct determination of the amount of radioactivity applied to the skin could not be accomplished reproducibly, since the moisture content of soap is variable and since the [^{14}C] TCC soap pellet was, in effect, diluted when it was dipped in water before application to the skin. Use of soap suspensions was undesirable because the TCC has a propensity to precipitate. Therefore, the mean disintegrations per minute of the rinse water aliquots, corrected for background and total rinse volume, when added to the disintegrations per minute deposited on the corresponding treatment site, were taken to equal the total amount of radioactivity applied to the site. In the studies that used tape stripping, the total deposited TCC was calculated as the sum of the radioactivity on the tape and the skin.

Radioactivity for all skin, tape, and rinse water samples was determined in a Beckman LS 100C scintillation counter. Counting efficiency was determined using commercially prepared quenched standards (Beckman) and the external standard ratio method.

Deposition of Triclocarban on Human Skin

The cellophane tape stripping method used on hairless mouse skin to quantitate residual TCC was used in a clinical study to quantitate TCC deposition on human skin as a function of a simulated wash with bar soap.

Materials and Methods
The same materials used in the preclinical studies were used in a clinical study.

Subjects. Twelve normal, healthy human volunteers, free of apparent skin disease and abnormalities participated.

Methods. The subjects were provided with a bar of placebo soap (no TCC) 5 days before the day of treatment and were asked to use it exclusively. They were also instructed to avoid application of lotions or perfumes to the site of TCC-soap application.

On the day of soap treatment a 1 X 3 cm area was marked on one volar forearm of each subject. Three subjects were randomly selected to receive an application of placebo soap on the opposite forearm.

The test or placebo soap was applied to the treatment sites as described for the preclinical studies. The material remained on the sites for a total of 2, rather than 10 min. The 2 min period was selected to facilitate conducting the study, and the amount of TCC deposited on hairless mouse skin had been found to be the same after 2-min as well as 10-min exposures (data not shown).

The rinsing, tape stripping and quantitation of radioactivity were the same as described earlier.

Results

To evaluate TCC deposition by a noninvasive procedure, the amount of TCC removed by stripping the skin of the hairless mouse with pressure-sensitive tape was determined. In addition, the amount of radioactivity left in the skin after the stripping procedure was determined by skin excision. Analysis of the tape strips and the corresponding skin samples revealed that approximately 85% (99% confidence intervals: 82-87%) of the radioactivity was removed via the tape strips. An estimate of 80% removal of $[^{14}C]$ TCC by tape stripping was used to calculate the amount deposited on human skin. This value was selected to err on the conservative side for purposes of estimating a systemic dose of TCC. Figure 1 shows the percent of the total tape disintegrations per minute on each tape strip versus strip number for hairless mice and humans. The pattern of removal of radioactivity was similar between the two species.

Preliminary studies conducted on skin obtained from shaved, clipped, or unclipped rats revealed that the amount of TCC deposited was directly related to the amount of hair left on the skin. The amounts of TCC deposited were 0.09, 0.25 and 0.68 µg per square centimeter of skin for shaved, clipped (only), and unclipped skin, respectively.

Experiments using hairless mice to determine the effect of chemical depilation on TCC skin deposition gave results suggesting that the depilatory had affected the stratum corneum (data not shown). Therefore, a depilatory was not used in subsequent experiments.

Because of the nonnormal distribution of data, a nonparametric statistical analysis was used to compare deposition of TCC between species. The median,

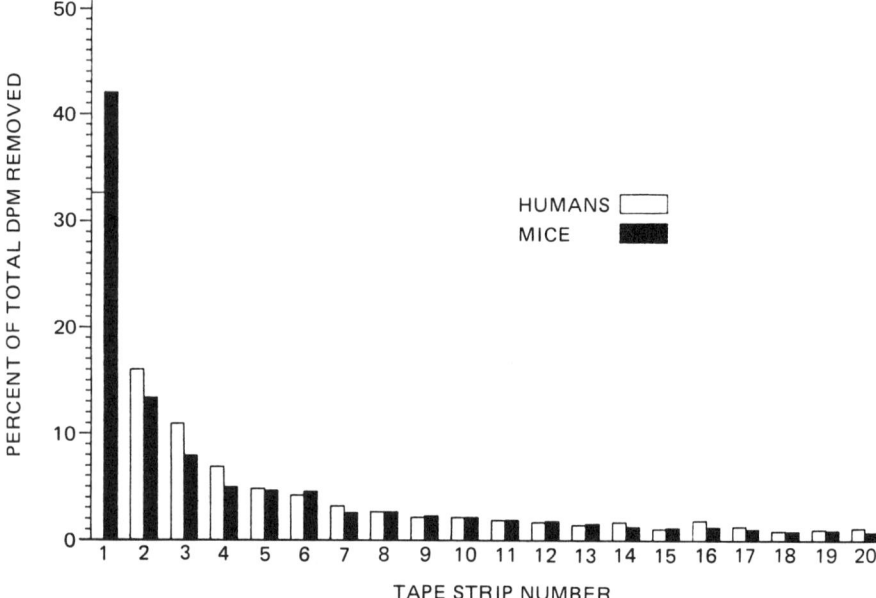

Figure 1 Pattern of [^{14}C]TCC removal by successive tape stripping of the skin of the hairless mouse (n=18) versus human (n=12).

Table 1 Deposition of TCC (micrograms per square centimeter of skin) on Rat, Hairless Mouse, and Human Skin

		Confidence levels	
Species (n)	Median	95%	99%
Rat (18)	0.8651[a,b]	0.7350, 1.1243	0.5398, 1.1299
Mouse (18)	0.1826[a,c,d]	0.1703, 0.2284	0.1608, 0.2533
Mouse (TS)[e] (18)	0.2147[d]	0.1819, 0.2456	0.1730, 0.2900
Human (TS)[e] (12)	0.3306[b,c]	0.2498, 0.4263	0.2423, 0.5836

[a]Statistically significant, p = 0.0001.
[b]Statistically significant, p = 0.0001.
[c]Statistically significant, p = 0.0006.
[d]No significant difference, p = 0.1892; Wilcoxon rank sum test (two sided).
[e]Tape stripping, corrected for recovery.
Source: Wilcoxon and Wilcox (1964).

Table 2 Deposition of TCC (micrograms per square centimeter of skin) on Hairless Mouse Skin Following Daily Washing with TCC-Soap[a]

Day	Immediate sacrifice	8-hr sacrifice	24-hr sacrifice
1	0.194 ±0.019	0.010 ±0.006[b]	0.015 ±0.004
2	0.181 ±0.023	0.041 ±0.032	0.0001 ±0
3	0.131 ±0.028	0.014 ±0.009	0.002 ±0.002
4	0.193 ±0.025	0.071 ±0.016	0.077 ±0.050

[a]Values represent the mean value for skin samples obtained from three animals at each sacrifice.
[b]Sacrificed at 12 hr.

95% and 99% confidence intervals, and the results of the Wilcoxon rank sum test (Wilcoxon and Wilcox, 1964) are shown in Table 1. The deposition of TCC was greatest in the rat, followed, in order, by the human and the mouse. The depositions of TCC on mouse skin that had been excised and on mouse skin that had been stripped and corrected for recovery did not differ significantly. Rinsing with water removed greater than 98% of the applied radioactivity from the skin of all species, including humans.

The potential for TCC to accumulate on the skin as the result of repeated washings with TCC-soap was evaluated in hairless mice. In one study, the mice were treated as described earlier once daily, a normal consumer use pattern, for 4 consecutive days. The amount of TCC in excised skin was determined immediately after removal of the soap and 8 and 24 hr later. Results are shown in Table 2. TCC did not accumulate on the skin over the 4-day period. In addition, the amount of TCC remaining on the skin 8 and 24 hr after each wash was negligible.

In another study, hairless mice were washed twice per day, a regimen that could also be expected to be followed by consumers, for 3 consecutive days. Skin was excised immediately after the final (sixth) wash and rinse. A mean value of 0.282 ±0.043 µg of TCC was deposited per square centimeter skin (n = 5).

PERCUTANEOUS PENETRATION

Howes and Black (1976) reported that of the amount of TCC deposited on rat skin following washing with a TCC-soap suspension, a mean of 22.7% TCC was absorbed during 48 hr. They also reported a mean of 12.7% absorption of TCC in the rat during 48 hr when it was applied to the skin in acetone (and not rinsed). Maibach (1967) reported a mean of 14% absorption of TCC in humans (based on the amount excreted over a 10-day period) following its application in acetone. However, Scharpf et al. (1975) found that individuals who showered with an 8% soap suspension containing 2% [^{14}C]TCC excreted only 0.23% of the applied radioactivity in feces after 6 days and 0.16% in urine after 2 days. Thus, the extent of percutaneous penetration is strongly influenced by the method of test material application. The most projectable results would be obtained under conditions that match most closely those of actual human use.

In Vivo Penetration of Triclocarban in Rats Following Washing with TCC-Soap

Materials and Methods

The test materials used in this study were the same as those used in the deposition experiments.

Animals. Six female Sprague-Dawley rats were used. Twenty-four hours before the washing procedure, the hair on the dorsal and lateral parts of the torso of each rat was clipped short. Each rat was placed in a Nalgene metabolism cage for 24 hr, during which time urine and feces were collected to determine the background radioactivity.

Methods. On the day of treatment, each rat was anesthetized with an intraperitoneal injection of sodium pentobarbital and a 5 cm × 6 cm treatment site was marked in the scapular area of the back. A 30-cm^2 area was selected to enhance the probability of detecting absorbed TCC.

The treatment site was evenly moistened with 1 ml of tap water and the [^{14}C] TCC-soap pellet applied directly to the skin as described for the deposition studies. Following rinsing, the sites were covered with gauze and the rats were restrained in a manner that prevented them from tampering with the treated area. They were returned to the metabolism cages.

Urine and feces were collected at 24, 48, and 72 hr. Following the 72-hr collection, the rats were sacrificed with CO_2 and the treatment sites excised. Skin, urine, and feces samples were stored frozen until analyzed for radioactivity. The gauze patches were stored in sealed vials. The amount of radioactivity recovered in the excreta following soap application was corrected for the amount excreted following intravenous administration (93% reported by Howes and Black, 1976).

A Packard 306 Sample Oxidizer was used to combust 1 ml samples of urine and 0.5 ml of Combustaid (Packard) and weighed samples (approximately 0.5 g) of well-mixed feces. The 30-cm^2 treatment sites were cut into 5-cm^2 sections. Each section was solubilized in 4 ml of NCS and prepared for counting as previously described. Each gauze patch was extracted with 20 ml of AAA alcohol over 4-hr. A 10-ml aliquot was taken and added to 10 ml of PCS scintillation cocktail. The samples were counted in a Packard model 4640 liquid scintillation counter. The counting efficiency of the samples was 75–80% (external standard ratio method).

Results

Albino rats washed once with a bar soap containing 1.5% TCC absorbed 0.16 µg of TCC per square centimeter in 72-hr. The amount of TCC deposited on the

Table 3 Percutaneous Penetration of TCC in Albino Rats Washed Once with 1.5% TCC Soap

Rat no.	TCC absorbed (μg/30 cm^2 skin)			Total TCC absorbed (μg/cm^2 skin)	Total TCC deposited (μg/cm^2 skin)	Percentage penetration
	0–24 hr	24–48 hr	48–72 hr			
248	0.67	3.48	3.75	0.26	0.88	29.9
254	0.06	0.63	5.38	0.20	1.79	11.3
258	0.15	0.51	0.90	0.05	0.95	5.5
263	0.17	1.26	0.98	0.08	0.63	12.8
267	0.10	0.22	4.35	0.16	1.26	12.4
271	0.18	3.20	2.66	0.20	0.85	25.5
Mean ± SD	0.22 ± 0.22	1.55 ± 1.43	3.00 ± 1.83	0.16 ± 0.08	1.06 ± 0.41	16.2 ± 9.4

treated site was calculated as the sum of the total skin residue (on 30 cm^2 of skin), the gauze residue, and the absorbed TCC. The percentage absorption was calculated as the micrograms of TCC absorbed per square centimeter per micrograms of TCC deposited per square centimeter × 100. The values are shown in Table 3. A mean of 16% of the deposited TCC was absorbed by the rat over the 72-hr period.

DISCUSSION

Quantitating the deposition, or substantitivity, of TCC on the skin of the rat and the hairless mouse using the methods described produced results that were consistent and reproducible. The results are supported by those of other investigators, despite the difference in the method of soap application. For example, Howes and Black (1976) reported 1-2 μg TCC/cm^2 deposited on rat skin when an 8% soap suspension containing 1% [^{14}C] TCC was applied to the skin and rinsed. In the studies described here, 0.9 μg TCC/cm^2 was deposited on rat skin following direct application of the soap pellet containing 1.5% [^{14}C] TCC. Black et al. (1975) reported 0.10 μg TCC/cm^2 deposited on human skin versus 0.33 μg TCC/cm^2 in the studies reported here.

Rutherford and Black (1969) speculated that observed differences in TCC deposition were largely dependent on the presence or absence of hair, and the findings described here substantiate this theory: the rat, which had the most hair despite clipping, had the largest amount of TCC residue. The hairless mouse proved to be an especially good model for predicting the deposition of TCC on human skin since it, like the human, has relatively little hair.

In repeat application experiments, the hairless mouse possesses a considerable advantage over other rodents. TCC-containing soap and undoubtedly other test materials may be applied on the hairless mouse in a manner and at a frequency that matches that of normal consumer use without regard to clipping. For example, when Black et al. (1975) evaluated the cumulative deposition of TCC on guinea pig skin over several days, they found no increase in TCC deposition after nine washes. However, the animals in their studies required repeated clipping, a procedure that by itself might have removed all or part of the TCC skin residue. The present results obtained from the experiments involving repeated washing of hairless mice indicated no significant accumulation of TCC on the skin. These results demonstrate that the lack of TCC accumulation seen in the studies of Black et al. (1975) was not an artifact of the repeated clipping. Although some of the TCC residue is undoubtedly absorbed, the major TCC loss (from the skin) between washings is probably the result of grooming and sloughing of the stratum corneum.

The rinsing procedure itself removes at least 98% of the TCC applied as the result of direct application of TCC-soap to the skin of the hairless mouse, rat, or human. Of the amount of TCC deposited, 16% is absorbed by the rat, a result comparable to those reported by Howes and Black (1976). If approximately 0.3 µg of TCC is deposited per square centimeter on human skin as a result of washing with a 1.5% TCC bar soap and the adult human skin surface area is approximately 18,000 cm^2, the topical dose of TCC is 6 mg per person. If approximately 16% of the deposited TCC is absorbed, as shown in the percutaneous penetration study involving rats, the systemic dose of TCC would be less than 1 mg per person. Thus, human exposure to TCC as the result of regular bathing or showering with TCC-soap is minimal. In fact, the percentage penetration of TCC, expressed as a fraction of the amount *applied*, would be 0.3% (2% of applied amount deposited × 16% of deposited amount absorbed). This value is supported by that obtained in the study by Scharpf et al. (1975): 0.39% penetration of TCC by the sixth day following a single shower.

The results described here confirm the minimal deposition and penetration of TCC providing an explanation for the low or nondetectable plasma levels of TCC following bathing (Hoar and Bowen, 1977; Hong et al., 1975; Scharpf et al., 1975). The results support the safe use of this germicide in bar soap by consumers.

ACKNOWLEDGMENTS

The skilled technical assistance of Patricia Wellington, Nell Melvin, and Dan Bucks and the cooperation of Drs. Howard Maibach and Ronald Wester are gratefully acknowledged. The authors thank Drs. D. I. Richardson, J. E. Heinze, and E. P. Seitz for their critical review of this manuscript and Shelly Alop Merzel for her valuable assistance in manuscript preparation.

REFERENCES

Black, J. G., Howes, D., and Rutherford, T. (1975). Skin deposition and penetration of trichlorocarbanilide. *Toxicology 3*: 253–264.

Hoar, D. R. and Bowen, M. H. (1977). GLC determination of free triclocarban in blood. *J. Pharm. Sci. 66*: 725–726.

Hong, H. S. C., Steltenkamp, R. J., and Smith, N. L. (1975). Quantitative analysis of triclocarban in blood. *J. Pharm. Sci. 64*: 860–861.

Howes, D. and Black, J. G. (1976). Percutaneous absorption of triclocarban in rat and man. *Toxicology 6*: 67–76.

Maibach, H. I. (1967). Skin penetration of hexachlorophene in living man. OTC Volume 020186 (part of U.S. Food and Drug Administration Over-the-Counter Topical Antimicrobial Products review).

Pinkus, H. (1951). Examination of epidermis by the strip method of removing horny layers. *J. Invest. Dermatol. 16*: 383–386.

Rutherford, T. and Black, J. G. (1969). The use of autoradiography to study the localization of germicides in skin. *Br. J. Dermatol. 81*: 85–87.

Scharpf, L. G., Hill, I. D., and Maibach, H. I. (1975). Percutaneous penetration and disposition of triclocarban in man. *Arch. Environ. Health 30*: 7-14.

Wilcoxon, F. and Wilcox, R. A. (1964). Some rapid approximate statistical procedures. Lederle Laboratories, Pearl River, N.Y.

12
Topical Pharmacokinetics of [^{14}C] Butylated Hydroxytoluene in the Guinea Pig

Sandrine I. Courtheoux* and Jacques L. Wepierre
Université Paris-Sud, Chatenay Malabry, France

Jean-Paul Marty
Université de Picardie, Amiens, France

Butylated hydroxytoluene (BHT) is a widely used antioxidant in foods, cosmetics, and drug products. Entire populations are exposed to BHT; but a recent review by Babich (1982) indicates that fewer than 10 studies have determined either the fate or the metabolism of BHT in man.

The pharmacokinetic profile of BHT in laboratory animals is well documented. Dacre (1961) showed that a rabbit dosed orally with BHT excreted about 54% in urine over 4 days. After an intraperitoneal injection of tritiated BHT (Golder et al., 1962) or [^{14}C] BHT (Ladomery et al., 1963) into the rat, a slow and incomplete rate of urinary output was found even after a week. Daniel and Gage (1965) found similar results and also noted a high fecal excretion. After a single oral dose of [^{14}C] BHT, these authors noticed that 80-90% of the administered dose was excreted 4 days later. In females, 40% of the dose was in the urine, versus only 25% in males. An appreciable proportion was excreted in bile, suggesting an extensive enterohepatic recirculation. This hypothesis was confirmed by Ladomery et al. (1967a).

No results were reported concerning the ability of BHT to diffuse through the skin. These studies were designed to provide useful data on the percutaneous absorption of BHT under realistic conditions.

EXPERIMENTAL

Animals

Dunkin Hartley and tricolor (for multiple dosing) guinea pigs of both sexes (400-500 g) were individually housed at 22°C in metabolic cages with urine and

---

*Present affiliation: International Drug Development, Paris, France

feces separators and collectors. Water and guinea pig pellets were given ad libitum.

Radioactive Compounds and Materials

Different formulations were prepared according to the route of administration. All solvents used were of analytical grade or French Pharmacopeia grade.

Intravenous: propylene glycol/ethanol solution (80/20, w/w)
Intramuscular: Labrafil 1980 (glyceryl oleic triesters, ethoxylated) solution
Topical: acetone solution and lipophilic vehicle, Labrafil 1980/Labrafil 2130 (55/45, w/w)

In each case, 5 mg of BHT was administered; the radiochemical dose was 5 μCi per guinea pig. Stock solutions of [^{14}C]BHT were formulated from [^{14}C]BHT (specific activity, 52 mCi/mmol) synthetized by C.E.A. (Saclay, France). Neat BHT was used for isotopic dilution.

Application Techniques

To correct the skin absorption data for incomplete urinary excretion, a parenteral control experiment was performed using intravenous injection.

For topical dosing, the compound was applied to the bald area located behind the guinea pig ear (Zackeim and Langs, 1962). A circular area of 1.5 cm^2 was demarcated behind each ear by pressing a ring against the skin surface. We first applied topically a single dose in acetone or Labrafil solution of [^{14}C]BHT (1.66 mg/cm^2, 5 μCi/guinea pig).

Multiple dosing was then undertaken. Two groups of five guinea pigs were dosed daily for 21 days with 25 μl of Labrafil solution over a 2 × 1.5 cm^2 skin area (1.66 mg/cm^2). On days 1, 8, and 15 the animals were dosed with [^{14}C]-BHT diluted in neat chemical (5 μCi/guinea pig). On the other days, the nonradioactive formulation was applied. Application was at 10 A.M. daily. One hour before dosing the application site of the first group was washed using cotton swab soaked in a soap/water solution (5/45, v/v). The procedure was: soap/water/soap/water/water (2 ml). The skin of the second group wasn't washed.

Analysis

Urine and feces were collected every 24 hr. The radioactivity in 1-ml aliquots of each urine sample was measured in 15-ml Picofluor 30 (Packard Instrumental) with a liquid scintillation septrophotometer (Packard Tricarb) using external standard correction for quenching. Dried feces were homogenized, and specimens (approximately 0.1 g) were combusted in an oxidizer (Kontron Intertechnique

Pharmacokinetics of [^{14}C] BHT in the Guinea Pig

1N 4101). The radioactive carbon dioxide was trapped in Carbomax (Kontron) and counted as described above.

Results were calculated as a percentage of the applied dose for each urine or feces collection using a programmed computer. The total absorption was determined, after correction for incomplete urinary excretion, using the correction factor obtained from the parenteral study; an alternative method involves addition of urine and feces values.

RESULTS

Table 1 shows the total excretion of BHT after intravenous (I.V.), intramuscular (I.M.), oral (P.O.), and percutaneous (cut.) administration. One week after one I.V. administration, only 74.5 ±8.5% of the dose appeared both in urine and feces. The fecal elimination is not negligible, representing 17.4 ±1.7%.

The total ^{14}C recovery after 7 days in feces roughly represents 17.5% of the dose, whatever the administration route might be. This value corresponds to

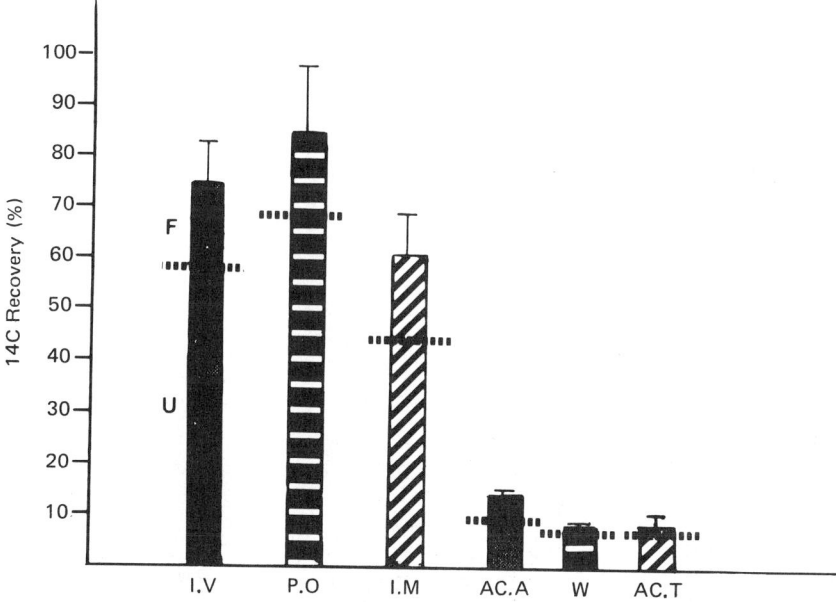

Figure 1 Total ^{14}C recovery (as a percentage of the applied dose) in urine and feces, after administration of BHT by different routes: I.V. = intravenous, I.M. = intramuscular, P.O. = oral, AC.M = percutaneous on albino strain of the acetone solution, W = percutaneous of the Labrafil solution with washing procedure, AC.T = percutaneous on tricolor strain of the acetone solution.

Table 1 ^{14}C Recovery in Urine After Single Parenteral (intravenous and intramuscular) Oral, and Cutaneous Administration[a]

Administration	Excretion rate (%/day)										Total recovery (%)
	Urine							Feces			
	0–1	1–2	2–3	3–4	4–5	5–6	6–7		0–5	5–7	
Intravenous[b] (n = 4)	16.52 (3.72)	15.38 (2.62)	10.01 (1.82)	6.60 (1.58)	5.32 (1.74)		3.29 (1.4)		15.58 (3.32)	1.79 (0.42)	74.49 (8.53)
Intramuscular[c] (n = 4)	20.61 (11.52)	7.79 (1.02)	5.48 (0.72)	3.53 (0.94)	2.2 (0.22)	1.66 (0.26)	1.71 (0.34)		14.84 (4.08)	2.98 (3.8)	60.80 (7.59)
Oral[b] (n = 4)	48.23 (6.64)	11.88 (3.26)	4.50 (0.58)	1.57 (0.66)	0.41 (0.24)	0.43 (0.5)	0.21 (0.24)		17.27 (0.94)	0.51 (0.18)	85.01 (12.60)
Percutaneous[d] (n = 5)	4.39 (0.98)	2.84 (0.4)	0.86 (0.08)	0.45 (0.11)	0.29 (0.04)	0.17 (0.02)	0.09 (0.01)		4.6 (0.64)	0.36 (0.04)	14.05 (0.71)

[a] Mean values ± SD, in parentheses.
[b] Propylene glycol vehicle.
[c] Labrafil vehicle.
[d] Acetone solution.

Table 2 Total Recovery of [^{14}C]BHT Excreted by Rats After Intramuscular and Oral Administration[a]

Adminis-tration	Excretion in urine (%/day)										Total recovery (%)
	0–1	1–2	2–3	3–4	4–5	5–6	6–7	7–8	8–9	9–10	
I.M.											
Female ($n = 5$)	9.01 (1.20)	9.15 (1.49)	9.39 (2.34)	6.34 (1.31)	6.65 (1.31)	4.36 (0.80)	3.65 (0.33)	3.51 (0.37)	2.52 (0.62)	1.62 (0.46)	55.95 (3.16)
Male ($n = 4$)	20.61 (11.52)	7.79 (1.02)	5.48 (0.72)	3.53 (0.94)	2.22 (0.22)	1.66 (0.26)	1.71 (0.34)	1.77 (1.4)	0.89 (0.26)	0.83 (0.26)	46.47 (9.12)
P.O.											
Female ($n = 3$)	60.65 (5.97)	13.51 (4.57)	2.71 (1.26)	0.66 (0.27)	0.25 (0.08)	0.13 (0.03)	0.06 (0.01)	0.04 (0.03)	—	—	78.01 (4.41)
Male ($n = 4$)	48.23 (6.64)	11.88 (3.26)	4.50 (0.58)	1.57 (0.66)	0.41 (0.24)	0.43 (0.5)	0.21 (0.24)	0.14 (0.14)	—	—	67.37 (7.28)

Adminis-tration	Excretion in feces (%/day)							Total recovery (%)
	0–1	1–2	2–3	3–4	4–5	5–6	6–10	
I.M.								
Female	0.67 (0.82)	1.33 (0.35)	1.27 (0.55)	0.65 (0.06)	0.79 (0.13)	0.77 (0.24)	2.16 (0.11)	7.64 (1.51)
Male	3.69 (2.96)		11.15 (3.8)			2.98 (0.7)	2.61 (1.36)	20.46[b] (3.6)
P.O.								
Female		11.46 (5.80)		1.70 (1.55)	0.42 (0.27)	0.18 (0.08)	0.23 (0.01)	13.99 (6.51)
Male		13.70 (8.32)		2.78 (11.68)	0.79 (0.64)	0.29 (0.18)	0.22 (0.16)	17.78 (10.14)

[a]Mean values ± SD in parentheses.
[b]Significance level $p < 0.01$.

Table 3 Percutaneous Absorption of $[^{14}C]$BHT After Single Topical Application in Labrafil Solution[a] to 5 Male Guinea Pigs

Condition	Dose absorbed (%/day)								Total absorbed (%)
	1	2	3	4	5	6	7	8	
No washing	2.25	3.11	1.56	0.57	0.31	0.28	0.23	0.19	8.5
	(0.66)	(0.44)	(0.26)	(0.08)	(0.06)	(0.11)	(0.04)	(0.04)	(1.42)
Washing	2.35	1.95	0.66	0.21	0.12	0.07	0.04	0.03	5.43[b]
	(0.71)	(0.33)	(0.24)	(0.04)	(0.02)	(0.01)	(0.01)	(0.01)	(0.80)

[a]Mean values ± SD in parentheses.
[b]Significance level $p < 0.001$.

Table 4 Percutaneous Absorption of [^{14}C]BHT, Multiple Dosing[a]

Daily dose	Radioactive dose	Dose absorbed (%/day)							Total absorbed (%)
		1	2	3	4	5	6	7	
No washing ($n = 5$)	First	1.57 (0.46)	1.47 (0.53)	0.67 (0.13)	0.3 (0.06)	0.18 (0.04)	0.13 (0.01)	0.12 (0.01)	4.44 (0.89)
	Second	2.76 (0.62)	2.25 (0.24)	1.35 (0.17)	0.80 (0.13)	0.41 (0.04)	0.22 (0.02)	0.09 (0.02)	7.88 (1.67)
	Third	3.05 (0.60)	2.85 (0.57)	1.52 (0.26)	0.69 (0.11)	0.45 (0.11)	0.35 (0.10)	0.16 (0.10)	9.07 (2.40)
Washing ($n = 4$)	First	1.30 (0.2)	1.28 (0.26)	0.48 (0.1)	0.27 (0.12)	0.12 (0.02)	0.08 (0.01)	0.06 (0.1)	3.59 (0.32)
	Second	3.60 (1.12)	2.77 (0.82)	1.38 (0.08)	0.69 (0.26)	0.38 (0.14)	0.21 (0.06)	0.09 (0.02)	9.12 (1.26)
	Third	3.65 (1.12)	3.13 (1.04)	1.66 (0.5)	0.85 (0.28)	0.48 (0.16)	0.32 (0.16)	0.46 (0.14)	10.23 (3.8)

[a]Mean values ± SD in parentheses.

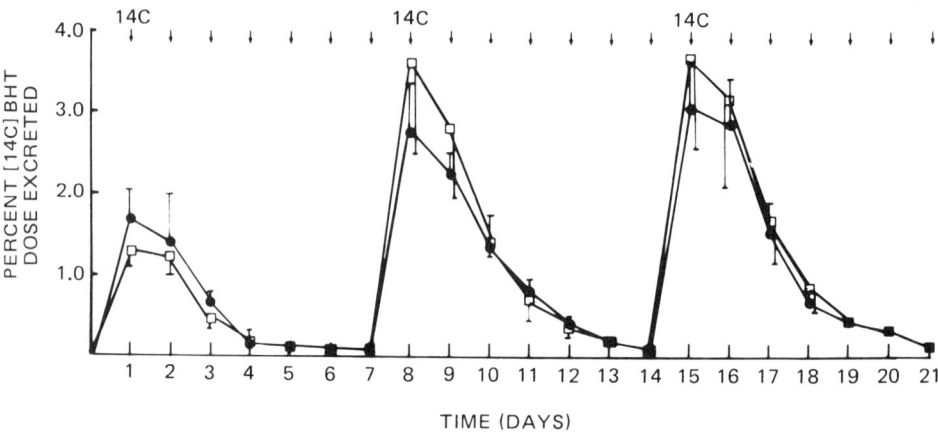

Figure 2 Percutaneous absorption of [^{14}C] BHT after long-term topical application in Labrafil vehicle. Arrows represent application of BHT (1.66 mg/cm^2) and ^{14}C when [^{14}C] BHT was applied. Each point is main value for four or five guinea pigs; bars represent ±SD. □, four guinea pigs washed daily; ●, five guinea pigs unwashed before new application.

21-29% of the total elimination at the end of the experiment (Fig. 1). During the first 24 hr the amount excreted in urine represents 31% (I.V.), 48% (I.M.), 71% (P.O.), and 48% (cut.) out of the total quantity excreted by the kidneys in 7 days. In all cases after 48 hr more than 50% of the total urinary output was recovered in the samples (56% I.V., 66% I.M., 89% P.O., and 79% cut.). The distribution and storage of [^{14}C] BHT were determined in the tissues of the guinea pig. One week after intravenous administration, the highest concentrations of ^{14}C were detected in bile (5.04 ±0.89 μg/g) and body fat (1.31 ±0.22 μg/g); little activity appeared in the brain and heart.

Table 2 reveals a sex difference in the main pathways for the elimination of BHT. Ten days after I.M. injection, males put out as much as 46 ±9% of the dose in urine and 20.5 ±3.6% in feces, whereas females excreted only 7.6 ±1.5% in feces and 56 ±3.2% in urine.

This observation was not confirmed after oral administration. The distribution and storage of the material was determined on the females on the fifteenth day following intramuscular injection. Important amounts of ^{14}C were detected in body fat (1.75 ±0.95 μg/g) and in bile (1.65 ±0.57 μg/g). Low quantities were recovered in liver (0.14 ±0.03 μg/g), kidneys (0.18 ±0.04 μg/g), and heart (0.2 ±0.01 μg/g). Even 37 days after I.M. injection, the urinary excretion determined on one female only was 0.068% of the administrated dose, showing a slow rate of elimination.

Table 5 Statistical Study Using Analysis of Variance[a] on the Urinary Elimination of BHT (and metabolites) According to Administration Route

	Intravenous	Intramuscular	Oral	Cutaneous
Intravenous	–	***	NS	***
Intramuscular	***	–	***	***
Oral	NS	***	–	***
Cutaneous	***	***	***	–

[a]Results: *** = $p < 0.001$, NS = not significant.

Urinary excretion rates following percutaneous administration are given in Table 3. After 8 days, an average of 8.5 ±1.4% of the applied dose was obtained for the unwashed group and 5.43 ±0.8% for the washed group. This difference appeared when the washing procedure was done on the second day. The values were not corrected for incomplete urinary recovery.

Table 4 and Figure 2 give the percutaneous absorption data following multiple BHT administration. In both cases, the total amounts absorbed on days 8 and 15 were greater than those absorbed on day 1. Therefore the percutaneous absorption of BHT increases when applied over the long term, that is, between the first and the second radioactive doses. It appears that the presence of cold BHT after the second radioactive dose has no effect on the excretion of radioactive material from the body.

Table 5 compares statistically elimination for the different groups.

DISCUSSION

BHT ingested by the oral route is well absorbed; we assume an important first-pass effect (previously suggested in man by Wiebe et al., 1978). Indeed 48 ±6.6% were eliminated on the first day after oral administration and 16.5 ±3.7% after intravenous injection. The first-pass effect induces metabolite formation; easily eliminated, this metabolism may occur more slowly with another route of administration.

After I.M. injection the material is slowly eliminated because the product, being lipophilic, is slowly distributed toward the liver and metabolized. Total amounts excreted are not significantly different from those obtained after I.V. injection. Urinary excretion is the main pathway for the elimination of BHT; nonnegligible amounts of the total radioactive are recovered in feces. The quantities in feces are similar for all routes of administration.

The method for ascertaining incomplete urinary excretion using the correction factor obtained from parenteral experiments assumes that urinary excretion constitutes the major metabolic pathway. Accepting this, we may calculate the absolute bioavailability of the percutaneous route from the cumulative urinary excretion or from the bulk cumulative excretion. The excretion correction factor for BHT applied topically is 1.75. The corrected value for percutaneous absorption from the acetone solution is 15.9 ±1.5%. When this value is calculated from the bulk elimination (urine and feces), the absolute bioavailability for this application route is 18.8 ±0.95%.

The importance of fecal excretion suggests a biliary secretion. This observation correlates well to earlier findings (Ladomery et al., 1967b). It is noteworthy that the hepatic metabolism is important (Gilbert and Golberg, 1967; Nakagawa et al., 1979; Shaw and Chen, 1972) and enterohepatic recirculation is possible. After I.M. injection and oral administration, the total amounts excreted in urine were not different for females and males. It is difficult to explain the difference obtained in feces between males and females after I.M. injection. In any event, coprophagia was avoided here. Tye et al. (1965) have shown that in the rat, the amounts excreted after an oral dose were greater in females' urine than males' urine. At the opposite extreme, after a subcutaneous injection the main radioactivity was found in feces. These results are scattered and no conclusion can be made about a sex difference in the main pathways for the elimination of BHT.

The corrected values for percutaneous absorption from Labrafil solution for the unwashed and washed groups respectively, were 14.8 ±2.4 and 9.5 ±1.4%. Those results are significantly different. During the first day, absorption was similar; washing the area produced a decrease in absorption. The total recovery when Labrafil solution was applied was significantly less important than when using an acetone vehicle. The relative bioavailability compared to the acetone vehicle is 59.7 ±17.3%. This is because Labrafil is a lipophilic vehicle and BHT is very soluble in lipids; thus the partition coefficient for BHT favors the vehicle rather than the stratum corneum. On the other hand, acetone solution will, by evaporation, increase the local concentration of BHT and so modify absorption.

The percutaneous penetration of BHT increases after long-term administration. Wester et al. (1980) found a similar increase with long-term application of hydrocortisone. This significant enhancement between the first and the second week (6.6 ±1.3% and 11.8 ±2.5% for the unwashed; 5.3 ±0.4 and 13.6 ±1.9% for the washed group) could be connected to the following conditions:

1. The slow elimination obtained after administration of a single dose
2. A pharmacological action in the skin
3. The possible tendency of multiple applications of the vehicle to modify lag time and diffusion rate

When the dosing interval is shorter than the time required for total elimination, an accumulative curve is obtained that does not increase indefinitely but levels off to a plateau (here, statistically, there is no difference in elimination between the second and the third weeks). After topical administration of BHT, comparison of the amount excreted during the first 24 hr for both groups (single dose and first dose in the multiple procedure) reveals no statistical difference. This result shows the absence of variation in percutaneous absorption between the two strain of guinea pigs (albinos and tricolor). The results obtained after one week's treatment with repeated application were lower than those obtained from a single dose. Adding cold BHT every day may cause an isotopic dilution, which could explain this difference. In contrast with the single dose, removing the BHT by washing the skin area every day did not statistically modify the total absorption.

CONCLUSION

After intravenous, intramuscular, or oral administration, two-thirds of the total radioactivity is eliminated in urine. The release is incomplete after a week; one month after intramuscular injection, the elimination still represented 0.07% of the dose. After percutaneous application, elimination follows the same pathways in the same proportions. Washing the area of application 24 hr after a single application decreases significantly the absorption. After application of multiple doses, the amounts absorbed during the second and the third weeks are greater than during the first week, regardless of whether the skin is washed.

REFERENCES

Babich, H. (1982). BHT: A review. *Environ. Res. 29*: 1-29.
Dacre, J. C. (1961). The metabolism of 3.5-di-*tert*-butyl-4-hydroxytoluene and 3.5-di-*tert*-butyl-4-hydroxybenzoic acid in the rabbit. *Biochem. J. 3*: 405-415.
Daniel, J. W. and Gage, J. C. (1965). The absorption and excretion of BHT in the rat. *Food Cosmet. Toxicol. 3*: 405-415.
Gilbert, D. and Golberg, L. (1967). BHT oxidase: A liver microsomal enzyme induced by treatment of rats with BHT. *Food Cosmet. Toxicol. 5*: 481-490.
Golder, W. S., Ryan, A. J., and Wright, S. E. (1962). The urinary excretion of tritiated butylated hydroxytoluene. *J. Pharm. Pharmacol. 14*: 268-271.
Ladomery, L. G., Ryan, M. J., and Wright, S. E. (1963). The urinary excretion of ^{14}C labeled butylated hydroxytoluene by the rat. *J. Pharm. Pharmacol. 15*: 771-774.
Ladomery, L. G., Ryan, A. J., and Wright, S. E. (1967a). The excretion of [^{14}C] BHT in rat. *J. Pharm. Pharmacol. 19*: 383-387.
Ladomery, L. G., Ryan, A. J., and Wright, S. E. (1967b). The bilary metabolites of BHT in the rat. *J. Pharm. Pharmacol. 19*: 388-394.
Nakagawa, Y., Hiraga, K., and Suga, T. (1979). Biological fate of BHT: Binding

in vitro of BHT to liver microsomes. *Chem. Pharm. Bull.* (Tokyo) *27*: 480–485.

Shaw, Y. S. and Chen, C. (1972). Ring hydroxylation of BHT by rat liver microsomal preparation. *Biochem. J. 128*: 1285–1291.

Tye, R., Engel, J. D., and Rapien, I. (1965). Disposition of BHT in the rat. *Food Cosmet. Toxicol. 3*: 547–551.

Wester, R. C., Noonan, P. K., and Maibach, H. I. (1980). Percutaneous absorption of hydrocortisone increases with long-term administration. *Arch. Dermatol. 116*: 186–188.

Wiebe, L. I., Mercer, J. R., and Ryan, A. J. (1978). Urinary metabolites of [BHT]^{13}C in man. *Drug Metab. Disposition* 6(3): 296–302.

Zackheim, H. S. and Langs, L. (1962). The bald area of the guinea pig. *J. Invest. Dermatol. 38*(6): 347–349.

13
Percutaneous Absorption
Computer Simulation Using Multicompartmented Membrane Models

Joel L. Zatz
Rutgers University College of Pharmacy, Piscataway, New Jersey

Simulation models are simplified representations of real systems, which may be complex. The simulation model can generate data that illustrate typical behavior. It is possible to get an indication of the effect of system variables on the dynamics of a process under study. By performing "experiments" using the model, it is possible to determine whether particular factors are likely to be of major significance to the process. Simulation is thus useful as an adjunct in teaching, in the design of experiments, and in the study of mechanisms underlying experimental results.

Percutaneous absorption studies are usually interpreted in terms of simple diffusional transfer. In many instances, experiments are designed to yield steady-state transport, to which a simple form of Fick's law [Eq. (1)] may be applied (Tregear, 1966).

$$J = \frac{PDC}{h} \tag{1}$$

In this equation, J represents the steady-state flux (amount penetrating per unit area per unit time); P is the barrier membrane/vehicle partition coefficient, which is dimensionless; D is the diffusion coefficient within the membrane, C is the concentration of permeant within the vehicle, and h is the membrane thickness. Experimental conditions must be chosen such that the concentration of permeant in the vehicle does not change during the experiment. Also, diffusion must take place into a chamber of negligible drug concentration (sink conditions). Use of Eq. (1) implies that the rate-limiting membrane is homogeneous and inert, assumptions that are at variance with the known properties of the stratum corneum.

Buerger (1967) criticized the application of Fick's laws to integumental penetration because the skin is an interactive tissue. He treated the barrier membrane as a series of spaces filled with immiscible liquids and assumed that transport from one space to another is a first-order process. He then showed, based on these assumptions and on the further assumption that back transport from the subintegumental tissues was negligible, that the overall transport process must be first order at steady state. Equation (1) has the form of a first-order relationship. Division of the skin into a series of spaces or compartments has been used in the analysis of penetration data. Wallace and Barnett (1978) utilized a simple compartment model to describe methotrexate absorption through hairless mouse skin.

Models similar to those suggested by Buerger have several advantages for simulation. For one thing, it is not necessary to limit conditions to those suitable for steady-state penetration. Of course, under appropriate circumstances, the penetration curves should exhibit steady-state behavior. Permeant concentrations in all spaces may be followed so that membrane concentration profiles can be constructed for any time interval. A variety of easily understood parameters may be manipulated to mimic corresponding changes in actual experiments. Although the models described here are relatively simple, it is possible to add elements to take additional parameters into account.

DESCRIPTION OF THE MODELS

The simulation models utilized represent the stratum corneum, the primary barrier layer of the skin, as a series of connected sections or compartments. In the model shown in Figure 1, stratum corneum has five sections. Each compartment is of equal volume, and transport between them is described by a single first-order rate constant, K. Other elements within this model represent the source of drug (DONOR), the tissues lying beneath the stratum corneum (AQ), and the blood (SINK).

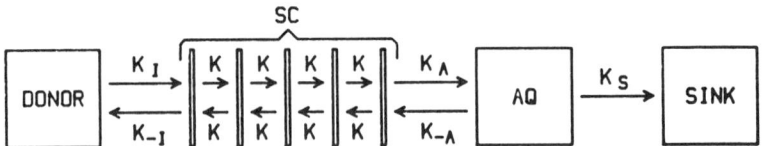

Figure 1 Schematic representation of a multicompartmented membrane model. Standard values for model parameters are listed in Table 1.

The DONOR (or vehicle) compartment contains the drug in solution; both volume and concentration must be specified. Complexities such as dissolution or diffusion rate limited absorption of suspended drugs within the vehicle are not considered, although more complex models could be developed to deal with such situations. The living portion of the epidermis as well as the portion of the dermis separating the stratum corneum from the capillaries are combined into the AQ compartment. These tissues are primarily aqueous. The SINK compartment, which represents the circulation, collects all drug molecules to reach it. Although the circulation is thought of as a perfect sink, this may not be true in all cases (Guy and Maibach, 1983); another compartment can be added to account for uptake by muscle tissue, for example.

All the transfer processes are assumed to be first order. A single rate constant is used to describe all transfers between stratum corneum compartments. This is equivalent to stating that the upper and lower sections of the stratum corneum are identical. Although it is possible to take into account differences in the stratum corneum depending on proximity to the living tissues by assigning different values to the stratum corneum transfer constants, this procedure would unduly complicate things at the present stage of model development.

In assigning transfer rate constants, it is necessary to consider that in the usual situation, transport through the stratum corneum is the rate-limiting step in skin penetration. The value of K should be smaller than that of the other rate constants to ensure that this will be true for the simulations as well. The effect of changing the various rate constants is explored in the next section.

To run a simulation, it is necessary to supply values for the various rate constants and the volumes of the compartments. The initial drug concentration in the donor must also be specified. A numerical integration procedure (McCracken and Dorn, 1964) is used to calculate drug amount in the compartments as a function of time.

SIMULATION STUDIES

Two general types of experimental condition were modeled. The first was the type leading to steady-state penetration after a period of time. Referred to as the "infinite dose" situation (Franz, 1978), it requires sufficient donor to ensure that the amount of drug lost by penetration is too small to change the donor concentration. For modeling purposes, a donor volume of 100 ml/cm^2 was selected. (Donor volumes of 10 or 1 ml led to essentially the same results.)

The second group of experiments utilized a much lower donor volume (0.002 ml) to provide some insight into situations in which the drug concentration within the donor might decrease during the experiment. This "finite dose" arrangement is thought to be more consistent with the conditions found in clinical dermatologic therapy (Franz, 1978). It is not surprising that finite dose

Table 1 Standard Values of Model Parameters

Parameter	Value	
	Infinite dose	Finite dose
Number of stratum corneum compartments	5	5
K	0.4	0.4
V	0.0002	0.0002
K_I	45	45
K_{-I}	1	1
K_A	2	2
K_{-A}	2	2
K_s	2	2
Donor concentration	10	10
Donor volume	100	0.002

systems and infinite dose systems responded somewhat differently to alteration of certain model parameters.

Model Parameters

A standard set of parameters was assigned to facilitate exploration of the characteristics of the models (Table 1). In simulation experiments, the values of one parameter were varied while the other parameter values were maintained constant. A model with five stratum corneum compartments was chosen. More compartments would provide better data on drug distribution within the stratum corneum, but this potential advantage is outweighed by the additional computer time required.

Infinite Dose Systems

Typical penetration curves, illustrating the effect of the value of K on amount penetrated, are shown in Figure 2. The steady-state flux is the single most important experimentally determined result for infinite dose conditions. The lag time, determined by extrapolating the linear portion of the penetration curve back to the time axis, is sometimes used for estimation of the diffusion coefficient.

Using the simulation model, it is possible to calculate drug concentration in various compartments. Concentration profiles within the stratum corneum for one set of model parameters are presented in Figure 3. After 1 hr, the stratum corneum compartment nearest the donor had a relatively high drug concentra-

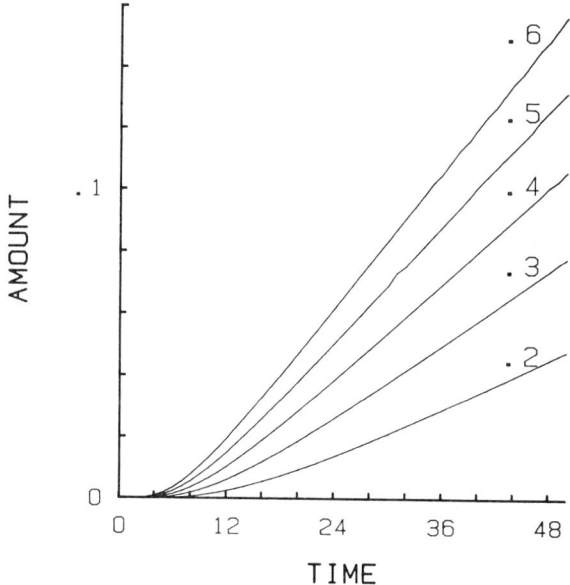

Figure 2 Penetration curves showing the effect of changing the value of K.

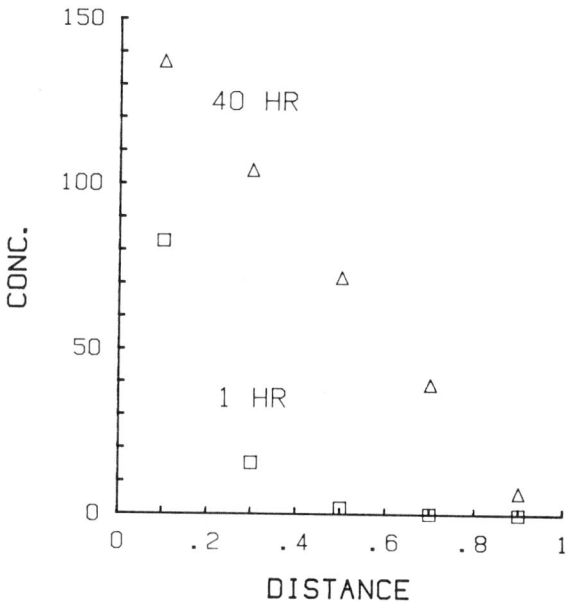

Figure 3 Concentration profiles calculated from stratum corneum (SC) compartment values at two different time periods for infinite dose situation, standard parameter values.

tion, but concentration fell off rapidly with distance from the donor. As time went on, more drug was transferred from the donor and there was further movement into other stratum corneum compartments. After steady state was reached, the concentration profile was essentially linear (see curve for 40 hr in Fig. 3). This result is in agreement with that predicted by the simple diffusional model (Tregear, 1966). Figure 4 shows the same data for 1 hr as a plot of the logarithm of concentration versus distance from the donor. This time the curve is linear. A similar pattern, obtained by stripping layers of the stratum corneum with tape, has been reported (Zesch and Schaefer, 1974).

By varying a single parameter while the others are maintained constant, it is possible to evaluate its effect on penetration characteristics. The effect of variations in the transport rate constant on steady-state flux (obtained from the curves in Fig. 2) is shown in Figure 5. An increase in the value of K results in a nearly proportional increase in steady-state flux.

The ratio of K_I to K_{-I} describes the membrane/donor partitioning tendency of drug molecules. Steady-state flux is proportional to K_I/K_{-I} (Fig. 6). Similarly, steady-state flux is directly proportional to V, the volume of each compartment making up the barrier membrane (Fig. 7).

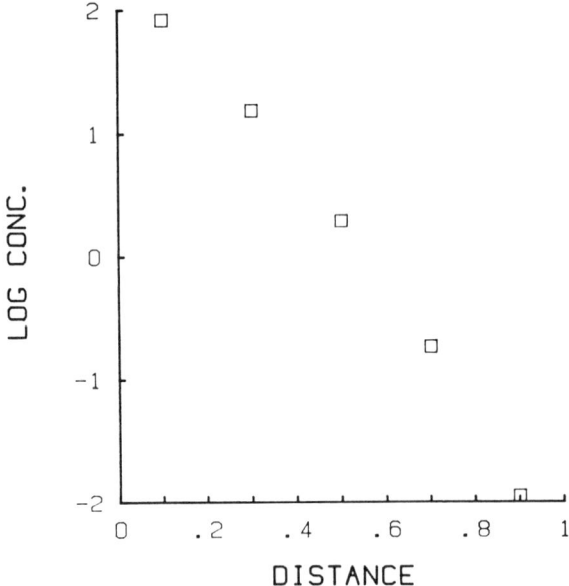

Figure 4 Concentration profile plotted on log scale for values at 1 hr for infinite dose situation, standard parameter values.

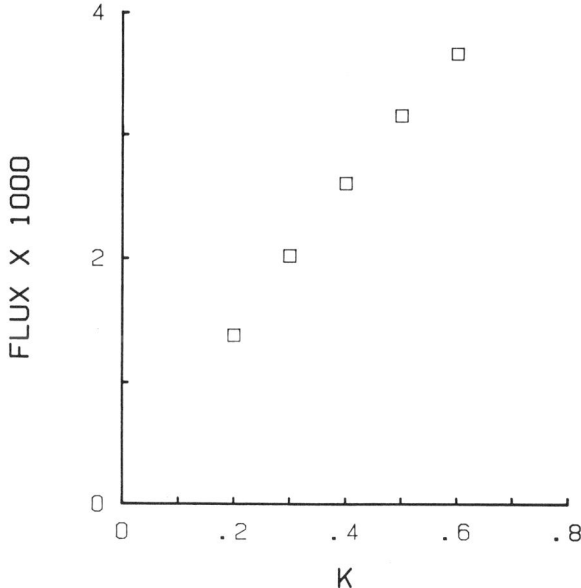

Figure 5 Relation between steady-state flux and value of K.

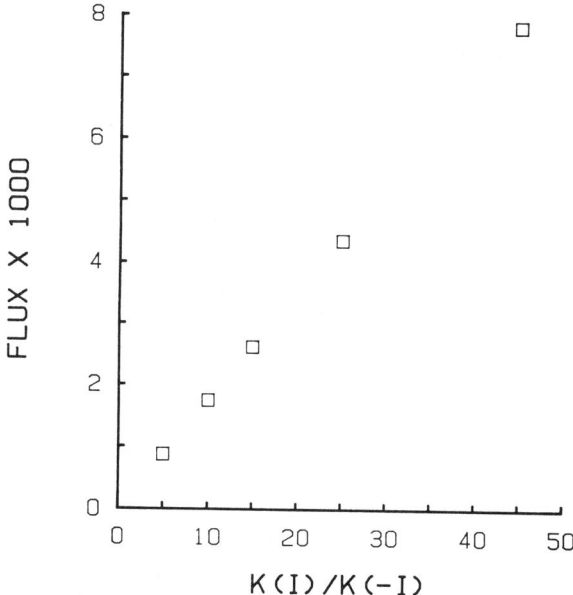

Figure 6 Relation between steady-state flux and value of K_I/K_{-I}.

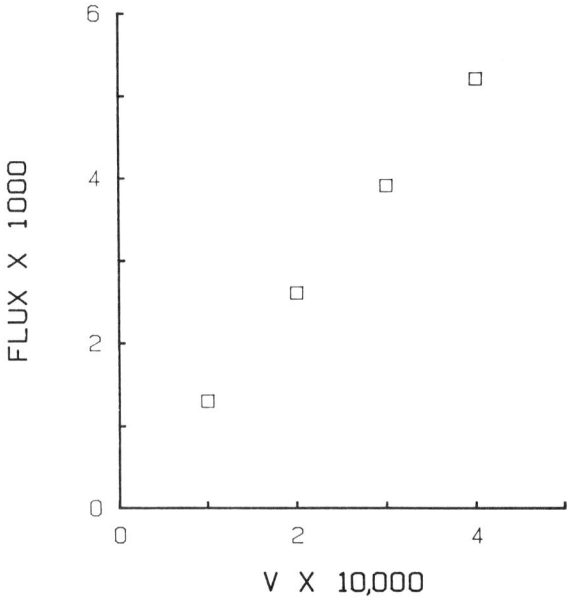

Figure 7 Relation between steady-state flux and value of V.

A change in the number of compartments comprising the stratum corneum is equivalent to utilizing a membrane of greater or lesser thickness but the same construction. Figure 8 shows that an increase in the number of compartments results in a decrease in steady-state flux. In fact, the reciprocal of the flux value is directly proportional to the number of compartments.

Table 2 summarizes the effect of variations in the value of K_A, the rate constant describing transfer from the last barrier membrane compartment into the AQ compartment. Reduction of the value of K_A causes a drop in the steady-state flux and the concentration in the AQ compartment, while the amount of drug retained within the stratum corneum increases. These changes are of relatively small magnitude, considering the rather large range of K_A considered.

The influence of K_s values on flux and drug concentration in the AQ compartment are summarized in Figure 9. Variation in K_s has essentially no effect on the steady-state flux. However, there is a linear correlation between concentration in the AQ compartment and the reciprocal of K_s.

In many ways the multicompartmented membrane models are similar to simple diffusional models. In the latter, the stratum corneum is considered to be an inert, uniform membrane. Under steady-state conditions, Eq. (1) applies. In Eq. (1), the P and C terms describe the concentration gradient across the

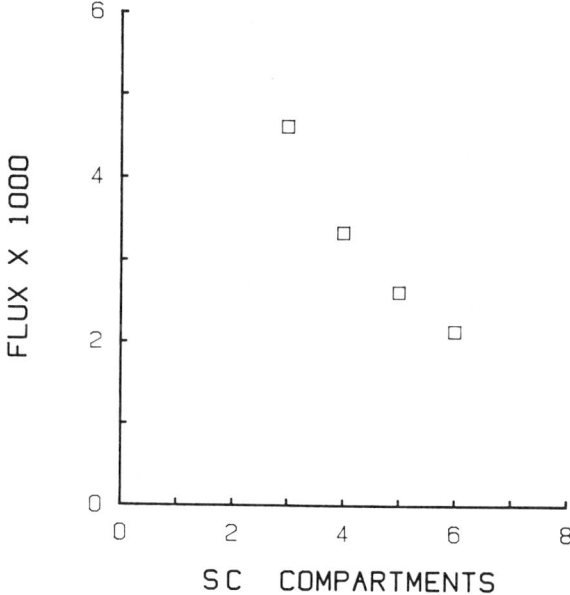

Figure 8 Relation between steady-state flux and the number of stratum corneum (SC) compartments.

membrane. The D and h terms describe the membrane's transport characteristics; membrane resistance may be defined as h/D, with units of hours per centimeter.

In the computer model, K_I/K_{-I} is analogous to P. Membrane resistance is given approximately by N/(VK) divided by area. The units are, again, hours per centimeter. The proportionality of flux to K_I/K_{-I} and K and the inverse proportionality to N are fully in accord with the simple diffusion model. The fact that

Table 2 Effect of K Values on Simulation Results at Steady State

K	Flux	AQ concentration	Amount in stratum corneum
4.0	0.00267	0.0666	0.0700
2.0	0.00261	0.0652	0.0718
1.0	0.00251	0.0624	0.0750
0.5	0.00230	0.0575	0.0808
0.2	0.00185	0.0462	0.0934
0.1	0.00137	0.0342	0.105

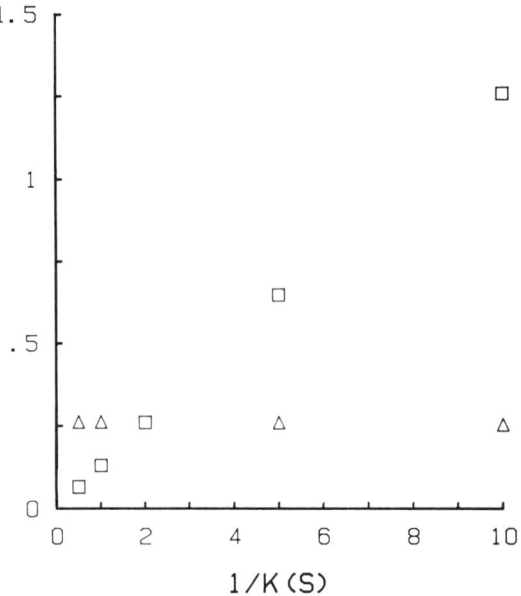

Figure 9 Effect of K_s value on steady-state flux (△) and AQ concentration (□).

flux increases in proportion to V requires some comment. On the face of it, increasing V seems to represent an increase in stratum corneum thickness, which might be expected to cause a lowering in flux. However, transfer between compartments is the actual process determining the overall movement through the membrane; transfer within each stratum corneum compartment is assumed to be instantaneous. In the model, increasing V means that the amount of drug in each compartment must be larger for the concentration to be the same, regardless of the value of V. This results in the increased flux. The permeability of skin is not necessarily related simply to stratum corneum thickness. The poor resistance to permeation of stratum corneum of the palm and sole relative to other locations is well known (Scheuplein and Blank, 1971).

Other parameters, namely K_A and K_s have minor influence on flux as long as they are not set to extremely small values, in which case the rate-limiting step in transport would be moved from the stratum corneum to some other location. However, while K_s does not particularly influence flux, it does exert considerable control over the concentration in the AQ compartment, which represents the skin's viable tissues. The AQ concentration is also a function of the rate of input to that comparement, which is essentially the rate of transport through the skin as a whole. Figure 10 shows the relation between AQ concentration and

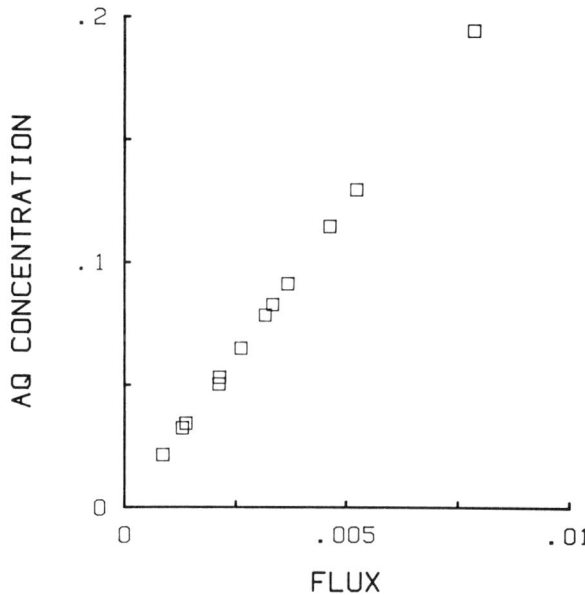

Figure 10   Relation between AQ concentration and steady-state flux.

flux. These values were taken from simulations in which K, K_I/K_{-I}, N, and V were varied. Drug concentration in AQ is thus a function of the factors that control barrier membrane resistance and entry into the barrier as well as the rate of loss to the sink. Model simulations therefore show that a knowledge of flux alone does not enable one to calculate viable tissue concentrations.

Finite Dose Systems

In a finite dose application, a small amount of material is applied to the skin surface. Several differences from infinite dose application are apparent. For one thing, the composition of the donor is kept constant following infinite dose application, so that evaporation does not occur to a significant extent. In the finite dose case, the solution is applied as a thin film from which evaporation can take place. Another difference is in the degree of skin hydration, particularly if the solvent is water. With the small amount of liquid used in finite dose application, and in view of evaporation, the tendency to hydrate the outer stratum corneum is greatly reduced. Hydration affects skin permeability, so that we might expect differences in the effective diffusion coefficient, depending on the mode of application. An important consequence of the deposition of a limited amount of active substance on the skin surface is that the donor concentration may drop as

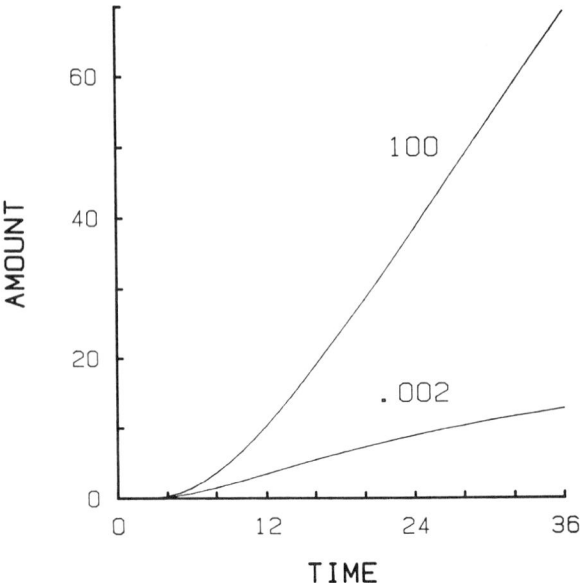

Figure 11 Penetration curves showing the effect of donor volume.

penetration proceeds, while donor concentration is maintained constant under infinite dose conditions.

In these computer experiments, all the rate constants and also the volume of the donor were assumed to remain constant during an experiment. This corresponds to the use of a nonvolatile, nonpenetrating solvent for the donor. Values of model parameters are listed in Table 1.

Figure 11 compares penetration curves generated under infinite dose conditions (donor volume = 100 ml/cm^2) and finite dose conditions (donor volume = 0.002 ml/cm^2). All other model parameters are the same for both situations. Penetration is reduced under finite dose conditions. This is better shown in Figure 12, which plots penetration flux values against time. With infinite dose application, the rate is small at first, then gradually increases to a limiting value. After finite dosing, the pattern for the first few hours is similar. However, instead of approaching a plateau, the flux curve reaches a peak and gradually drops as time goes on. This is due to a continuous reduction in the drug concentration in the donor, which reduces the gradient across the membrane. This loss of drug, which is due to absorption into the membrane as well as penetration through it, causes important differences between the behavior of infinite and finite dose systems.

Figure 13 shows the effect of changes in the value of K on penetration flux. All three curves have the same general shape. However, the curve representing

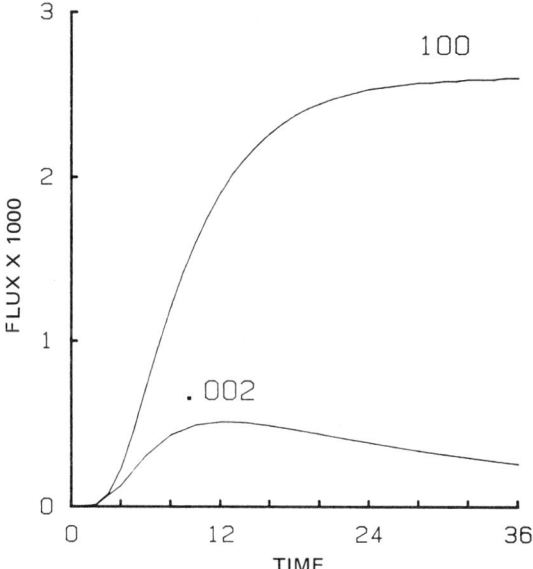

Figure 12 Effect of donor volume on penetration flux.

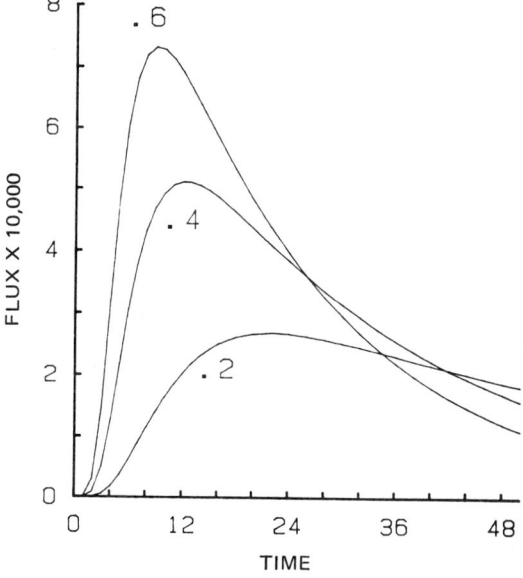

Figure 13 Dependence of penetration flux on value of K in finite dose system.

Table 3 Effect of Variation in K and K_I/K_{-I} on Skin Penetration Under Finite Dose Conditions

K	K_I/K_{-I}	Peak flux $\times 10^4$	Time for peak flux	Donor concentration at $t = 3$
0.4	15	5.11	12	2.83
0.2	15	2.68	22	3.25
0.6	15	7.32	9	2.56
0.4	5	3.57	15	5.78
0.4	45	5.97	11	1.05

the highest transfer coefficient has the highest peak flux value, the earliest peak, and the sharpest peak. As the value of K is reduced, peak values drop and occur later, and the curves become more rounded. Peak flux is approximately proportional to the value of K (Table 3).

The influence of K_I/K_{-I} is shown in Figure 14. Since this ratio is a measure of partitioning, we would anticipate that flux would be positively correlated with it. This is the case; however, the effect is surprisingly small. A three times increase in partitioning results in much less than a three times increase in peak flux. This can be explained by considering that while a high value of K_I/K_{-I} should produce a correspondingly high gradient across the barrier membrane, there is also a significant loss of material from the donor, which is the source of the drug. Because the donor and the first stratum corneum compartment are linked reversibly, there is a tendency toward a pseudoequilibrium distribution in which the actual transmembrane gradient is not as large as would be expected on the basis of the value of the K_I/K_{-I} ratio (see Table 3).

A similar result is found for the effect of V (Fig. 15). The three curves shown in this figure are relatively close together, despite the differences in V. The explanation is the same as for the K_I/K_{-I} situation.

Figure 16 shows how changing the number of stratum corneum compartments influences the flux curves. A reduction in the number of compartments lowers the membrane resistance to transport. Here, the effects are significant.

It seems that depletion of the drug within the donor can be a significant factor in permeation. Changing K_I/K_{-I} or V had a smaller impact on flux than changing K or N, whereas under steady-state conditions all these parameters had equal weight. These results suggest that comparisons made at steady state using infinite dose application may not apply directly to situations in which donor depletion must be taken into account. When making comparisons of formulations, for example, knowledge of the mechanism by which changes in flux are effected is an important consideration in deciding whether extrapolation to non-steady-state conditions may be justified.

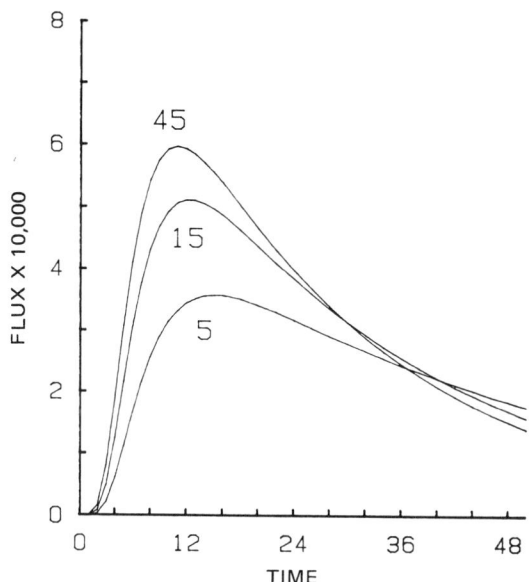

Figure 14 Dependence of penetration flux on value of K_I/K_{-I} in finite dose system.

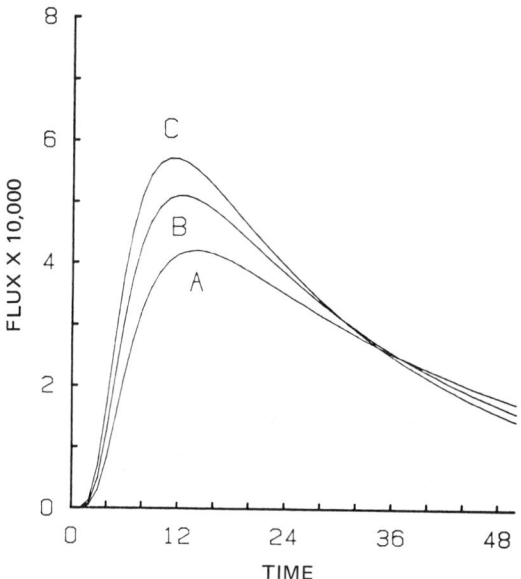

Figure 15 Dependence of penetration flux on value of V in finite dose system: (A) 0.0001 ml, (B) 0.0002 ml, and (C) 0.0004 ml.

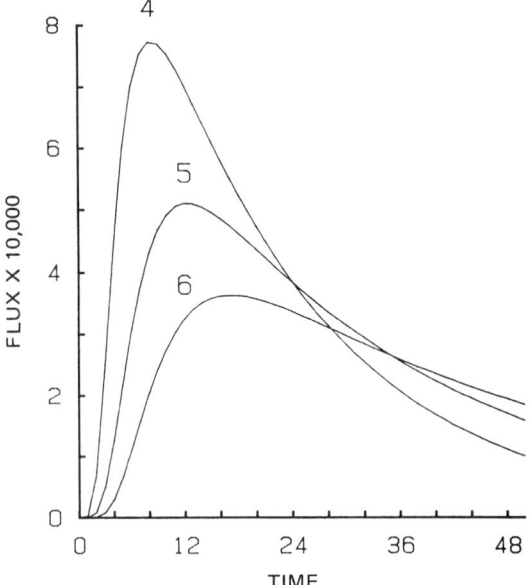

Figure 16 Dependence of penetration flux on number of stratum corneum compartments.

CONCLUSIONS

Simulation experiments with multicompartmented membrane models produce results closely related to a widely accepted diffusional model and to experimental data. An advantage of the new models is that it is possible to study conditions under which the simple form of Fick's law does not apply. By making the donor volume small, finite dose conditions were simulated. Calculated results provide new insight into the factors that may be involved under finite dose conditions.

The models can be made more complex, if necessary, to study other variables. For example, it is possible to introduce tissue binding as one of the model parameters and to study its effect on skin permeation. The versatility of these models and the correspondence of simulation results to laboratory findings suggest that they can function as useful adjuncts in teaching and research.

ACKNOWLEDGMENTS

This work was supported by the Rutgers University Faculty Academic Study Program and by a grant from the Rutgers University Research Council.

REFERENCES

Buerger, A. A. (1967). A theory of integumental penetration. *J. Theor. Biol. 14*: 66-73.

Franz, T. J. (1978). The finite dose technique as a valid in vitro model for the study of percutaneous absorption in man. *Curr. Probl. Dermatol. 7*: 58-68.

Guy, R. H. and Maibach, H. I. (1983). Drug delivery to local subcutaneous structures following topical administration. *J. Pharm. Sci. 72*: 1375-1380.

McCracken, D. D. and Dorn, W. S. (1964). *Numerical Methods and FORTRAN Programming*. Wiley, New York.

Scheuplein, R. J. and Blank, I. H. (1971). Permeability of the skin. *Physiol. Rev. 51*: 702-747.

Tregear, R. T. (1966). *Physical Functions of Skin*. Academic, New York.

Wallace, S. M. and Barnett, G. (1978). Pharmacokinetic analysis of percutaneous absorption: Evidence of parallel penetration pathways for methotrexate. *J. Pharmacokinet. Biopharm. 6*: 315-325.

Zesch, A. and Schaefer, H. (1974). Penetration kinetics of four drugs in the human skin. *Acta Dermatovenereol.* (Stockholm) *54*: 91-98.

14
Influence of Age on Percutaneous Absorption of Drug Substances

Charanjit R. Behl
Hoffmann-LaRoche, Inc., Nutley, New Jersey

Nancy H. Bellantone
Pfizer, Inc., Groton, Connecticut

Gordon L. Flynn
University of Michigan College of Pharmacy, Ann Arbor, Michigan

There are no published reports that describe systematically designed studies to determine how ageing alters chemical penetration through the skin over the entire life span of human or animal. There are several reasons for this deficiency. It is difficult to obtain "normal" human skin specimens for in vitro studies or to have access to human skin for in vivo studies covering desired age groups. Large intersubject and site-to-site variabilities have been experienced. Lack of suitable methods to study percutaneous absorption and difficulties in the interpretation of experimental data have contributed to the problem.

This chapter refers briefly to literature reports on the influence of aging on the in vivo and in vitro aging skin permeabilities of some substances. Greater emphasis is given to recent systematic in vitro studies in hairless mice.

IN VIVO PERCUTANEOUS ABSORPTION STUDIES

The first indication of age-related differences in percutaneous absorption might be traced as early as 1886, when Rayner reported a sudden onset of significant cyanosis in infants, which was attributed to freshly stamped diapers. In cases of this type reported by several other investigators, the poisoning could have been due to absorption through the infant skin (Gottschall and Bunney, 1940; Graubarth et al., 1945; Kagan et al., 1949; Neuland, 1921; Scott et al., 1946; Stevens, 1928; Wiemberg, 1931; Zeligs, 1929). There were more than 60 cases reported. It was suggested in many of these reports that the observed toxicities might be due to the unusually high permeability of infant skin, especially that of preterm infants. Cases of pentachlorophenol poisoning in nurseries for newborn infants have been reported by Robson et al. (1969) and Armstrong et al. (1969).

Clinicopathologic studies in infants who were washed in hexachlorophene and rinsed off by immersing in water revealed substantial brain damage attributed to this agent. The level of the brain damage was about five times higher in babies who were born at 8 months gestational age than in full-term babies (Shuman et al., 1975). Since hexachlorophene has been shown to be absorbed dermally, the systemic availability of the chemical can be a factor in the observed brain damage. This work was followed by similar studies performed in rhesus monkey (Marzulli and Maibach, 1975). The newborn monkeys washed with hexachlorophene developed brain effects, whereas monkeys 4 to 7 years old did not.

Perhaps the first controlled study to assess the effect of age on skin permeability was reported by Nachman and Esterly in 1971. They studied the percutaneous absorption of Neosynephrine·HCl in infants of gestational ages ranging from 28 through 42 weeks. The extent of absorption was determined by measuring the time of blanching. They found that the skins at about 7 months were substantially more permeable than at full term.

Wester et al. (1977) studied the percutaneous absorption of testosterone in newborn and adult rhesus monkeys. They normalized the absorption data with respect to the body weight to account for differences in the systemic accumulations. When accounting for the surface area to body weight differences, the systemic absorption in the newborn was found to be three times that of the adult.

A more recent study (Harpin and Ratter, 1982) has shown that the skins of preterm infants (27 weeks gestational age) can be very susceptible to simple alcohol because of the high skin permeability at this age. Some more direct approaches have been taken by others. Christophers and Kligman (1964) studied the percutaneous absorption of testosterone through the dorsal skins of two age groups, old and young. The method of Malkinson (1958) was used in these studies. A suitable volume of radiolabeled drug in ethylene glycol/monomethyl ether was placed on a 1.8-cm^2 section of the dorsum and the extent of absorption was assessed by monitoring the residual drug in 24 hr. The results (Table 1) indicated rather large intersubject variability in the aged group. The absorption in the young subjects (average age was 24 years) was about 38%, compared to about 13% absorption in the older subjects (average age, 75 years). These results were noted to be in contradiction to their earlier in vitro studies.

Similarly, Malkinson and Ferguson (1955) studied the percutaneous absorption of [^{14}C]hydrocortisone in two age groups, namely, 41 and 58 years. The drug was applied in the form of an ointment (2.5% in petrolatum), and the absorption was assessed by monitoring hydrocortisone appearance in the urine. They found that only 1–2% of the dose was absorbed, and there was no age-related difference in these skin populations. Later, Feinblatt et al. (1966) studied the percutaneous absorption of hydrocortisone in young subjects ranging

Table 1 Percutaneous Absorption of Testosterone

	Young			Aged	
Subject	Age (years)	Percentage absorbed in 24 hr	Subject	Age (years)	Percentage absorbed in 24 hr
1	22	30.4	1	76	10.0
2	26	62.9	2	76	11.8
3	22	50.1	3	71	13.2
4	23	33.2	4	82	14.7
5	26	38.2	5	76	1.1
6	27	26.8	6	71	22.7
7	26	44.1	7	80	7.0
8	19	40.5	8	75	12.1
9	22	35.8	9	72	8.0
10	30	17.1	10	72	25.2
Average ± SD.	24 ±3	37.9 ±12.7		75 ±4	12.6 ±7.1

Source: Christophers and Kligman (1964).

from 2 to 22 months. The ^{14}Carbon-labeled drug was applied in the form of a 1% water-soluble cream. Their results indicated about 22% absorption, as estimated from the urine samples. Although the two studies were carried out about a decade apart with different methodologies, the results were revealing. There is a strong indication that the skin of infants is more permeable than that of adults. Similar interpretations can be implicated in other case reports, which have suggested that topical corticosteroids are more dangerous to use on children than in adults (Benson and Pharoah, 1960; Fanconi, 1962; Feiwel et al., 1969; Munro, 1976).

Studies by Wildnauer and Kennedy (1970) indicated a slower transepidermal water loss in newborns than in adults (Table 2). A similar observation has been reported by Kligman (1979), who studied the rate of transepidermal water loss in young (19-26 years old) and in old (66-81 years old) subjects using the lateral leg and the dorsal forearm sites (Table 2). The rate was found to be about 2.5 times higher in the leg site of old subjects compared to the young subjects. A reverse trend was observed in the case of the forearm site. These results do not provide a clear age dependence of water permeability through the skin, but they do show that differences exist. Hammarlund and Sedin (1979) determined the transepidermal water loss in newborn infants and related it with the gestational

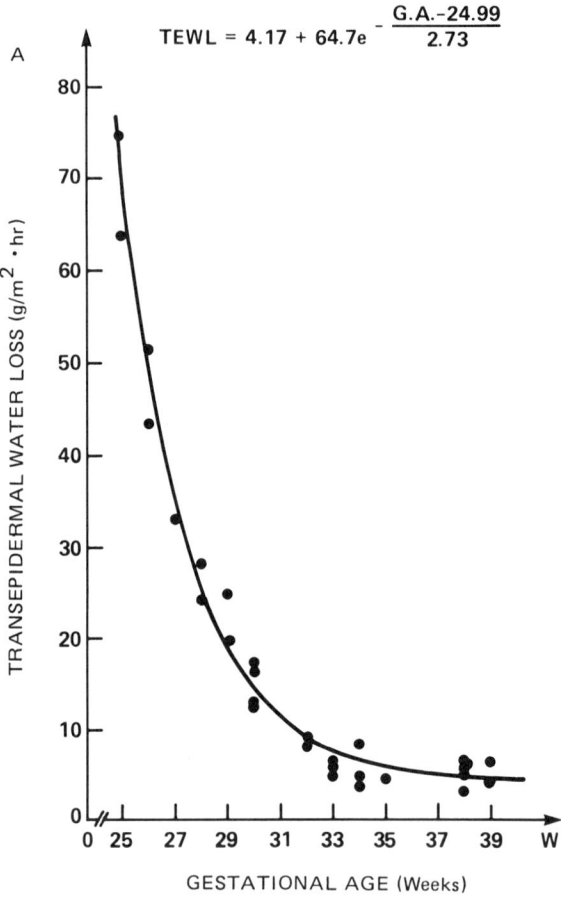

Figure 1 (A)Transepidermal water loss (TEWL) as a function of gestation age (G.A.); W = completed weeks of gestation. (From Hammarlund and Sedin, 1979.) Plot of excised rat skin permeability to 5% triethyl phosphate as a function of age. (From Tregear, 1966.)

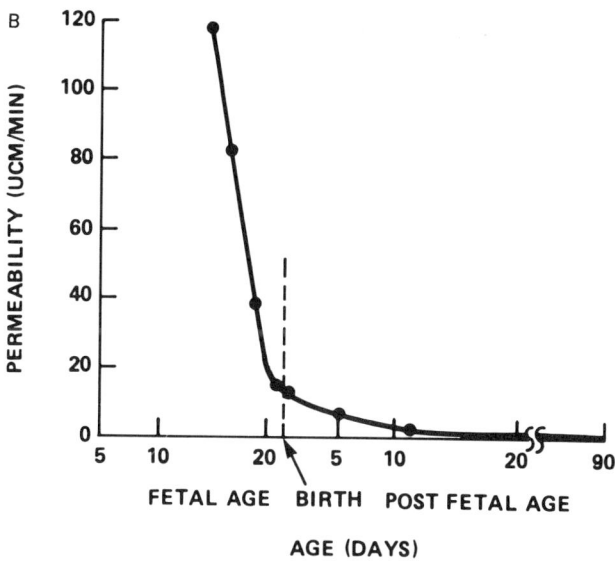

Table 2 Transepidermal Water Loss Data

Age	Site	Water loss (mg/cm² /hr ± SD)
Newborn[a]	Upper back	0.18 ± 0.06
Newborn[a]	Rump	0.17 ± 0.04
Adult[a]	Upper back	0.27 ± 0.04
19-26 yr[b]	Leg (lateral)	0.05 ± 0.03
	Forearm (dorsal)	0.16 ± 0.06
66-81 yr[b]	Leg (lateral)	0.12 ± 0.06
	Forearm (dorsal)	0.10 ± 0.03

[a] Data of Wildnauer and Kennedy (1970).
[b] Data of Kligman (1979).

age. They found that between 25 and 39 weeks of gestational age, the rate of transepidermal water loss declined exponentially with gestational age (Fig. 1A). Actually one should be careful in using the measurement of transepidermal water loss as a criterion to determine the effect of aging on the skin permeability unless other factors such as age-altered eccrine activity, which plays an important role in the loss of water, are ruled out.

Behavior similar to that observed for water has been seen in the emission rates of carbon dioxide in newborns and adults. Wilson and Maibach (1982) found that the rate of carbon dioxide emission was not different from the back and forearm skins of neonates and adults. Since carbon dioxide loss can also be affected by sweating, it may also be inappropriate to reflect aging influences on the skin permeability to other chemicals unless sweating is absent.

IN VITRO SKIN PERMEATION STUDIES

General

The major resistance to skin permeation resides in the stratum corneum (Marzulli, 1962; Marzulli and Tregear, 1961). The stratum corneum maintains its characteristic barrier properties after it is fully formed from the underlying epidermal cells. This is true despite the fact that the horny layer continuously undergoes the process of turnover. The stratum corneum is composed of biologically dead and keratinized cells, which undergo little change upon isolation from the body. Therefore, the in vitro and in vivo permeation rates should be of the same order of magnitude under comparable circumstances (Ainsworth, 1960). According to Christophers and Kligman (1964), once having crossed the horny layer barrier, a permeant finds no important obstacle to its inward diffusion to the circulation through the epidermis, basement membrane, and superficial dermis. Therefore, penetration in vitro may be a valid measurement of the permeability characteristics of the horny layer in vivo. While this has been accepted as true for most part, the issue of in vitro/in vivo correlation needs further investigation. Studies are presently underway to examine this aspect in detail, using test permeants and hairless mouse and fuzzy rat as the model systems (Behl et al., 1981a, 1983a-c).

Using excised skin samples, Marzulli determined the steady-state penetration rates of tri-n-propyl phosphate (TNPP) through various anatomical sites of humans of ages ranging from 3 through 57 years. While the sample size was too small to draw any firm quantitative conclusions, the data showed a general trend of decreasing skin permeability with increasing age. For example, the average penetration rates per minute in 57-year-old, full-thickness skin (regardless of the anatomical site) and in 3-year-old skin are 1.6 and 3.9 $\mu g/cm^2$ respectively (Table 3). Table 3 shows that the sectioned skins are generally more permeable than the intact skins.

Table 3 Steady-State Rates of Penetration of Tri-n-propyl Phosphate Through Skin and Its Components at 10–20 hr After Application of 2 mg to 0.2 cm^2 Surface

Age (years)	Site	Penetration rates (μg/cm^2/min)				
		Full skin	Stripped skin	Dermis	Epidermis	Stratum corneum conjunctum
3	Chest, midline	4.70	2.41	4.30	2.13	0.83
3	Chest, side	3.15	2.80	3.62	0.60	1.90
Adult	Chest, side	0.30	1.50	1.80	0.27	0.40
Adult	Chest, side	1.83	2.84	2.57	0.41	0.37
34	Chest, midline	3.50	4.04	5.15	4.01	0.70
57	Leg above ankle (outer)	0.98	3.55	2.43	0.89	1.40
57	Leg above ankle (inner)	2.40	3.85	3.25	0.90	0.65
57	Foot, dorsum	0.91	2.49	4.05	0.18	0.78
57	Ankle, inner	1.70	1.82	3.82	0.30	0.47
57	Abdomen, midline	2.15	1.64	3.45	0.23	0.50
	Mean rates:	2.16	2.69	3.44	0.99	0.80

Source: Marzulli (1962).

The effect of two age groups, young and aged, on the permeation of water through the skin was investigated by Christophers and Kligman (1964). They used diffusion chambers and procedures similar to those used by Blank (1952). Briefly, the epidermis was sealed over water in diffusion chambers and was maintained at 37°C in a desiccator. The water permeation was determined by the daily weight loss of the chambers over 6 days. The observed average permeation rates for the aged and young skin, respectively, are 0.74 and 0.80 mg/hr·cm^2 for the young skin, indicating a lack of aging effect on in vitro water transport (Table 4). Lack of definite correlation between in vivo transdermal water loss and age was reported by Wildnauer and Kennedy (1970). This reaffirms the statement made earlier in this chapter that perhaps the permeability of the skin to water is not totally reflective to age-related permeability differences.

By using modified diffusion apparatus (two-compartment permeation cell), Christophers and Kligman (1964) extended their efforts to the study of sodium fluorescein permeation as a function of age. The results indicate that aged skin is

Table 4 Transepidermal Water Loss Data

	Aged			Young	
Subject	Age (years)	Water loss (mg/hr·cm^2)	Subject	Age (years)	Water loss (mg/hr·cm^2)
1	77	0.67	1	22	0.82
2	74	0.76	2	28	1.05
3	73	0.59	3	23	0.60
4	73	0.62	4	27	0.83
5	69	1.63	5	26	1.03
6	68	0.50	6	24	0.68
7	68	1.07	7	25	0.90
8	75	0.40	8	22	0.47
9	76	0.51	9	25	0.81
10	82	0.73	10	21	0.79
11	74	0.77	11	23	1.00
12	75	0.59			
Average ± SD:	74 ±4	0.74 ±0.33		24 ±2	0.82 ±0.18

Source: Christophers and Kligman (1964).

about seven times more permeable than young skin (Table 5). The data show a high degree of variability for the aged skin, an observation consistent with the fact that the aged skins are more variable in their histologic characteristics. These data and the in vitro/in vivo water permeation data suggest that permeation through the skin of water and chemicals may not follow identical mechanisms.

Permeation of some test compounds (ethanol, benzyl alcohol, decanol, and cetyl alcohol) through neonatal and adult skins was studied by McCormack et al. (1982). The neonatal skins were noted to be more permeable than either the full-term or the adult skins. When the studies were repeated with fatty acids (e.g., caprylic, oleic, stearic, and lauric), the data did not reveal age-related differences. The available information in these reports is insufficient to define the reasons behind this different behavior.

Tregear (1966) carried out an interesting study of the skin permeability of triethyl phosphate using excised skin samples of rats ranging in age from several weeks preterm to about 3 months (postnatal). As shown in Figure 1B, the permeability sharply falls from about 15 days of fetal age to birth, then drops more gradually up to about 3 months after birth. These results can be compared with those of Hammarlund and Sedin (1979) (Fig. 1A). Although the two

Table 5 In Vitro Penetration of Sodium Fluorescein

	Young			Aged	
Subject	Age (years)	Penetration ($\mu g/hr \cdot cm^2$)	Subject	Age (years)	Penetration ($\mu g/hr \cdot cm^2$)
1	29	1.17	1	72	7.3
2	24	1.10	2	69	10.3
3	26	0.23	3	70	22.1
4	25	0.88	4	68	6.3
5	26	1.76	5	72	3.9
6	24	0.68	6	71	3.8
7	21	0.82	7	67	1.1
			8	78	1.9
			9	74	4.4
Average ± SD:	25 ±2	0.95 ±0.47		71 ±3	6.79 ±6.39

Source: Christophers and Kligman (1964).

studies are not identical, the similarity in the initial rapid declines in the rate of transepidermal water loss in human (Fig. 1A) and the in vitro skin permeability of rat fetus (Fig. 1B) cannot be overlooked. The associated implication of in vitro/in vivo correlation is a significant observation in reaffirming the reliability of in vitro skin permeation data.

Skin Permeation Studies Using the Hairless Mouse

The permeability characteristics of the skin of the hairless mouse skin to *n*-alkanols (Behl et al., 1980b; Durrheim et al., 1981; Flynn et al., 1981) are comparable to those of the human skin (Scheuplein and Blank, 1971). Both skins offer *three* major mechanisms for the in vitro permeation of *n*-alkanols. These include (1) an aqueous pore-type pathway, which may occur through the appendages or microchannels in the stratum corneum (region I of Fig. 2), (2) partitioning through the lipoidal components of the stratum corneum (region II of Fig. 2), and (3) diffusion through the aqueous strata, viable epidermis, and dermis (region III of Fig. 2). On a relative scale, polar, moderately nonpolar, and nonpolar solutes follow regions I, II, and III, respectively (Behl, 1979).

Recent studies were carried out to investigate the influence of age on the in vitro permeability of test compounds water, methanol, ethanol, butanol, hexanol, and octanol through the abdominal and the dorsal skins of male and female hairless mice (Behl, 1983d, 1984). The homologous series of alcohols was

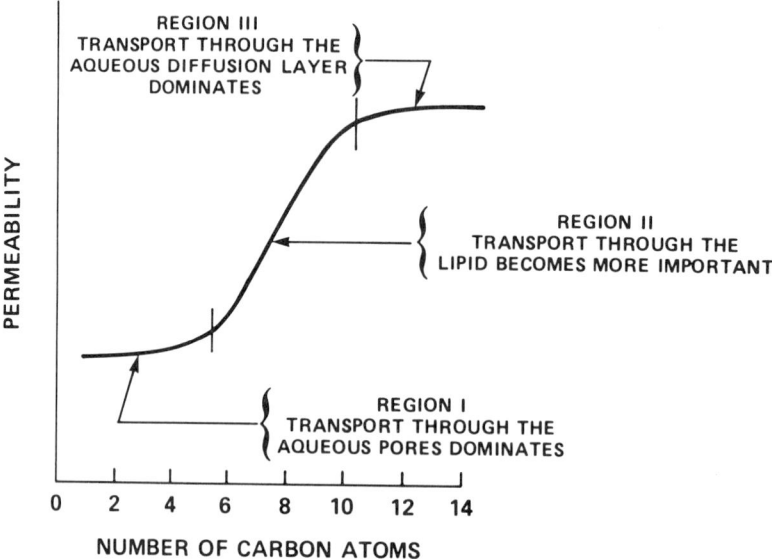

Figure 2 Schematic representation of biological membrane permeability as a function of the alkyl chain length of n-alkanols. (From Behl, 1979.)

chosen because these simple, straight-chain neutral molecules represent an approximate 100-fold spread in lipophilicity. The hairless mouse was selected as the animal model because its skin permeability characteristics appear similar to those of the human skin, it is readily available, and its whole life span is relatively short (about 1.5 years). The methods used were those reported earlier (Behl et al., 1980b; Durheim et al., 1981). Briefly, the skin samples were excised from the abdominal or dorsal sites of freshly sacrificed animals and were sandwiched between the cell halves of the two-compartment permeation cells. The permeation was studied from saline solution (0.9% NaCl) at 37°C by monitoring the permeant concentration in the receiving chamber as a function of time. Permeability coefficients were calculated from steady-state fluxes.

Anatomical and Histological Changes in the
Hairless Mouse with Age

Visual and histological changes as a function of age can be of great value in explaining the age-permeation data. Such properties of laboratory animals have been extensively studied (Brooke, 1926; Chase and Montagna, 1951; Chase et al., 1953; Crew and Mirskaia, 1931; David, 1932, 1934; Dry, 1926; Mann, 1971; Mann and Straik, 1961; Montagna et al., 1952; Orwin et al., 1967; Wolbach, 1951; Yun and Montagna, 1961). At birth the mice are glabrous, but the follicular appendages rapidly develop. The skin is taut, smooth, pinkish, and delicate, characteristics also seen in the skin of the newborn human. The skin of the mouse is rapidly covered with a dense white fur by about 2 weeks of age. Except for the human scalp, this is an obvious and exaggerated departure from the development of the human integument. Starting in the third week the animal begins to lose hair caudally and by the beginning of the fourth week, it appears fully hairless. Before this hair loss begins, the hairless mouse is visually indistinguishable from strains such as the Swiss mouse.

Young adult hairless mice have smooth, pinkish skins, with a visual resemblance to the skin of the human preadolescent. Histologically this mouse skin is punctuated with cystic follicular appendages. These cysts become more prominent and more numerous with further aging. Usually, there is a sparse distribution of prominent hairs, most notably about 2 months after birth, which represents a highly incomplete secondary cycle of hair. Of great importance, the gross anatomical construction of the hairless mouse skin past the initial hair cycle is similar to the human skin (hairy regions excluded) in aspects that relate to the skin's chemical barrier properties. Specifically, there is follicular presence but no prominent hair. Exact dimensions aside, the compositions of the epidermises are similar; each is overlayered by tightly compacted layers of horny cells. Even the kinetics of turnover of the epidermises are similar if viewed in proportion to the masses of the respective tissues. Furthermore, blemishing, wrinkling, and textural changes occur with aging in both hairless mouse and man, albeit the root causes may be substantially different. In the mouse skin the increasingly stippled appearance of the skin during aging is the result of increased prominence of the follicular cysts. In addition, the animal's weight increases to an asymptote of 36-38 g at about the age of 140 days, approximately one third to one fourth of the mean animal life span. When put in terms of fractional age, even attainment of full adult size and weight is comparable to the human.

Skin Thickness Versus Age and Hair Cycle

In some cases the follicular cycles have been related to changes in the dimensions of the skin. For instance, Chase et al. (1953) reported precise data on thickness of the whole skin and the skin's individual strata (epidermis, dermis, and adipose layers) during the first hair cycle of the Swiss mouse. The overall skin thickness expands to its maximum during the anagen phase of follicle growth, there is contraction during the catagen phase, and a minimum is reached in skin width during the telogen phase. The decrease in full skin thickness during the telogen phase is concurrent with thickening of the epidermis.

The general development of hairless mouse skin in terms of its full thickness during the early hair cycle is substantially the same as reported by Chase et al. (1953) for the Swiss strain. The skin thickness of the abdominal and the dorsal skins of hairless mice was measured over the first year of age. An excised piece

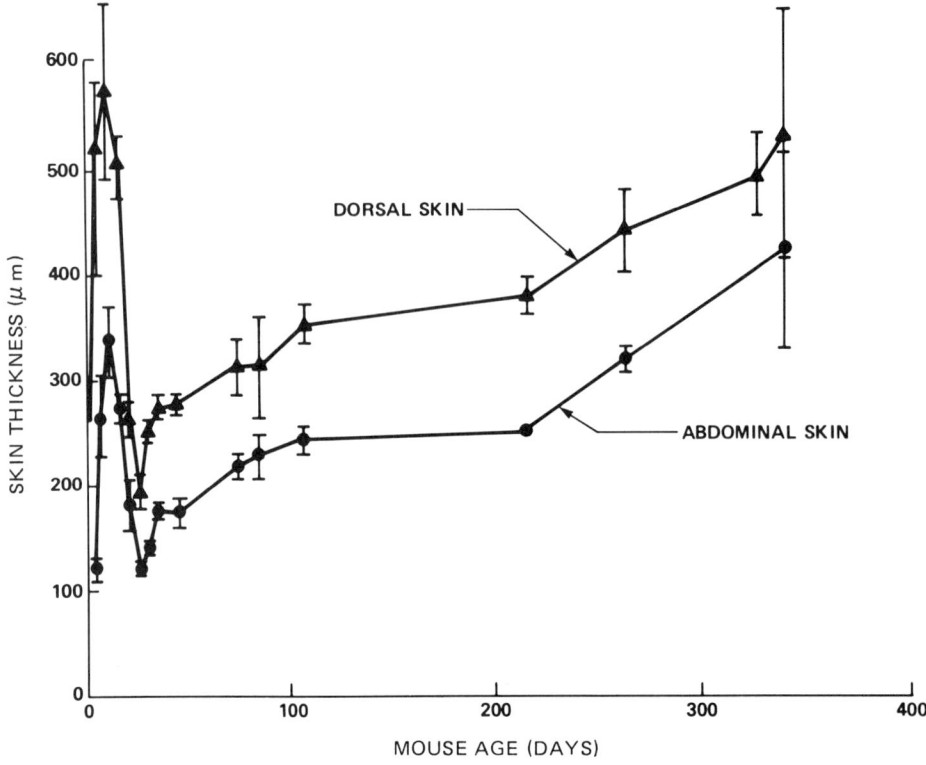

Figure 3 Plots of average skin thickness of male hairless mouse as a function of age. (From Behl et al., 1983d.)

of skin several square centimeters in area was sandwiched between glass microscope slides. Using a micrometer, the thickness of the sandwich was measured with and without skin, the difference being the net thickness of the skin. The measurements were made in triplicate and were found to be unaffected by varying pressure of the micrometer on the glass plates.

The data displayed in Figure 3 show the dorsal skin thickness to be greater than that of the abdomen at all ages. However, the complex patterns of change in thickness over the age span are qualitatively the same between the two sites. There are marked increases in thickness associated with the development of hair, approximately extending to 10 days. Loss of hair and atrophy of the follicles is accompanied by a sharp decline in skin thickness. The thickness reaches a minimum value for either site by the twenty-fifth day of age, which occurs approximately when the mouse becomes hairless. Past this age the skin systematically thickens, a process that is relatively rapid up to 45 days and gradual thereafter.

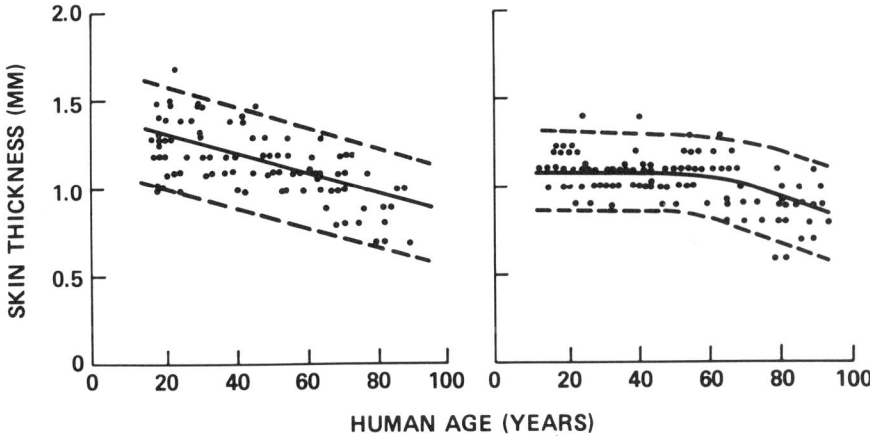

Figure 4 Plots of human skin thickness as a function of age. (From Shuster et al., 1975.)

This measured thickening may be due to the continued development of the follicular cysts, which form layers beneath the skin surface. These profiles of age versus thickness are in contradiction to what is known in the human skin. Human skin may thin with age (Black, 1969; Meema et al., 1964; Montagna et al., 1952; Shuster et al., 1975). The results of one such study are shown in Figure 4.

The data reported in Figure 3 are the thicknesses of the whole skins. The individual stratum thicknesses were not measured. Since the thicknesses of the epidermis of adult hairless mouse is about 40 μm (Yu, 1978), it can be safely assumed that the variations in thickness of the whole skin are far too large to be strictly epidermal in origin and must therefore represent changes occurring in the dermal layer. This is in agreement with the observations made by Chase and Montagna (1951).

Permeability Versus Age

Figure 5 contains age-permeability profiles for water, methanol, ethanol, butanol, hexanol, and octanol. All these plots show a general pattern. The skin permeability increases to reach a maximum value around 25 days, declines rather sharply up to about 60 days of age, and remains more or less invariant thereafter. During the hair cycle, there seems to be a three- to fivefold change in the permeability coefficients. For all these compounds, the dorsal skins are more permeable than the abdominal skins. It is important to note that the dorsal skins are more permeable only up to about 60 days, and the two sites' permeabilities converge thereafter. Octanol data show exception to this observation in that permeation rates for octanol are about the same through either site throughout the ages

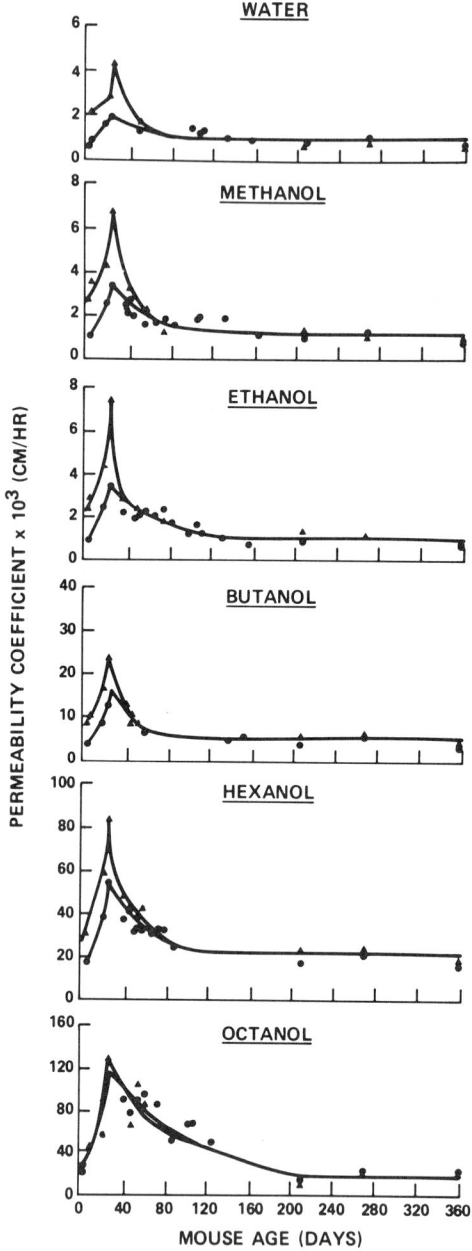

Figure 5 Plots of permeability coefficients of male hairless mouse skin as a function of age: ▲, dorsal skin; ●, abdominal skin. (From Behl et al., 1983d.)

studied. Note that the dorsal skins are consistently thicker than the abdominal skins (Fig. 3). These results are understandable, since for water and polar alkanols the rate-controlling mechanism has been shown to be permeation through the stratum corneum (Flynn et al., 1980; Behl, et al., 1980b; Meyer et al., 1981).

In separate studies the effects of aging on the permeabilities of hairless mouse skin to hydrocortisone and phenol were investigated (Behl et al., 1983e,f). The observed age-permeability profiles are qualitatively similar to those of water and n-alkanols (Figs. 6 and 7). This shows the usefulness of using test permeants in studying the factors that affect percutaneous absorption.

Alkyl Chain Length Influences Versus Age

The permeability coefficients are plotted semilogarithmically as a function of the alkyl chain length for ages 4, 5, 20, 25, 53, 210, 270, and 360 days (Fig. 8). These plots demonstrate a sigmoidal shape showing the three regions discussed earlier (Fig. 2), namely, the lower plateau, the exponentially increasing middle region, and the second plateau. The data for the two sites are qualitatively comparable. The middle exponentially linear portion is due to the alkyl chain length

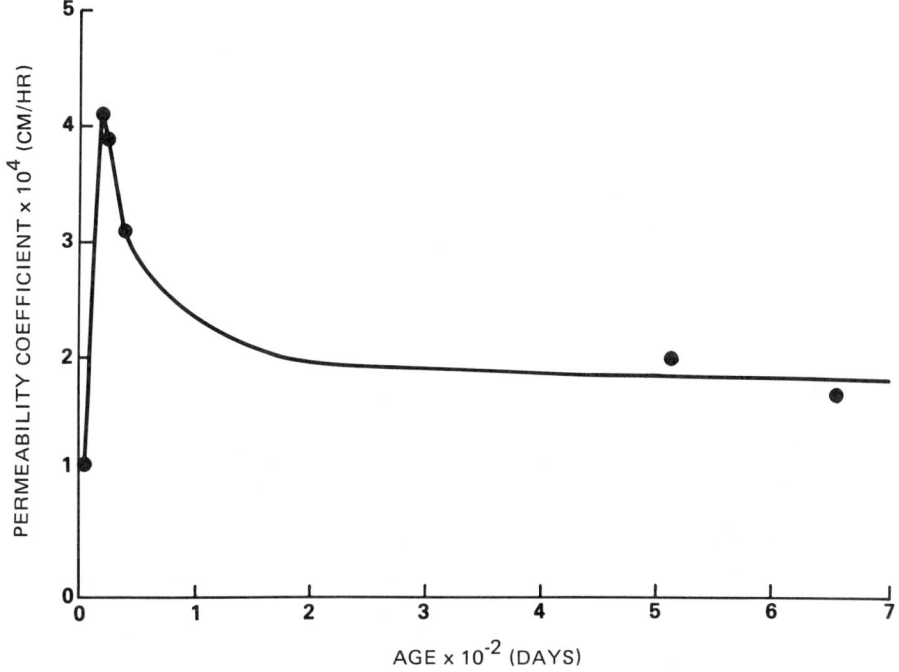

Figure 6 Plot of permeability coefficients of tritiated hydrocortisone through male hairless mouse skin as a function of age. (From Behl et al., 1983e.)

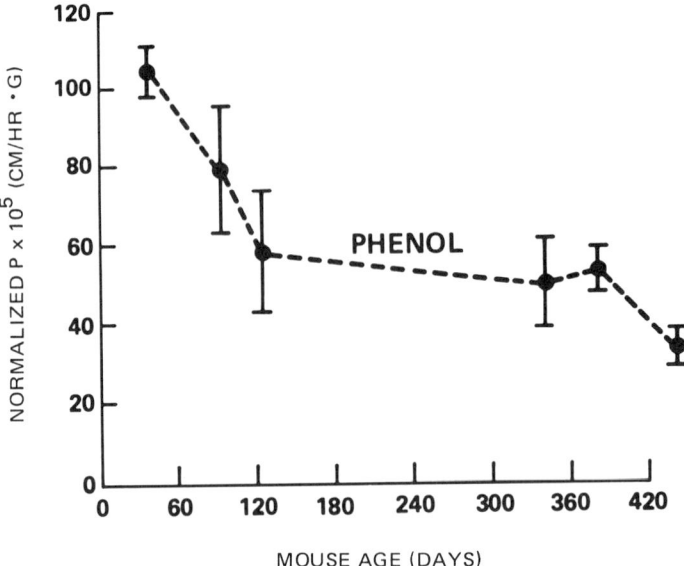

Figure 7 Plot of normalized permeability coefficients P of phenol through male hairless mouse skin as a function of age. (From Behl et al., 1983f.)

partitioning dependency of the permeability coefficients. The slope of this portion is called methylene group sensitivity and is designated as π. The π values were determined and are plotted as a function of age separately for the abdominal and the dorsal sites (Fig. 9). The π values are constant between the ages of 53 and 360 days, indicating that the alkyl chain length sensitivities and the underlying transport mechanisms for these ages are uniform. However, there appears to be a slight irregularity in the π values during the hair cycle, with a minimum value observed at 25 days. Recall that the permeability versus age profiles indicated a maximum value at 25 days (Fig. 5), the skin thickness versus age profile had shown a minimum at the same age (Fig. 3), and the animals were observed to become fully hairless around 25 days of age. All the available anatomical and histological observations indicate that the hairless mouse skin contains a maximum number of fully developed and active hair follicles around the age of 25 days. In view of all this information it is difficult not to attach at least some significance to the possibility that the contribution of the transfollicular pathway varies with age during the hair cycle and may be partly responsible for the observed minimum in the π versus age plot.

Influence of Age on Percutaneous Absorption

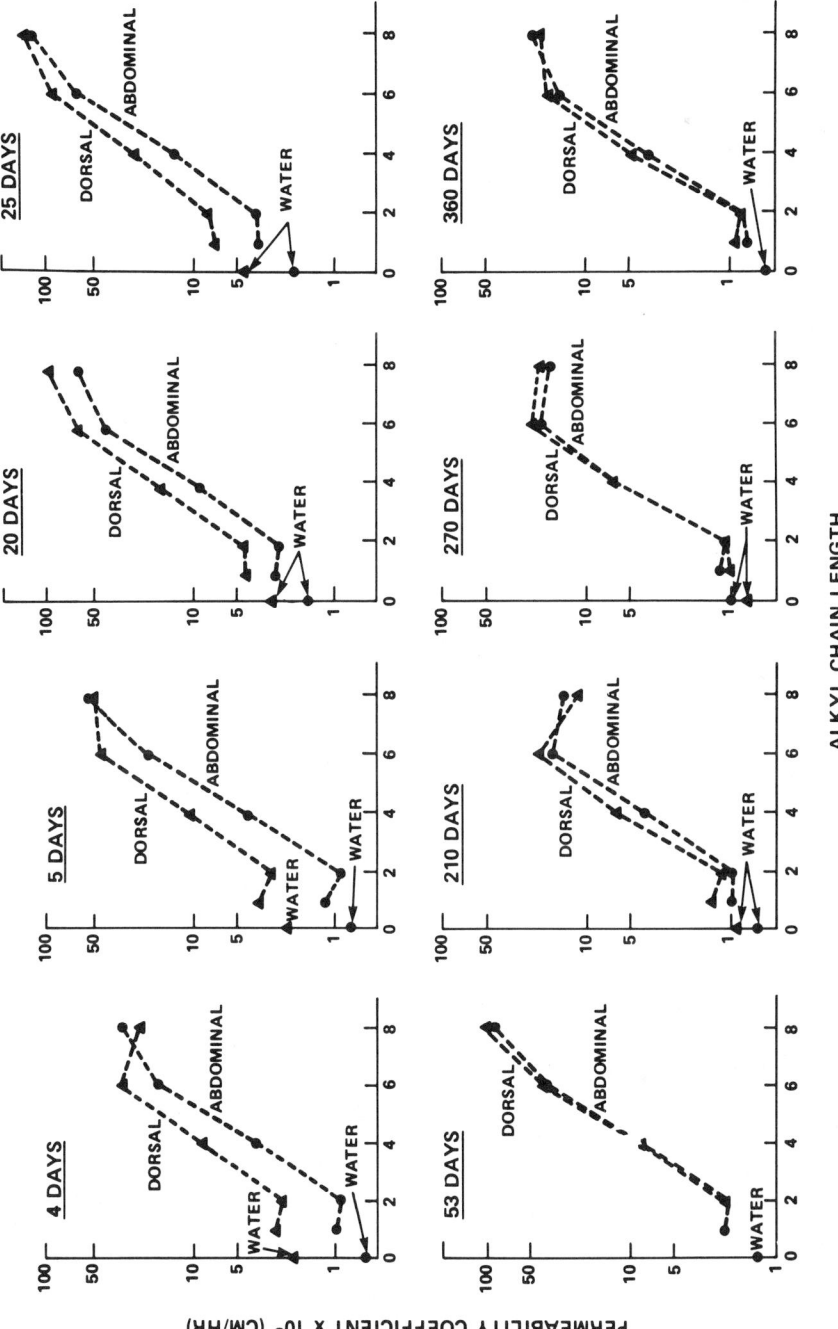

Figure 8 Semilogarithmic plots of permeability coefficients of n-alkanols through the abdominal and the dorsal skins of male hairless mice of different ages as a function of alkyl chain length. (From Behl et al., 1983d.)

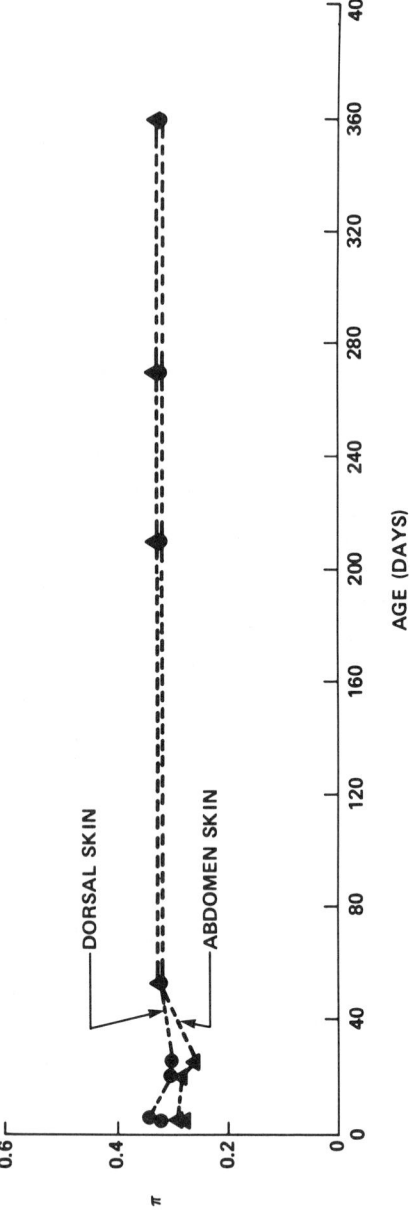

Figure 9 Plot of π values versus age of male hairless mouse. (From Behl et al., 1983d.)

Normalization of the Permeability Data

Wester et al. (1977) reported that the ratio of body surface area to body weight changes with age and has a significant effect on the systemic accumulation of topically applied chemicals. The method recommended by these investigators to demonstrate the increased risk to younger animals is to normalize the permeabilities to body weight. Using this approach, our data on alkanols (Behl et al., 1983d) were normalized, and the resulting profiles are presented in Figure 10 for water, methanol, ethanol, butanol, hexanol, and octanol, for both the abdominal and the dorsal skin sites. The normalized permeabilities are large in the beginning and fall rather rapidly until about 60 days of age, to remain invariant thereafter. Even in the absence of any real age-related permeability differences, these profiles indicate that young animals will systematically accumulate topically applied chemicals about 10 times faster than adults. Comparable weight differences are seen between human infants and adults, which implies that when treating infants one must be careful to limit the area of application to the minimum that is necessary.

Effect of Sex on Profiles of Age Versus Thickness and Age Versus Permeability

The results reported thus far pertain to the skins of the male hairless mice. The entire study was repeated in female hairless mouse skins to determine the effect of sex on the skin thickness and the skin permeability as a function of age, using skins from both the abdominal and the dorsal sites, and alkanols as test permeants (Behl et al., 1984). The results indicated that there are *no* substantial sex-related differences in the aging influences on skin thickness versus age profiles (cf. Fig. 11 with Fig. 3), skin permeability versus age profiles (cf. Fig. 12 with Fig. 5), the alkyl chain length effects as a function of age (cf. Fig. 13 with Fig. 8; Fig. 14 with Fig. 9), or normalized permeability versus age profile (cf. Fig. 15 with Fig. 10).

Significance of the Hairless Mouse Study

The skin of the hairless mouse undergoes dramatic visual and histological changes especially, during the first 60 days of age. Some of these changes, schematically depicted in Figure 16, make this animal a unique model because the experimentally observed data can be related to them to make some mechanistic interpretations.

Is the increase in permeation rates during the skin's metamorphosis directly due to the increased follicular presence? Additionally, can the lower plateau in the semilogarithmic plot of permeability versus alkyl chain length be explained in terms of the follicular pathway? Certainly the follicles enlarge and the opportunity for transfollicular passage is expanded. A rise in rates of three- to fivefold is not entirely unreasonable. *This* hypothesis is especially attractive for defining

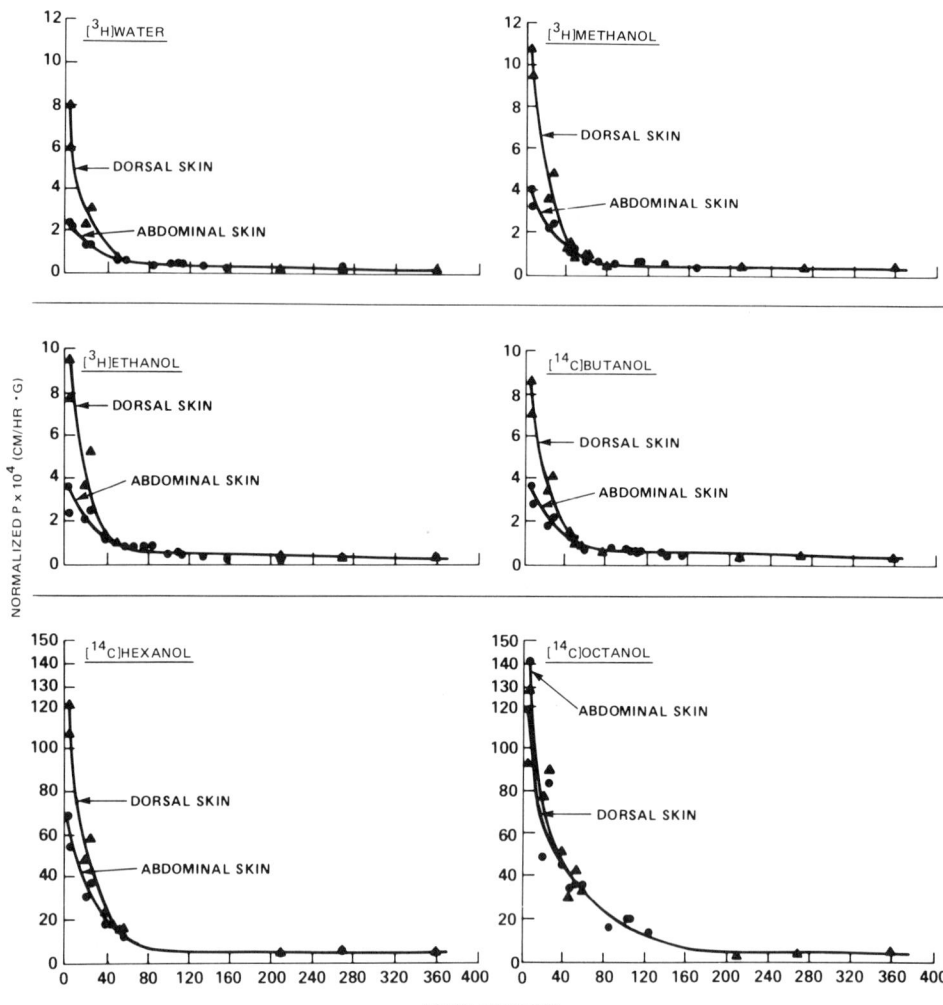

Figure 10 Plots of weight-normalized permeability coefficients of the abdominal and the dorsal skins of male hairless mice as a function of age. (From Behl et al., 1983d.)

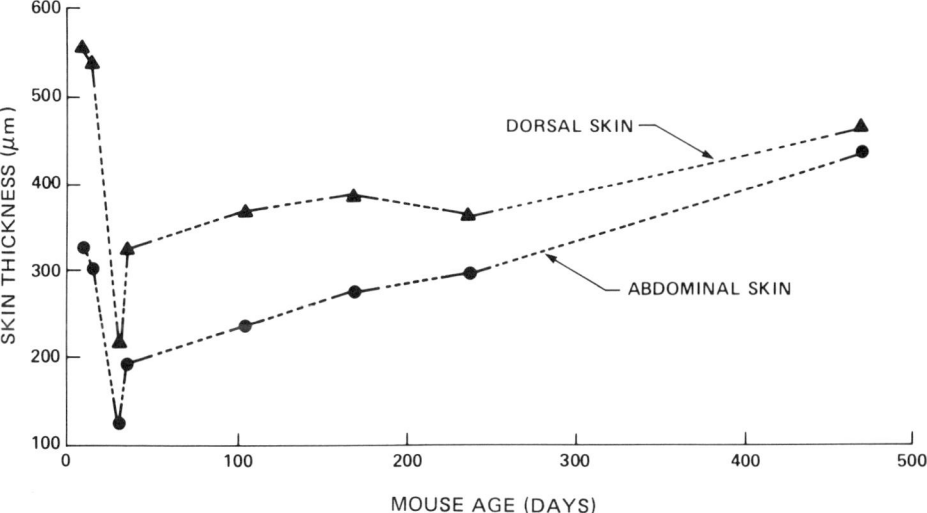

Figure 11 Plots of average thickness of female hairless mouse skin as a function of age. (From Behl et al., 1984.)

the stepped-up role of the aqueous shunt route, provided the follicular pore is filled with a heterogeneous medium of lipid and water. Such a medium might offer an aqueous conduit by bypassing the stratum corneum and an alternate lipid route as well. It should be noted that the orifice of the follicle is the only histologically demonstrated pore portal of entry through the skin. Unfortunately the nature of the sebum in hairless mouse skin immersed in saline is not known.

An *alternate* hypothesis is that concurrent changes in the stratum corneum accompany the follicular developments and may cause the stratum corneum to be either thinner or diminished in barrier competency. Lipogenesis by the keratinocytes might be depressed, for instance, during the period when the tissue becomes involved in the formation of hair, with a general loss in integrity of the horny tissue. As in the previous follicular case, both lipoidal and aqueous pathways would have to be similarly affected, considering that the increases in permeability are similar for polar and nonpolar solutes. Under the circumstances that the passage is transepidermal, the nature of the shunt route remains ill defined.

Unfortunately, not enough is known concerning the biology of the hairless mouse skin and how it changes during the hair cycle to permit unequivocal

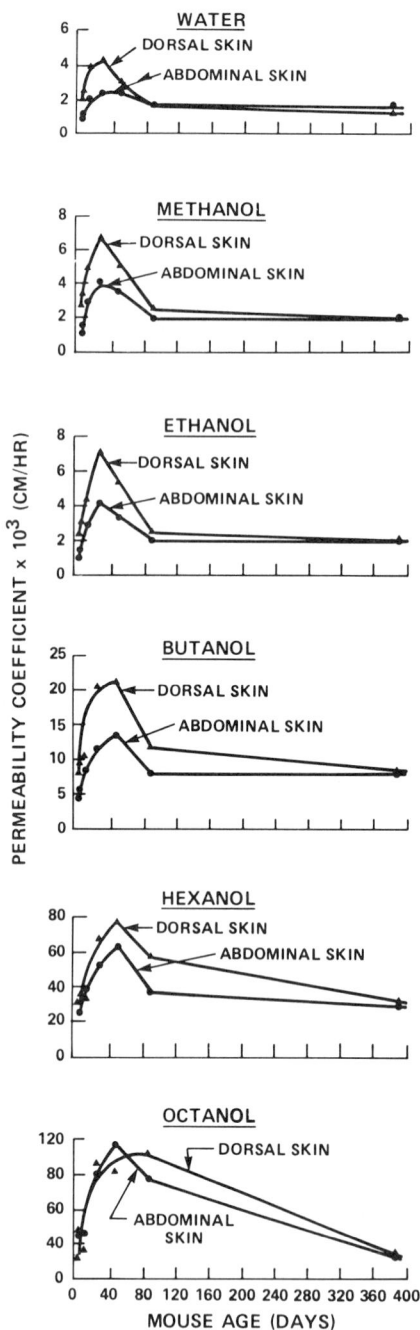

Figure 12 Plots of permeability coefficients of female hairless mouse skin as a function of age. (From Behl et al., 1984.)

assignment of the observed phenomena to one or another of the mechanisms or acceptance of some combination of the two. Like others (Blank, 1963; Scheuplein and Blank, 1973), Behl et al. (1980b, 1983d) and Flynn et al. (1981) also tend to favor the transepidermal explanation for the middle chain length homologs where the partitioning dependence is evident. The origin of the shunt route, however, must be further studied in detail. Ongoing studies may provide some additional insight into the issue.

The more gradual decline in permeability coefficient for octanol (possibly to a lesser extent for hexanol as well) would seem to be related to changes taking place in phases of the tissue other than the stratum corneum. Octanol's permeability is not strictly controlled by the stratum corneum, and the thickness of the full skin gradually increases throughout mouse life, except of course the first 25 days of age. Increased thickness of the dermis phase (Fig. 3) and increased filimentation of the true dermis together would cause steady decreases in the P values, which are sensitive to mass transfer across strata beneath the horny layer.

Irrespective of mechanism, one factor clearly demonstrated in these studies and extrapolatable to the human situation is the increased liability of systemic toxicity by the topical route. When the permeability coefficients are normalized with respect to body weight, young animals are seen to be substantially more subject to systemic accumulation than are adults. This factor is over and above considerations of the shifting permeability patterns, and it offers significant clinical implications.

There are certain experimentally important observations in these data for those who use the hairless species in toxicological and drug delivery investigations or for other purposes that involve percutaneous absorption. The skin of the young hairless mouse undergoes a rapid transformation in its permeability properties and, based on the alkanol data, it is not until about 100 days of age that these effects are essentially stabilized. Moreover, up to about 60 days the dorsal skin is more permeable than the abdominal skin to most of the test compounds studied. It appears, then, that investigators must be careful to fix the age of the animals used in their studies and to excise skin sections from clearly defined sites to minimize variability. A general technique where the dorsal surface is traumatized and the abdominal surface is used as the control for permeation studies has been developed (Behl et al., 1980a, 1981b). In this case, it is important to wait to an age of about 60 days, when the permeability coefficients of the two sites tend to converge, to make comparisons of the normal and treated surfaces.

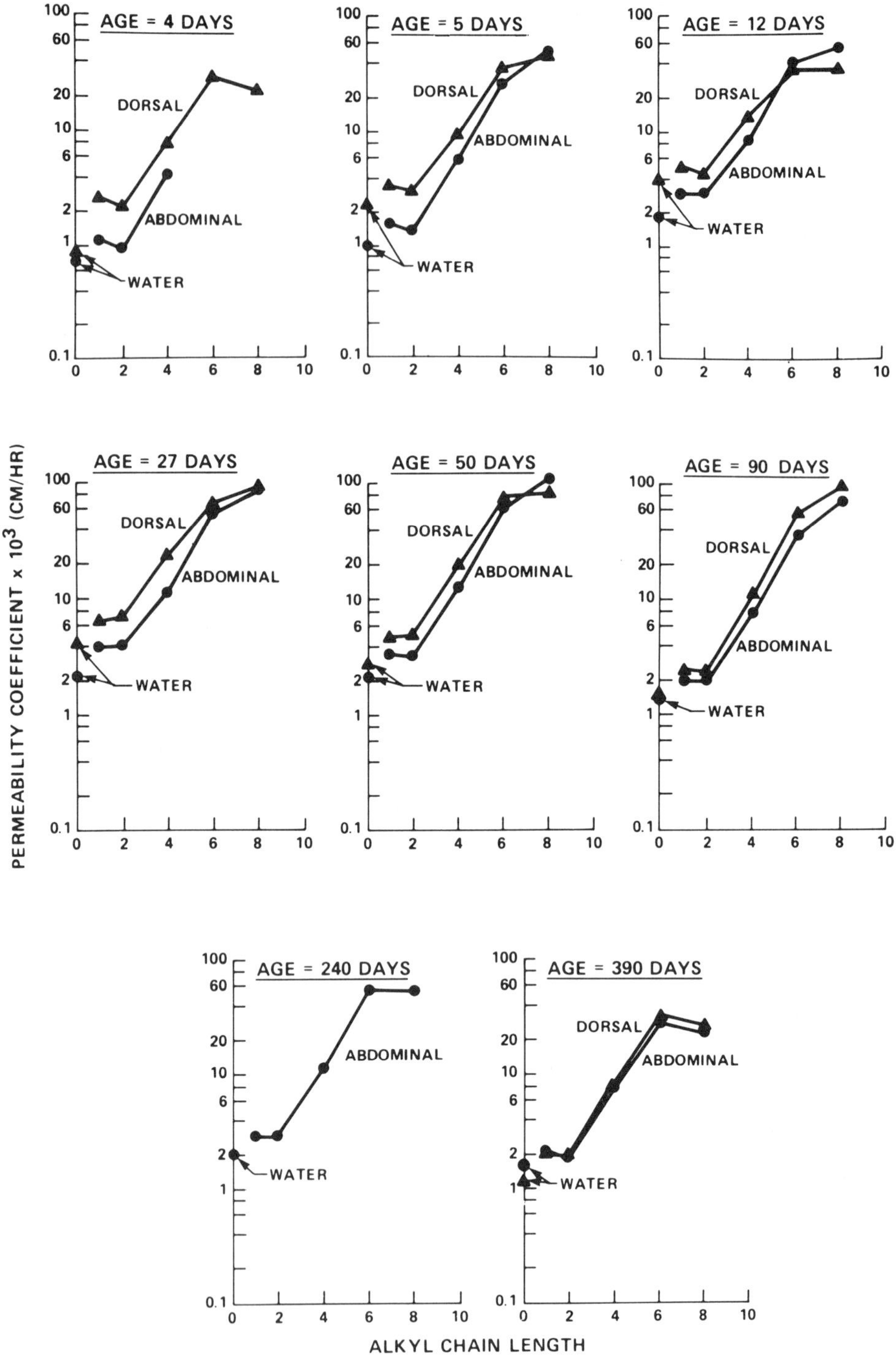

AGE = 4 DAYS
AGE = 5 DAYS
AGE = 12 DAYS
AGE = 27 DAYS
AGE = 50 DAYS
AGE = 90 DAYS
AGE = 240 DAYS
AGE = 390 DAYS
DORSAL
ABDOMINAL
WATER
PERMEABILITY COEFFICIENT x 10^3 (CM/HR)
ALKYL CHAIN LENGTH

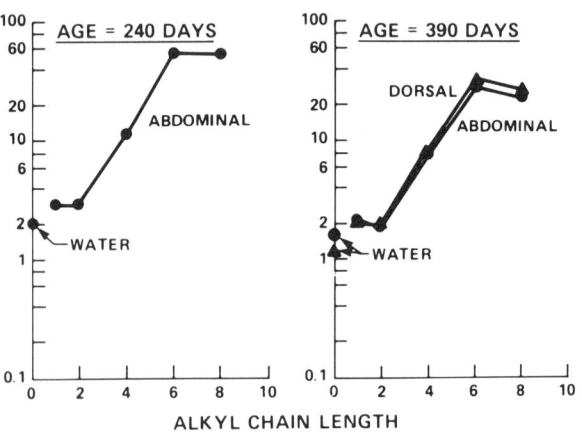

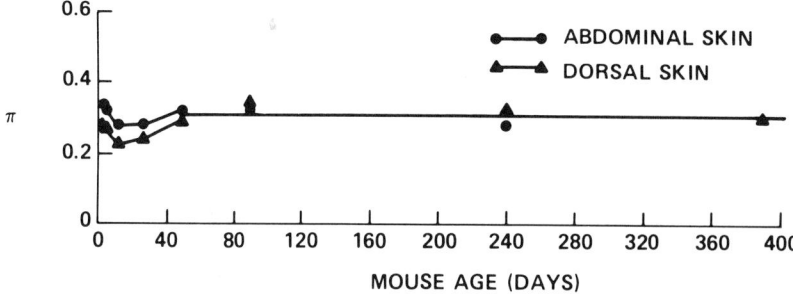

Figure 14 Plot of π values versus age of female hairless mouse. (From Behl et al., 1984.)

Figure 13 Semilogarithmic plots of permeability coefficients of n-alkanols through the abdominal and the dorsal skins of female hairless mice of different ages as a function of the alkyl chain length. (From Behl et al., 1984.)

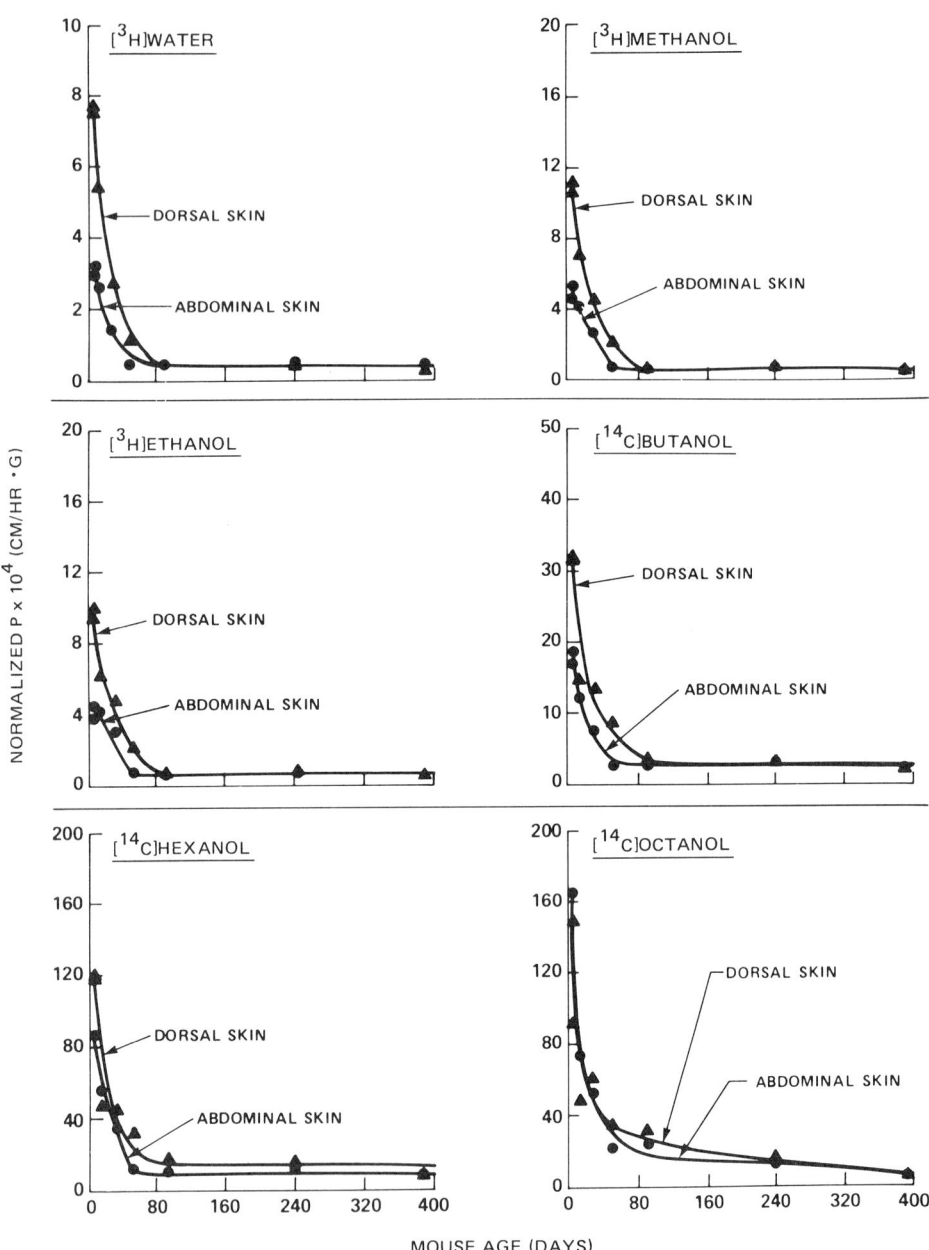

Figure 15 Plots of weight-normalized permeability coefficients P of the abdominal and the dorsal skins of female hairless mice as a function of age. (From Behl et al., 1984.)

Influence of Age on Percutaneous Absorption 209

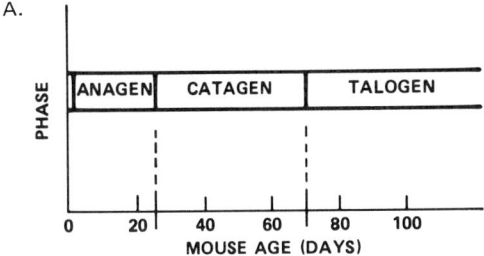

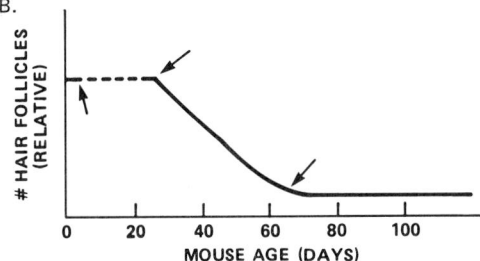

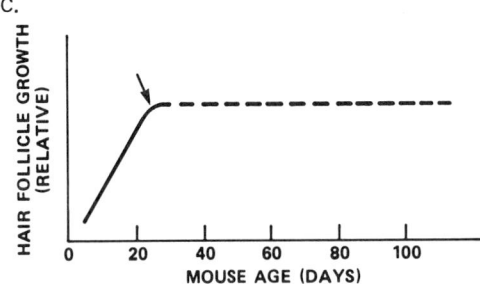

Figure 16 Schematic representation of certain anatomical and histological changes in the hairless mouse skins as a function of age. (A) The three biological phases. (B) Number of hair follicles. (C) Hair follicle growth.

REFERENCES

Armstrong, R. W., Eichner, E. R., Klein, D. E., Barthel, W. F., Bennett, J. V., Johnson, V., Bruce, H., and Loveless, L. E. (1969). *J. Pediatr.* 75: 317.

Behl, C. R. (1979). Systems approach to the study of vaginal drug absorption in the rhesus monkey. Ph.D. thesis, University of Michigan, Ann Arbor.

Behl, C. R., Flynn, G. L., Kurihara, T., Smith, W. M., Gatmaitan, O., Higuchi, W. I., Ho, N. F. H., and Pierson, C. L. (1980a). *J. Invest. Dermatol.* 75: 340.

Behl, C. R., Flynn, G. L., Kurihara, T., Harper, N., Smith, W. M., Higuchi, W. I., Ho, N. F. H., and Pierson, C. L. (1980b). *J. Invest. Dermatol.* 75: 346.

Behl, C. R., Meyer, R., and Flynn, G. L. (1981a). Percutaneous absorption by the living mouse—Uptake of water and *n*-alkanols across normal and stripped skins. Presented at the 128th Annual Meeting of the American Pharmaceutical Association, April 1981, St. Louis. Basic Pharmaceutics Abstract 22.

Behl, C. R., Flynn, G. L., Barrett, M., Walters, K. A., Linn, E. E., Mohamed, Z., Kurihara, T., and Pierson, C. L. (1981b). *Burns* 7: 389.

Behl, C. R., Pei, J., Bellantone, N. H., and Matluck, M. (1983a). Correlation of in vitro and in vivo permeation of propranolol through hairless mouse skin. Comparisons with Swiss mouse and Silastic data. Presented at the 130th Annual Meeting of the American Pharmaceutical Association, April 1983, New Orleans. Basic Pharmaceutics Abstract 10.

Behl, C. R., Bellantone, N. H., and Pei, J. (1983b). Effects of the alkyl chain length and anatomical site on the alkanol permeation through fuzzy rat skins. Presented at the 130th Annual Meeting of the American Pharmaceutical Association, April 1983, New Orleans. Basic Pharmaceutics Abstract 32.

Behl, C. R. and Bellantone, N. H. (1983c). Influence of the alkyl chain length on the in situ permeation of *n*-alkanols through fuzzy rat skins and comparison with the in vitro data. Presented at the 31st National Meeting of the Academy Pharmaceutical Science, November 1983, Miami, Fla. Basic Pharmaceutics Abstract 38.

Behl, C. R., Flynn, G. L., Kurihara, T., Smith, W. M., Bellantone, N. H., Gatmaitan, O., Pierson, C. L., Higuchi, W. I., and Ho, N. F. H. (1983d). Age and anatomical site influences on permeation of skin of male hairless mouse. *J. Soc. Cosmet. Chem.* In press.

Behl, C. R., Flynn, C. R., Linn, E. E., and Smith, W. M. (1983e). *J. Pharm. Sci.* In press.

Behl, C. R., Linn, E. E., Flynn, G. L., and Pierson, C. L. (1983f). *J. Pharm. Sci.* 72:391.

Behl, C. R., Flynn, G. L., Kurihara, T., Smith, W. M., Bellantone, N. H., Gatmaitan, O., Pierson, C. L., Higuchi, W. I., and Ho, N. F. H. (1984). Aging and anatomical site influences on the permeation of water and *n*-alkanols through female hairless mouse skin. Presented at the 131st Annual Meeting of the American Pharmaceutical Association, May 1984. Basic Pharmaceutics Abstract 2.

Benson, P. F. and Pharoah, P. O. D. (1960). *Guy Hosp. Rep.* 109: 212.

Black, M. M. (1969). *Br. J. Dermatol.* 81: 661.

Blank, I. H. (1952). *J. Invest. Dermatol. 18*: 433.
Blank, I. H. (1963). *J. Invest. Dermatol. 43*: 415.
Brooke, H. (1926). *J. Hered. 17*: 173.
Chase, H. B. and Montagna, W. (1951). *Proc. Soc. Exp. Biol. Med. 76*: 35.
Chase, H. B., Montagna, W., and Malone, J. D. (1953). *Anat. Rec. 116*: 75.
Christophers, E. and Kligman, A. M. (1964). Percutaneous absorption in aged skin. In *Advances in the Biology of the Skin*, Vol. VI. Edited by W. Montagna. Pergamon, New York, p. 163.
Crew, F. A. F. and Mirskaia, L. (1931). *J. Genet. 25*: 17.
Curley, A., Hawk, R. E., Kimbrough, R. D., and Finberg, L. (1971). *Lancet 2*: 296.
David, L. T. (1932). *Z. Zell. Mikrosk. Anat. 14*: 616.
David, L. T. (1934). *J. Exp. Zool. 68*: 501.
Dry, F. W. (1926). *J. Genet. 16*: 287.
Durrheim, H., Flynn, G. L., Higuchi, W. I., and Behl, C. R. (1981). *J. Pharm. Sci. 69*: 781.
Fanconi, V. G. (1962). *Helv. Paediatr. Acta 17*: 267.
Feinblatt, B. I., Aceto, T., Beckhorn, G., and Bruck, E. (1966). *Am. J. Dis. Child. 112*: 218.
Feiwel, M., James, V. H. T., and Barnet, E. S. (1969). *Lancet 1*: 485.
Flynn, G. L., Durrheim, H., and Higuchi, W. I. (1981). *J. Pharm. Sci. 70*: 52.
Gottschall, R. Y. and Burney, W. E. (1940). *J. Immunol. 38*: 345.
Graubarth, M., Bloom, C. J., Coleman, F. C., and Solomon, H. N. (1945). *JAMA 128*: 1155.
Hammarlund, K. and Sedin, G. (1979). *Acta Paediatr. Scand. 68*: 795.
Harpin, V. and Ratter, N. (1982). *Arch. Dis. Child. 57*: 477.
Kagan, B. M., Mirman, B., Calvin, J., and Lunden, E. (1949). *J. Pediatr. 34*: 574.
Kligman, A. M. (1979). *J. Invest. Dermatol. 73*: 39.
Malkinson, F. D. and Ferguson, E. H. (1955). *J. Invest. Dermatol. 25*: 281.
Malkinson, F. D. (1958). *J. Invest. Dermatol. 31*: 29.
Mann, S. J. (1971). *Anat. Rec. 170*: 485.
Mann, S. J. and Straile, W. E. (1961). *Anat. Rec. 140*: 97.
Marzulli, F. N. (1962). *J. Invest. Dermatol. 39*: 387.
Marzulli, F. N. and Maibach, H. I. (1975). Relevance of animal models: The hexachlorophene story. In *Animal Models in Dermatology*. Edited by H. I. Maibach. Churchill-Livingstone, New York, p. 156.
Marzulli, F. N. and Tregear, R. T. (1961). *J. Physiol. 157*: 52.
McCormack, J., Biosits, E. K., and Fisher, L. B. (1982). An in vitro comparison of the permeability of adult versus neonatal skin. In *Neonatal Skin, Structure, and Function*. Edited by H. I. Maibach and E. K. Boisits. Dekker, New York, p. 149.
Meema, H. E., Sheppard, R. H., and Rapopart, A. (1964). *Radiology 82*: 411.
Meyer, R., Behl, C. R., and Flynn, G. L. (1981). Influences of anatomical site on the permeabilities of water and n-alkanols through stripped skins of hairless mice. *J. Pharm. Sci.* Submitted.

Montagna, W., Chase, H. B., and Melaragno, H. P. (1952). *J. Invest. Dermatol. 19*: 83.
Munro, D. D. (1976). *Br. J. Dermatol. 94*: 67.
Nachman, R. L. and Esterly, N. B. (1971). *J. Pediatr. 79*: 628.
Neuland, W. (1921). *Med. Klin. 17*: 906.
Orwin, D. F. G., Chase, M. B., and Silver, A. F. (1967). *Am. J. Anat. 121*: 489.
Raynar, W. (1886). *Br. Med. J. 1*: 294.
Robson, A. M., Kissane, J. M., Elvick, N. H., and Pundavela, L. (1969). *J. Pediatr. 75*: 309.
Scheuplein, R. J. and Blank, I. H. (1971). *Physiol. Rev. 51*: 702.
Scheuplein, R. J. and Blank, I. H. (1973). *J. Invest. Dermatol. 60*: 286.
Scott, E. P., Prince, G. E., and Rotondo, C. C. (1946). *J. Pediatr. 28*: 713.
Shuman, R. M., Leech, R. W., and Alvord, E. C. (1975). *Arch. Neurol. 32*: 320.
Shuster, S., Black, M. M., and Mevitie, E. (1975). *Br. J. Dermatol. 93*: 639.
Stevens, A. N. (1928). *JAMA 90*: 116.
Tregear, R. T. (1966). Molecular movement. The permeability of skin. In *Theoretical and Experimental Biology*, Vol. 5, *Physical Functions of the Skin*. Academic, London, p. 13.
Weimberg, A. A. (1931). *Am. J. Obstet. Gynecol. 21*: 104.
Wester, R. C., Noonan, P. K., Cole, M. P., and Maibach, H. I. (1977). *Pediatr. Res. 11*: 737.
Wildnauer, R. H. and Kennedy, R. (1970). *J. Invest. Dermatol. 54*: 483.
Wilson, D. and Maibach, H. I. (1982). Carbon dioxide emission rate in the newborn. In *Neonatal Skin, Structure and Function*. Edited by H. I. Maibach and E. K. Boisits. Dekker, New York, p. 111.
Wolbach, S. B. (1951). *Ann. N.Y. Acad. Sci. 53*: 517.
Yu, C.-d. (1978). Prodrug-based topical delivery: Simultaneous skin transport and bioconversion. Ph.D. Thesis, University of michigan, Ann Arbor.
Yun, J. S. and Montagna, W. (1961). *Anat. Rec. 140*: 77.
Zeligs, M. (1929). *Arch. Pediatr. 46*: 502.

15
In Vitro Studies on the Permeability of Infant Skin

Louis B. Fisher
Mary Kay Cosmetics, Inc., Dallas, Texas

Damaging effects due to the percutaneous absorption of toxic compounds in the newborn range from dermal atrophy (Keipert, 1971) through a variety of more severe changes (Feinblatt et al., 1966; Feiwel, 1969; Kagan et al., 1949; Powell et al., 1973; Shuman et al., 1975) to death (Armstrong et al., 1969; Brown, 1970; Harpin and Rutter, 1982). Mostly, these involved either diseased skin (where it is reasonable to assume increased penetration) or low birth weight infants. Generally, clinical systemic effects were recorded but no distinction was made between differences in barrier function and differences due to individual size. It is important to recognize that the latter exist. This is an effect due to the surface to volume ratio; that is, a child has less body volume per unit area of skin than an adult and consequently any material that penetrates will be more concentrated and thus will have a greater systemic effect. This has been reviewed by West et al. (1981), who also point out the probable lack of maturity in cutaneous metabolic and detoxification pathways at this age.

Results obtained from in vivo applications of testosterone to rhesus monkeys led Wester et al. (1977) to conclude that in the newborn rhesus the barrier function to this steroid resembles that of the adult. Although excretion rates of the labeled material in the newborn monkey were higher than in the adult, the differences were entirely attributed to the greater surface to volume ratio of the younger animal. Attempts to specifically measure percutaneous absorption in the human newborn are sparsely documented. Parmley and Seeds (1970) demonstrated a decrease in water permeability correlated with the histological appearance of a stratum corneum in the human, and they reported "no detectable diffusion" through the skin of older fetuses. Nachman and Esterley (1971) noted an inverse correlation between gestational age and the blanching response to topical Neo-Synephrine, while Wildnauer and Kennedy (1970) suggested that the barrier function of the healthy newborn may be even better than that of the adult with regard to transepidermal water loss (TEWL). However, Cunico et al. (1977) have suggested that these differences may be due to the immaturity of the infant sweat glands; that is, more of the water loss in the adult may be due to sweating—a function not fully developed in the newborn (Foster et al., 1969).

The purpose of the work described in this chapter, carried out at Johnson & Johnson Baby Products Company, in conjunction with Dr. E. Boisits and J. McCormack, was to clarify this situation via the development of an in vitro method for evaluating skin barrier properties of infants with respect to a variety of materials.

MATERIALS AND METHODS

Although baby skin was available via autopsies, the quantity was minimal. We developed an in vitro cell that required only small amounts of tissue. The penetration cell developed is similar to cells previously described only inasmuch as it holds a piece of skin in a way that allows liquid to be applied to both sides (Fig. 1). It consists of a plastic block with a depression where the tissue is placed. A watertight seal is obtained by placing a Teflon gasket over the skin, and this is held down with a knurled plug. The gasket and plug are penetrated by 3-mm holes (A), which allow application of liquid to the skin surface. Below the skin, the plastic block has three intersecting channels. One channel provides access to the general circulation for the purpose of taking samples. The other two are joined by plastic tubing, which passes through a peristaltic pump. Thus the fluid below the skin continuously circulates rather than being stirred. The total fluid volume is 0.5 ±0.1 ml. Cells were permanently marked and a record of the exact reservoir volume kept for use in the calculations (see below).

In any one experiment, a rack of 10 cells was used, all run from the same peristaltic pump. Although this setup was used for the initial studies some modification was made following the experiments using tritiated water. The channel accessing the area below the skin sample (and previously used for sampling) was closed. The circulation between the remaining two channels was broken, and the circulating fluid (water) was continuously fed from a reservoir, across the lower surface of the skin via the peristaltic pump, and directly into a scintillation vial. The pump was used to provide a flow rate of 2 ml/15 min. This resulted in an automated system providing samples at 15-min intervals without concerns for sampling errors, without introducing bubbles with the sampling needle, and with no need for continuous count corrections.

All the skin samples used were abdominal, obtained at autopsy; they were frozen immediately and kept at −70°C until used. The only distinction was based

Permeability of Infant Skin

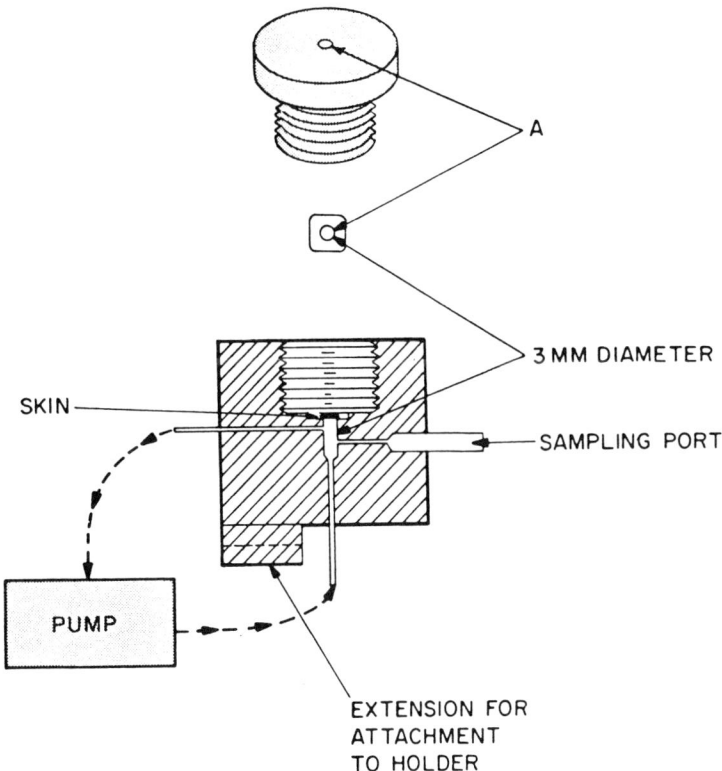

Figure 1 The penetration cell, machined from Lexan, showing the holes (A) through which material is applied to the skin surface and the working diameter.

on age: adult (50-76 years), full-term infant (37-40 weeks gestation; 1-3 days postnatal), and premature infant (26-30 weeks gestation; 1-3 days postnatal). The adult and full-term infant skin was keratotomed to a depth of 0.3 mm to prevent excess dermis blocking the circulation. However the premature infant skin (total thickness about 0.5 mm) was too small to keratotome.

Radiolabeled material in 50-μl portions was applied to the epidermal surface using a microsyringe. In the initial studies with tritiated water, 50-μl samples were removed at intervals from the circulating fluid with a microsyringe and replaced with fresh fluid. Care had to be taken that no air bubbles were introduced during either operation. Each 50-μl sample removed was placed in a glass vial with 10 ml of Instagel scintillation fluid. In the later automated system, samples were collected in the scintillation vials directly from the penetration cell. Next, 50-μl of stock tritiated water (equal to the amount applied to the skin surface) was also placed in a vial with Instagel. All samples were counted in a Hewlett-Packard scintillation counter model 3330. External standardization was used to allow for quench correction.

CALCULATIONS

Much of the following applies only to the initial closed-circulation system in which the penetration of water was investigated. Counts were corrected to disintegrations per minute (dpm) using a quench correction curve. A further correction had to be made for all counts removed before taking any sample (closed-circulation system only). Thus the true number of dpm penetrated was:

$$(C_N - Bkg) \times \frac{V_R}{V_S} + \sum_0^{N-1} C = C_T$$

where C_N is the actual dpm obtained from the sample, Bkg is background, V_R is the total reservoir volume (fixed for each cell), V_S is the sample volume (= 50 μl), and $\sum_0^{N-1} C$ is the sum of all previously removed dpm. The permeability coefficient (K_p) is obtained from:

$$\frac{Q_T}{C_0 \times T} = K_p$$

where $Q_T = C_T/A$, A is the membrane area (0.07 cm^2), C_0 is the total dpm of the material initially applied to the skin surface, and T is the time in minutes. This is obtained by plotting Q_T/C_0 against time and finding the slope. The K_p is shown for the water studies so that a comparison can be made directly with the literature and thus validate the system. In the clinical setting, a steady state may be established for only a short time. Consequently the bulk of the data are expressed here as percentage penetration per unit time, since this has more direct clinical relevance. In addition, since the automated technique was used, these data did not need the volume corrections indicated above.

RESULTS

The water results show a mean K_p for adult skin of 4.9×10^{-5} cm/min, which is similar to published values (e.g., Scheuplein, 1977, gives 1.5×10^{-5} cm/min). Full-term infants averaged 6.6×10^{-5} cm/min, while in contrast the premature infant skin averaged 4.6×10^{-4} cm/min. The data are plotted in Figure 2, which shows that while adult and full-term infant results fall in the same range, there is minimal overlap with the premature data. This difference is seen more clearly in

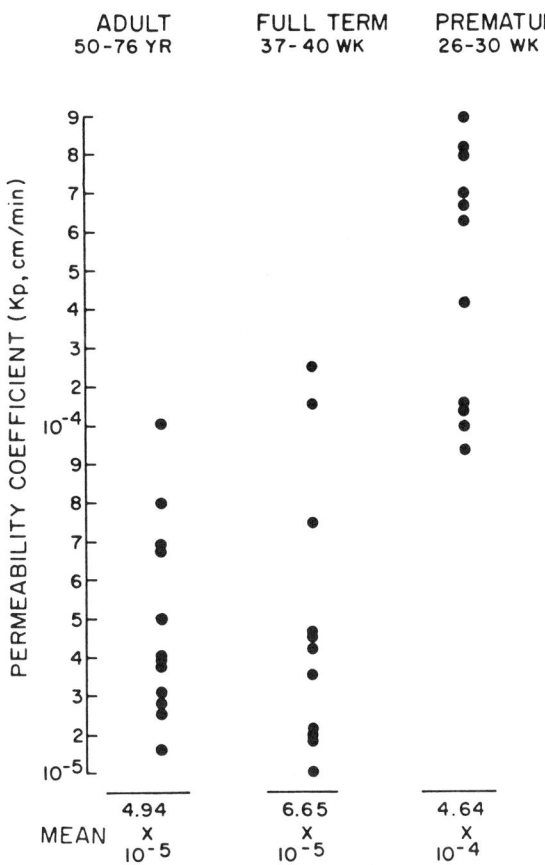

Figure 2 Plot of permeability coefficient versus age.

Figure 3, where Q_T/C_0 is plotted against time for individual samples from each age range. Clearly, the premature data are close to the result of an equal thickness of dermis where there is no stratum corneum barrier. In the subsequent alcohol studies, rather than try to prevent evaporation of the volatile materials, a correction was made. Studies were repeated with the addition of aluminum foil underneath the skin sample to completely prevent penetration of the radioactivity. At the completion of the usual study period (6 hr) the recovery was determined from the cell, the skin, and the foil. Ethanol was the only material of which more than 95% was not recovered. Only 33% of the ethanol was recovered, and a correction was applied to the permeability data. Data obtained from the four alcohols (ethanol, benzyl alcohol, decanol, and cetyl alcohol) were relative-

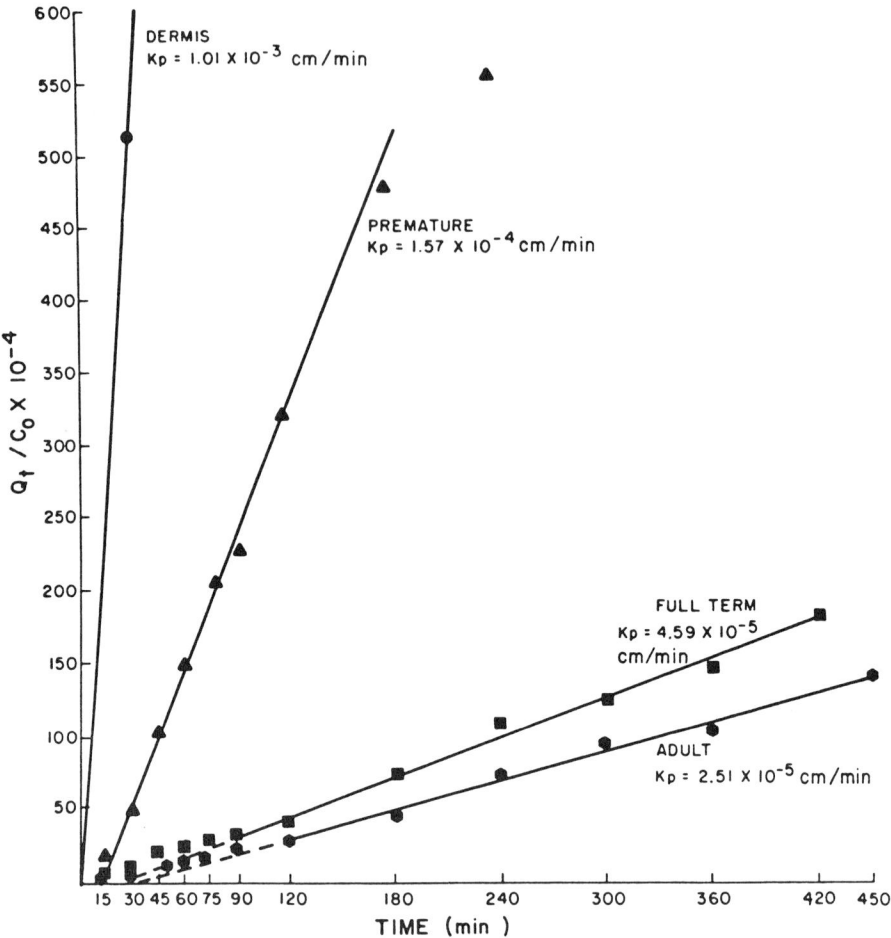

Figure 3 Plot of penetration of tritiated water versus time for single skin samples: ●, dermis; ▲, premature infant skin; ■, full-term infant skin; ●, adult skin.

ly similar to that for water with respect to age. In all instances the permeability of full-term baby skin was very similar to that of adult skin, while the skin of the premature infant was much more permeable (Table 1).

The fatty acid series (lauric acid, caprylic acid, oleic acid, and stearic acid) was different in that there was no consistency (Table 2). In general, it seems as though adult skin is less permeable than that of babies of either age. The lack of

Table 1 Comparative Penetration of Alcohols Through Human Skin[a]

	Adult	Infants	
		Full-term	Premature
Decanol	0.0247 ± 0.0036	0.0158 ± 0.0057	0.0259 ± 0.057
$n =$	10	10	10
Cetyl alcohol	0.0045 ± 0.0001	0.023 ± 0.002	0.0418 ± 0.03
$n =$	11	11	11
Ethanol	1.3 ± 0.3	1.6 ± 0.3	4.8 ± 1.5
$n =$	14	18	17
Benzyl alcohol	1.42 ± 0.94	0.73 ± 0.48	35.5 ± 5.6
$n =$	16	12	14

[a]Data represent the total percentage of the applied dose (± SD) penetrating during the 0–6 hr period of study.

Table 2 Comparative Penetration of Fatty Acids Through Human Skin[a]

	Adult	Infants	
		Full-term	Premature
Caprylic acid	0.96 ± 0.81	2.94 ± 0.60	1.75 ± 0.99
$n =$	10	10	10
Oleic acid	0.0093 ± 0.0009	0.088 ± 0.016	0.101 ± 0.056
$n =$	10	10	10
Stearic acid	0.014 ± 0.004	0.011 ± 0.005	0.014 ± 0.010
$n =$	10	10	10
Lauric acid	0.114 ± 0.050	0.285 ± 0.111	0.648 ± 0.514
$n =$	10	10	10

[a]Data represent the total percentage of the applied dose (± SD) penetrating during the 0–6 hr period of study.

consistency in penetration patterns may, at least in part, be due to the fact that a solvent (acetone or hexane) was needed to apply these materials. Once the application had been made, a gentle stream of warm air was blown over the surface of the sample to evaporate the solvent. However, we do not know the effect of this short-term contact.

DISCUSSION

The data obtained on adult skin using tritiated water indicates that the miniaturized cell, as described, is reliable for routine testing of skin permeability because it agrees with previously published work (Galey et al., 1976; Scheuplein, 1977). Of major importance is that the working diameter of the described cell is only 3 mm. Permeability data can be obtained from samples as small as 5-mm punch biopsies or blister tops, which solves the problem of the limited availability of infant tissue.

The data obtained from premature skin suggest that there is little or no barrier to water penetration at this age. This does not entirely agree with the results of Parmley and Seeds (1970), although it is likely that the differences are due to their lack of data at older ages (two samples at 24 weeks) and to the fact that measurements were made on the scalp, where keratinization is most advanced at that age. Our data agree with the clinical findings of Nachman and Esterley (1971) within both age groups, as well as a number of studies comparing the transepidermal water loss of infants of different ages (Rutter and Hull, 1979; Stornowski and Hornchen, 1981; Wilson and Maibach, 1980). Parmley and Seeds (1970) suggested that a drop in permeability correlated with the appearance of the stratum corneum. We would not disagree with that generalization, although this may not be as simple as it sounds. There is little stratum corneum in the earlier age group, while the full-term infants exhibit a histological stratum corneum that is, if anything, thicker than that of the adult. Thus, given equal penetration at the two ages, the thicker stratum corneum in the infant suggests the possibility of some degree of immaturity in the chemicophysical structure at this age.

Structural studies by Holbrook (1982) suggested to her that the epidermis of the full-term infant is similar to that of the adult, and that both of these are different from the epidermis of the premature infant. However, the dermis of the full-term infant seems to be in a transitional state between the adult and the premature infant, and it is certainly possible that the epidermal lipid content may show a similar variability. Variation in these parameters could explain the differences we have seen in penetration patterns between the two groups of materials we have investigated. In any case, it is apparent that a well-nourished, full-term infant has a skin barrier to water at least functionally equal to that of.the adult. However, we are not implying that this will hold for all materials applied to the skin. In fact the fatty acid data described above suggest that this is not true. Nevertheless, it does appear that the barrier properties of the full-term infant may be every bit as good as those of the adult with respect to at least some materials.

It is important to remember, however, that the application procedures for topical products can and do influence penetration. The factors involved in this with respect to the neonate have been reviewed by Wester and Maibach (1982). We believe that data presented here should be treated from an academic rather than a clinical point of view at this time. There is no question that the detoxification mechanisms, even in the full-term infant, are immature, and there is much to be learned concerning the potential metabolism of topically applied products by the infant skin. Even assuming adult skin barrier properties, the surface to volume ratio of the infant is such that the systemic concentration of any material that has penetrated may reach toxic proportions. Although there may not be an immediate practical application for these data, the results of this and future studies should prove useful in gaining a better understanding of the maturation of the epidermal barrier to penetration.

REFERENCES

Armstrong, R. W., Eichner, E. R., Klein, D. E., Bartel, W. F., Bennett, J. V., Jonsson, V., Bruce, H., and Loveless, L. E. (1969). Pentachlorophenol poisoning in a nursery for newborn infants. II. Epidemiologic and toxicologic studies. *J. Pediatr. 75*: 317-325.

Brown, B. W. (1970). Fatal phenol poisoning from improperly laundered diapers. *Am. J. Public Health 60*: 901-902.

Cunico, R. L., Maibach, H. I., Kahn, H., and Bloom, E. (1977). Skin barrier properties in the newborn: Transepidermal water loss and carbon dioxide emission rates. *Biol. Neonate 32*: 177-182.

Feinblatt, B. I., Aceto, T., Beckhorn, G., and Bruck, E. (1966). Percutaneous absorption of hydrocortisone in children. *Am. J. Dis. Child. 112*: 218-224.

Feiwel, M. (1969). Percutaneous absorption of topical steroids in children. *Br. J. Dermatol. 81* (Suppl. 4): 113-116.

Foster, K. G., Hey, E. N., and Katz, G. (1969). The response of the sweat glands of the newborn baby to thermal stimuli and intradermal acetylcholine. *J. Physiol. 203*: 13-29.

Galey, W. R., Lonsdale, H. K., and Nacht, S. (1976). The in vitro permeability of skin and buccal mucosa to selected drugs and tritiated water. *J. Invest. Dermatol. 67*: 713-717.

Harpin, V. and Rutter, N. (1982). Percutaneous alcohol absorption and skin necrosis in a preterm infant. *Arch Dis. Child. 57*: 477-479.

Holbrook, K. A. (1982). A histological comparison of infant and adult skin. In *Neonatal Skin: Structure and Function*. Edited by H. I. Maibach and E. K. Boisits. Dekker, New York, pp. 3-31.

Kagan, B. M., Mirman, B., Calvin, J., and Lundeen, E. (1949). Cyanosis in premature infants due to aniline dyes. *J. Pediatr. 34*: 574-578.

Keipert, J. A. (1971). The absorption of topical corticosteroids with particular reference to percutaneous absorption in infancy and childhood. *Med. J. Aust. 1*: 1021-1025.

Nachman, R. L. and Esterley, N. B. (1971). Increased skin permeability in preterm infants. *J. Pediatr. 79*: 628-632.

Parmley, T. H. and Seeds, A. E. (1970). Fetal skin permeability to isotopic water (THO) in early pregnancy. *Am. J. Obstet. Gynecol. 108*: 128-131.

Powell, H., Swarner, O., Gluck, L., and Lampert, P. (1973). Hexachlorophene myelinopathy in premature infants. *J. Pediatr. 82*: 976-981.

Rutter, N. and Hull, D. (1979). Water loss from the skin of term and preterm babies. *Arch. Dis. Child. 54*: 858-868.

Scheuplein, R. J. (1977). Permeability of the skin. In *Handbook of Physiology*, Sect. 9, *Reaction to Environmental Agents*. Edited by D. H. K. Lee. American Physiological Society, Bethesda, pp. 299-322.

Shuman, R. M., Leech, R. W., and Alvord, E. C. (1975). Neurotoxicity of hexachlorophene in humans. II. A clinicopathological study of 46 premature infants. *Arch. Neurol. 32*: 320-325.

Stornowski, C. and Hornchen, H. (1981). Transepidermaler Wasserverlust bei Fruh und Neugeborenen. *Monatsschr. Kinderheilkd. 129*: 239-244.

West, D. P., Worobec, S., and Solomon, L. M. (1981). Pharmacology and toxicology of infant skin. *J. Invest. Dermatol. 76*: 147-150.

Wester, R. C. and Maibach, H. I. (1982). Percutaneous absorption: Neonate compared to the adult. In *Environmental Factors in Human Growth and Development*. Edited by W. R. Hunt, M. K. Smith, and D. Worth. Cold Spring Harbor Press, Cold Spring Harbor, N.Y., pp. 3-15.

Wester, R. C., Noonan, P. K., Cole, M. P., and Maibach, H. I. (1977). Percutaneous absorption of testosterone in the newborn rhesus monkey. Comparison to the adult. *Pediatr. Res. 11*: 737-739.

Wildnauer, R. H. and Kennedy, R. (1970). Transepidermal water loss of human newborns. *J. Invest. Dermatol. 54*: 483-486.

Wilson, D. R. and Maibach, H. I. (1980). Transepidermal water loss in vivo: Premature and term infants. *Biol. Neonate 37*: 180-185.

16
Predictability of In Vitro Diffusion Systems
Effect of Skin Types and Ages on Percutaneous Absorption of Triclocarban

Ronald C. Wester, Howard I. Maibach, John Surinchak, and Daniel A. W. Bucks
University of California School of Medicine, San Francisco, California

Our objective was to determine the predictive ability of in vitro percutaneous absorption for triclocarban (TCC) using several skin sources. The in vivo percutaneous absorption of TCC was 7.0 ±2.8% of applied dose. In the static diffusion cell, percutaneous absorption for all skin types (human adult, newborn, and infant abdominal skin, and rhesus monkey abdominal skin) were 30-fold less than in vivo absorption. This was attributed to the design of the static diffusion system, because a continuous flow system gave values equal to the in vivo absorption. Differences were attributed to lack of TCC solubility in the small receptor volume of the static system.

Human newborn foreskin is used as a supply of human skin for in vitro diffusion studies. Absorption in newborn foreskin was 10-fold greater than in human abdominal skin. This was attributed to age (newborn) rather than site (foreskin) because absorption in adult foreskin was closer to adult abdominal skin than to newborn foreskin.

INTRODUCTION

Triclocarban (TCC) is a bacteriostatic agent used in antimicrobial toilet soap. Its present wide use and future potential for even wider utilization necessitate accurate estimates of its percutaneous absorption for safety and efficacy evaluation. Wider use of TCC might involve its incorporation into additional baby products, and it is in the infant where the greatest potential for topical toxicity can exist (Wester and Maibach, 1982).

Marty and Wepierre (1979) determined the in vitro percutaneous absorption of TCC in human skin to be extremely low. This corroborated the work of Scharpf et al. (1975), where the absorption of TCC in vivo in man under showering conditions was also low. Our initial objective was to ascertain whether the percutaneous absorption of TCC also is low in newborn and infant skin. For this we used the common in vitro static diffusion system used by others, including Marty and Wepierre (1979). However, in the course of our study, we discovered that our standard diffusion data were not predictive of our in vivo human absorption data. The disparity was traced to the inability of TCC to solubilize in the diffusion saline of the static system. A new continuous flow system gave results that were predictive of man in vivo.

MATERIALS AND METHODS

Abdominal, full-thickness skin sections were obtained from human and rhesus monkey cadavers within 24 hr of death. Subcutaneous fat and muscle were removed with a scalpel and the skin samples stored in plastic bags at $-15°C$. Foreskin samples obtained from infant and adult circumcisions were stored under similar conditions. The newborn abdominal sections were obtained from a 5-day-old female donor; the infant samples were obtained from a 9-month-old male. Adult abdominal sections were obtained from male and female donors 60–70 years old.

After a storage period ranging from 1 to 8 weeks, the skin sample was allowed to thaw at room temperature before separation of the epidermis. Epidermal separation was achieved by immersing the skin in $60°C$ water for 3 min and subsequently teasing the epidermis away from the dermis. The epidermis was placed on top of diffusion cells and sealed in place with Teflon O-rings. Degassed saline was used as the perfusion medium. Four μl of $[^{14}C]$ TCC in acetone, at a concentration of 27 $\mu g/cm^2$, was applied to the surface of the epidermis with a Hamilton microliter syringe. An open cap was fastened to the top of the cell with a spring-loaded clamp.

Glass diffusion cells were either of static (Crown Glass Co., Somerville, N.Y.) or flow design. The static cells had a volume of 3.77 ml and an epidermal surface area of 0.126 cm^2. The flow cells had the same surface area and a flow rate of 15 ml/hr. Flow cells were at an ambient temperature of $23°C$ and the static cells at either ambient temperature or $37°C$. Saline in the static cells was changed every 2 hr for the first 12 hr and at approximately 10-hr intervals thereafter for the 48 hr of each study. Flow cells emptied into scintillation vials housed in a fraction collector, which advanced hourly.

A 5-ml aliquot of the perfusion medium was mixed with 14 ml of PCS scintillation fluid (Amersham/Searle Corp., Chicago) and radioactivity content determined. Nonaqueous samples such as O-rings, caps, and digested epidermis were counted in a toluene/PPO cocktail. Epidermal samples were digested in NCS solution (Amersham/Searle) for an hour before addition of the cocktail and subsequent counting. An internal standard was added to each vial to determine quench. Data were calculated as total cumulative absorption (percentage of dose) for comparison to in vivo data. At the end of each experiment, the residual activity in the skin and the diffusion cells was determined for balance.

In vivo percutaneous absorption in man was determined from intravenous and topical administration of [^{14}C] TCC to man. One microcurie of [^{14}C] TCC was dissolved in 1 ml of acetone and applied topically over 500 cm^2 of skin area of five subjects. Final topical concentration was 4 µg/cm^2. Urine was collected for 10 days and percutaneous absorption was determined by the ratio of ^{14}C excreted in urine following topical and intravenous administration.

RESULTS AND DISCUSSION

Table 1 summarizes the results on the in vitro and in vivo percutaneous absorption of triclocarban. A series of multiple, nonpaired t tests indicated significant differences between flow and static systems ($p < 0.01$), between adult abdominal skin and foreskin ($p < 0.025$), between newborn abdominal skin and foreskin ($p < 0.005$), and between adult and newborn foreskin ($p < 0.02$).

Table 1 In Vitro Percutaneous Absorption of Triclocarban in Adult and Newborn Abdominal and Foreskin Epidermis

Type	Dose absorbed (%, ± SD)
Static system, 37°C	
Human adult abdominal (n = 14)	0.23 ± 0.15
Human newborn abdominal (n = 6)	0.26 ± 0.28
Human infant abdominal (n = 4)	0.29 ± 0.09
Monkey adult abdominal (n = 6)	0.25 ± 0.09
Human adult foreskin (n = 4)	0.60 ± 0.25
Human newborn foreskin (n = 7)	2.5 ± 1.6
Static system, 23°C	
Human adult abdominal (n = 8)	0.13 ± 0.05
Continuous flow system, 23°C	
Human adult abdominal (n = 12)	6.0 ± 2.0
Man in vivo (n = 5)	7.0 ± 2.8

The total amount of residual radioactivity in each diffusion cell and skin was determined for balance. In each, 90% or more of the applied dose was accounted for. Most of the radioactivity resided with the skin. It was not determined whether the skin radioactivity was on the skin surface or on the skin.

The in vitro absorption using the static diffusion system was 0.23 ±0.15% of applied dose for human adult abdominal skin. Similar results were obtained for newborn (0.26 ±0.28%), infant (0.29 ±0.09%), and adult rhesus abdominal skin (0.25 ±0.09%). The results suggest no difference in percutaneous absorption of these skin types.

Human newborn foreskin is used as a source of human skin for in vitro diffusion studies. The in vitro absorption for newborn foreskin was 2.5 ±1.6%. This was 10-fold greater than human abdominal skin. Human adult foreskin absorption was 0.60 ±0.25%, suggesting that the newborn foreskin difference was possibly due to age (newborn) rather than site (foreskin), although probably both age and site contributed to the 10-fold difference.

Another variable in an in vitro diffusion system is solubility of chemical in the receptor fluid. If the chemical diffusing through skin is not soluble in the receptor fluid, the rate of diffusion is very slow and the chemical remains in the skin. This was ascertained for TCC, which has high lipid solubility and low water solubility (< 50 μg/liter) (Scharpf et al., 1975). In the static diffusion system set at room temperature (23°C), the absorption with human adult abdominal skin was 0.13 ±0.05%. With a continuous flow system absorption increased to 6.0 ±2.0%. The continuous flow system provides a larger sink (more volume) for the diffusing chemical to solubilize in. This is more analogous to the continual perfusion of blood in the in vivo situation. The percutaneous absorption of TCC in man was 7.0 ±2.8%. The continuous flow system, not the static diffusion system, would be predictive of TCC in vivo percutaneous absorption in man.

REFERENCES

Marty, J.-P. and Wepierre, J. (1979). Evaluation de la toxicité d'agents d'activité cosmétique, cas du trichlorocarbanilide. *Labo-Pharma-Problems Techn. 286*: 306-310.

Scharpf, L. G., Jr., Hill, I. D., and Maibach, H. (1975). Percutaneous penetration and disposition of triclocarban in man. *Arch. Environ. Health 30*: 7-14.

Wester, R. C. and Maibach, H. I. (1982). Comparative percutaneous absorption. In *Neonatal Skin, Structure and Function*. Edited by H. Maibach and E. Boisits. Dekker, New York, pp. 137-147.

17
In Vivo Percutaneous Absorption of Paraquat from Hands, Legs, and Forearm of Man

Ronald C. Wester, Howard I. Maibach, and Daniel A. W. Bucks
University of California School of Medicine, San Francisco, California

Michael B. Aufreret†
Standard Oil Company of California, Richmond, California

This study determines the in vivo percutaneous absorption of paraquat in man. Three skin sites of application were used in a crossover manner for six subjects. The percentages (± SD) of applied dose (9 $\mu g/cm^2$) absorbed were 0.29 ±0.2 for the leg, 0.23 ±0.1 for the hand, and 0.29 ±0.1 for the forearm. This gives an in vivo absorption rate of 0.03 $\mu g/cm^2$ for the 24-hr exposure. Paraquat can be absorbed in vivo through the skin of man, however it is considered to be a minimally absorbed chemical. Paraquat toxicity from dermal exposure has been reported; our findings confirm the possible systemic availability of paraquat from this route of exposure.

INTRODUCTION

Paraquat, used widely as a herbicide in agriculture, is highly toxic when taken orally; however, little information exists concerning its absorption through the skin. Bismuth and co-workers (1982, 1983), in reporting paraquat poisoning cases in France, suggested that body routes of entry other than ingestion may be significant. They refer specifically to the inhalation of paraquat, but Howard (1983) suggests that inhalation was not likely to have occurred. Paraquat dermal absorption thus appears a possible route for subsequent dermal toxicity. Newhouse (1978) reported the death and striking cutaneous lesions of a middle-aged woman after cutaneous contact with paraquat. Athanaselis et al. (1983) described

---

Reprinted from *J. Toxicol Environ. Health 14:* 759-762, 1984 with permission of the publisher.
†Deceased.

the death of a 64-year-old spray operator whose knapsack sprayer leaked 0.5% paraquat solution down his back for 3.5 hr. Other fatal and nonfatal intoxications attributed to dermal absorption have been reported (Athanaselis et al., 1983). Thus, safety hazard assessment of paraquat is necessary for dermal exposure, and for this the percutaneous absorption of paraquat in man needed to be determined.

MATERIALS AND METHODS

A stock solution of [^{14}C]paraquat (obtained from Chevron Standard Oil Company of California) was formulated in distilled water. Six volunteers were dosed with a volume of 50-μl paraquat solution spread over 70 cm^2 of skin surface area for a dose of 9 μg/cm^2 (5.3 μCi/mmol specific activity) bilaterally to the back of the legs, the ventral forearm, or the back of the hands in a crossover design. Volunteers were instructed not to wash the site for 24 hr. There were 2 weeks of washout between applications.

Urine samples were collected at 4, 8, and 12 hr the first day; then every 24 hr for 5 days. A 5-ml aliquot of each urine sample was mixed with 14 ml of PCS (Amersham/Searle, Chicago). A ^{14}C internal standard was added to a triplicate vial of each sample to determine the extent of quenching.

The percutaneous absorption of paraquat was determined by the ratio of ^{14}C urinary excretion following parenteral and topical application (Wester and Maibach, 1983). The risk of parenteral paraquat administration to man was considered; therefore paraquat was parenterally administered to rhesus monkeys, and the amount of urinary ^{14}C excretion in the monkey was used to correct for that amount of the dose that was excreted by other routes (feces, etc.) or retained in the body. In the rhesus, 58.6% of the parenterally administered dose was excreted in the urine; this value was used for man.

RESULTS

Table 1 gives the percutaneous absorption of paraquat in man following topical application to the legs, hands, and forearm. Total doses absorbed were 0.28 ±0.2% from the legs, 0.23 ±0.1% from the hands, and 0.29 ±0.1%, from the forearm, giving an in vivo absorption rate of 0.03 μg/cm^2 for the 24-hr exposure. Therefore, paraquat can be absorbed in vivo through the skin of man; however, it must be considered to be a low-absoring chemical. There was no difference in absorption ($p > 0.05$) with the different sites of application.

Table 1 Percutaneous Absorption of Paraquat in Man

Time (hr)	Dose absorbed (%, ± SD)		
	Leg	Hand	Forearm
0-4	0.02 ±0.02	0.04 ±0.02	0.03 ±0.01
4-8	0.02 ±0.02	0.03 ±0.02	0.01 ±0.01
8-12	0.02 ±0.01	0.02 ±0.02	0.02 ±0.01
12-24	0.01 ±0.01	0.03 ±0.02	0.04 ±0.01
24-48	0.04 ±0.04	0.05 ±0.03	0.04 ±0.02
48-72	0.06 ±0.06	0.02 ±0.01	0.04 ±0.02
72-96	0.06 ±0.05	0.02 ±0.01	0.04 ±0.01
96-120	0.06 ±0.05	0.02 ±0.02	0.04 ±0.01
Total	0.29 ±0.2	0.23 ±0.1	0.29 ±0.1

DISCUSSION

Dugard (1983) determined the in vitro percutaneous absorption rate of paraquat in human skin to be 0.5 µg per square centimeter of skin surface over an initial 24-hr period, the rate slowing to less than 0.1 µg/cm^2 thereafter. By comparison, the in vivo rate is 0.03 µg/cm^2. These results placed paraquat at the slow extreme of the range of absorption. An in vitro permeability constant of 0.73 × 10^5 cm^{-1}/hr for human skin was determined (M. Walker, P. H. Dugard, and R. C. Scott, personal communication, 1983). Values in other species studied (rat, hairless rat, nude rat, mouse, hairless mouse, rabbit, guinea pig) were 40-1460 times greater, suggesting that these animal models were not predictive of human skin. Maibach and Feldmann (1974) reported that the in vivo percutaneous absorption in the forearm of man of the closely related chemical diquat was 0.4% of applied dose when the site was open. This increased to 1.4% with occlusion, and to 3.8% when the skin site was damaged.

The reports above generally agree with our conclusion that paraquat is a minimally absorbed chemical in man. However, it is also obvious that paraquat can become systemically available through the skin and that the factors that affect percutaneous absorption (e.g., occlusion and skin damage, as mentioned for diquat) can enhance absorption (Wester and Maibach, 1983). Thus, paraquat toxicity is possible from dermal exposure; hence, appropriate precautions in handling the chemical should lead to decreased hazard.

Hayes (1967) summarized the general toxicity of paraquat in animal and man. In rat, the LD$_{50}$ was 110 mg/kg, while the 90-day LD$_{50}$ was 20.5 mg/kg, a chronicity factor of 5. We do not know whether the percutaneous absorption of single-dose paraquat is the same as for chronic-dose exposure.

Wester and Maibach (1983) presented an overview of the regional (anatomical) variation in percutaneous absorption. This study presents the first in vivo human data for the legs and hands compared to the forearm.

REFERENCES

Athanaselis, S., Qammaz, S., Alevisopoulos, G., and Koutselinis, A. (1983). Percutaneous paraquat intoxication. *J. Toxicol. Cutan. Ocul. Toxicol. 20*: 3-5.

Binns, C. W. (1976). A deadly cure for lice. A case of paraquat poisoning. *Papua New Guinea Med. J. 19*: 105.

Bismuth, C. (1983). Response by the authors: Letter to the editor. *J. Toxicol. Clin. Toxicol. 20*: 195-196.

Bismuth, C., Garnier, R., Dally, S., Fournier, P. E., and Scherrmann, J. M. (1982). Prognosis and treatment of paraquat poisoning: A review of 28 cases. *J. Toxicol. 19*: 461-474.

Hayes, W. (1967). The 90-day LD_{50} and chronicity factor as a measure of toxicity. *Toxicol. Appl. Pharmacol. 11*: 327-335.

Howard, J. K. (1983). The myth of paraquat inhalation as a route for human poisoning. *J. Toxicol. Clin. Toxicol. 20*: 191-193.

Maibach, H. I. and Feldmann, R. (1974). Systemic absorption of pesticides through the skin of man. In Occupational Exposure to Pesticides: Report to the Federal Working Group on Pest Management from the Task Group, pp. 120-127.

Newhouse, M., McEvoy, D., and Rosenthal, D. (1978). Percutaneous paraquat absorption. *Arch. Dermatol. 114*: 1516-1519.

Walker, M., McEvoy, D., and Rosentha., D. (1978). Percutaneous paraquat absorption. *Arch. Dermatol. 114*: 1516-1519.

Wester, R. C. and Maibach, H. I. (1983). Cutaneous pharmacokinetics: 10 steps to percutaneous absorption. *Drug Metab. Rev. 14*: 169-205.

18
Influence of Hydration on Percutaneous Absorption

Ronald C. Wester and Howard I. Maibach
University of California School of Medicine, San Francisco, California

Water plays an extremely important role in the rate of absorption of materials through skin. Water can act as a common vehicle and as the stratum corneum's endogenous plasticizer. Under normal conditions, the stratum corneum is always partially hydrated. A gradient in water concentration exists through the tissue corresponding to an average water concentration of approximately 0.9 g per gram of dry tissue weight. This amount of water in in vitro studies increases the rate of absorption of the stratum corneum approximately 10-fold over its value when perfectly dry (Scheuplein, 1978). Upon additional contact with liquid water, the stratum corneum can ultimately absorb three to five times its own weight in water. This further hydration results in an additional approximate two- to threefold increase in the rate of absorption to water and other polar molecules. Figure 1 illustrates the increase in steroid absorption observed in vitro when water vapor is allowed to come into contact with dry stratum corneum having a surface deposit of cortisone. The initial rate of absorption (J_s) with "dry" stratum corneum was 2.64×10^{-11}. The introduction of water vapor increased the rate to 3.62×10^{-10}, a logarithmic increase in rate of absorption. The reintroduction of Drierite and subsequent decrease in water content decreased the rate to 2.7×10^{-11}.

EARLY STUDIES

Stoughton (1965) studied the in vivo and in vitro rates of absorption of ethyl nicotinate for skin hydrated by warm or cold water immersion. Excised human skin is mounted over a well containing saline and the stratum corneum of the

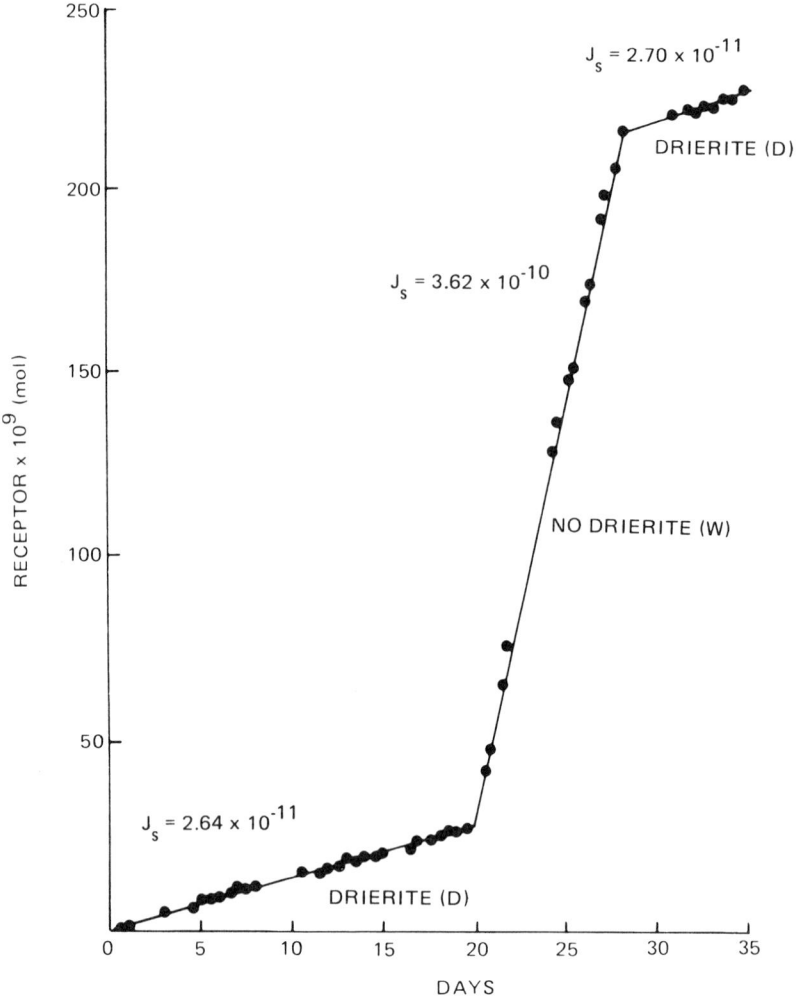

Figure 1 Effect of water vapor and the permeation of cortisone through stratum corneum. (From Scheuplein, 1978.)

epidermis remains exposed to the air. Ethyl nicotinate labeled with ^{14}C is applied to the epidermis surface, and the rate of appearance of radioactivity in the saline below taken as the rate of absorption of ethyl nicotinate. Table 1 indicates that hydrated skin allowed about five times as much ethyl nicotinate to pass through as skin not previously hydrated. Table 2 expresses results obtained when determining the minimum concentration of ethyl nicotinate necessary to produce

Table 1 Penetration of Ethyl Nicotinate After Hydration of the Skin (30-min period for penetration)

	Number of subjects	Average penetration (%)
Warm water	4	5.80
Cold water	4	5.88
Control	8	0.98

Source: Stoughton (1965).

erythema on the forearms of human volunteers. One forearm was soaked in warm or cool water for 30 min before the application of graded concentrations of ethyl nicotinate. The nonhydrated arm required about 5-10 times the concentration of ethyl nicotinate to produce erythema as did the hydrated arm. The author concluded that the increased rate of absorption with hydration caused the clinical changes in the epidermis.

Munies and Wurster (1965) examined the rate of absorption of methyl ethyl ketone from hydrated stratum corneum. Figure 2 shows the data obtained in comparing the absorption from a normal skin surface to that of a hydrated surface in the same individual. The upper curve shows the concentration under hydrous conditions after only 40 sec. The influence of moisture is great. After only 40 sec the expiration of methyl ethyl ketone was 13.5 μg per/liter of expired

Table 2 In Vivo Hydration of Human Skin Factor: Difference in End-Point Concentrations of Ethyl Nicotinate Giving Erythema on Hydrated and Nonhydrated Arms

Warm water hydration (30 min; 22 subjects)	
Hydrated arm average	0.0017
Nonhydrated arm average	0.02
Factor difference = 12	
Cool water hydration (30 min; 15 subjects)	
Hydrated arm average	0.003
Nonhydrated arm average	0.02
Factor difference = 6	

Source: Stoughton (1965).

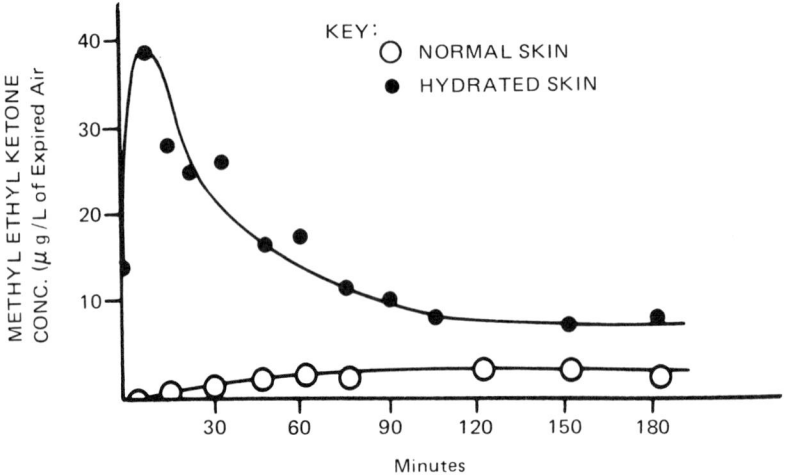

Figure 2 Expired air data showing the influence of moisture on the percutaneous absorption of methyl ethyl ketone. (From Munies and Wurster, 1965.)

air, which is much greater than the plateau value of normal skin. Figures 3 and 4, extensions of the work by Munies and Wurster (1965), show that hydration continued to enhance the rate of absorption of methyl ethyl ketone in man.

Piotrowski (1967) studied the effects of temperature and humidity on the rate of absorption of nitrobenzene vapor through skin. Table 3 shows the influence of humidity on the rate of absorption of nitrobenzene. With the temperature kept constant at 25°C, a humidity increase of 35-67% increased the rate of absorption of nitrobenzene through human skin from 0.25 to 0.38 mg/hr. Thus, the humidity (i.e., water vapor) increased the rate of absorption of nitrobenzene.

Wurster and Kramer (1961) measured the rate of absorption of acetylsalicylic acid through skin. When the tissue was hydrated, the rate of absorption of the most water-soluble ester increased more than that of the other esters studied. This work was extended by Fritz and Stoughton (1963). Full hydration of the keratin (accomplished by layering water over acetylsalicylic acid on the epidermal surface) dramatically increased the rate of absorption when compared to conditions of lower humidity at the same temperature.

The early work of McKenzie and Stoughton (1962) showed the importance of hydration on skin by employing occlusive plastic film in steroid therapy. They showed that the rate of absorption of corticoid steroids could be increased substantially by occluding the site of application. This prevents the loss of water vapor from the skin and thus hydrates the stratum corneum. Vehicles may also affect skin penetration by their ability to reduce water vapor loss from the skin

Hydration and Percutaneous Absorption 235

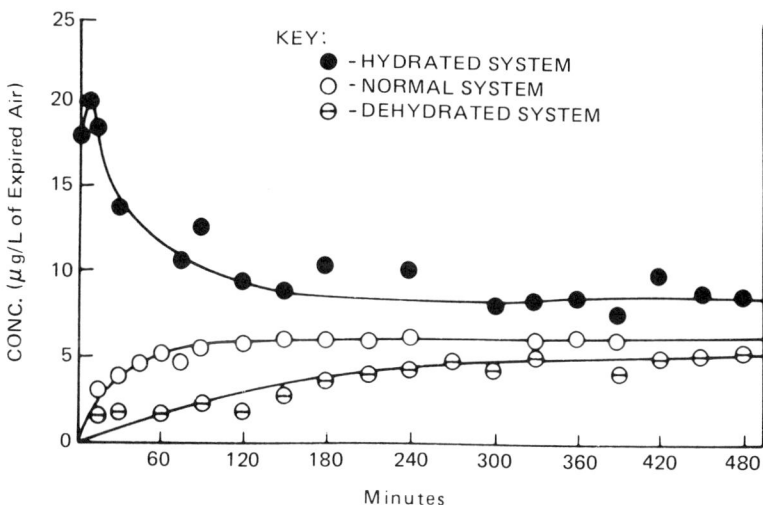

Figure 3 Individual expired air elimination data showing the influence of hydration and dehydration on the percutaneous absorption of methyl ethyl ketone. (From Munies and Wurster, 1965.)

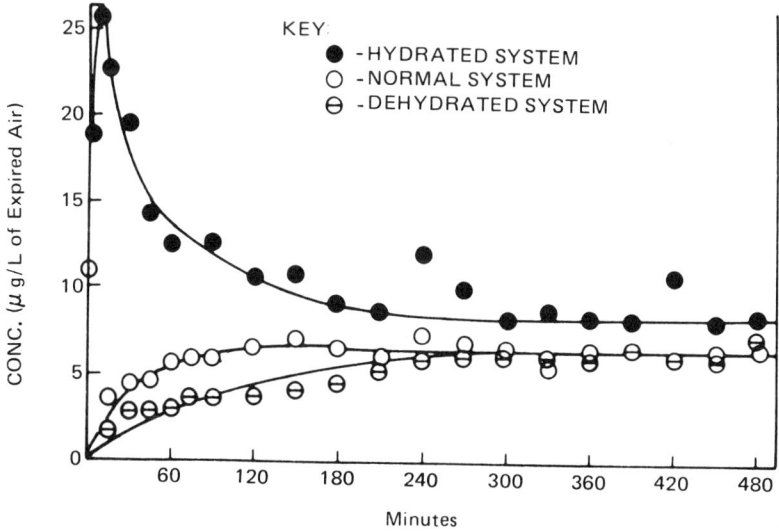

Figure 4 Average expired air elimination data showing the influence of hydration and dehydration on the percutaneous absorption of methyl ethyl ketone. (From Munies and Wurster, 1965.)

Table 3 Effects of Temperature and Humidity on the Absorption of Nitrobenzene Vapor Through the Skin[a]

Series	Number of experiments	Temperature (°C)	Humidity (%)	Absorbed doses of nitrobenzene (mg)[b]	Absorbed rate per unit of concentration (mg/hr:μg/liter)
3	3	25	35	19, 16, 10 (15)	0.25
5	3	30	25	13, 16, 10 (13)	0.22
6	4	25	67	18, 34, 18, 24 (23)	0.38

[a]Other conditions were as follows: air concentration, to μg/liter, persons naked; time of exposure, 6 hr.
[b]Mean values are shown in parentheses.
Source: Piotrowski (1967).

surface. Of the common vehicles, paraffin bases have shown the greatest effect on suppressing a transepidermal water diffusion. Most vehicles develop a high degree of occlusion and thus increase the rate of absorption of materials.

RECENT WORK

Behl and co-workers (1980) studied the influence of hydration on alkanol permeation through the skin of the hairless mouse. The skin was immersed in saline for up to 30 hr and a steady-state rate of permeation was established in several minutes. These circumstances allowed multiple sequential runs over a period in which the permeability coefficients of some chemicals were gradually changing. The permeabilities of water, methanol, and ethanol were slightly affected by hydration. However, there was a doubling of the permeability coefficient of butanol and hexanol during the first 10 hr of immersion. More hydrophobic alkanols seem to be less sensitive to the aqueous conditioning. Table 4 and Figure 5 illustrate the results of the study.

Behl and Barrett (1981) examined the possible effects of hydration on barrier integrity of Swiss mouse skin using water, methanol, ethanol, and butanol as permeants, and the previously described procedure involving multiple sequential permeation runs on skin. The permeation rate of water increased almost linearly up to 30 hr of hydration, then tended to level off. Transport rates of methanol and ethanol increased, and then plateaued at about 15 hr. These results contrast with the earlier findings of hairless mouse skin, where the permeabilities of these three compounds were unaffected by aqueous immersion. The permeation rate of butanol also increased during the first 15 hr of hydration, then gradually declined over the next 25 hr. The results again contrast with the hairless mouse species, in which butanol permeability doubled in 10 hr and then plateaued. The results of this study are summarized in Table 5, showing the hydration effects on water, methanol, ethanol, and butanol. Thus, we see the influence of a second variable (source of skin) on data of hydration and skin.

A recent study examined the effect of multiple-dose applications on malathion in vivo percutaneous absorption in the guinea pig (J.-P. Marty, personal communication, 1984). The sites of skin application were either washed or not washed between daily malathion applications. Figure 6 shows that daily malathion applications without daily wash produced no change in percutaneous absorption. However, when daily skin washes were included, percutaneous absorption increased as the multiple dose (and multiple washings) increased.

Table 4 Summary of the Average Permeability Coefficients P ($\times 10^4$ cm/hr $\pm$ SD) and Average Ratios as a Function of Hydration Time

Hydration time (hr)	[^{3}H]Water, 8 skins	[^{14}C]Ethanol, 8 skins	Average ratio $\pm$ SD[a] $[Pc_2 + PH_2O]$
0.5	1.6 $\pm$ 0.6	2.1 $\pm$ 0.7	1.4 $\pm$ 0.1
5.5	1.5 $\pm$ 0.5	2.2 $\pm$ 0.6	1.6 $\pm$ 0.2
10.5	1.4 $\pm$ 0.5	2.3 $\pm$ 0.7	1.6 $\pm$ 0.2
15.5	1.3 $\pm$ 0.4	2.2 $\pm$ 0.6	1.8 $\pm$ 0.2
20.5	1.3 $\pm$ 0.4	2.1 $\pm$ 0.6	1.7 $\pm$ 0.2
25.5	1.2 $\pm$ 0.4	2.0 $\pm$ 0.6	1.8 $\pm$ 0.3
29.5	1.1 $\pm$ 0.3	1.9 $\pm$ 0.6	1.8 $\pm$ 0.2
	[^{3}H]Methanol, 4 skins	[^{14}C]Ethanol, 4 skins	$[Pc_2 + Pc_1]$
0.3	1.8 $\pm$ 0.3	2.0 $\pm$ 0.4	1.1 $\pm$ 0.0
5.8	1.6 $\pm$ 0.4	2.0 $\pm$ 0.5	1.3 $\pm$ 0.1
9.8	1.7 $\pm$ 0.6	2.1 $\pm$ 0.7	1.2 $\pm$ 0.1
13.8	1.9 $\pm$ 0.7	2.3 $\pm$ 0.8	1.2 $\pm$ 0.1
17.8	1.8 $\pm$ 0.6	2.1 $\pm$ 0.6	1.2 $\pm$ 0.1
26.3	1.8 $\pm$ 0.5	2.2 $\pm$ 0.4	1.2 $\pm$ 0.2
	[^{3}H]Methanol, 4 skins	[^{14}C]Butanol, 4 skins	$[Pc_4 + Pc_1]$
0.3	2.9 $\pm$ 0.6	6.5 $\pm$ 0.9	2.3 $\pm$ 0.2
4.3	2.6 $\pm$ 0.5	8.2 $\pm$ 0.9	3.3 $\pm$ 1.0
7.8	2.3 $\pm$ 0.5	11.8 $\pm$ 2.0	4.7 $\pm$ 0.7
11.3	2.8 $\pm$ 0.7	12.4 $\pm$ 2.4	4.5 $\pm$ 0.7
14.3	2.5 $\pm$ 0.9	11.9 $\pm$ 3.3	4.8 $\pm$ 0.3
26.3	2.4[b]	11.5[b]	4.8[b]
0.3	1.7 $\pm$ 0.6	4.2 $\pm$ 1.2	2.6 $\pm$ 0.3
5.8	1.6 $\pm$ 0.6	6.8 $\pm$ 2.2	4.4 $\pm$ 0.7
9.8	1.5 $\pm$ 0.6	7.3 $\pm$ 2.0	5.2 $\pm$ 0.6
13.8	1.5 $\pm$ 0.5	7.5 $\pm$ 2.0	5.3 $\pm$ 0.6
17.8	1.4 $\pm$ 0.5	7.3 $\pm$ 2.0	5.2 $\pm$ 0.5
26.3	1.5 $\pm$ 0.5	7.9 $\pm$ 2.1	5.3 $\pm$ 0.5

Table 4 (Continued)

Hydration time (hr)	[^{3}H]Methanol, 8 skins	[^{14}C]Hexanol, 8 skins	Average ratio ± SD[a] $[Pc_2 + P_1]$
0.8	2.1 ± 1.0	19.4 ± 7.8	9.6 ± 1.2
5.0	1.8 ± 0.7	28.6 ± 9.6	16.4 ± 3.9
10.0	1.9 ± 0.8	38.6 ± 12.3	21.3 ± 2.0
15.0	1.9 ± 0.8	37.4 ± 11.2	21.1 ± 3.4
20.0	1.9 ± 0.9	37.4 ± 11.9	20.8 ± 3.5
28.0	2.0 ± 0.9	38.1 ± 11.5	20.4 ± 3.4
	[^{3}H]Methanol, 4 skins	[^{14}C]Heptanol, 4 skins	$[Pc_6 + Pc_1]$
0.5	6.1 ± 1.9	65.9 ± 24.4	10.9 ± 1.2
5.0	5.7 ± 1.6	80.7 ± 39.4	13.8 ± 3.4
10.0	5.2 ± 1.6	101.4 ± 24.2	19.8 ± 1.8
15.0	6.0 ± 1.8	97.9 ± 27.2	16.6 ± 1.8
20.0	6.3 ± 1.9	102.6 ± 23.9	16.8 ± 2.0
25.0	6.2 ± 1.7	101.5 ± 22.0	16.8 ± 1.5
30.0	5.8 ± 1.6	99.4 ± 22.6	17.4 ± 1.7
	[^{3}H]Methanol, 8 skins	[^{14}C]Octanol, 8 skins	$[Pc_8 + Pc_1]$
0.8	2.3 ± 0.9	78.2 ± 10.8	36.3 ± 9.1
6.2	2.2 ± 0.7	120.8 ± 11.9	61.5 ± 25.1
10.0	2.2 ± 0.7	94.5 ± 14.8	48.2 ± 22.2
15.0	2.3 ± 0.8	93.1 ± 16.7	45.0 ± 19.8
22.0	2.5 ± 1.0	94.8 ± 10.8	45.3 ± 22.2
27.0	2.6 ± 1.0	97.0 ± 17.7	43.6 ± 21.0

[a]Ratio averages are the average of the individually computed ratios, not the ratio of the averaged values.
[b]Three skins were damaged.
Source: Behl et al. (1980).

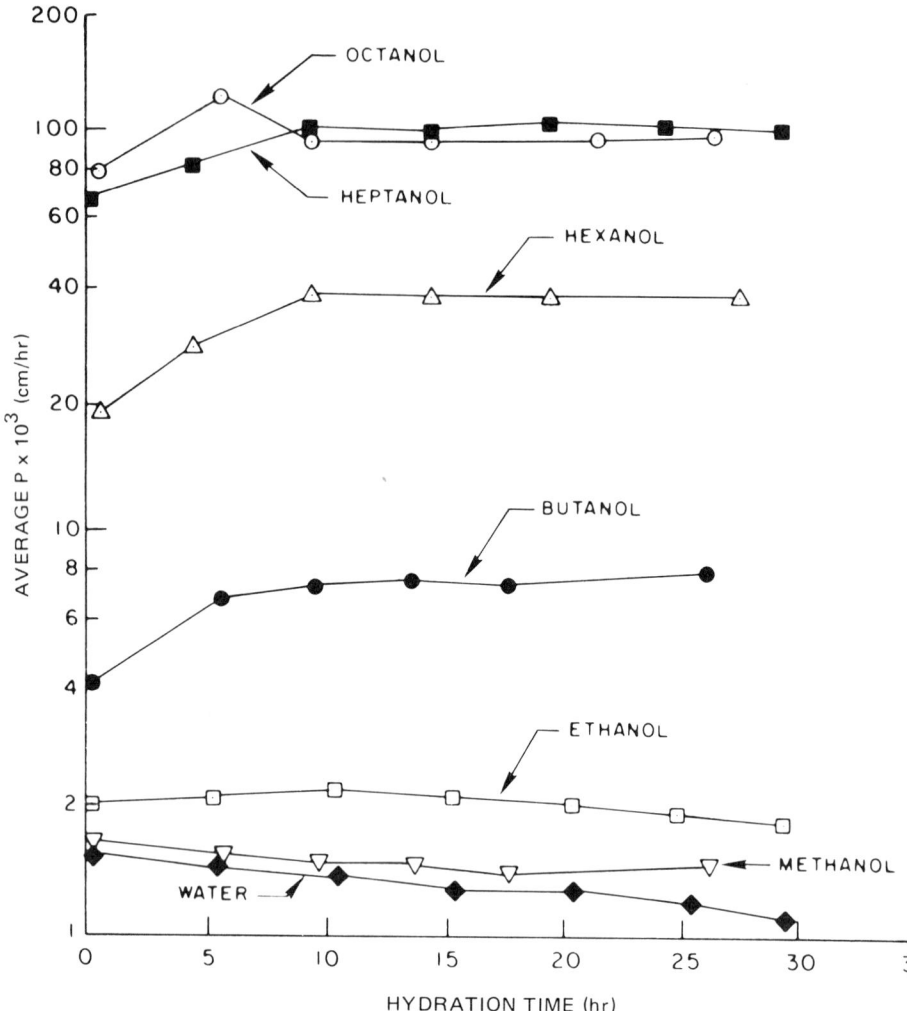

Figure 5 Semilogarithmic display of a consecutive set of averaged permeability coefficients (P_{avg}) for each compound studied. The values span a range from slightly over 1×10^3 cm/hr for heptanol and octanol. Hydration effects are easily distinguishable for butanol and hexanol, even on the logarithmic scale. (From Behl et al., 1980.)

Table 5 Summary of Hydration Effects

Hydration time (hr)	Hydration effect (%)[a]			
	Water	Methanol	Ethanol	Butanol
0	0.0	0.0	0.0	0.0
5	27.5	20.4	31.3	61.8
10	50.0	37.0	46.9	77.6
15	85.0	66.7	71.9	114.5
20	122.5	74.1	81.3	105.3
25	140.0	81.5	87.5	101.3
30	172.5	75.9	96.9	94.7
43[b] or 48[c]	192.5	81.5	84.4	81.6

[a] Percentage hydration effect $= \dfrac{P \text{ (at a given hydration time)} - P \text{ (at zero hydration)}}{P \text{ (at zero hydration)}} \times 100$

[b] Methanol and butanol.
[c] Water and ethanol.
Source: Behl and Barrett (1981).

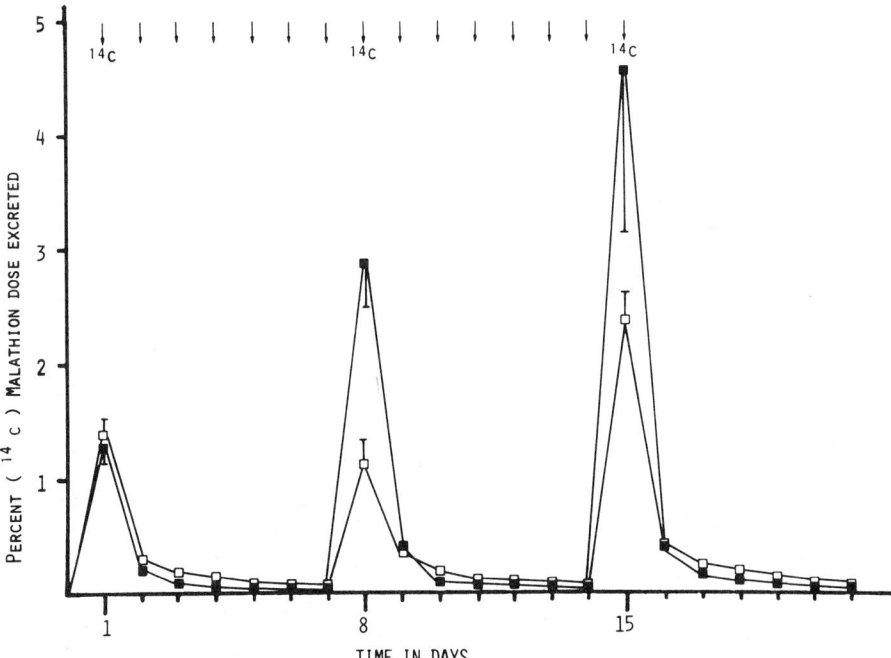

Figure 6 Percutaneous absorption of malathion in the guinea pig following multiple daily applications with (■) and without (□) multiple daily skin washing. Arrow represents malathion dose application; ^{14}C indicates where radiolabeled malathion was used. (From J. P. Marty, Personal Communication.)

DIRECTIONS FOR FUTURE WORK

The manner in which hydration increases the rate of absorption through the stratum corneum has not been determined. Water-soluble extractive substances compose 20-40% of normal stratum corneum by weight. The strongly hydroscopic properties of these water-soluble compounds suggest a prominent role for them in regulating the water content of stratum corneum cells. The removal of some of these substances following excessive exposure to water may compromise barrier cell permeability. Excessive water uptake may further impede barrier function in the stratum corneum by facilitating intracellular passage through otherwise tightly packed keratin and perhaps by inducing swelling or even bursting of cell membranes. Also, the enhanced water content of extracellular nucleopolysaccharide substances might impair intracellular adhesiveness. Certainly the gross irritability of the stratum corneum is significantly increased by excessive hydration (Malkinson, 1965).

We believe that understanding the mechanisms involved in hydrating effects on skin must lead to new pharmacological potential.

REFERENCES

Behl, C. R. and Barrett, M. (1981). Hydration and percutaneous absorption. II. Influence of hydration on water and alkanol permeation through Swiss mouse skin; Comparison with hairless mouse. *J. Pharm. Sci. 10*(11): 1212-1215.

Behl, C. R., Flynn, G. L., Kurihara, T., Harper, N., Smith, W., Higuchi, W. I., Ho, N. F. H., and Pierson, C. L. (1980). Hydration and percutaneous absorption. I. Influence of hydration on alkanol permeation through hairless mouse skin. *J. Invest. Dermatol. 75*: 346-352.

Fritz and Stoughton, R. B. (1960). *J. Invest. Dermatol. 82*: 24.

Fritz, W. F. and Stoughton, R. B. (1963). The effect of temperature and humidity on the penetration of ^{14}C acetylsalicylic acid in excised human skin. *J. Invest. Dermatol. 41*: 307-312.

Malkinson, F. D. (1965). Industrial problems relating to the stratum corneum. *Arch. Environ. Health 11*: 538-545.

McKenzie, A. W. and Stoughton, R. B. (1962). Method for comparing percutaneous absorption of steroids. *Arch. Dermatol. 86*: 608-610.

Munies, R. and Wurster, D. D. (1965). Factors influencing percutaneous absorption. II. Absorption of methyl ethyl ketone. *J. Pharm. Sci. 54*: 554-556.

Piotrowski, J. (1967). Further investigations on the evaluation of exposure to nitrobenzene. *Br. J. Ind. Med. 24*: 60-65.

Scheuplein, R. J. (1978). Site variations and permeability. In *The Physiology and Pathophysiology of the Skin*, Vol. 5. Edited by A. Jarrett. Academic, New York, pp. 1731-1752.

Stoughton, R. B. (1965). Percutaneous absorption. *Arch. Environ. Health 11*: 551-554.

Wurster, D. E. and Kramer, S. F. (1961). Investigation of some factors influencing percutaneous absorption. *J. Pharm. Sci. 50*: 288-293.

METHODOLOGY

19
In Vivo Methods for Percutaneous Absorption Measurements

Ronald C. Wester and Howard I. Maibach
University of California School of Medicine, San Francisco, California

IMPORTANCE OF IN VIVO PERCUTANEOUS ABSORPTION

There is a persistent belief that skin viability has little importance in percutaneous absorption. This concept of skin as a passive membrane has led to the domination of the study of percutaneous absorption by laws of mass action and physical diffusion. This concept has also led investigators to use skin excised from cadavers (human and animal) and then to physically (e.g., by freezing or heat separation) and chemically isolate skin sheets or sections and determine chemical diffusion across these treated tissues.

A consequence of this earlier concept was the designation of the stratum corneum as the barrier to percutaneous absorption. Many compounds such as low molecular weight alcohols were studied, and the barrier properties of the isolated stratum corneum were demonstrated for these chemicals. It has then been assumed that the stratum corneum is the primary barrier for all compounds.

The need to study percutaneous absorption has its reality in dermatoxicity, where compounds pose a threat to human health, and to dermatopharmacology, where drugs need to be delivered into and through the skin to treat disease both locally (skin disease) and systemically (transdermal delivery). Most compounds and defined drugs that are of interest and concern in dermatotoxicology and dermatopharmacology are lipophilic. The stratum corneum, the supposed barrier to percutaneous absorption, is a lipid-saturated tissue that is like a sink to topically applied lipotropic materials; its function more closely approximates that of a sponge capable of absorbing a quantity of material, limited only by the solubility of the chemical in sebaceous and epidermal lipids.

The chemical and physical properties of the topical vehicle and the barrier/sink properties of the living stratum corneum determine the initial absorption of compounds into the skin. The vitality of the living skin will determine the metabolism, distribution, and excretion of the compounds through the skin and the body.

We cannot in this chapter define and discuss all the factors that determine the nature of in vivo percutaneous absorption. That is the mission of this book, and many of the important aspects of in vivo percutaneous absorption have their own chapters. We discuss only some of the methodology and its limitations, only pointing out the steps of in vivo percutaneous absorption as we understand them.

IN VIVO METHODS

Radioactivity in Excreta

Percutaneous absorption in vivo is usually determined by the indirect method of measuring radioactivity in excreta following topical application of the labeled compound. In human studies plasma levels of compound are extremely low following topical application, often below assay detection level, so it is necessary to use tracer methodology. The compound, usually labeled with ^{14}C or tritium, is applied and the total amount of radioactivity excreted in urine or urine plus feces determined. The amount of radioactivity retained in the body or excreted by some route not assayed (CO_2, sweat) is corrected for by determining the amount of radioactivity excreted following parenteral administration. This final amount of radioactivity is then expressed as the percentage of applied dose that was absorbed (Feldmann and Maibach, 1969, 1970, 1974).

The equation used to determine percutaneous absorption is:

$$\text{Percent} = \frac{\text{total radioactivity following topical administration}}{\text{total radioactivity following parenteral administration}} \times 100$$

The limitation on determining percutaneous absorption from urinary and/or fecal radioactivity is that the methodology does not account for metabolism by skin. The radioactivity in urine is a mixture of parent compound and metabolites. This type of information is useful in defining the total disposition of the applied topical dose. Because the nature of the radioactivity is undefined, kinetic interpretation should be severely limited.

Radioactivity in Blood

Plasma radioactivity can be measured and the percutaneous absorption determined by the ratio of the areas under the plasma concentration versus time curves following topical and intravenous administration (Wester and Noonan,

1978). Note that radioactivity in blood can include both the applied compound and metabolites, thus, the same limitations discussed for excreta also apply here. This method has given results similar to those obtained from urinary excretion (Wester et al., 1983).

Surface Recovery

Another approach to finding in vivo percutaneous absorption is to determine the loss of material from the surface as it penetrates into the skin. Skin recovery from an ointment or solution application is difficult because total recovery of compound from the skin is never assured. With topical application of a transdermal delivery device, the total unit can be removed from the skin and the residual amount of drug in the device determined. It is assumed that the difference between applied dose and residual dose is the amount of drug absorbed.

Surface Disappearance

Related to surface recovery, it is possible to monitor the disappearance of ^{14}C from the surface of skin using appropriate instrumentation. The limitation on this methodology is that the disappearance is due both to movement of ^{14}C-labeled chemical into the skin and to the quenching effect of the skin on the β rays bouncing back to the instrument. This can be simply demonstrated by applying a quantity of radiolabeled chemical on a surface, placing a sheet of stratum corneum over the radiolabeled chemical, and then measuring the radioactivity with an external device. The device will record some radioactivity (β rays penetrating total stratum corneum), yet the radiolabeled chemical is on the other side of the stratum corneum. The degree of quench of chemical in the various cell layers of the skin has not been defined.

Biological/Pharmacological Response

Another in vivo method of estimating absorption is to use a biological/pharmacological response (McKenzie and Stoughton, 1962). Biological assay is substituted for a chemical assay, and absorption is estimated. An obvious disadvantage is that biological responses are limited to compounds that elicit responses that can be measured easily and accurately. An example of a biological response would be the vasoconstrictor assay when the blanching effect of one compound is compared to a known compound. This method is more qualitative than quantitative.

Other qualitative methods of estimating in vivo percutaneous absorption include whole body autoradiography and fluorescence. While body autoradiography provides an overall picture of the dermal absorption followed by the involvement of other body tissues.

Table 1 Absolute Bioavailability of Topical Nitroglycerin

Method	Mean bioavailability (%)
Plasma nitroglycerin AUC[a]	56.6 ± 2.5
Plasma total radioactivity AUC[a]	77.2 ± 6.7
Urinary total radioactivity[b]	72.7 ± 5.8

[a]Absolute bioavailability of nitroglycerin and ^{14}C:
$$\text{Percent} = \frac{\text{AUC (ng/hr·ml)}}{\text{topical dose}} \bigg/ \frac{\text{AUC (ng/hr·ml)}}{\text{intravenous dose}} \times 100$$
[b]Percent =
$$\frac{\text{total }^{14}\text{C excretion after topical administration}}{\text{total }^{14}\text{C excretion after intravenous administration}} \times 100$$
Source: Adapted from Wester et al. (1983).

Absolute Topical Bioavailability

The only way to determine the absolute bioavailability of a topically applied compound is to measure the compound by specific assay in blood or urine following topical and intravenous administration. This is extremely difficult to do in plasma, since concentrations after topical administration are often low. However, when advances in analytical methodology bring forth more sensitive assays, estimates of absolute topical bioavailability will become a reality.

A comparative example of three methods (Wester and Noonan, 1978) was done using [^{14}C] nitroglycerin in the rhesus monkey (Table 1). Topical bioavailability estimated from urinary excretion was 72.7 ±5.8%. This was similar to the 77.2 ±6.7% estimated from plasma total radioactivity AUC (area under curve of plasma concentration versus time). The absolute bioavailability estimated from plasma nitroglycerin unchanged compound AUCs was 56.6 ±2.5%. The estimates from plasma ^{14}C and urinary ^{14}C were in good agreement. Also the difference in estimate between that of the absolute bioavailability (56.6%) and that of ^{14}C (72.7-77.2%) is the percentage of compound metabolized in the skin as the compound was being absorbed. For nitroglycerin this is about 20% (Wester and Maibach, 1983).

FACTORS AND STEPS IN PERCUTANEOUS ABSORPTION

Wester and Maibach (1983) defined the steps (Table 2) that require consideration when determining in vivo percutaneous absorption. Many of these individual steps have been expanded into chapters of this book. Each step is important, and in vivo percutaneous absorption is a summation of all these steps.

Table 2 10 Steps to Percutaneous Absorption

1. Vehicle release
2. Absorption kinetics
   a. Skin site of application
   b. Individual variation
   c. Skin condition
   d. Occlusion
   e. Drug concentration and surface area
   f. Multiple dose application
3. Excretion kinetics
4. Effective cellular and tissue distribution
5. Substantivity (nonpenetrating surface adsorption)
6. Wash and rub resistance/decontamination
7. Volatility
8. Binding
9. Anatomic pathways
10. Cutaneous metabolism

Source: Wester et al. (1983).

REFERENCES

Feldmann, R. J. and Maibach, H. I. (1969). Percutaneous penetration of steroids in man. *J. Invest. Dermatol.* 52: 89-94.

Feldmann, R. J. and Maibach, H. I. (1970). Absorption of some organic compounds through the skin in man. *J. Invest. Dermatol.* 54: 399-404.

Feldmann, R. J. and Maibach, H. I. (1974). Percutaneous penetration of some pesticides and herbicides in man. *Toxicol. Appl. Pharmacol.* 28: 126-132.

McKenzie, A. W. and Stoughton, R. B. (1962). Method for comparing percutaneous absorption of steroids. *Arch. Dermatol.* 86: 608-610.

Wester, R. C. and Noonan, P. K. (1978). Topical bioavailability of a potential antiacne agent (SC-23110) as determined by cumulative excretion and areas under plasma concentration-time curves. *J. Invest. Dermatol.* 70: 92-94.

Wester, R. C. and Maibach, H. I. (1983). Cutaneous pharmacokinetics: 10 steps to percutaneous absorption. *Drug Metab. Rev.* 14: 169-205.

Wester, R. C., Noonan, P. K., Smeach, S., and Kosobud, L. (1983). Pharmacokinetics and bioavailability of intravenous and topical nitroglycerin in the rhesus monkey. Estimate of percutaneous first-pass metabolism. *J. Pharm. Sci.* 72: 745-748.

20
In Vivo Animal Models for Percutaneous Absorption

Ronald C. Wester and Howard I. Maibach
University of California School of Medicine, San Francisco, California

The ideal way to determine the penetration potential of a compound in man is to do the actual study in man. Mechanisms and parameters of percutaneous absorption elucidated in vivo with human skin are most relevant to the clinical situation. However, many compounds are potentially too toxic to test in vivo in man and so their percutaneous absorption must be done in animals. Likewise, until more complete animal to human validation studies become available, not all investigators will have access to human volunteers. Mechanism studies and studies on parameters affecting absorption must therefore be explored using animals and in vitro techniques. This chapter discusses the validity of animal models for percutaneous absorption.

COMPARATIVE IN VIVO STUDIES

The basic data for in vivo human percutaneous absorption, to which animal models are compared, were obtained from Feldmann and Maibach (1969a,b, 1974). In these clinical studies a specific concentration of radioactive compound (4 $\mu g/cm^2$) was applied to a specific anatomical site (ventral forearm); the area was not occluded, and subjects were requested not to wash the area for 24 hr. The radioactive compounds were applied to the skin in an acetone solution and the acetone quickly evaporated with a gentle stream of air. Urine was collected for 5 days and assayed for radioactivity. A tracer dose was also given parenterally, and the percentage of radioactivity in the urine following parenteral adminis-

---

Reprinted from *Models in Dermatology*, vol. 2. Edited by H. I. Maibach and F. N. Marzulli. Copyright © 1985, Karger, Basel, pp. 159-169, with permission of the publisher.

tration was used to correct for compound that might be excreted by some other route and for compound that might be retained within the body.

Bartek et al. (1972) undertook a comparative study of percutaneous absorption in rats, rabbits, miniature swine, and man. Methodology in the animals was similar to that in man except that in animals the compounds were applied to the skin of the back and the site of application was shaved. Radioactive compounds were applied to the skin in the same manner that had been used in man. A nonoccluding device was used to keep the animal from removing the applied compound.

Haloprogin, a topical antifungal agent, was completely absorbed in the rat and rabbit. Penetration through the skin of pigs and man was similar and much slower than it was through rat and rabbit skin. Penetration of acetylcysteine was minimal in all species. Cortisone, a minimal penetrant through the skin of man and miniature swine, was well absorbed in the rat and rabbit. Caffeine readily penetrated the skin of all species. Penetration of butter yellow through rabbit skin was much greater than through the skin of the other three species. Testosterone penetration was greatest in the rabbit, followed closely by the rat, and then the pig, which was closest to man. This study showed rabbit skin to be the most permeable to topically applied compounds, followed closely by rat skin. In contrast, it appears that the permeability of the skin of the miniature swine is closer to that of human skin (Table 1). Clearly, percutaneous absorption in the rabbit and rat would not be predictive of that in man. It is not known whether the subtle differences seen between pig and human skin were due to methodology (site of application, shaving) or to the skin itself. However, generally the pig appears to be a good predictor of percutaneous absorption in man. Figure 1 summarizes the results.

Bartek and La Budde (1975) also studied the percutaneous absorption of pesticides in the rabbit, pig, and squirrel monkey and compared the results with

Table 1 Percutaneous Absorption of Several Compounds by Rat, Rabbit, Pig, and Man (in vivo)

Penetrant	Dose absorbed (%)			
	Rat	Rabbit	Pig	Man
Haloprogin	95.8	113.0	19.7	11.0
Acetylcysteine	3.5	2.0	6.0	2.4
Cortisone	24.7	30.3	4.1	3.4
Caffeine	53.1	69.2	32.4	47.6
Butter yellow	48.2	100.0	41.9	21.6
Testosterone	47.4	69.6	29.4	13.2

Source: Bartek et al. (1972).

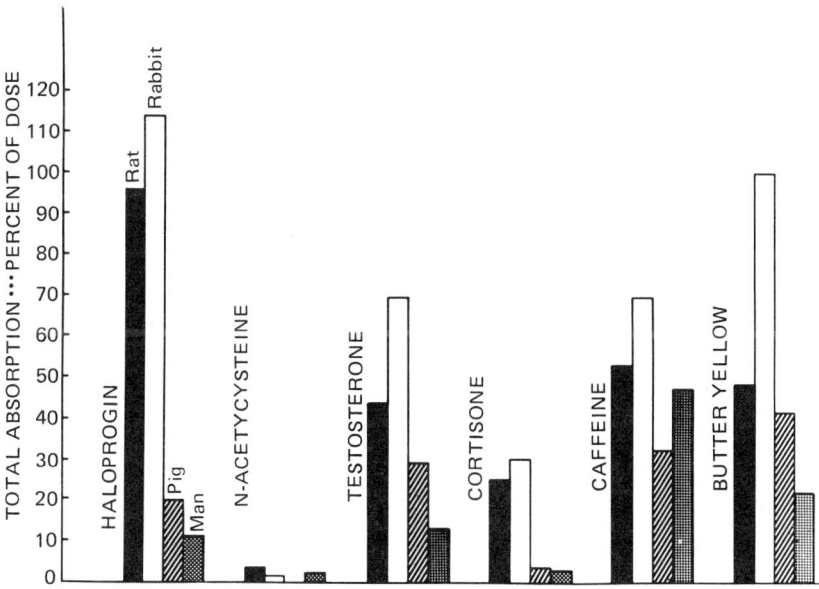

Figure 1 Percutaneous absorption of several chemicals in rat, rabbit, weanling pig, and man. (From Bartek et al., 1972.)

the absorption obtained in man. The methodology used was the same as in their previous studies. The compounds were also applied to the back of the squirrel monkey. The results were compared to man, where the site of application was the ventral forearm. DDT was a minimal penetrant in man, whereas in the rabbit and pig penetration rates were considerably greater. Absorption in the squirrel monkey was very low; however, the value reported was uncorrected with parenteral control data. Penetration of lindane, parathion, and malathion in the rabbit exceeded that in the other species. Penetration of lindane in the squirrel monkey was closer to that in man, whereas parathion penetration in the pig was closest to that in man. Penetration of malathion was similar in the squirrel monkey and the pig, and could be predictive of that in man. It appears that the in vivo percutaneous absorption of pesticides in the rabbit was again much greater than in man, whereas penetration in the pig and squirrel monkey was closer to that in man (Table 2).

Several comparisons of percutaneous absorption in the rhesus monkey and in man were made by Wester and Maibach (1975a,b, 1976, 1977, 1979) and Wester et al. (1979). Methodology and the site of application (ventral forearm) were the same for both species. The site of application was lightly clipper shaved in the monkey. A direct comparison of unshaven and lightly clipper-shaved skin showed no difference in absorption (Wester and Maibach, 1975a). Table 3 summarizes

Table 2 Percutaneous Absorption of Several Pesticides by Rabbit, Pig, Squirrel Monkey, and Man (in vivo)

Pesticide	Dose absorbed (%)			
	Rabbit	Pig	Monkey	Man
DDT	46.3	43.4	1.5	10.4
Lindane	51.2	37.6	16.0	9.3
Parathion	97.5	14.5	30.3	9.7
Malathion	64.6	15.5	19.3	8.2

Source: Bartek and La Budde (1975).

the results of these studies. In vivo percutaneous absorption of hydrocortisone, testosterone, and benzoic acid was similar for the rhesus monkey and man. Also, the dose-response curve was similar in the two species (Fig. 2).

In a related study Wester et al. (1977a) studied the percutaneous absorption of testosterone in the newborn rhesus monkey. The results showed that the percentage dose absorbed in the newborn rhesus was similar to that in the adult rhesus and adult man (Fig. 3). The study also showed that the ratio of surface

Table 3 Percutaneous Absorption of Increased Topical Doses of Several Compounds in the Rhesus Monkey and Man (in vivo)

Penetrant	Dose ($\mu g/cm^2$)	Dose absorbed (%)	
		Rhesus	Man
Hydrocortisone	4	2.9	1.9
	40	2.1	0.6
Benzoic acid	4	59.2	42.6
	40	33.6	25.7
	2000	17.4	14.4
Testosterone	4	18.4	13.2
	40	6.7	8.8[a]
	250	2.9	
	400	2.2	2.8
	1600	2.9	
	4000	1.4	

[a] $30 \mu g/cm^2$.
Source: Wester and Noonan (1980).

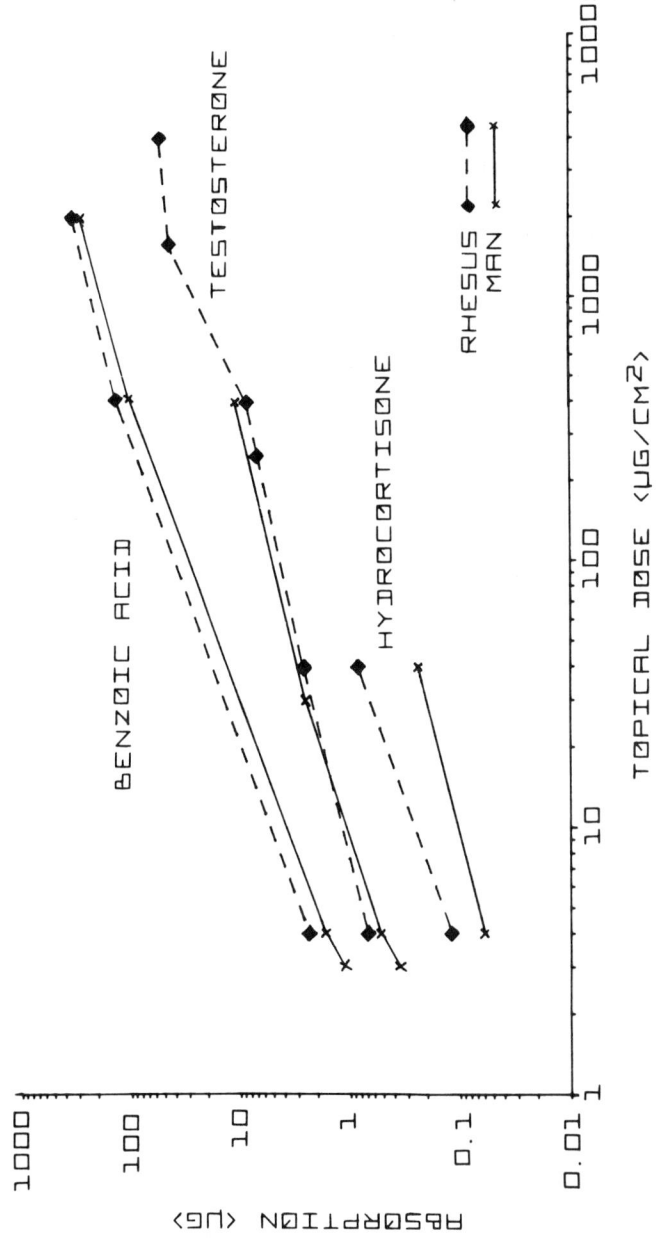

Figure 2 Dose response percutaneous absorption for benzoic acid, testosterone and hydrocortisone in rhesus monkey and man. (From Wester and Maibach, 1976.)

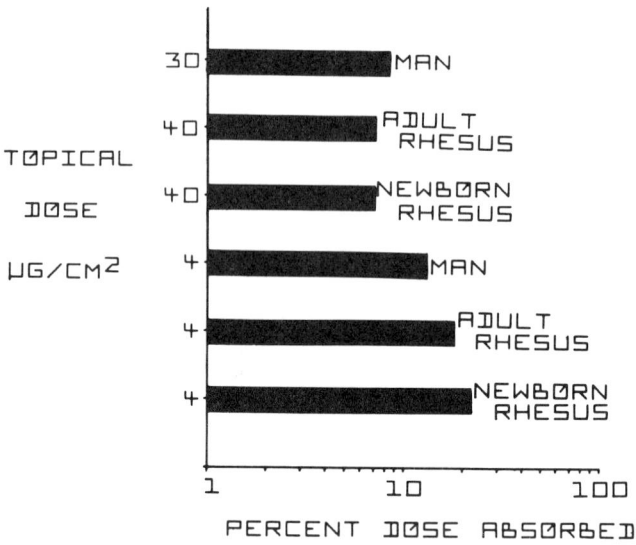

Figure 3 Percutaneous absorption of testosterone in the newborn rhesus monkey compared to adult rhesus and adult man. (From Wester et al., 1977a.)

area to body weight in the newborn is greater than that of an adult. The therapeutic ratio is probably lower in the newborn than in the adult when the compound is applied topically. The newborn rhesus monkey may be a good animal model for studying percutaneous absorption in the neonate.

Andersen et al. (1980) determined the percutaneous absorption of hydrocortisone, testosterone, and benzoic acid in the guinea pig and compared the results to man. A concentration of 4 μg/cm^2 of the ^{14}C-labeled compound was applied to the shaved backs of the animals and percutaneous absorption determined from urinary and fecal excretion. Absorption of hydrocortisone and benzoic acid was similar to published human absorption data. However, testosterone was absorbed to a greater extent in guinea pigs than in man. The absorption value for testosterone in the guinea pig was closer to man if the radioactivity excretion in urine and feces were measured, rather than just the radioactivity excretion in urine alone. If a large proportion of the radioactivity is excreted in the feces, a more accurate estimate of the percutaneous absorption can be obtained by determining the radioactivity excretion in both urine and feces (Wester and Noonan, 1978).

Hunziker et al. (1978) studied the percutaneous absorption of ^{14}C-labeled benzoic acid, progesterone, and testosterone in the Mexican hairless dog, and compared the absorption data, with those obtained in man. Total absorption and

Table 4 Comparative Percutaneous Absorption
of Testosterone in Several Species

Species	Dose absorbed (%)
Rat	47.4
Rabbit	69.6
Guinea pig	34.9
Pig	29.4
Rhesus monkey	18.4
Man	13.2

Source: Wester and Noonan (1980).

maximum absorption rates were greater in man than in the hairless dog. Surface counting experiments showed that benzoic acid and progesterone persisted on the dog skin far longer than on human skin.

In several of the preceding studies the percutaneous absorption of testosterone was determined. In these studies the same topical concentration, 4 $\mu g/cm^2$, was used. Additionally, the same method of analysis, determination of urinary ^{14}C excretion, was used. Table 4 and Figure 4 summarize the results. Absorption of testosterone in the rat, rabbit, and guinea pig was high compared to man. Absorption in the pig was approximately twice that in man, and that in the rhesus monkey was closest to man. Even when the method and applied dose were the same, however, there were other differences besides species. The site of application in the rat, rabbit, guinea pig, and pig was the back, whereas in the rhesus monkey and man the site of application was the ventral forearm. Percutaneous absorption of testosterone in the rhesus monkey and man has been shown to vary with the site of application (Feldman and Maibach, 1967; Maibach et al., 1971; Wester et al., 1980a). It is not known what proportions of the variation in the comparison above are due to species and to site of application, respectively. However, the data indicate that when a difference is found, it could be a sum of the many variables in the study.

Table 5 gives the topical bioavailability of hair dyes in guinea pig, rhesus monkey, and man. The percentage of applied dose absorbed for the three hair dyes (resorcinol, 2-nitro-*p*-phenylenediamine, 4-amino-2-nitrophenol) was similar in all species, suggesting that the efficiency of absorption (percent) was the same. Obviously, the human scalp area is larger than the scalp area of the monkey. Thus, more mass (microgram) would enter the human body than the monkey's body. However, for efficiency of absorption, the monkey and guinea pig appear to be predictive animal models for these hair dyes.

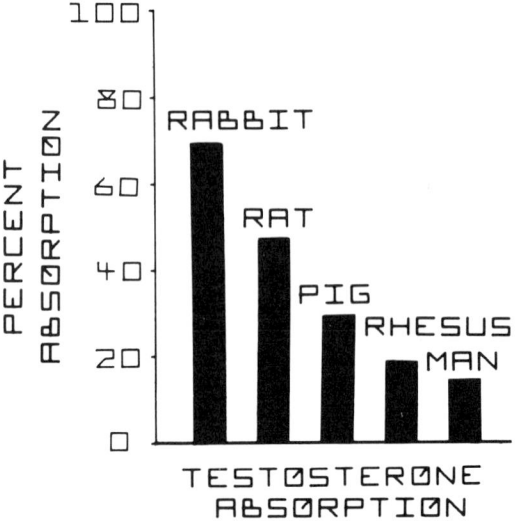

Figure 4 Percutaneous absorption of testosterone in rabbit, rat, weanling pig, rhesus monkey and man. (From Wester and Noonan, 1980.)

McMaster and co-workers (1984) studied the effect of rubbing or spreading a cream on the skin, using the guinea pig and rhesus monkey as animal models. Cortisone was the test chemical, and Feldmann and Maibach (1969a) had previously determined that the percutaneous absorption of cortisone (in acetone vehicle) was 3.4 ±1.6% of applied dose (Table 6). The absorption of cortisone spread on monkey skin was 5.3 ±3.3% (similar to man), while that in the guinea pig was fourfold that of man and the rhesus monkey and guinea pig.

Table 7 gives the in vivo and in vitro dermal absorption of paraquat and water through human and laboratory animal skin. The permeability rate of paraquat through human skin was some 10-fold less in vivo than in vitro. Comparison of

Table 5 Topical Bioavailability of Hair Dyes

Species	Applied dose absorbed (%)		
	Resorcinol	2-Nitro-p-phenylenediamine	4-Amino-2-nitrophenol
Guinea pig	0.065	0.111	0.694
Monkey	0.016	0.508	—
Man	0.071	0.127	0.236

Table 6 Effect of Rubbing Cream on Dermal Absorption of Cortisone: Comparison of Rhesus Monkey and Guinea Pig to Man

	Cortisone dose absorbed (% ± SD)	
	Rub	Spread
Man	—	3.4±1.6[a]
Rhesus monkey	6.2±2.7	5.3±3.3[b]
Guinea pig	20.0±3.7	20.1±4.3[b]

[a] Acetone vehicle.
[b] Cream vehicle.
Source: Feldmann and Maibach (1969a).

Table 7 Absorption of Paraquat and Water Through Human and Laboratory Animal Skin

In vivo/in vitro	Paraquat permeability rate ($\mu g/cm^2$)	
Human (in vivo)[a]	0.03	
Human (in vitro)[b]	0.5	

In vitro[c]	Permeability constant (cm/hr × 10^5)[d]	
	Water	Paraquat
Human	93	0.7
Rat	103	27.2*
Hairless rat	130	35.3*
Nude rat	152	35.5*
Mouse	164	97.2*
Hairless mouse	254*	1065.0*
Rabbit	253*	92.9*
Guinea pig	442*	196.0*

[a] Wester et al. (1984).
[b] Dugard (1984).
[c] Walker et al. (1983).
[d] Asterisk indicates value significantly different from human.

in vitro permeability constants for water and paraquat show that most laboratory animal skin is not predictive of human skin.

In general, the comparative in vivo data that have been reviewed demonstrate that percutaneous absorption in the pig and monkey (rhesus and squirrel) is in most cases similar to that in man, whereas in the rat, and especially in the rabbit, skin penetration is greater than that observed in man. The skin of the Mexican hairless dog has permeability characteristics significantly different from those of human skin. Absorption in the guinea pig was similar to man for hydrocortisone and benzoic acid, but high for testosterone and cortisone.

COMPARATIVE IN VITRO STUDIES

Percutaneous absorption can be determined using the in vitro cell diffusion technique. Table 8 summarizes the ranking of skin permeability of different species, as determined in vitro by several investigators (Marzulli et al., 1969; McGreesh, 1965; Tregear, 1966). Allowing for the different compounds used in each study to rank the species and the differences in origin of the skin sample (back forearm), the studies generally show that the skin of common laboratory animals (rabbit, rat, and guinea pig) is more permeable than the skin of man. Skin from the pig and the monkey more generally approximates the permeability of human skin. Not surprisingly, this general ranking is in close agreement with the in vivo data discussed earlier.

Table 8 Ranking of Skin Permeability of Different Species, Decreasing Order of Permeability, as Determined in Vitro

Tregear (1966)	Marzulli et al. (1969)	McGreesh (1965)
Rabbit	Mouse	Rabbit
Rat	Guinea pig	Rat
Guinea pig	Goat	Guinea pig
Man	Rabbit	Cat
	Horse	Goat
	Cat	Monkey
	Dog	Dog
	Monkey	Pig
	Weanling pig	
	Man	
	Chimpanzee	

Campbell et al. (1976) investigated the permeation of scopolamine in vitro through rat, rabbit, and human skin. The results indicated that human skin is the least permeable of the species tested, and the relative order of rat and rabbit skin permeabilities depends both on skin location (back and side) and the method used to remove the hair.

In the study of Marzulli et al. (1969), mouse skin was the most permeable, certainly much more permeable than human skin. In contrast, studies by Stoughton (1975) using human and hairless mouse skin in vitro showed remarkable similarities in absorption for the skin of the two species for many compounds.

Table 9 summarizes the in vitro and in vivo percutaneous absorption of triclocarban (TCC) in adult (human and rhesus monkey) and newborn abdominal foreskin epidermis. A series of multiple, nonpaired t tests indicated significant differences between flow and static systems ($p < 0.01$), between adult abdominal skin and foreskin ($p < 0.025$), between newborn abdominal skin and foreskin ($p < 0.005$), and between adult and newborn foreskin ($p < 0.02$).

The in vitro absorption using the static diffusion system was 0.23 ±0.15% of applied dose for human adult abdominal skin. Similar results were obtained for newborn (0.26 ±0.28%), infant (0.29 ±0.09%), and adult rhesus abdominal skin (0.25 ±0.09%). The results suggest no difference in percutaneous absorption of these skin types.

Table 9 In Vitro Percutaneous Absorption of Triclocarban in Adult and Newborn Abdominal and Foreskin Epidermis

	Dose absorbed (% ± SD)
Static system, 37°C	
Human adult abdominal (n = 14)	0.23 ± 0.15
Human newborn abdominal (n = 6)	0.26 ± 0.28
Human infant abdominal (n = 4)	0.29 ± 0.09
Monkey adult abdominal (n = 6)	0.25 ± 0.09
Human adult foreskin (n = 4)	0.60 ± 0.25
Human newborn foreskin (n = 7)	2.5 ± 1.6
Static system 23°C	
Human adult abdominal (n = 8)	0.13 ± 0.05
Continuous flow system, 23°C	
Human adult abdominal (n = 12)	6.0 ± 2.0
Man in vivo (n = 5)	7.0 ± 2.8

Human newborn foreskin is used as a source of human skin for in vitro diffusion studies. The in vitro absorption for newborn foreskin was 2.5 ±1.6%. This was 10-fold greater than human abdominal skin. Human adult foreskin absorption was 0.60 ±0.25%, suggesting that the newborn foreskin difference was possibly due to age (newborn) rather than site (foreskin), although probably both age and site contributed to the 10-fold difference.

Another variable in an in vitro diffusion system is solubility of chemical in the receptor fluid. If the chemical diffusing through skin is not soluble in the receptor fluid, diffusion is stopped and the chemical remains in the skin. This was ascertained for TCC, which has high lipid solubility and low water solubility (< 50 µg/liter). In the static diffusion system set at room temperature (23°C), the absorption with human adult abdominal skin was 0.13 ±0.05%. With a continuous flow system absorption increased to 6.0 ±2.0%. The continuous flow system provides a larger sink (more volume) for the diffusing chemical to solubilize in. This is more analogous to the continual perfusion of blood in the in vivo situation. The percutaneous absorption of TCC in man was 7.0 ±2.8%. The continuous flow system, not the static diffusion system, would be predictive of TCC in vivo percutaneous absorption in man.

THE IN VITRO MODEL

Kligman (1983) recently pontificated that in vitro data are more credible than in vivo data, and that if differences do exist, the in vivo data are suspect. Until recently the only comparative data available came from the work of Franz (1975), who evaluated the permeability of 12 organic compounds in vitro using excised human skin and compared the results to those obtained previously by Feldmann and Maibach in living man. Care was taken to ensure that his in vitro conditions closely followed those used in vivo, although it was necessary to use human abdominal skin for the in vitro studies. Additionally, the doses employed ranged from 4 to 40 µg/cm^2, with the assumption that the percentage of applied dose absorbed would not be dose dependent. Quantitatively, the in vitro and in vivo data did not agree. The in vitro method was of value to the extent that it tended to distinguish compounds of low permeability from those of high permeability. However, there are notable differences such that the in vitro method alone would not always be a reliable or accurate predictor of percutaneous absorption in living man.

Table 7 on paraquat absorption and Table 9 on triclocarban absorption give additional in vivo/in vitro comparisons for human skin. For each chemical the difference was at least 10-fold. With triclocarban the difference was due to the in vitro diffusion cell mechanism, where the chemical was not soluble in the low volume of diffusion media. This was corrected with a continuous flow system, which increased the volume of diffusion media and thus the solubility. The in vitro system was then relevant to in vivo absorption. Until these in vivo/in vitro discrepancies cease to appear, in vivo determinations must be continued and the in vitro systems must remain as experimental models, urgently needing further validation for relevance to man.

DISCUSSION

The overriding theory of percutaneous absorption has been Fick's law of diffusion, which has been used to explain all aspects of percutaneous absorption including species differences. Fick's law would account for species differences by the differences in skin thickness (Kligman, 1983). However, measurements of skin thickness such as in Table 10 do not correlate with specie differences in percutaneous absorption. A theory presented by Elias and co-workers (1980, 1981) is that the lipid content of skin represents the barrier to percutaneous absorption and that differences in species (or other aspects such as site variation) are due to differences in lipid content.

In reviewing studies comparing percutaneous absorption between animals and man, care must be taken to ascertain what influences the methodology may have had on the data. Differences in results can be due to different techniques used in the studies. This becomes very important when the data from an animal study are compared to published literature values on absorption in man. Subtle differences in technology may not be readily expressed in the printed methodology.

When comparing the percutaneous absorption of species, it becomes obvious that differences do exist. Some of these differences are due to the species themselves and some of the differences are to techniques used in the study. Various parameters affect percutaneous absorption (Wester and Maibach, 1983; Wester

Table 10 Human and Animal Skin Thickness Measurements

Type of skin (number of sections)	Measurements[a]		
	Stratum corneum (μm)	Epidermis (μm)	Whole skin (mm)
Human (16)	16.8 ± 0.7	46.9 ± 2.3	2.97 ± 0.28
Pig (35)	26.4 ± 0.4	65.8 ± 1.8	3.43 ± 0.05
Rat (9)	18.4 ± 0.5	32.1 ± 1.3	2.09 ± 0.07
Hairless mouse (12)	8.9 ± 0.4	28.6 ± 0.9	0.70 ± 0.02
Mouse (9)	5.8 ± 0.3	12.6 ± 0.8	0.84 ± 0.02

[a]Values are means ± SE of the thickness of the number of sections. Three to six sections were taken from each skin sample.
Source: Bronaugh et al. (1982).

and Noonan, 1980). It becomes important that in any species comparative study, the methods and techniques used be as close to each other as possible. Some of the parameters, such as site of application, occlusion, dose concentration, surface area, and vehicle, can be controlled by the investigator. Some parameters, such as skin metabolism, skin age, and skin condition, may, in part, be difficult for an investigator to control.

The perfect comparative study probably cannot be done; however, the data in the literature suggest that differences in percutaneous absorption exist between species. Compared to absorption in man, absorption in common laboratory animals (rat and rabbit) is high. Absorption in the pig and the monkey (squirrel and rhesus) appears to be more predictive of that in vivo, whereas the comparative in vitro studies done with skin from different species favorably agree with the in vivo results.

Thus it appears that the animal models most predictive of percutaneous absorption in man are the weanling pig and monkey. It may be difficult to have access to monkeys and weanling pigs. This then does not mean that the investigator has to do meaningless studies in vitro or in vivo with rats and rabbits. What it means is that the results obtained must be carefully explained within the scope of the methods and species used. Correlations and predictions of results to man must be done with utmost care.

REFERENCES

Andersen, K. E., Maibach, H. I., and Ango, M. D. (1980). The guinea pig: An animal model for human skin absorption of hydrocortisone, testosterone and benzoic acid? *Br. J. Dermatol. 102*:447-453.

Bartek, M. J. and La Budde, J. A. (1975). Percutaneous absorption in vitro. In *Animal Models in Dermatology*. Edited by H. I. Maibach. Churchill-Livingstone, New York, pp. 103-120.

Bartek, M. J., La Budde, J. A., and Maibach, H. I. (1972). Skin permeability in vivo: comparison in rat, rabbit, pig and man. *J. Invest. Dermatol. 58*: 114-123.

Bronaugh, R. L., Stewart, R. F., and Congdon, E. R. (1982). Methods for in vitro percutaneous absorption studies. II. Animal models for human skin. *Toxicol. Appl. Pharmacol. 62*:481-488.

Campbell, P., Watanabe, T., and Chandrasekaran, S. K. (1976). Comparison of in vitro skin permeability of scopolamine in rat, rabbit and man. *Fed. Proc. (Fed. Am. Soc. Exp. Biol.) 35*:639.

Elias, P. M., Brown, B. E., and Ziboh, V. A. (1980). The permeability barrier in essential fatty acid deficiency: Evidence for a direct role for linoleic acid in barrier function. *J. Invest. Dermatol. 73*:230-233.

Elias, P. M., Cooper, E. R., Korc, A., and Brown, B. E. (1981). Percutaneous transport in relation to stratum corneum structure and lipid composition. *J. Invest. Dermatol. 76*:297-301.

Feldmann, R. J. and Maibach, H. I. (1967). Regional variation in percutaneous penetration of [^{14}C]cortisone in man. *J. Invest. Dermatol. 48*: 181-183.

Feldmann, R. J. and Maibach, H. I. (1969a). Percutaneous penetration of steroids in man. *J. Invest. Dermatol. 52*:89-94.

Feldmann, R. J. and Maibach, H. I. (1969b). Absorption of some organic compounds through the skin in man. *J. Invest. Dermatol. 54*:339-404.

Feldmann, R. J. and Maibach, H. I. (1974). Percutaneous penetration of some pesticides and herbicides in man. *Toxicol. Appl. Pharmacol. 28*:126-132.

Franz, T. J. (1975). Percutaneous absorption. On the relevance of in vitro data. *J. Invest. Dermatol. 64*:190-195.

Franz, T. J. (1979). The finite dose technique as a valid in vitro model for study of percutaneous absorption in man. Presented at the Society of Cosmet. Chemists Annual Scientific Seminar, Dallas, Tex., May.

Hunziker, N., Feldmann, R. J., and Maibach, H. I. (1978). Animal models of percutaneous penetration: Comparison in Mexican hairless dogs and man. *Dermatologica 156*:79-88.

Kligman, A. M. (1983). A biological brief on percutaneous absorption. *Drug Dev. Ind. Pharm.* 521-560.

Maibach, H. I., Feldmann, R. J., Melby, T. H., and Serat, W. F. (1971). Regional variation in percutaneous penetration in man. *Pesticides Arch. Environ. Health 23*: 208-211.

Marzulli, F. N., Brown, D. W. C., and Maibach, H. I. (1969). Techniques for studying skin penetration. *Toxicol. Appl. Pharmacol.* Suppl. 3:79-83.

McGreesh, A. H. (1965). Percutaneous toxicity. *Toxicol. Appl. Pharmacol.* Suppl. 2:20-26.

McMaster, J., Maibach, H. I., Wester, R. C., and Bucks, D. (1984). Does rubbing enhance in vivo dermal absorption?

Stoughton, R. B. (1975). Animal models for in vitro percutaneous absorption. In *Animal Models in Dermatology*. Edited by H. I. Maibach. Churchill-Livingstone, New York, p. 121.

Tregear, R. T. (1966). *Physical Function of Skin*. Academic, New York.

Walker, M., Dugard, P. H., and Scott, R. C. (1983). In vitro percutaneous absorption studies: A comparison of human and laboratory species. *Hum. Toxicol. 2*:561.

Wester, R. C. and Maibach, H. I. (1975a). Percutaneous absorption in the rhesus monkey compared to man. *Toxicol. Appl. Pharmacol. 32*:394-398.

Wester, R. C. and Maibach, H. I. (1975b). Rhesus monkey as an animal model for percutaneous absorption. In *Animal Models in Dermatology*. Edited by H. I. Maibach. Churchill-Livingstone, New York, pp. 133-137.

Wester, R. C. and Maibach, H. I. (1976). Relationship of topical dose and percutaneous absorption in rhesus monkey and man. *J. Invest. Dermatol. 67*: 518-520.

Wester, R. C. and Maibach, H. I. (1977). Percutaneous absorption in man and animal: A perspective. *Cutaneous Toxicity*. Edited by V. Drill and P. Lazar. Academic, New York, pp. 111-126.

Wester, R. C. and Maibach, H. I. (1983). Cutaneous pharmacokinetics: 10 steps to percutaneous absorption. *Drug Metab. Rev. 14*:169-205.

Wester, R. C. and Noonan, P. K. (1978). Topical bioavailability of a potential antiacne agent (SC-23110) as determined by cumulative excretion and areas under plasma concentration-time curves. *J. Invest. Dermatol. 70*:92-94.

Wester, R. C. and Noonan, P. K. (1980). Relevance of animal models for percutaneous absorption. *Int. J. Pharm. 7*:99-110.

Wester, R. C., Noonan, P. K., Cole, M. P., and Maibach, H. I. (1977a). Percutaneous absorption of testosterone in the newborn rhesus monkey: Comparison to the adult. *Pediatr. Res. 11*:737-739.

Wester, R. C., Noonan, P. K., and Maibach, H. I. (1977b). Frequency of application on percutaneous absorption of hydrocortisone. *Arch. Dermatol. 113*: 620-622.

Wester, R. C., Noonan, P. K., and Maibach, H. I. (1979). Recent advances in percutaneous absorption using the rhesus monkey model. *J. Soc. Cosmet. Chem. 30*:297-307.

Wester, R. C., Noonan, P. K., and Maibach, H. I. (1980a). Variations in percutaneous absorption of testosterone in the rhesus monkey due to anatomic site of application and frequency of application. *Arch. Dermatol. Res. 267*: 229-235.

Wester, R. C., Noonan, P. K., and Maibach, H. I. (1980b). Percutaneous absorption of hydrocortisone increases with long-term administration: In vivo studies in the rhesus monkey. *Arch. Dermatol. 116*:186-188.

21
Determination of Percutaneous Absorption by In Vitro Techniques

Robert L. Bronaugh
Food and Drug Administration, Washington, D.C.

The rather recent awareness that the skin is an important portal of entry of chemicals into the body has stimulated an intense interest in the study of the percutaneous absorption process. From a toxicological standpoint, potentially toxic compounds that come in contact with the body from cosmetic products or exposure in the workplace are of concern. In addition, the pharmaceutical industry has seen an opportunity to use the skin as a means of delivering rather potent drugs for systemic effects at a slow, steady-state rate. This interest has been encouraged by the success of topical nitroglycerin products.

The barrier properties of the skin reside primarily in the stratum corneum (Blank and Scheuplein, 1969). This thin layer (15 μm in humans) on the surface of the skin is composed of nonliving tissue. Its protein framework and high lipid composition are the result of the keratinization process of the dermal epithelium. For lipophilic compounds, substantial barrier properties are also due to the predominantly aqueous tissue of the viable epidermis and dermis. Absorption appears to be a passive diffusion process, and the rate of entry into the skin would therefore be unaffected by metabolic processes.

In choosing a means to measure the absorption of chemicals through the skin, a number of factors need to be considered. In vitro procedures allow the determination of rate of absorption directly below the skin membrane, where it is physiologically important. Errors in extrapolating from rates of urinary excretion are avoided. For highly toxic compounds, in vitro methodology may be the only means of obtaining percutaneous absorption data with human skin, and, as we will see, the skin is unique and no animal model is entirely suitable. Finally, in vitro experiments can be done with much less effort and therefore in greater numbers because of the simplicity in methodology.

IN VITRO METHODOLOGY

In many of the early percutaneous absorption studies, the diffusion of chemicals through skin was measured under rigorous physicochemical conditions. Two-chambered diffusion cells were used so that a chemical could be applied in solution on one side of the membrane and its rate of permeation could be obtained from sampling the identical solvent (usually water or saline) on the other side (Blank and Scheuplein, 1969). The donor side as well as the receptor side of the cell was sometimes stirred to ensure homogeneity of the solutions. From the standpoint of studying absorption under "use" conditions, one-chambered cells (receptor beneath skin) are now more commonly chosen. This approach enables the investigator to apply the test compound to the skin in a vehicle of choice and also maintains the surface of the skin at ambient conditions of hydration.

The static cell of Franz (1975) has been widely used, and there are many of similar design (Bronaugh et al., 1981). Flow-through cells (Bronaugh and Stewart, 1985) offer the advantage of automatic collection and may increase the solubility in the receptor solution of hydrophobic compounds.

Regardless of the cell one chooses, the preparation of the skin is a critical step. In humans, pigs, rats, and guinea pigs, the dermis is 2-3 mm thick compared to the epidermis, which is approximately 50-100 μm. If full-thickness skin is used in the diffusion cell studies, the thick dermal tissue can present an artificial barrier, particularly for water-insoluble compounds. Compounds that are absorbed through skin in vivo are taken up by blood vessels directly beneath the epidermis, so they are not required to penetrate the full thickness of the skin.

For hairless skin, the preparation of an epidermal membrane by heat separation has been a convenient solution to the problem of skin thickness (Bronaugh et al., 1981). Haired animal skin cannot be separated by this technique because the shafts of hair leave holes in the epidermis when it is peeled away. The need for split-thickness animal skin was the impetus for our use of a dermatome (Padgett Electrodermatome, Kansas City, Mo.) in the preparation of rat skin for diffusion studies (Bronaugh and Stewart, 1984). A layer thickness of 350 μm was chosen so that a section of skin containing the whole epidermis and the upper papillary dermis was removed. I now use the dermatome for the preparation of human skin because of the more "physiological" layer obtained and also to avoid any unknown detrimental effects of heat treatment of the skin.

In studies with animal skin that is relatively thin (1 mm or less) such as the mouse, hairless mouse, and the rabbit, the preparation of a section using a dermatome is not only a major effort, it is probably not necessary. The dermal tissue is of course much thinner in the skin of these animals.

IN VIVO/IN VITRO COMPARISONS

Because the absorption process is one of passive diffusion through a primary barrier of nonliving tissue, it is not surprising that in vivo and in vitro absorption comparisons have generally been favorable. Because of the difficulty in doing in vivo human studies, most of the comparisons thus far have been made with animal skin.

Some years ago, Burch and Winsor (1944) observed that the permeation of water through excised human skin in diffusion cells was similar to water permeation through intact living skin. The most thorough comparison of human data was made by Franz (1975, 1978), who compared his in vitro results to those of the in vivo absorption values obtained for 12 organic compounds by Feldmann and Maibach (1970). Although the initial comparison (Franz, 1975) showed evidence of discrepancies with a few compounds, his additional studies (1978) demonstrated that these differences were due simply to experimental variation.

Comparisons with animal skin are more numerous. Ainsworth (1960) observed a similarity in tributyl phosphate penetration through rabbit and pig skin using excised and intact living skin. Sekura and Scala (1972) found similar fluxes of alkyl methyl sulfoxides with in vivo and in vitro experiments using rabbit skin. Identical in vivo/in vitro absorption was obtained through the stratum corneum of rabbit ear for water and tripropyl phosphate (Creasey et al., 1978). We compared the absorption of three compounds with differing permeability properties through excised and intact rat skin (Bronaugh et al., 1982). The in vitro absorption (Fig. 1) was nearly identical to the in vivo absorption (Fig. 2).

Additional studies, particularly with human skin, are needed to make available comparative data on compounds from a greater number of chemical classes.

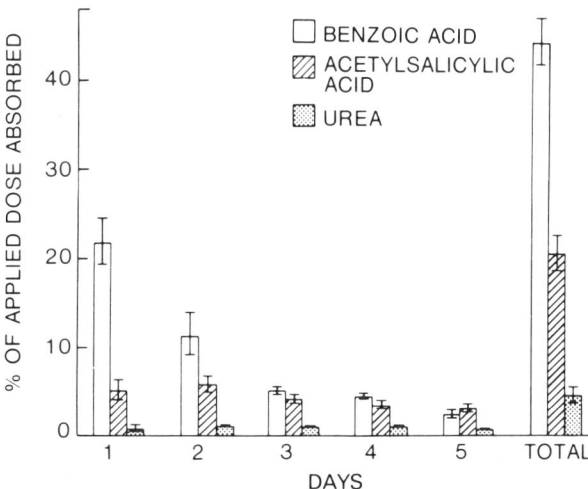

Figure 1 Percutaneous absorption in the rat in vitro. Values are the mean ±SE of four to eight determinations. (From Bronaugh et al., 1982. Reprinted with permission of the publisher.)

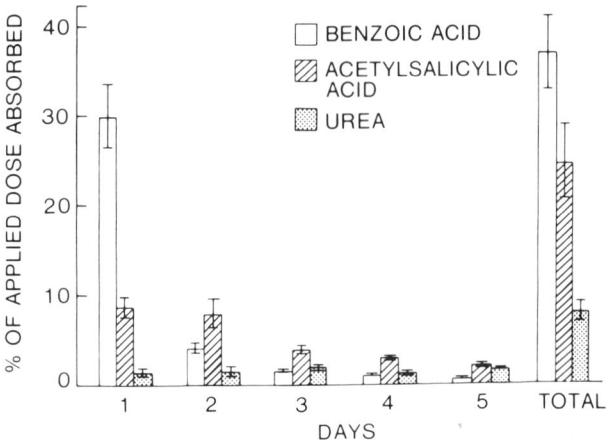

Figure 2 Percutaneous absorption in the rat in vivo. Values are the mean ±SE of five to eight determinations. (From Bronaugh et al., 1982. Reprinted with permission of the publisher.)

HYDROPHOBIC COMPOUNDS

A compound with limited water solubility must be examined carefully when using in vitro diffusion cell techniques. This type of substance may seem to penetrate skin only slightly, when, in fact, the limiting step is not penetration into the skin but the partitioning from skin into the aqueous diffusion cell receptor fluid.

Under in vivo conditions, hydrophobic compounds that penetrate the skin are taken up and carried away by blood in the capillary loops immediately below the epidermis. However, in vitro, if normal saline or physiological buffer solution is used in the diffusion cell receptor, the compound may remain in the skin rather than partition into the receptor solution.

This potential problem has been alluded to in the past. Franz (1975) omitted from his study highly water-insoluble compounds to avoid results that were "artificially limited due to insolubility in the dermal bathing solution." Brown and Ulsamer (1975) found that the skin permeation of the hydrophobic compound hexachlorophene increased twofold when normal saline was replaced with 3% bovine serum albumin (in a physiological buffer) in the diffusion cell receptor. In a recent study (Hoelgaard and Mollgaard, 1982), a nonionic surfactant (Poloxamer 188) was used to enhance the solubility of linoleic acid. Tsuruta (1977) suggested that differences between his in vivo and in vitro absorption data of chlorinated solvents might be due to their respective solubility differences in body fluids (in vivo) and in normal saline (in vitro).

We have recently extensively examined the effect of a variety of receptor fluids on the permeation of two hydrophobic compounds, cinnamyl anthranilate and acetyl ethyl tetramethyltetralin (AETT), using a petrolatum vehicle and rat skin (Bronaugh and Stewart, 1984). The effect of the different agents on the integrity of the barrier properties of the skin was determined using a second radiolabeled compound, [^{3}H] cortisone, as a control compound in the same experiments. The thin layer of skin obtained with the dermatome was required for the enhancement in absorption of cinnamyl anthranilate by the nonionic surfactant oleth 20 (Volpo 20, Croda, New York) (Table 1). Maximum in vitro absorption without an increase in the permeation of the control compound was obtained with a 6% solution in water of oleth 20. Rabbit serum and 3% bovine serum albumin were less effective in increasing absorption of the hydrophobic

Table 1 Effect of Diffusion Cell Conditions on the Absorption of Cinnamyl Anthranilate, I (cortisone control)[a]

Receptor fluid	I (% absorbed in 5 days)	Cortisone permeability constant $\times 10^5$
Normal saline (4)[b]	5.0 ± 0.3	3.8 ± 0.7
1.5% Oleth 20 (4)[b]	5.4 ± 0.9	–
Normal saline (4)	5.8 ± 0.4	7.1 ± 0.5
1.5% Oleth 20 (10)	15.5 ± 1.2[c]	6.1 ± 0.5
6% Oleth 20 (8)	27.9 ± 1.8[c,d]	7.0 ± 0.9
20% Oleth 20 (8)	18.3 ± 1.8[c]	9.3 ± 0.9
Rabbit serum (4)	8.8 ± 0.6[c]	6.8 ± 0.8
3% Bovine serum albumin (4)	12.1 ± 1.2[c]	5.4 ± 0.2
50:50 Methanol/water (4)	27.1 ± 2.0[c]	17.2 ± 0.2[c]
1.5% Octoxynol 9 (4)	17.9 ± 1.1[c]	10.8 ± 0.5[c]
6% Octoxynol 9 (4)	38.4 ± 2.9[c]	14.5 ± 1.3[c]
6% Poloxamer 188 (4)	7.3 ± 1.3	9.8 ± 0.6[c]

[a]Values are the mean ±SE of the number of determinations in parentheses. For most experiments, a 350-μm section from the surface of whole rat skin was prepared with a dermatome. Compounds were applied to the skin in a petrolatum vehicle. In vivo absorption of I was 45.6%.
[b]Whole skin.
[c]Significant increase when compared to results from saline (dermatome section) by one-tailed Student's t test, $p < 0.05$.
[d]Significant increase when compared to results from all receptor fluids except methanol/water and 6% octoxynol 9; by one-tailed Student's t test, $p < 0.05$.

Table 2 Comparison of Solubility Properties and the Effect of Oleth 20 on Percutaneous Absorption

Compound	Water solubility (mg/liter)	Partition coefficient for octanol/water, K	Skin permeability ratio, 6% oleth 20/ saline[a]
Urea	1×10^6	0.002	1.1[b]
Cortisone	280	44	1.2[c]
Testosterone	11	2089	2.3[d]
Cinnamyl anthranilate	0.23	652	3.1[c]
Acetyl ethyl tetramethyltetralin	0.012	3589	30.0[e]

[a]The skin permeability ratio was determined by comparing the amount of compound absorbed in experiments using the two receptor fluids.
[b]Water vehicle, 43 hr.
[c]Acetone vehicle, 5 days.
[d]Acetone vehicle, 43 hr.
[e]Petrolatum vehicle, 5 days.

compound, but they also did not damage the skin barrier. Methanol solution and octoxynol 9 (Triton X-100, Rohm & Haas, Philadelphia) increased both cinnamyl anthranilate and cortisone absorption. Since in vivo absorption of the test compound was 45.6% (Table 1), apparently the use of oleth 20 did not completely facilitate the partitioning from the skin and therefore further improvements in this technique may be needed.

The solubility and permeability properties of selected compounds are compiled in Table 2 as a guide to indicate when the lack of water solubility may reduce the accuracy of an in vitro skin permeability study. Urea and cortisone have sufficient water solubility so that the oleth 20/saline permeability ratio is close to unity. Testosterone appears to have borderline water solubility, as increased absorption begins to be seen with the oleth 20 solution. Testosterone has a water solubility of about 10 mg/liter and is much more soluble in oil (octanol). With cinnamyl anthranilate and AETT, absorption markedly increased when saline was replaced with the surfactant solution. Preliminary results seem to indicate that the absorption of compounds that lack both water and oil solubility is not as much in error when saline is used in the receptor. This is probably because the compounds do not penetrate very well and also do not have a significantly stronger affinity for skin than the receptor solution.

ANIMAL MODELS FOR HUMAN SKIN

Since enough human skin for large numbers of permeability experiments is usually not available, it is important to study and compare the permeability of human and animal skin. Recent articles (Bronaugh and Maibach, 1983, 1985) have summarized current knowledge, with particular emphasis on studies by in vitro techniques. The skin of the rabbit and the mouse is usually most permeable. The permeability of hairless mouse skin has been reported to be similar to human skin for some compounds (Durrheim et al., 1980; Stoughton, 1975), but Bronaugh et al. (1982a) have shown that this may depend on the nature of the compound and is certainly not always the case. Similarly, with the rat, Bartek et al. (1972) concluded that the permeability of the skin is not similar to human skin; however, others (Bronaugh et al., 1982a; Walker et al., 1983) have found that for a number of compounds it indeed has very similar permeability properties to human skin. These apparent discrepancies can be explained by the structural differences between human and animal skin. Human skin is unique in its stratum corneum thickness and hair follicle density. Bronaugh et al. (1982a) have shown that rat skin has a stratum corneum that is in fact as thick as that of human skin. For compounds that penetrate rapidly and do not rely on appendageal diffusion, rat skin may be a good model for human skin, but its many hair follicles may make it a poor model for other compounds. The reverse argument holds for the inconsistent agreement between absorption through hairless mouse and human skin. Hairless mouse skin has a similar hair follicle density, but the stratum corneum is thinner than human skin (Bronaugh et al., 1982a) and so it is often more permeable. A sex difference exists in the thickness and permeability properties of rat skin (Bronaugh et al., 1983). The thicker male back skin (Table 3) is dependent on androgens—castrated male weanling rats had skin at

Table 3 Rat Skin Thickness Measurements from Frozen Sections[a]

Type of skin[b]	Skin thickness		
	Stratum corneum (um)	Whole epidermis (um)	Whole skin (mm)
Male			
Back	34.7 ± 2.3	61.1 ± 3.0	2.80 ± 0.08
Abdomen	13.8 ± 0.7	30.4 ± 1.5	1.66 ± 0.06
Female			
Back	18.2 ± 1.0	31.2 ± 1.5	2.04 ± 0.05
Abdomen	13.7 ± 0.6	34.8 ± 1.8	0.93 ± 0.02

[a]Values are the mean ± SE of 36 measurements for each layer of skin.
[b]Osborne-Mendel rats, Camm Research Animals.
Source: Bronaugh et al. (1983). Reprinted with permission of the publisher.

Table 4 Effect of Sex and Body Site on the Permeability of Rat Skin[a]

	Male		Female	
Compound	Permeability constant (cm/hr × 10^4)	Lag time (hr)	Permeability constant (cm/hr × 10^4)	Lag time (hr)
Water				
Back	4.9 ± 0.4	2.4 ± 0.1 (7)	9.3 ± 1.1	2.0 ± 0.1 (4)
Abdomen	13.1 ± 2.1	1.7 ± 0.2 (4)		
Urea				
Back	1.6 ± 0.5	15.0 ± 1.8 (6)	4.8 ± 1.3	11.1 ± 0.6 (3)
Abdomen	18.8 ± 5.5	16.5 ± 4.3 (4)		
Cortisone				
Back	1.7 ± 0.4	33.4 ± 4.4 (8)	4.7 ± 1.1	20.0 ± 2.6 (3)
Abdomen	12.2 ± 0.6	32.9 ± 2.4 (4)		

[a]Values are the mean ± SE of the number of determinations in parentheses. Compounds were applied to excised skin in a water vehicle. Rats were obtained from Camm Research Animals.
Source: Bronaugh et al. (1983). Reprinted with permission of the publisher.

maturity with thickness and permeability properties comparable to those of female rats. The differences in the permeability of male and female rat back skin (Table 4) clearly reflect the observed differences in thickness of the stratum corneum.

The skin of the monkey at the sites of testing (abdomen and ventral forearm) is relatively sparsely haired in comparison to other areas of the body. Wester and Maibach (1975) found monkey skin to be a good model for human skin in numerous in vivo studies. Recently Bronaugh and Maibach (1985a) compared the absorption of five nitroaromatic compounds in humans and monkeys using both in vivo and in vitro techniques (Table 5). Except for the highly volatile compound nitrobenzene, no significant differences were found in the four groups of data. Extensive evaporation of nitrobenzene occurred (approximately 80% of that applied to skin), and it was therefore speculated that the increased absorption in the in vitro studies was due to reduced evaporation caused by the short walls on the diffusion cell tops.

The absorption of fragrance ingredients in cosmetics has been compared through human and monkey skin (Bronaugh et al., 1985) (Fig. 3). The in vitro absorption measurements of cinnamyl anthranilate and safrole required the use of 6% oleth 20 in the receptor fluid. Again, increased in vitro absorption of

Table 5 Percutaneous Absorption of Nitroaromatic Compounds[a]

Compound	Applied dose (%)			
	Human		Monkey	
	In vivo	In vitro	In vivo	In vitro
p-Nitroaniline		48.0 ± 11.0 (9)	76.2 ± 8.4 (4)	62.2 ± 6.1 (6)
4-Amino-2-nitrophenol		45.1 ± 8.0 (5)	64.0 ± 6.2 (6)	48.2 ± 7.8 (5)
2,4-Dinitrochlorobenzene	53.1 ± 6.2 (4)	32.5 ± 8.7 (8)	52.5 ± 4.3 (4)	48.4 ± 3.9 (11)
2-Nitro-p-phenylenediamine		21.7 ± 2.6 (7)	29.9 ± 6.9 (3)	29.6 ± 4.3 (5)
Nitrobenzene	1.5 ± 0.3 (6)	7.8 ± 1.2 (6)	4.2 ± 0.5 (4)	6.2 ± 1.0 (6)
		41.1 ± 2.0 (3)[b]		

[a]Values are the means ± SE of the number of determinations in parentheses. Only with nitrobenzene were there significant differences (Student's two-tailed t test, $p < 0.05$) between the values determined for the compounds by the four different methods; the value for the human in vivo study was significantly different from the results from the other three procedures, and there also were significant differences between the human in vitro and the monkey in vivo values.
[b]Diffusion cell tops covered with Parafilm.

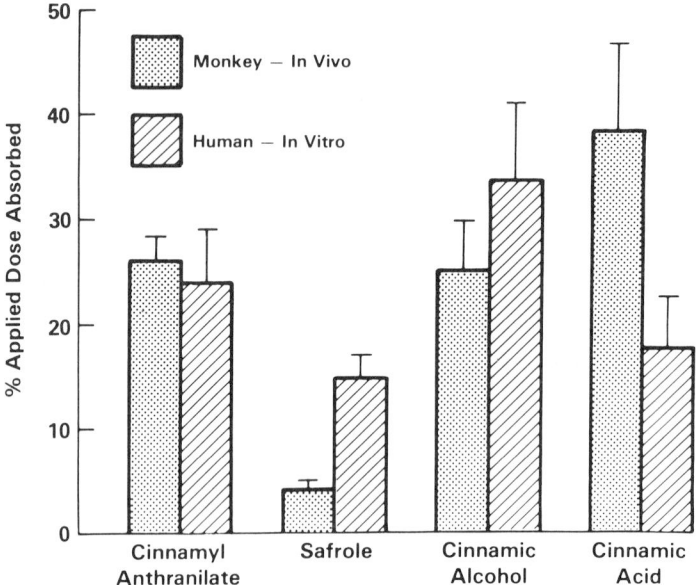

Figure 3 Percutaneous absorption of fragrances with human and monkey skin. Values are the mean + SE of four to nine determinations.

safrole might have been due to the high volatility of this compound. Cinnamic acid appeared to be absorbed through monkey skin more readily. No significant differences were found between human and monkey skin permeability for cinnamyl anthranilate and cinnamic alcohol.

SOLUBILITY PROPERTIES OF PENETRANT

The physicochemical properties of a molecule, in particular its solubility properties in oil and water, have been compared with permeability data in hope of finding correlations. Usually the solubility is expressed as an oil/water ratio (or its logarithm); the octanol/water partition coefficients for a number of compounds have been published by Hansch and Leo (1979).

Reasonably good correlations of permeability and oil/water partition coefficients have been obtained with some homologous series of compounds. If compounds are applied as dilute solutions in aqueous vehicles, positive correlations have resulted (Roberts et al., 1977; Scheuplein, 1965; Treherne, 1956). This result is due, at least in part, to an increased driving force from the aqueous vehicle caused by increasing lipid solubility. Of course, the absolute solubility in the aqueous vehicle is critical to permeation but is ignored in expressing solubility data as partition coefficients.

When compounds are applied undiluted, a number of studies have found that the best correlations have been positive with water solubility (Marzulli et al., 1965; Scheuplein, 1977; Tsuruta, 1975). Under these conditions, the importance of a molecule's water solubility in promoting good skin permeation is emphasized rather than its ability to partition from water into oil.

Application of compounds in a saturated solution should, in theory, overcome the influence of the vehicle on percutaneous absorption. When the permeation of a structural variety of compounds was determined from saturated aqueous solutions, no correlation of skin absorption with mineral oil/water partition coefficients was seen (Michaels et al., 1975). It is likely that relying on partitioning data to estimate percutaneous absorption will often be misleading, since other determinants such as the effect of the vehicle and skin binding are not considered.

The importance to the absorption process of the binding of chemicals to skin is covered in detail in Chapter 3. We have seen that binding of chemicals to skin in some cases may be of experimental interest only and not important under conditions applicable during the skin absorption process (Bronaugh and Congdon, 1984). For a series of hair dyes, permeability constants from an aqueous vehicle were, in general, ranked in the same order as measured octanol/water partition coefficients. However, initial stratum corneum/water partition coefficients (K_m) did not correlate with these findings. Binding to stratum corneum at the low concentrations used in the K_m studies gave higher values for some dyes than the values that were subsequently obtained using concentrations of dye applied in the permeability studies. The binding sites were saturated, giving K_m values in agreement with the other permeability data.

CONCLUSIONS

Increasing evidence apparently supports the contention that in vitro permeability studies can accurately predict in vivo absorption. This is true only if studies take into account potential problem areas. Cadaver skin should be used cautiously; the permeability should be checked with a standard compound. Use of full-thickness human or animal skin may result in an artificial reduction in permeation, particularly for compounds with high lipid solubility. The absorption of hydrophobic compounds must be measured with an appropriate receptor fluid. At this time, prediction of percutaneous absorption from solubility data seems useful only in the sense of furnishing a crude estimation, which must be substantiated by other means.

REFERENCES

Ainsworth, M. (1960). Methods for measuring percutaneous absorption. *J. Soc. Cosmet. Chem. 11*: 69–78.

Bartek, M. J., LaBudde, J. A., and Maibach, H. I. (1972). Skin permeability in vivo: Comparison in rat, rabbit, pig, and man. *J. Invest. Dermatol. 58*: 114–123.

Blank, I. H. and Scheuplein, R. J. (1969). Transport into and within the skin. *Br. J. Dermatol. 81* (Suppl. 4): 4–10.

Bronaugh, R. L. and Congdon, E. R. (1984). Percutaneous absorption of hair dyes: Correlation with partition coefficients. *J. Invest. Dermatol. 83*: 124–127.

Bronaugh, R. L. and Maibach, H. I. (1983). In vitro percutaneous absorption. In *Dermatotoxicology*. Edited by F. N. Marzulli and H. I. Maibach. Hemisphere, Washington, D.C., pp. 117–129.

Bronaugh, R. L. and Maibach, H. I. (1985). In vitro models for human percutaneous absorption. In *Models in Dermatology*. Edited by H. I. Maibach and N. J. Lowe. Karger, Basel, pp. 178–188.

Bronaugh, R. L. and Maibach, H. I. (1985a). Percutaneous absorption of nitroaromatic compounds. *J. Invest. Dermatol.* In press.

Bronaugh, R. L. and Stewart, R. F. (1984). Methods for in vitro percutaneous absorption studies. III. Hydrophobic compounds. *J. Pharm. Sci. 73*: 1255–1258.

Bronaugh, R. L. and Stewart, R. F. (1985). Methods for percutaneous absorption studies. IV. The flow-through diffusion cell. *J. Pharm. Sci. 74*: 64–67.

Bronaugh, R. L., Congdon, E. R., and Scheuplein, R. J. (1981). The effect of cosmetic vehicles on the penetration of N-nitrosodiethanolamine through excised human skin. *J. Invest. Dermatol. 76*: 94–96.

Bronaugh, R. L., Stewart, R. F., and Congdon, E. R. (1982a). Methods for in vitro percutaneous absorption studies. II. Animal models for human skin. *Toxicol. Appl. Pharmacol. 62*: 481–488.

Bronaugh, R. L., Stewart, R. F., Congdon, E. R., and Giles, A. L., Jr. (1982b). Methods for in vitro percutaneous absorption studies. I. Comparison with in vivo results. *Toxicol. Appl. Pharmacol. 62*: 474–480.

Bronaugh, R. L., Stewart, R. F., and Congdon, E. R. (1983). Differences in permeability of rat skin related to sex and body site. *J. Soc. Cosmet. Chem. 34*: 127–135.

Bronaugh, R. L., Wester, R. C., Bucks, D., Stewart, R. F., Anderson, J., and Maibach, H. I. (1985). Comparison of percutaneous absorption of fragrances in humans and monkeys. *Food Chem. Toxicol. 23*: 111–114.

Brown, D. W. C. and Ulsamer, A. G. (1975). Percutaneous penetration of hexachlorophene as related to receptor solutions. *Food Cosmet. Toxicol. 13*: 81–86.

Burch, G. E. and Winsor, T. (1944). Rate of insensible perspiration locally through living and dead human skin. *Arch. Intern. Med. 74*: 437–444.

Creasey, N. H., Battensby, J., and Fletcher, J. A. (1978). Factors affecting the permeability of skin. *Curr. Probl. Dermatol. 7*: 95–106.

Durrheim, H., Flynn, G. L., Higuchi, W. I., and Behl, C. R. (1980). Permeation of hairless mouse skin. I. Experimental methods and comparison with human epidermal permeation by alkanols. *J. Pharm. Sci. 69*: 781-786.

Feldmann, R. J. and Maibach, H. I. (1970). Absorption of some organic compounds through the skin in man. *J. Invest. Dermatol. 54*: 399-404.

Franz, T. J. (1975). Percutaneous absorption. On the relevance of in vitro data. *J. Invest. Dermatol. 64*: 190-195.

Franz, T. J. (1978). The finite dose technique as a valid in vitro model for the study of percutaneous absorption. *Curr. Probl. Dermatol. 7*: 58-68.

Hansch, C. and Leo, A. (1979). *Substituent Constants for Correlation Analysis in Chemistry and Biology*. Wiley, New York, pp. 171-330.

Hoelgaard, A. and Mollgaard, B. (1982). Permeation of linoleic acid through skin in vitro. *J. Pharm. Pharmacol. 34*: 610-611.

Marzulli, F. N., Callahan, J. F., and Brown, D. W. C. (1965). Chemical structure and skin penetrating capacity of a short series of organic phosphates and phosphoric acid. *J. Invest. Dermatol. 44*: 339-344.

Michaels, A. S., Chandrasekaran, S. K., and Shaw, J. E. (1975). Drug permeation through human skin: Theory and in vitro experimental measurements. *AIChE J. 21*: 985-996.

Roberts, M. S., Anderson, R. A., and Swarbrick, J. (1977). Permeability of human epidermis to phenolic compounds. *J. Pharm. Pharmacol. 29*: 677-683.

Scheuplein, R. J. (1965). Mechanism of percutaneous absorption. I. Routes of penetration and the influence of solubility. *J. Invest. Dermatol. 45*: 334-346.

Scheuplein, R. J. (1977). Permeability of the skin. In *Handbook of Physiology: Reactions to Environmental Agents*. Edited by D. H. K. Lee. Williams & Wilkins, Baltimore, pp. 299-322.

Sekura, D. and Scala, J. (1972). The percutaneous absorption of alkyl methyl sulfoxides. In *Pharmacology and the Skin*. Edited by W. Montagna, E. Van Scott, and R. Stoughton. Appleton-Century-Crofts, New York, pp. 257-269.

Stoughton, R. B. (1975). Animal models for in vitro percutaneous absorption. In *Animal Models in Dermatology*. Edited by H. I. Maibach. Churchill-Livingstone, New York, pp. 121-132.

Treherne, J. E. (1956). The permeability of skin to some non-electrolytes. *J. Physiol. 133*: 171-180.

Tsuruta, H. (1975). Percutaneous absorption of organic solvents. I. Comparative study of the in vivo percutaneous absorption of chlorinated solvents in mice. *Ind. Health 13*: 227-236.

Tsuruta, H. (1977). Percutaneous absorption of organic solvents. II. A method for measuring the penetration rate of chlorinated solvents through excised rat skin. *Ind. Health 15*: 131-139.

Walker, M., Dugard, P. H., and Scott, R. C. (1983). In vitro percutaneous absorption studies: A comparison of human and laboratory species. *Hum. Toxicol. 2*: 561-562.

Wester, R. C. and Maibach, H. I. (1975). Percutaneous absorption in the rhesus monkey compared to man. *Toxicol. Appl. Pharmacol. 32*: 394-398.

22
Localization of Compounds in Different Skin Layers and Its Use as an Indicator of Percutaneous Absorption

Wolfgang Schalla and Hans Schaefer
Centre International de Recherches Dermatologiques, Valbonne, France

In pharmacokinetics a given systemically administered drug is usually characterized by the concentration changes with time in serum and in various organs as well as the quantities eliminated in urine and feces. These compartments are important for understanding systemic effects after a drug has been applied topically. Except for percutaneous systemic therapy developed recently with special delivery devices (e.g., the Transdermal Therapeutic System), measurements of such compartments serve to explain the side effects of topical application. However for the local action of the drug in the skin, the target organ, they give only indirect evidence of what will happen in the skin. Therefore, additional information should be obtained by measuring the pharmacokinetic behavior in the skin itself, since its easy access, its enormous surface compared to the samples needed, and its resistance to postoperational or postmortem changes (the horny layer is usually dead!) are factors conducive to such studies. We discuss some methods for direct skin compartment measurements and the additional information one can obtain.

METHODS

The various in vitro and in vivo methods used for pharmacokinetic studies after topical application have been recently reviewed (Schaefer et al., 1982). Some of the methods useful for localization and distribution within the skin are summarized.

Dedicated to Prof. G. Stüttgen, Freie Universität Berlin, on the occasion of his 65th birthday.

Diffusion into the Horny Layer

Stripping
The stratum corneum as the outermost skin layer can be removed by repetitive application of adhesive tape to the same skin surface area. The drug amount can be measured in each single tape, giving a concentration profile within the horny layer.

The stripping technique can be used to measure drug concentrations after topical application as well as after systemic administration under in vitro and in vivo conditions. It also can be used to analyze pharmacodynamic activity thus taking into account binding, decomposition, and metabolism of a given drug (e.g. antifungal effects: Knight, 1974).

Skin Surface Biopsy
Cyanoacrylate is applied to a glass slide (or a tape strip) and pressed on the skin surface, and the slide is removed after the glue has polymerized (Marks and Dawber, 1971). This technique allows one to quantitate the amount of drug found after various application times in the horny layer (Finlay and Marks, 1982). Because the hair follicle also is removed with this method, a differentiation between the transepidermal and the transfollicular routes of penetration is not possible.

Diffusion into and Through the Horny Layer and Epidermis

Epidermal Sheets for in Vitro Studies
Different methods are available to separate the epidermis, including the horny layer, from the underlying dermis (Kligman and Christophers, 1963; Polano et al., 1972; van Scott, 1952). Sheets obtained by one of these methods can be mounted in diffusion cells, and the diffusion of compounds may be followed (Dugard and Scheuplein, 1973; Schulze, 1971; Smeenk and Polano, 1965).

Suction Blister Technique
Using a partial vacuum of 150-300 mmHg below atmospheric pressure, blisters can be raised that separate the epidermis from the dermis in vivo (Kiistala, 1968, 1976). For pharmacokinetic studies, 10 or more blisters are formed; then the drug is applied epicutaneously or systemically, and the blister fluid is taken after various time intervals. We use 250 mmHg of negative pressure and capsules with five holes, 8 mm in diameter. The time needed for blister formation is in the order of 1-3 hr on the lower abdomen. In addition to the fluid, the drug concentration in the blister roof (= epidermis) and the blister base (= dermis) can be measured after sampling by forceps and punch biopsy, respectively, followed by homogenization and extraction. For such additional compartment analysis, epicutaneously applied drugs should be formulated in vehicles such as films, which allow the complete removal of the drug excess.

The suction blister technique is becoming more popular; some drawbacks should be considered. The blister fluid corresponds roughly to the interstitial fluid (Rossing and Worm, 1981; Vermeer et al., 1979). The protein content is one half to one fifth that of serum according to the molecular size; that is, the vascular endothelium retains its sieve effect on normal skin (Kiistala, 1976; Rossing and Worm, 1981; Vermeer et al., 1979; Volden et al., 1980). Therefore, the blister fluid should be checked for the presence of blood cells, which indicate that the values obtained should be treated with extreme caution. On the other hand, no increase of extracellular potassium could be seen after UV irradiation, suggesting that the blister fluid is a filtrate of the serum rather than true interstitial fluid (Volden et al., 1980).

In diseased skin, particularly if the epidermis is altered, the blister fluid is modified (e.g., the protein content changes, usually cells are found, and the blister fluid penetrates more easily into the surrounding tissue). In parakeratotic dermatoses, blisters often cannot be raised properly; that is, there is secretion into the capsule with or without bursting of the blister roof. The standardization on diseased skin is far from optimal.

Distribution in the Skin

Skin Sections

Skin sections can be used in vivo and in vitro. The radiolabeled drug in its galenical formulation is applied to a small surface area of skin (2-7 cm^2). After a defined penetration period, the horny layer is removed by stripping, and the single tape strips are measured by scintillation counting. The skin is excised under anesthesia, and three punch biopsies 6 mm in diameter are taken, frozen by carbon dioxide evaporation, and sectioned parallel to the skin surface by a cryomicrotome. The 10- or 40-μm thick sections are analyzed separately or in groups after solubilization by liquid scintillation counting. A concentration gradient can thus be obtained from the skin surface to the subcutis (Schaefer et al., 1982). The method takes into account neither the undulations of the dermoepidermal junction nor privileged penetration routes. Therefore, a combination with histoautoradiography or the skin surface biopsy technique gives additional information. Differentiation between the original drug and its metabolites is possible if the highly sensitive detection methods available are used after extraction of the sections.

Histoautoradiography

Using the common techniques in histoautoradiography, the bound compounds are preferentially detected. Quantitative estimates are therefore problematic, but conclusions about the mode of action can be drawn to some extent from the distribution. For pharmacokinetic studies, the "dry" techniques have some advantages.

The most intensive labeling after epicutaneous application is usually found in the horny layer. Therefore, the frozen tissue blocks must be cut from the subcutis to the skin surface, and the knife must be cleaned after each section. In some sections the skin appendages are also seen. It is advisable to remove the horny layer in one series, by stripping before exposure to the radiosensitive film or emulsion so that the exposure time can be prolonged to allow better observation of the distribution in viable layers and the skin appendages.

Binding and Drug Metabolism in the Skin

An ideal topical drug should penetrate into the skin in an inactive form to reach the target structures, where it is transformed into the active form and inactivated afterward within the skin or, at least, immediately on reaching the blood. The most obvious approach would be to take advantage of metabolism from a prodrug to the active drug within the skin, and further transformation to inactive metabolites thereafter. For such a process, the epidermal sheet, suction blister, and skin section are useful, but often larger skin samples are needed. Fresh skin specimens are necessary when using in vitro diffusion cells.

For total binding, small pieces of whole skin, separated epidermis, or dermis weighing 0.5-10 mg are placed in 2 ml of PBS, containing the desired drug concentration. After equilibration (e.g., after 36 hr at 4°C) the concentration difference of the drug in the PBS corresponds to the drug amount taken up by the tissue (Artuc et al., 1979; Menczel and Maibach, 1972). Subcellular fractions can be handled in a similar manner (Slaga et al., 1977).

Larger amounts of skin are needed for receptor-binding studies. They are therefore done on animal skin (Adachi, 1974), human skin from plastic surgery or amputations (Epstein and Bonifas, 1982), or cultures of fibroblasts or keratinocytes (Gazith et al., 1982).

DRUG CONCENTRATIONS IN THE SKIN

The skin consists of heterogeneous structures that are unevenly distributed three dimensionally rather than as a two-dimensional, uniform membrane with a unique diffusional resistance. The latter simplified model of the skin is useful for some pharmaceutical and systemic toxicity studies, but it has only limited value for a better understanding of skin pharmacology and skin toxicity. How drugs or other substances are distributed in the three dimensions is considered in the subsections that follow.

Topical Application

After epicutaneous application, a concentration gradient from the skin surface to the subcutis is formed. The steepness of this gradient depends only on the diffusional resistance of the various skin structures because there is no eivdence of any kind of an active transport mechanism in the skin.

Horny Layer

The horny layer is known to be the most important barrier against diffusion. Whether the substances pass the stratum corneum transcellularly or intercellularly, and whether there are differences between the various substances, are still matters of discussion. Recent findings seem to indicate that the intercellular pathway is more important than had been thought (brick wall model) (Elias, 1981, 1983).

Using the stripping technique and a semilogarithmic plot, a linear decrease of drug concentration can usually be observed (Fig. 1), although the amount of horny layer that sticks to each consecutive tape strip decreases (Tregear, 1966; Zesch and Schaefer, 1974). Stripping does not remove all the horny layer (Holyo-Tomoka and Kligman, 1972). This might be why data obtained with this method suggest a uniform resistance of each layer of horny cells rather than

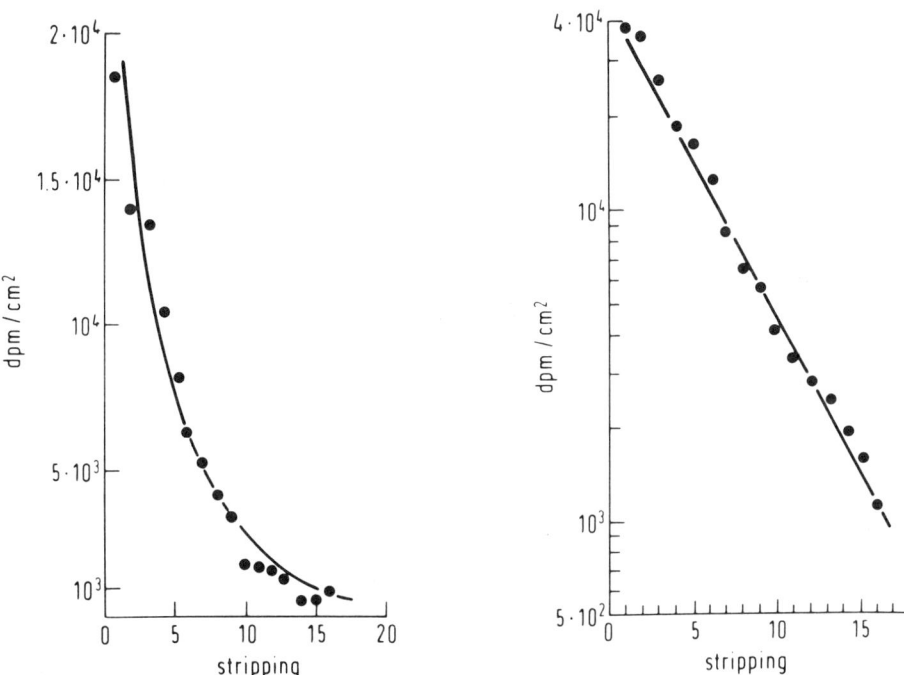

Figure 1 Distribution of radioactivity in the horny layer after topical application of 4-chlortestosterone acetate. (A) Linear plot. (B) Semilogarithmic plot. (From Schaefer et al., 1982.)

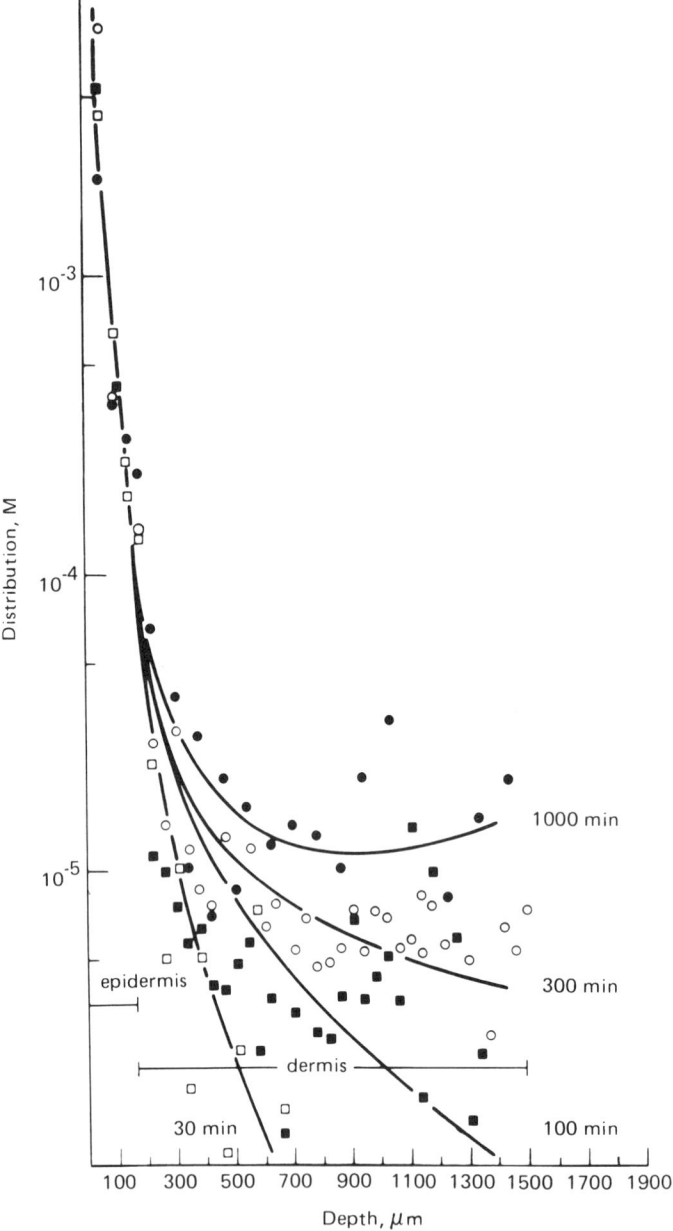

Figure 2 Distribution of triphenylstibine sulfide in the skin relative to the penetration period: □, 30 min; ■, 100 min; ○, 300 min; ●, 1000 min. (From Schaefer et al., 1982.)

supporting the existence of a stratum compactum, claimed by Szakall (1958) and recently by Bowser and White (1983), which would be situated in the lower part of the stratum corneum. For a detailed discussion about the horny layer as permeability barrier, see Elias (1981, 1983) and Schaefer et al. (1982).

Viable Skin Layers

The concentration decreases further in the epidermis and dermis. Under in vitro conditions the gradient between the superficial and the deeper parts of the skin diminishes with time (Fig. 2), whereas in vivo a steady state is obtained after a certain time. The difference between in vitro and in vivo skin concentrations is caused by resorption into the blood and lymph vessels. Therefore, the difference can be seen in the dermis, but not in the epidermis (Fig. 3). Nevertheless, a

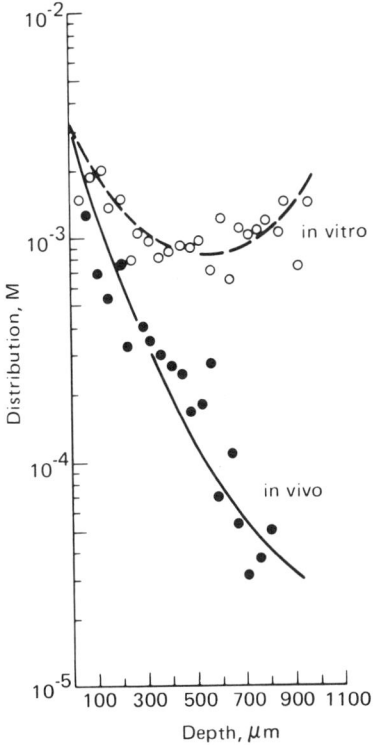

Figure 3 Molar distribution of hydrocortisone in human skin in vitro (○) and in vivo (●); 1% hydrocortisone in polyethylene glycol ointment; 1000-min penetration period. (From Zesch and Schaefer, 1975.)

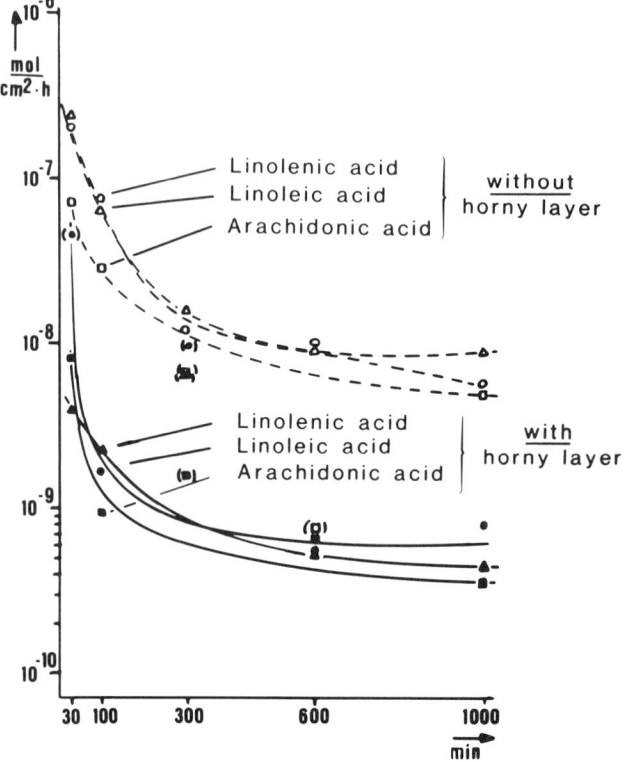

Figure 4 Influx of essential fatty acids (EFA) into the viable portion of intact and stripped skin layers versus application period in vitro; 6% (w/w) EFA preparations in peroxide free soybean oil. (From Schalla, 1978.)

steady state is also found in in vitro experiments (Fig. 4). Enrichment in the subcutaneous fat of lipophilic drugs, usually used for topical therapy, can sometimes be observed. Such an enrichment is often masked in vivo because of the overlying concentration gradient, but it can be seen after prolonged application periods (Fig. 5).

Skin Appendages

The distribution in the skin after epicutaneous application does not follow a simple concentration gradient in two (horny layer and viable part of the skin) or three (horny layer, epidermis, and dermis) membranes of different thicknesses. In addition, the blood flow for clearance of the skin of a penetrated substance and the uneven distribution in the skin and the skin appendages must be taken

Localization of Compounds in Skin Layers

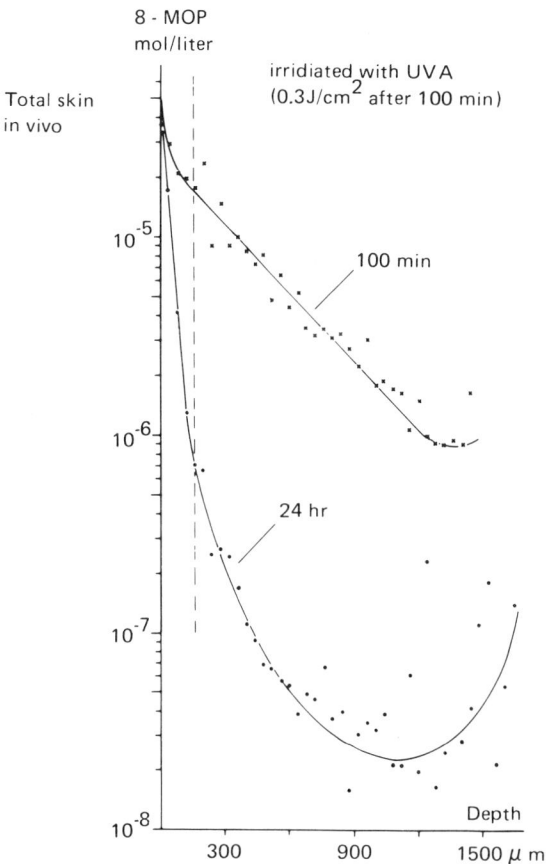

Figure 5 Penetration of 0.1% tritiated 8-methoxypsoralen (8-MOP) in oil into normal human skin in vivo, UV irradiation, 0.3 J/cm^2 after 100 min. Upper curve, 100-min penetration time; lower curve, 24-hr penetration time; left of vertical bar, epidermis; right, dermis. (From Schaefer et al., 1978.)

into account. Using histoautoradiography, an enrichment of drugs in the follicular channel (Fig. 6) and in the sweat glands (Fig. 7) can be found. Scheuplein (1967) claimed in his elegant article that the penetration route via these skin appendages plays a role only in the very first minutes after application. On the other hand, it is far from clear whether the assumptions made there holds true for clinical conditions. At least, the drug concentrations in those skin appendages are much higher even after prolonged application periods.

The nail plate has a low permeability for the lipophilic drugs currently used in topical therapy.

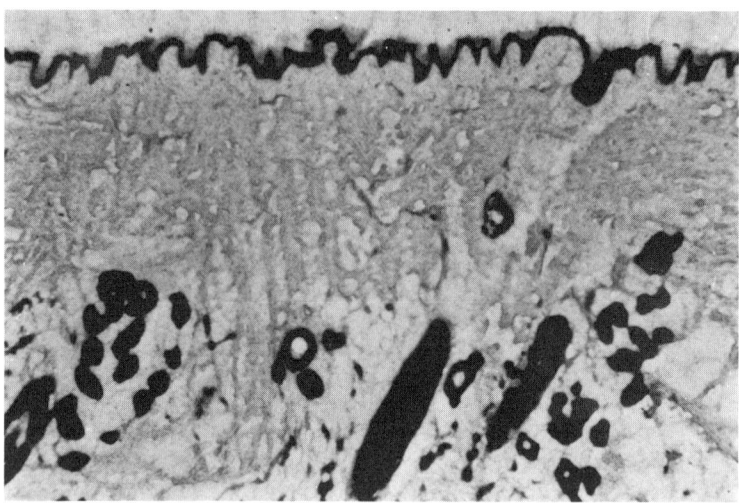

Figure 6 Overview of an autoradiograph of desoxymethasone after topical application in vivo. Application for 1 hr was performed under occlusion (0.25% tritium-labeled 17-α-desoxymethasone; specific activity, 17.4 μCi/g of cream base). (From Kukita et al., 1973.)

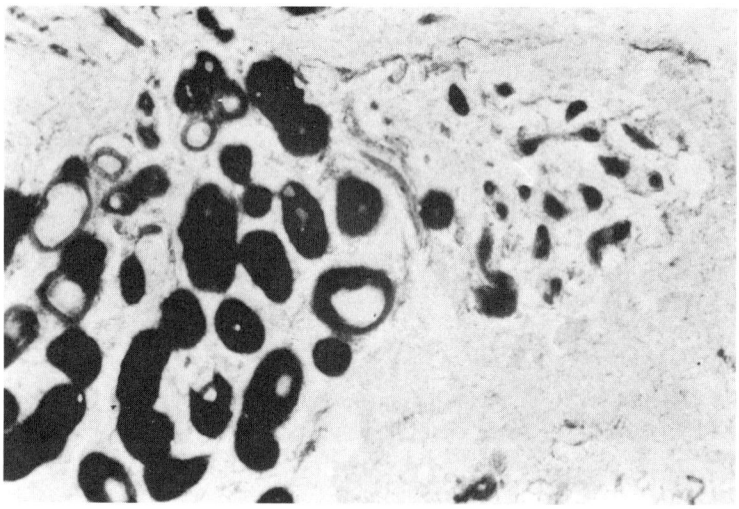

Figure 7 High magnification of the apocrine glands from the autoradiograph of Fig. 6. (From Kukita et al., 1973.)

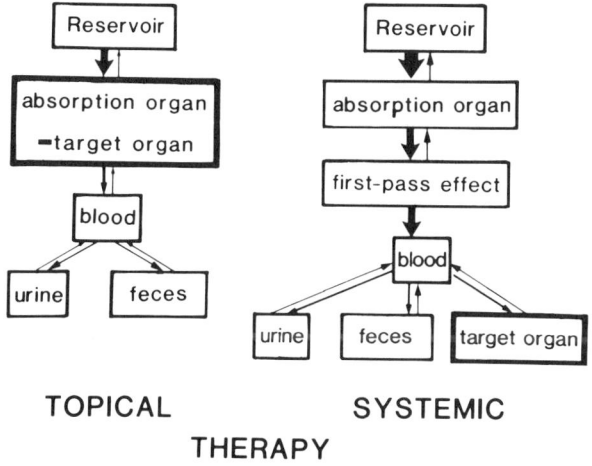

Figure 8 Comparison of topical and systemic therapies using a simple pharmacokinetic compartment model. (From Schalla and Schaefer, 1984.)

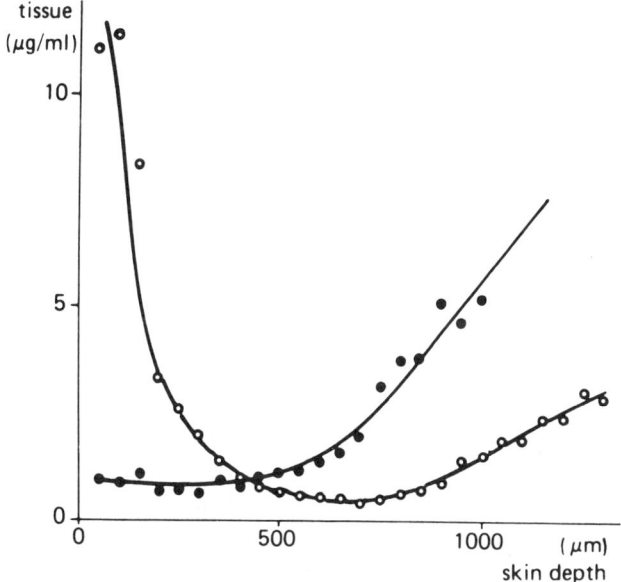

Figure 9 Cyproterone acetate distribution in the skin as a function of skin depth after local and oral administration of equal doses to rats. Oral dose: 7 × 0.4 mg per 200-g rat; topical dose: 7 × 4 mg/16 cm² skin. (From Täuber, 1982.)

Systemic Administration

After systemic administration a drug is at first distributed in all the body compartments accessible for that drug (Fig. 8); that is, it is diluted in a larger volume and therefore only a lower concentration is obtained in the skin when the same dose is administered. Hence, the whole body load of a drug is much higher after systemic administration for equivalent responses in the skin compared to topical administration.

In addition, the distribution within the skin itself differs dramatically (Fig. 9). The concentration after systemic administration falls from the deeper part of the dermis to the skin surface, in contrast to the gradient after topical application.

DRUG CONCENTRATION IN DISEASED SKIN

Diseases modify pharmacokinetics in many ways. For example, changes in blood flow and vascular permeability may alter the drug concentration in the target organ itself, gastrointestinal disorders may disturb the absorption after oral uptake, and hepatic or renal insufficiency may modify metabolism and elimination.

Dermatoses

In the topical therapy of dermatoses, changes of the barrier function will also influence the topical bioavailability of a drug (for definition see Schalla and Schaefer, 1984), in addition to the factors mentioned above. Therefore, all skin diseases with abnormal keratinization are potential candidates for such modifications in pharmacokinetics. Whereas after topical therapy abnormal keratinization will influence the influx of a drug into the skin, the blood flow and vascular permeability will only modify the efflux to the rest of the body, in contrast to systemic therapy.

Psoriasis

This common skin disease is characterized by abnormal keratinization (parakeratosis, absence of the granular layer) and abnormal microcirculation (elongated, tortuous capillaries, increased blood flow). The concentration of drugs within the involved skin is higher compared to the uninvolved skin of the same patients. This holds true for some corticoids (Schaefer et al., 1977, 1982; Schalla et al., 1980a; Zesch and Schaefer, 1975) (Fig. 10). The elimination into the urine was faster and higher (Winkler, 1966; Zesch and Schaefer, 1975). Only in one study did the increased elimination into the urine fail to reach a significant level in involved skin of psoriatic patients, compared with normal skin of healthy volunteers (Wester et al., 1983).

Other Diseases

Skin permeability also could be increased in some other dermatoses that may be associated with parakeratosis, such as eczema and superficial fungal infections.

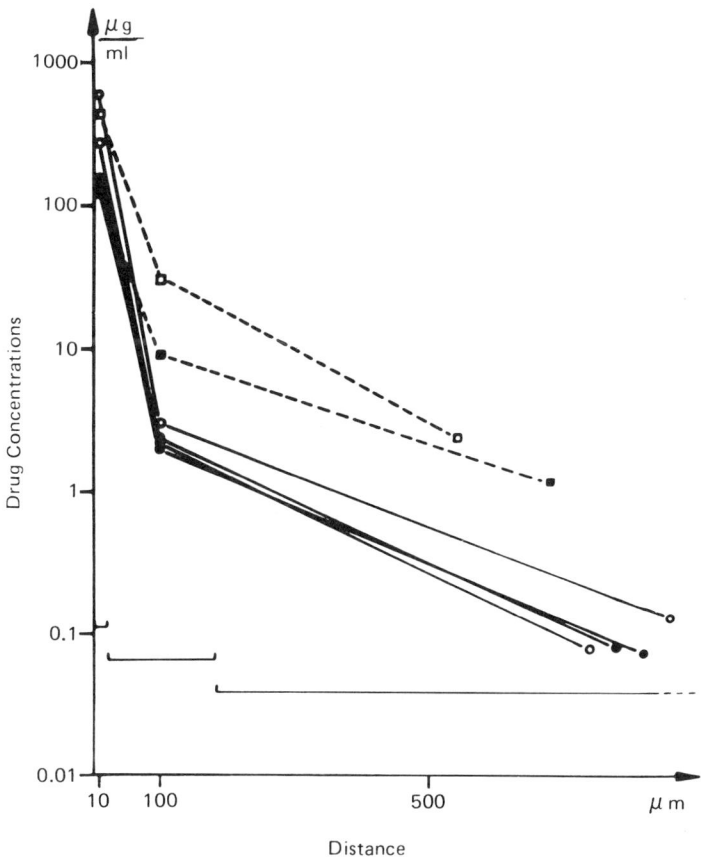

Figure 10 Drug concentrations in involved (– – –) and uninvolved (——) psoriatic skin after topical application of 0.05% (open symbols) and 0.25% (closed symbols) desoxymethasone ointment in vivo versus distance from the skin surface (mean values for the different skin layers, which are indicated on the bottom of the graph). Thicknesses used for calculations: stratum corneum = 0.02 mm, epidermis = 0.16 mm, dermis = according to the number of sections. (From Schalla et al., 1980a.)

At least for some types of eczema there is much indirect evidence that this is the case.

Increased thickness of the horny layer (hyperkeratosis) should be correlated with diminished permeability. This could be demonstrated for the plantar and to a lesser extent for the palmar skin (Feldmann and Maibach, 1967), but it should also be valid for callosities. On the other hand, the situation in hyperkeratotic disorders of keratinization, such as the various types of ichthyosiform dermatoses, is far from being clear because the thickened horny layer is an indicator for an abnormal keratinization.

Models for Skin Diseases

To overcome some of the problems encountered with patients in pharmacokinetic studies, human and animal models were developed to mimic dermatoses with a defective barrier function and/or an increased uptake by the skin vessels.

Stripping

Using the stripping technique, the horny layer can be partially or nearly completely removed according to the number of strips and the adhesive tape used. This causes a manifold increase in the concentration of various drugs in the skin (reviewed in Schaefer et al., 1982). In general, the lower the penetration into normal skin, the larger the increase by removal of the horny layer. Partial removal of the horny layer is itself sufficient for this effect if *lipophilic* substances are used (Fig. 11). This is in contrast to the claimed enhanced resistance against diffusion of *water* in the deeper part of the horny layer and the granular layer (see the "Horny Layer" section).

Ultraviolet Irradiation

With the removal of the stratum corneum by stripping, other properties of this layer can also be lost. Therefore, other models in which this barrier is disturbed but not removed may give additional information.

Forty-eight hours after UVC irradiation, the permeability of hairless mouse skin was increased in vitro (Solomon and Lowe, 1979). An increase in permeability could also be found in vivo in hairless rats 72 hr after UVB irradiation (Lamaud and Schalla, 1984). Interestingly enough, in both cases the penetration was increased only for a few hours.

Chemically Induced Barrier Dysfunction

A number of chemicals are known to modify the composition of the horny layer and thereby the penetration (Schaefer et al., 1982). The effect is quite often short lived, so that this approach does not seem to offer any advantages over UV irradiation.

Magnesium Ion Deficiency in the Hairless Rat

The skin symptoms of magnesium ion deficiency appear after 1 week, reach a maximum shortly afterward, and regress over the next few days. Skin permeability is increased, but this effect is detectable only by the increased urinary elimination, whereas the concentrations of drugs in the different skin layers remain unchanged after topical application (Schalla, Lambrey, and Lamaud, in preparation).

Essential Fatty Acid Deficiency in the Hairless Mouse and Rat

The skin symptoms of essential fatty acid deficiency and the increase in water evaporation develop more slowly, but, on the other hand, are stable over long

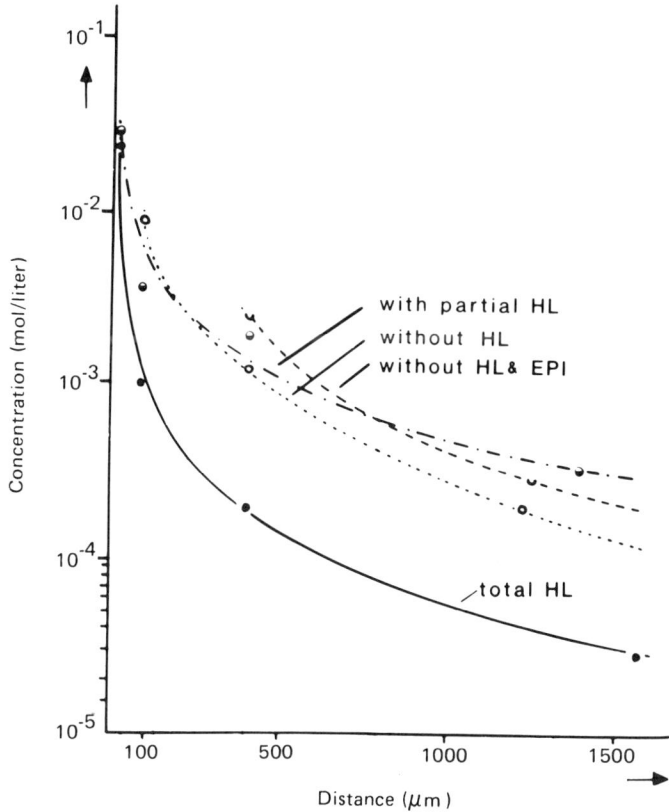

Figure 11 Influence of different degrees of skin damage on the concentrations in the different skin layers. Mean values of sections 10 and 40 μm thick for the epidermis and upper and lower dermis ($n = 2$); 10% linoleic acid in peroxide-free soybean oil; application period of 1000 min in vitro; HL = horny layer, EPI = epidermis. (From Schalla, 1978.)

periods. The skin permeability for lipophilic drugs is also increased (Lambrey, Lamaud, and Schalla, in preparation; Solomon and Lowe, 1978).

INFLUX INTO THE SKIN AND EFFLUX INTO THE BODY

Steady State

As mentioned before, the skin concentrations may be changed without corresponding changes in the urinary elimination, and vice versa. To study such questions it is important to differentiate between the early phase of penetration and

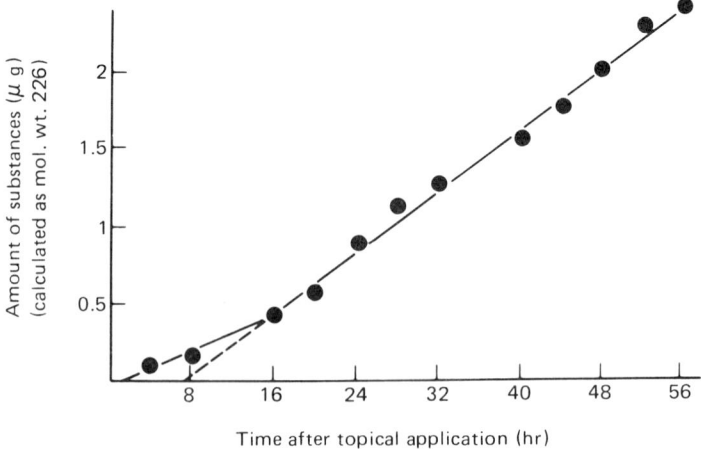

Figure 12 Cumulative urinary excretion of tritium-labeled substances calculated as 226 molecular weight after a single topical application of 0.1% anthralin in petrolatum to 28 cm² of skin surface in vivo. (From Schalla et al., 1981.)

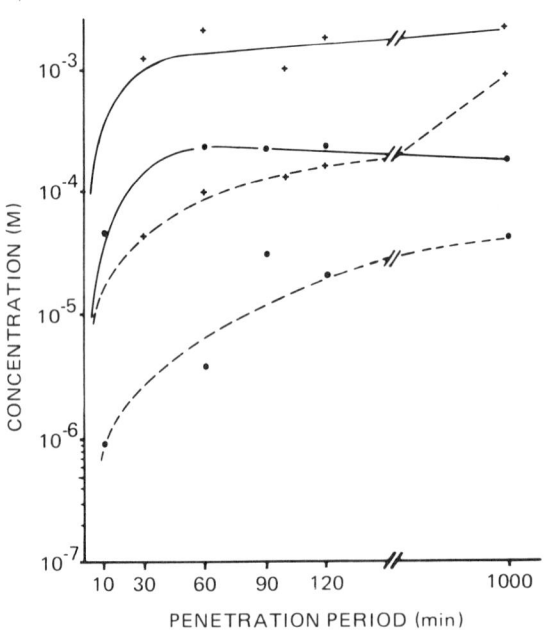

Figure 13 Molar concentrations of tritium-labeled anthralin; 0.1% (●) and 1% (+) in petrolatum in the epidermis (defined as 160 μm skin thickness following removal of the horny layer) in relation to the penetration period (– – –) with and (———) without horny layer; in vitro.

Localization of Compounds in Skin Layers

steady-state conditions and between in vitro and in vivo experiments. The reservoir formed in the horny layer and in the hair follicles and the slow influx into the skin imply that the steady state is usually reached after several hours and lasts for half a day or more for the lipophilic drugs in topical therapy (Figs. 4, 12, and 13). Applied to practical therapy, this means that topical treatment once daily is often sufficient because this holds true for both intact and disturbed barrier function. This conclusion could be validated by the unchanged urinary elimination in rhesus monkeys (Wester et al., 1977) and by the constant concentrations in the different skin layers using various application frequencies over a constant total period of 1000 min (Schalla, 1978) as well as by clinical trials (Eaglstein et al., 1974; Fredriksson et al., 1980; Hauss and Proppe, 1977; Sudilovsky et al., 1981).

Short Contact Therapy

Regarding the early phase of penetration, there is an important difference between involved and uninvolved parakeratotic skin, namely, more drug enters

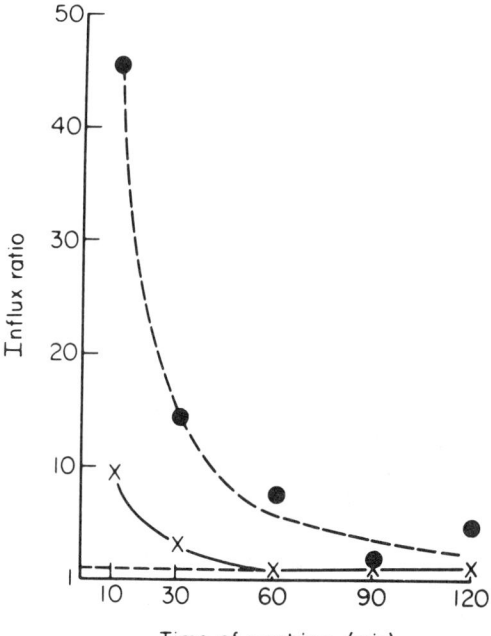

Figure 14 Ratio of the skin influx, noninfluenced, to that influenced by washing off the excess drug at different times with intact (– – –) and damaged (———) barrier function, of 0.1% tritium-labeled anthralin; total penetration period always 1000 min; in vitro.

more rapidly into diseased areas. This led us to the concept of short contact therapy (Schaefer et al., 1980; Schalla et al., 1980b, 1981): Removal of the drug excess from the skin surface after 10-60 min particularly diminishes the permeation in the uninvolved skin within the following hours compared to continuous application for the same total period, whereas there is no or only minor reduction in the involved areas (Fig. 14). This treatment regimen based on pharmacokinetic considerations could be confirmed in clinical studies (Runne and Kunze, 1982; Schaefer et al., 1980).

CALCULATIONS OF PERCUTANEOUS RESORPTION

For systemic pharmacological and toxic effects only resorption by blood and lymph vessels is of interest from the entire percutaneous absorption process (for definitions see Schaefer et al., 1978). Usually the resorption is measured by serum kinetics or in the elimination compartments. Nevertheless, there are two possibilities for calculating resorption using the skin compartments alone.

Calculations from the Skin Concentrations of in Vitro Studies

The equation below allows a rough estimation of the quantities absorbed in a given time—usually 24 hr—under steady-state conditions. Because of the assumptions made, the value represents an overestimation. Therefore, this calculation is of toxicological interest for epicutaneous application, particularly if the "no-effect level" of the substance after intravenous or subcutaneous injection is already known. Using human skin in vitro, this method then informs us whether systemic toxicity can be neglected or whether additional studies are necessary to rule out such a risk.

If only the amount of a given substance and/or its decomposition products/metabolites found in the acceptor phase after diffusion in vitro through full-thickness skin specimens is taken into account, important material still in the skin may be overlooked. On the other hand, the amount that has not yet passed the horny layer under steady-state conditions or has remained on the skin surface should not be included in the calculations. Therefore, the influx density or the specific influx will be defined for the inhomogeneous three-dimensional membrane skin from a practical point of view as follows:

$$\phi = \frac{Q_{VS} + Q_{AP}}{\text{mol wt} \times t} = \frac{Q_E + Q_{UD} + Q_{LD} + Q_{SF} + Q_{AP}}{\text{mol wt} \times t}$$

where ϕ is the specific influx into the skin (mol/cm^2/hr) and Q is the quantity (g) in the compartments indicated by the subscripts:

VS (viable skin layers)
E (epidermis)
UD and LD (upper and lower dermis, respectively)
SF (subcutaneous fat)
AP (acceptor phase)

If the steady state (ss) is reached (usually the 16- and 24-hr experiments can be used), the quantity resorbed (Q_r) after epicutaneous application can be overestimated by:

$$Q_r = \phi ss \times mol\ wt \times 24\ hr\ (g/day)$$

Calculations from Horny Layer Strips

Recently, Rougier et al. (1983) applied various compounds topically for 30 min and followed the invasion, distribution, and excretion over 96 hr in hairless rats. They demonstrated that the concentrations found in the first six horny layer strips were closely correlated to the total amount penetrating within the 96-hr period. For the hairless rat, this correlation was characterized by the equation $y = 1.644 \times x - 0.536$ ($r = 0.998$). If this were confirmed in human skin, the amount penetrating could be predicted using the simple stripping technique.

CONCLUSIONS AND SUMMARY

The following general rules pertain for the localization and the pharmacokinetics of topically applied drugs:

1. Percutaneous absorption is a passive diffusion process that may be modified by skin metabolism.
2. The main barrier against free diffusion is the stratum corneum.
3. The entire stratum corneum acts as a multilayer membrane for lipophilic drugs (brick wall model) in intact skin, in contrast to hydrophilic compounds such as water, for which an inner stratum compactum and an outer stratum disjunctum of the horny layer have been claimed.
4. Recent studies seem to indicate that the granular layer may act as an additional barrier.
5. The other viable skin layers are of minor or no importance in terms of diffusional resistance.
6. Enrichment in the subcutaneous fat is possible because of the partitioning between dermis and this tissue and perhaps also binding in some cases, although this often is of minor importance because of the low concentrations in the lower dermis.

7. The role of the skin appendages is not fully understood, although it is assumed that they play a role only in the early phase of penetration because of their small surface area compared to the interfollicular and interporous skin. Nevertheless, high concentrations can be found in hair follicles and sweat glands after long application periods.
8. In vitro methods are relevant for kinetics within the horny layer. If the application period is less than about 5 hr this also applies to the epidermis, whereas the dermal concentration measured in vitro are higher compared to in vivo studies.
9. The concentration gradient formed after topical application of lipophilic drugs means that the drug concentration in the epidermis and upper dermis is usually higher compared to systemic administration.
10. In cases of disturbed barrier function, drugs enter faster and in greater amounts into the skin. The risk for side effects on uninvolved skin and for other organs can be diminished, taking advantage of the difference between involved and uninvolved skin, by using short-contact therapy.
11. Calculations from skin compartments are available that allow one to verify whether a compound passes the "no-effect level" and also to quantitate the amount that will penetrate, at least for hairless rats.

REFERENCES

Adachi, K. (1974). Receptor proteins for androgen in hamster sebaceous glands. *J. Invest. Dermatol.* 62: 217–223.

Artuc, M., Stüttgen, G., Schalla, W., Schaefer, H., and Gazith, J. (1979). Reversible binding of 5- and 8-methoxypsoralen to human serum proteins (albumin) and to epidermis in vitro. *Br. J. Dermatol.* 101: 669–677.

Bowser, P. A. and White, R. J. (1983). Isolation and characterisation of the stratum compactum—A distinct region of the stratum corneum. *Br. J. Dermatol.* 109: 700.

Dugard, P. H. and Scheuplein, R. J. (1973). Effects of ionic surfactants on the permeability of human epidermis: An electrometric study. *J. Invest. Dermatol.* 60: 263–269.

Eaglstein, W. H., Farzad, A., and Capland, L. (1974). Topical corticosteroid therapy: Efficacy of frequent application. *Arch. Dermatol.* 110: 955.

Elias, P. (1981). Membranes, lipids, and the epidermal permeability barrier. In *The Epidermis in Disease*. Edited by R. Marks and E. Christophers. MTP, Lancaster, pp. 1–30.

Elias, P. (1983). Epidermal lipids, barrier function, and desquamation. *J. Invest. Dermato.* 80 (Suppl.): 44s–49s.

Epstein, E. H. and Bonifas, J. M. (1982). Glucocorticoid receptors for normal human epidermis. *J. Invest. Dermatol.* 78: 144–146.

Feldmann, R. J. and Maibach, H. I. (1967). Regional variation in percutaneous penetration of [^{14}C] cortisol in man. *J. Invest. Dermatol.* 48: 181–183.

Finlay, A., and Marks, R. (1982). Determination of corticosteroid concentration profiles in the stratum corneum using the skin surface biopsy technique. *Br. J. Dermatol. 107* (Suppl. 22): 33.

Fredriksson, T., Lassus, A., and Bleekes, J. (1980). Treatment of psoriasis and atopic dermatitis with halcinonide cream applied once and three times daily. *Br. J. Dermatol. 101*: 575–577.

Gazith, J., Cavey, M. T., Elena, P. P., Shroot, B., and Reichert, U. (1982). β-Adrenergic and histamine receptors in cultured skin fibroblasts and keratinocytes. *J. Invest. Dermatol. 78*: 329.

Hauss, H. and Proppe, A. (1977). Kortikoidsparende Behandlungsweisen in der Dermatologie. *Therapiewoche 27*: 5340–5352.

Holyo-Tomoka, M. T., and Kligman, A. M. (1972). Does cellophane tape stripping remove the horny layer? *Arch. Dermatol. 106*: 767–768.

Kiistala, U. (1968). Suction blister device for separation of viable epidermis from dermis. *J. Invest. Dermatol. 50*: 129–137.

Kiistala, U. (1976). The suction blister method for the in vivo separation of epidermis from dermis in human skin. Thesis, Helsinki.

Kligman, A. M. and Christophers, E. (1963). Preparation of isolated sheets of human skin. *Arch. Dermatol. 88*: 702–705.

Knight, A. G. (1974). The activity of various topical griseofulvin preparations and the appearance of oral griseofulvin in the stratum corneum. *Br. J. Dermatol. 91*: 49–55.

Kukita, A., Matsuzawa, T., and Takeda, Y. (1973). Percutaneous absorption of topically applied corticosteroids: An autoradiographic study. In *Proceedings of the Fourteenth International Congress on Dermatology*. Edited by F. Flarer and F. Serri. Excerpta Medica, Amsterdam, pp. 976–980.

Lamaud, E. and Schalla, W. (1984). Influence of UV-irradiation on penetration of hydrocortisone–In vivo study in the hairless rat skin. *Br. J. Dermatol.* (Suppl. 27): 152–157.

Marks, R., and Dawber, R. P. R. (1971). Skin surface biopsy: An improved technique for the examination of the horny layer. *Br. J. Dermatol. 84*: 117–123.

Menczel, E. and Maibach, H. I. (1972). Chemical binding to human dermis in vitro–Testosterone and benzyl alcohol. *Acta Dermatovenereol.* (Stockholm) *52*: 38–42.

Polano, M. K., Ponec, M., Smeenk, G., and Hendrikse, J. M. C. (1972). Factors influencing the penetration of corticosteroids through the epidermis. In *Advances in Biology of the Skin*, Vol. XII, *Pharmacology and the Skin*. Edited by W. Montagna, R. B. Stoughton, and E. van Scott. Appleton, New York, pp. 325–328.

Rossing, N. and Worm, A. M. (1981). Interstitial fluid: Exchange of macromolecules between plasma and skin interstitium. *Clin. Physiol. 1*: 275–284.

Rougier, A., Dupuis, D., Lotte, C., Rouguet, R., and Schaefer, H. (1983). In vivo correlation between stratum corneum reservoir function and percutaneous absorption. *J. Invest. Dermatol. 81*: 275–278.

Runne, U. and Kunze, J. (1982). Short duration ("minutes") therapy with dithranol for psoriasis: A new out-patient regimen. *Br. J. Dermatol. 106*: 135–139.

Schaefer, H., Zesch, A., and Stüttgen, G. (1977). Penetration, permeation and absorption of triamcinolone acetonide in normal and psoriatic skin. *Arch. Dermatol. Res. 258*: 241-249.

Schaefer, H., Stüttgen, G., Zesch, A., Schalla, W., and Gazith, J. (1978). Quantitative determination of percutaneous absorption of radiolabeled drugs in vitro and in vivo by human skin. In *Current Problems in Dermatology*, Vol. 7. Edited by J. H. W. Mali. Karger, Basel, pp. 80-94.

Schaefer, H., Farber, E. M., Goldberg, L., and Schalla, W. (1980). Limited application period for dithranol in psoriasis. *Br. J. Dermatol. 102*: 571-573.

Schaefer, H., Zesch, A., and Stüttgen, G. (1982). *Skin Permeability.* Springer, Berlin. (Reprinted from *Handbuch der Haut- und Geschlechtskrankheiten, Erg.-Werk,* Vol. I/4b, pp. 541-896.)

Schalla, W. (1978). Penetration von essentiellen Fettsäuren und Triglyzeriden in die menschliche Haut beim Säugling und Erwachsenen—In vitro- und in vivo Daten und ihre klinische Bedeutung. Thesis, Berlin.

Schalla, W., Bauer, E., and Schaefer, H. (1980a). Beinflussungsgrössen der Penetration von Steroidexterna. *Aktuel. Dermatol. 6* (Suppl. 1): 3-11.

Schalla, W., Bauer, E., Wesendahl, C., Goldberg, L., Farber, E. M., and Schaefer, H. (1980b). Penetration studies in short-term therapy with dithranol. *Arch. Dermatol. Res. 267*: 203.

Schalla, W., Bauer, E., and Schaefer, H. (1981). Skin permeability of anthralin. *Br. J. Dermatol. 105* (Suppl. 20): 104-108.

Schalla, W. and Schaefer, H. (1984). Lokalapplikation—Pharmakokinetik, therapeutische Systeme und Kurzzeit- (Minuten-) Therapie. In *Klinische Pharmakologie—Grundlagen, Methoden, Therapie.* Edited by H.-P. Kuemmerle, P. Hitzenberger, and G. Spitzy. Ecomed, Munich, pp. II-2.8.1-2.8.11.

Scheuplein, R. J. (1967). Mechanism of percutaneous absorption. II. Transient diffusion and the relative importance of various routes of skin penetration. *J. Invest. Dermatol. 48*: 79-88.

Schulze, W. (1971). Modellversuche an isolierter Epidermis zur Prüfung der Permeabilität der menschlichen Haut und der Kinetik des Penetrationsvorgangs. *Fette Seifen Anstrichm. 73*: 319-324.

Slaga, T., Thompson, S., and Schwarz, J. A. (1977). Binding of dexamethasone by the subcellular fractions of mouse epidermis and dermis. *J. Invest. Dermatol. 68*: 307-309.

Smeenk, G. and Polano, M. K. (1965). Methods for comparative estimations of the irritancy of various detergents on human skin. *Trans. St. Johns Hosp. Dermatol. Soc.* (London) *51*: 220-221.

Solomon, A. E. and Lowe, N. J. (1978). Percutaneous absorption in experimental epidermal proliferation. *Arch. Dermatol. 114*: 1029-1030.

Solomon, A. E. and Lowe, N. J. (1979). Percutaneous absorption in experimental epidermal disease. *Br. J. Dermatol. 100*: 717-722.

Sudilovsky, A., Muir, J. G., and Bocobo, F. C. (1981). A comparison of single and multiple applications of halcinonide cream. *Int. J. Dermatol. 20*: 609-613.

Szakall, A. (1958). Experimentelle Daten zur Klärung der Funktion der Wasserbarriere in der Epidermis des lebenden Menschen. *Berufsdermatosen 6*: 171–192.

Täuber, U. (1982). Metabolism of drugs on and in the skin. In *Dermal and Transdermal Absorption*. Edited by R. Brandau and B. H. Lippold. Wissenschaftliche Verlagsgesellschaft, Stuttgart, pp. 133–151.

Tregear, R. T. (1966). *Physical Functions of the Skin*. Academic, New York.

van Scott, E. J. (1952). Mechanical separation of the epidermis from the corium. *J. Invest. Dermatol. 18*: 377.

Vermeer, B. J., Reman, F. C., and van Gent, C. M. (1979). The determination of lipids and proteins in suction blister fluid. *J. Invest. Dermatol. 73*: 303–305.

Volden, G., Thorsrud, A. K., Bjornson, I., and Jellum, E. (1980). Biochemical composition of suction blister fluid determined by high resolution multicomponent analysis (capillary gas chromatography–mass spectrometry and two-dimensional electrophoresis). *J. Invest. Dermatol. 75*: 421–424.

Wester, R. C., Noonan, P. K., and Maibach, H. I. (1977). Frequency of application on percutaneous absorption of hydrocortisone. *Arch. Dermatol. 113*: 620–622.

Wester, R. C., Bucks, D. A. W., and Maibach, H. I. (1983). In vivo percutaneous absorption of hydrocortisone in psoriatic patients and normal volunteers. *J. Am. Acad. Dermatol. 8*: 645–647.

Winkler, K. (1968). Steroiduntersuchungen im Blut und Harn bei Anwendung von Fluocortolon- und Hydrocortisonsalbe. *Arch. Klin. Exp. Dermatol. 232*: 39–55.

Zesch, A. and Schaefer, H. (1975). Penetration of radioactive hydrocortisone in human skin from various ointment bases. II. In vivo experiments. *Arch. Dermatol. Res. 252*: 245–256.

Zesch, A., Schaefer, H., Hoffmann, W. (1973). Barriere- und Reservoirfunktion der menschlichen Haut für lokal aufgetragene Arzneimittel. *Arch. Dermatol. Res. 246*: 103–107.

23
Evaporation and Penetration from Skin

William G. Reifenrath
Letterman Army Institute of Research, San Francisco, California

Thomas S. Spencer
S. C. Johnson & Son, Inc., Racine, Wisconsin

MODES OF LOSS FROM THE SKIN SURFACE

Three types of material commonly contact the skin surface: (1) cosmetics and toiletries (hand and body lotions or perfume products), (2) drug products (steroids, sunscreens, or antiperspirants), and (3) toxicants that inadvertently contaminate the skin (certain laboratory chemicals or pesticides in agricultural situations). Components of all three classes of products evaporate from the skin, penetrate into the skin, and form reservoirs. However, in each class the relative importance of evaporation, penetration, or skin reservoir effect may vary.

Evaporation

In the case of toiletry products, evaporation produces a familiar cooling sensation on the skin as high-volatility compounds such as ethanol or isopropanol evaporate from the lotion. The rapid evaporation from a hand and body lotion gives a perception of quick absorption into the skin (actually evaporation from the skin). Some products contain compounds of lower volatility, which evaporate slowly over a longer period. Low-volatility compounds include perfumes and mosquito repellents, where evaporation is desirable or beneficial for the product effect.

Citation of trade names in this chapter does not constitute an official endorsement or approval of the use of such items. The opinions or assertions contained herein are the private view of the author(s) and are not to be construed as official or as reflecting views of the Department of the Army or the Department of Defense (AR 360-5).

For drug products, such as topical creams or lotions containing steroids, local anesthetics, or sunscreens, evaporation of an active ingredient would be undesirable. On the other hand, evaporation of a carrier or water from a formulation increases the surface concentration and may promote transdermal delivery of a drug for systemic effect. In the case of toxicants, the hazards associated with percutaneous absorption are well recognized. Evaporation is desirable in that it reduces the amount of compound available for skin penetration. However, evaporation creates an inhalation hazard to the exposed individuals as the toxicant vaporizes from the skin.

In summary, evaporation can be the major purpose for a topical formulation applied to the skin, evaporation may improve the transdermal delivery of a drug by concentrating a formulation or changing the relative components in a formulation, or evaporation may be a complicating factor when skin is exposed to environmental hazards.

Surface Reservoir Removal

For a period of time after topical application, a compound may form a surface reservoir on top or in the upper layers of the skin. In addition to potential losses of compound from this reservoir by evaporation and penetration into deeper layers of the skin, the reservoir itself can be removed chemically or mechanically. Contact of the skin reservoir with other surfaces such as the rubbing against clothing or abrading surface layers of the stratum corneum are examples of mechanical removal. Chemical removal may be effected by emulsification or solvation of the compound and subsequent removal by rinsing or by use of absorbents such as fuller's earth. If the compound itself is chemically unstable in the environment of the skin, hydrolysis, oxidation, or enzymatic degradation could contribute to its own removal process. In some cases, the skin surface is treated with chemicals (e.g., nucleophiles or oxidants) to speed this process. The normal sloughing of the stratum corneum could contribute a biological form of removal of surface reservoir. Whether chemical, mechanical, or biological means are operative, the fate of the surface reservoir must be taken into account to understand the processes of skin evaporation and penetration.

Penetration

For many compounds, penetration into the skin is a significant mode of loss from the skin surface. The penetration process is complicated by the possibility of concomitant degradation or metabolism and the formation of reservoirs in various internal layers of the skin. Circulation in the viable layers of the skin can remove the applied compound, its metabolites or breakdown products to varying degrees depending on relative affinity. In some cases, the compound can bind to the skin by formation of a covalent bond (e.g., aldehydes).

A complete discussion of skin penetration is beyond the scope of this chapter; however, it is important to understand that this process competes with other modes of loss from the skin surface. Although it is difficult or impossible to control or measure all the modes of loss simultaneously, events that directly affect one mode have indirect effects on the others.

METHODS

Evaporation/Penetration Cells

A design of cells used to measure evaporation of chemicals from the skin surface and penetration through the skin is shown in Figure 1 (Laboratory Glass Appara-

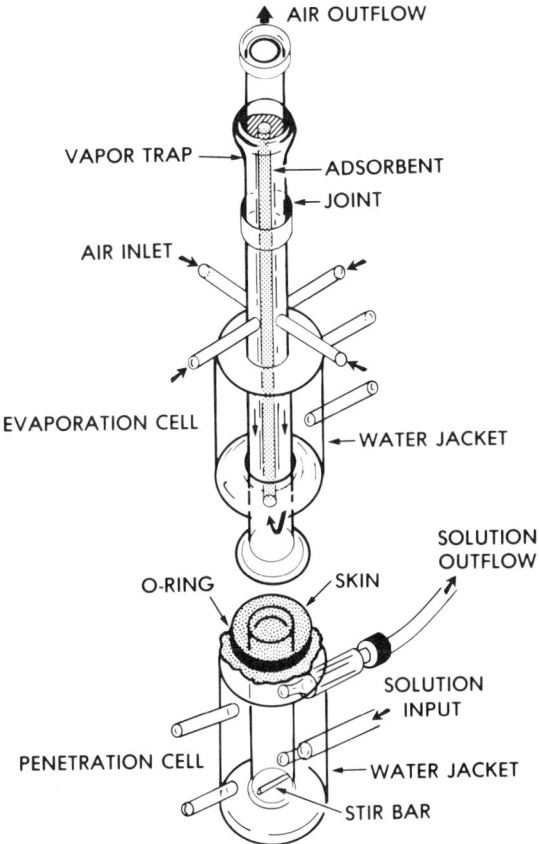

Figure 1 Skin penetration/evaporation cells.

tus, Berkeley, Calif.). The cells are essentially those described previously (Reifenrath and Robinson, 1982), but with the addition of water jackets to both evaporation and penetration cells, an O-ring mount for attaching the skin to the penetration cell, and an adapter for connecting the solution outflow port of the penetration cell to teflon tubing.

In operation, the cells are connected as shown in Figure 2. Skin is mounted, visceral side down, on the penetration cell and the cell filled with solution so that the visceral side of the skin is in contact with solution and no air bubbles are present. Solution is then pumped through the penetration cell from a reservoir to a collector so that chemical penetrating through the skin is carried away. The outflow of fluid can be fractionated into time intervals to obtain plots of percutaneous penetration versus time. The concentration of chemical in a given outflow sample is an average of concentration in the penetration cell over the time the sample was collected; however, if the flow of solution through the penetration cell is sufficient, a reasonably accurate description of the penetration process is obtainable.

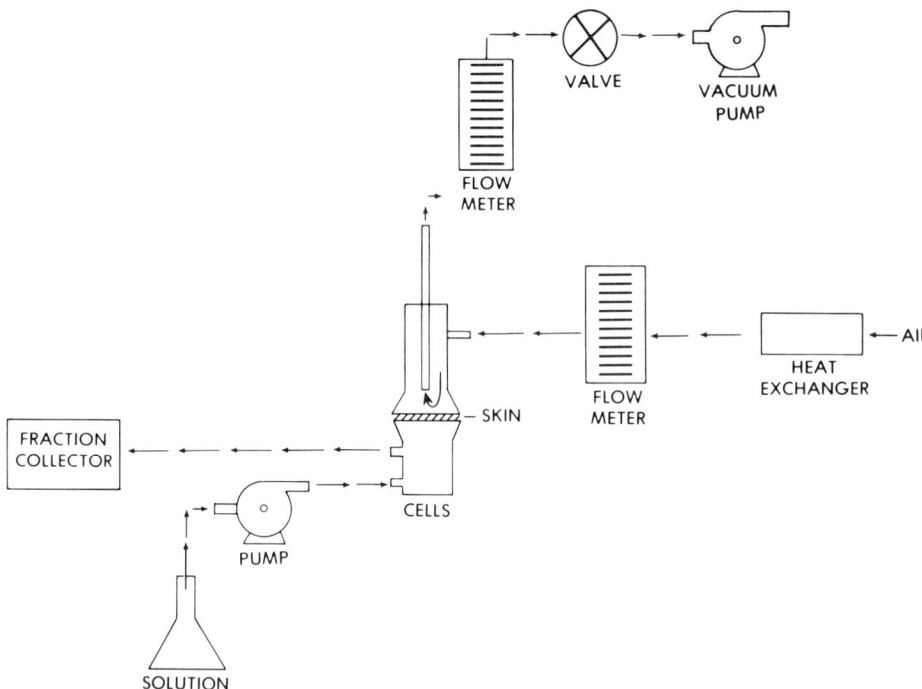

Figure 2 Diagram of apparatus for measurement of skin penetration and evaporation.

Air is drawn into the inlets of the evaporation cell, over the skin surface, and through a vapor trap. The vapor trap is connected to an air pump via a valve to control the flow of air through the evaporation cell. Chemical evaporating from the skin surface is entrained in the air flow and collected in the absorbent in the vapor trap tube. Vapor traps can be changed at intervals of time to obtain plots of evaporative loss vs time. Air temperature control is achieved before entry into the evaporation cell by passing air through a coil immersed in the water bath used to supply the jacket of the evaporation cell. Variations of the apparatus shown in Figures 1 and 2 were used in specific experiments discussed in the sections that follow. When significant, these variations will be noted.

Types of Skin

Animal Models and Anatomical Variation

Measurements of skin disposition of chemicals ideally would be done on human skin. However, the restrictions of conducting in vivo studies with human volunteers and the limited availability of human skin for in vitro studies necessitate animal models. The subject of animal models for human skin in permeability determinations has been reviewed (Meyer et al., 1978; Wester and Maibach, 1977); based on available data from in vitro and in vivo comparisons of skin permeability of various animals and man, the skin from the monkey and pig appeared to be better models for human skin than skin from rodents. More recently (Reifenrath et al., 1984a), the skin permeability properties of the female weanling Yorkshire pig were compared to man by determining the skin permeability of nine compounds (caffeine, benzoic acid, N,N-diethyl-m-toluamide, progesterone, testosterone, fluocinolone acetonide, parathion, malathion, and lindane) in these animals and comparing values obtained to published data for these compounds on the forearm of man (Bartek and LaBudde, 1975; Feldmann and Maibach, 1969, 1970). A significant correlation ($r = 0.83, p < 0.05$) was found between the values obtained for the weanling pig and man. When the skin permeability values of these nine compounds were determined on split-thickness skin from man and weanling pig grafted to the athymic nude mouse, reasonable agreement was found between the two types of skin, considering the variability of these determinations (Reifenrath et al., 1984a). Furthermore, a significant correlation ($r = 0.77, p < 0.05$) has been found between skin permeability values of 10 compounds determined on weanling pig skin in vitro versus previously published values on man (Hawkins and Reifenrath, 1984). Based on the foregoing and because of the limited availability and expense of monkey skin, the skin of the weanling pig was utilized when human skin was not available.

Because of previous reports of anatomical variation in skin permeability (Scheuplein, 1978), skin samples used in experiments described in the following sections were always harvested from the middorsal region of Yorkshire pigs. To eliminate possible variations due to age and sex with this animal model, only female weanling pigs were used. Human skin for in vitro determinations was obtained at autopsy from the abdomen. Because it was not possible to obtain this skin at times corresponding to experiments, skin was held frozen for periods up to 2 months. Frozen storage can affect the evaporation and penetration of a compound on the skin, as discussed below.

Skin Preparation

Pig skin used for in vitro measurements was either full thickness or split thickness. Full-thickness skin was obtained by removal of subcutaneous fat with a dermatome set at 1.9 mm. Split-thickness skin was obtained by removal of approximately 1 mm of dermis from the full-thickness skin, again by use of a dermatome. Full-thickness human skin used for in vitro measurements was prepared by removal of subcutaneous fat by scraping.

Procedures for Quantifying Evaporation from Skin and Penetration Through Skin

In Vitro Determinations

Method I. The dermal or visceral side of the skin samples (fresh or thawed from frozen storage) was placed on the penetration cell and the cell filled with solution. The evaporation cell (Fig. 1) was fitted and the system allowed to equilibrate. The evaporation manifold was then removed and radiolabeled compound applied to the skin. The evaporation cell was refitted, airflow above the skin and solution flow beneath the skin were started, and the sampling regime begun.

By changing the replaceable vapor traps (Fig. 1) filled with absorbent (Tenax GC, Alltech Associates, Arlington Heights, Ill.), vapor arising from the skin could be fractionated to allow determination of evaporation rate ($\mu gEq/cm^2/hr$) versus time. Absorbent was removed from the vapor traps and placed in scintillation counting vials, and disintegrations per minute (dpm) determined on a scintillation spectrometer. The percentage of the applied radioactive dose appearing in the vapor traps over the duration of the experiment was termed "total percent evaporation."

Outflow from the penetration cell was fractionated into hourly or bihourly samples. Aqueous counting solution was added to the fractions for scintillation counting. The percentage of applied radioactive dose appearing in fluid perfused through the penetration cell over the duration of the experiment was termed "total percent percutaneous penetration."

At the completion of each experiment, the stratum corneum side of the skin samples was rinsed with counting solution to remove compound from the skin surface. The skin was then oxidized and liberated $[^{14}C]CO_2$ or (^3H) H_2O determined as previously described (Reifenrath and Robinson, 1982). Penetration and evaporation cells were each rinsed with counting solution to remove any residual activity. Total recoveries of approximately 90% of the applied radioactive dose were routinely achievable.

Unless specifically noted, determinations of skin penetration and evaporation were conducted over a 50-hr period with fresh whole skin, Tyrode's solution perfusing the penetration cell, dry air at 24°C flowing through the evaporation cell at 60 ml/min, and the tip of the vapor trap tube positioned 9.5 mm above the skin surface. Three to four replicate determinations were obtained.

Method II. Method II differed from method I in that an evaporation cell of significantly different design was employed (T. S. Spencer et al., 1979), and trapping and fractionation procedures for vapor were different. Specifically, 6-cm collection tubes (syringes) containing dry cotton as an absorbent were attached to an evaporation cell. This cell was fashioned such that the tip of the vapor collection tube was 1.5 mm above the skin surface. The effect of this placement is discussed in the section on factors affecting the evaporation and penetration process. The cotton from the tube and the rinses were placed in a scintillation counting vial for determination of radioactivity. Alternately, this evaporation cell could be connected to a bubbler trap containing counting solution so that air passing over the skin was then caused to flow through the bubbler. The temperature of tubing from the evaporation cell to the bubler was raised above the temperature of air entering the evaporation cell to reduce condensation of evaporated compound before it reached the bubbler trap. The bubbler trap was equipped with solenoid-activated valves to allow automatic emptying and filling so that evaporation could be fractionated.

In Vivo Determinations

The in vivo experiments were performed using an evaporation cell (T. S. Spencer et al., 1979) with its water jacket maintained at 32°C. N,N-Diethyl-m-toluamide, a widely used mosquito repellent, was applied to the forearm using ethanol as a vehicle. A second site on the forearm received only ethanol. Thirty minutes after application, the evaporation cell was placed on the application site and a dry nitrogen gas source was connected to the inlet port of the evaporation cell. For determinations described in this section the evaporation cell discussed in connection with method II was used. Using Teflon tubing, the gas outflow from the evaporation cell was connected to a flame ionization detector. The reported results are the difference between the values for sites treated with N,N-diethyl-m-toluamide/ethanol and sites treated with ethanol only.

An alternate method involved ^{14}C-labeled N,N-diethyl-m-toluamide application to the forearm. A chemical dose of 25 μg/cm^2 and a radioactive dose of 0.01 μCi were used. After the site had been allowed to dry in air for 1 min, the evaporation cell was placed on the site and held in place using a strap (Velcro). Procedures for trapping and quantifying radioactive compound evaporation from the skin involved use of dry cotton packed tubes as discussed under method II.

When vapor collections were terminated, the skin surface was swabbed with toluene-soaked cotton balls to recover surface residue. Penetration into the superficial layers of the skin was assessed by stripping layers of stratum corneum from the application site by use of cellphane tape. The cotton swab and cellophane tape were placed directly into counting vials filled with scintillation fluid. This procedure was not found to affect counting efficiency.

COMPARISON OF SKIN PENETRATION AND EVAPORATION IN VITRO AND IN VIVO

For comparison of in vitro and in vivo evaporation and penetration from the skin, the topical insect repellent N,N-diethyl-m-toulamide is used as a model compound, since significant amounts of the compound are lost from the skin surface by both modes.

A direct comparison of in vitro and in vivo evaporation at 25 $\mu g/cm^2$ (the minimum effective dose of repellent necessary to repel mosquitoes) was carried out by T. S. Spencer et al. (1979). Evaporation in the in vitro cell afforded an evaporation rate of 4.0 $\mu g/cm^2/hr$ at a dose of 25 $\mu g/cm^2$. The same cell applied to the skin surface with the same airflow rate afforded an evaporation rate of 3.5 $\mu g/cm^2/hr$. A third method of measurement in which the effluent was passed directly into a flame ionization detector provided an evaporation rate of 3.5 $\mu g/cm^2/hr$ versus an ethanol control. Therefore, the three methods demonstrated good correlation between in vitro and in vivo evaporation rates.

In separate experiments, reasonable agreement has also been found between total percutaneous penetration values of N,N-diethyl-m-toulamide determined in vitro and in vivo when all experiments were conducted at a topical dose of 4 $\mu g/cm^2$. Specifically, Hawkins and Reifenrath (1984) report a value of 14 ±4% of the applied dose with pig skin in vitro versus in vivo values of 9 ±4% for the pig (Reifenrath et al., 1984a), and 17 ±5% for man (Feldmann and Maibach, 1970).

With the current limited data base, it appears that in vitro methodologies with appropriate skin and carefully designed cells can provide a good approximation for evaporation and penetration processes in vivo. Additional chemicals must be studied to verify if this trend will continue to hold.

FACTORS AFFECTING THE EVAPORATION AND PENETRATION PROCESS

Experimental Conditions

Skin Storage Conditions
The effect of frozen storage of skin on the evaporation and penetration processes has been examined with N,N-diethyl-m-toluamide (Hawkins and Reifenrath,

1984). The percutaneous penetration and the evaporation of the compound on pig skin were determined in triplicate on skin from five different pigs. Samples of the same skin were used fresh and again after freezing at $-80°C$ for 1-6 weeks. Pig skin held frozen for longer than 1 week was more permeable (Fig. 3). A significant correlation ($r = 0.87$, $p < 0.05$) was found between mean total percent percutaneous penetration and the number of weeks that the skin was held frozen. When the mean total percent percutaneous penetration values using fresh skin were subtracted from the mean total percent percutaneous penetration values obtained after freezing, the differences obtained correlated with the number of weeks of frozen storage ($r = 0.87$, $p = 0.05$). Although a significant correlation was not found between total evaporation values and weeks of frozen storage, total evaporation values decreased ($r = 0.92$, $p < 0.05$) when the penetration values were found to increase. These findings may not be relevant for all compounds or types of skin, but they suggest that skin storage conditions could be a factor in these determinations.

Vapor Collection Technique

The evaporation cells and associated vapor traps described were designed to capture chemicals from a stream of air that passed over the skin in an evaporation cell. An increase in the velocity of air over the skin surface increased evaporative loss of a compound (Table 1). The geometry of the evaporation cell, specifically the position of the tube drawing air from the cell relative to the skin, will increase

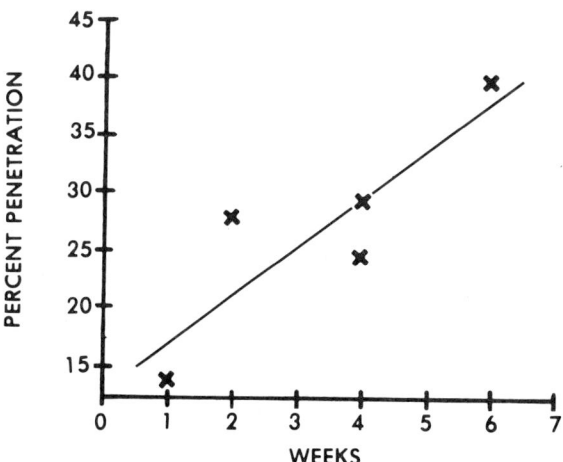

Figure 3 Linear regression line and plot of mean percent percutaneous penetration (percentage of applied radioactive dose) of N,N-diethyl-m-toluamide (320 $\mu g/cm^2$) versus frozen storage time of skin samples before use. (From Hawkins and Reifenrath, 1984.)

Table 1 The Influence of Airflow Rate on the Evaporation of N,N-Diethyl-m-Toluamide (30 μg/cm^2) from Pig Skin in Vitro[a]

Airflow rate (ml/min)	Percent of applied radioactive dose		Evaporation rate (μg/cm^2/time interval)[b]			
	Total evaporation	Total penetration	0–10 min	10–25 min	25–40 min	40–55 min
30	45±4	20±5	0.08 ±0.01	0.17 ±0.09	0.16 ±0.02	0.23 ±0.05
60	54±2	15±4	0.3 ±0.1	0.4 ±0.2	0.4 ±0.2	0.4 ±0.1

[a]Standard test conditions, except that split-thickness skin (1 mm total thickness) was used, tissue culture media (RPM I, Gibco Laboratories, Santa Clara, Calif.) perfused the penetration cell, and air was at 32°C and ambient relative humidity (approximately 40%).
[b]Microgram equivalents (μg Eq) of radioactivity recovered in the vapor traps at the times intervals designated.

Table 2 The Influence of Vapor Trap Position on the Evaporation of N,N-Diethyl-m-Toluamide from Pig Skin in Vitro[a]

Distance above skin surface (mm)	Total evaporation (mean ± SD)[b]	Evaporation rate[c] ($\mu g/cm^2/hr$)		n
		Initial	Final	
6.5	15±1	8±1	4±2	5
9.5	9±1	3±1	3±1	3

[a]N,N-Diethyl-m-toluamide was applied to full-thickness fresh pig skin at a chemical dose of 320 $\mu g/cm^2$. Ringer's solution was used to perfuse the penetration cell.
[b]Values were measured over 8 hr post application.
[c]Microgram equivalents (μg Eq) of radioactivity recovered in vapor traps averaged from hours 1 and 2 (initial) and hours 7 and 8 (final) post application periods.

air velocity over the skin as the distance between the skin and the tip of the tube decreases. Such a change increased evaporative loss (Table 2).

Vapor Pressure

Evaporative loss from the skin surface was expected to increase as the vapor pressure of a compound increased (Gabel et al., 1976). The overall trend shown in Table 3 is consistent with this expectation. Some error is introduced in this comparison because values for vapor pressure were obtained from a variety of sources. Differences in penetration into and through the skin may account for part of this discrepancy. For example, evaporative loss of benzoic acid was lower than for lindane and malathion, compounds with lower vapor pressures. But higher percutaneous penetration was found for benzoic acid versus lindane, and somewhat higher recovery of radioactivity was found for benzoic acid versus malathion by oxidation of the skin (Table 3).

Air Temperature and Humidity

The influence of air temperature on the percutaneous penetration and evaporation of N,N-diethyl-m-toluamide on pig skin was examined (Hawkins and Reifenrath, 1984). These experiments were conducted at a dose of 320 $\mu g/cm^2$, a standard repellent dosage (Hill et al., 1979). Triplicate determinations were made with air temperatures of 20, 24, and 32°C.

The temperature of air flowing through the evaporation manifold had a significant effect on both evaporation and percutaneous penetration (Figs. 4 and 5). When the temperature was increased from 20 to 24°C, a moderate increase in skin evaporation and a corresponding decrease in penetration were observed. (The 20°C evaporation plot was deleted in Fig. 4 for clarity, since it was nearly

Table 3 Comparison of Vapor Pressure and Disposition of Radioactivity After Topical Application of Radiolabeled Control Compounds to Pig Skin Under Standardized Conditions[a]

Compound	Vapor pressure (mm × 10^{-5} at 20°C)[c]	Percent of applied radioactive dose (mean ± SD)[b]				
		Evaporation	Percutaneous penetration	Skin oxidation	Skin wash	Total recovery[d]
DDT	0.015	4±5	0.2±0.2	47±7	35±4	93±1
Parathion	0.47	7.0±0.6	1.3±0.5	53±4	20±4	88±4
Malathion[e]	0.55	17±6	19±14	42±1	9±2	89±5
Lindane	3.3	26±5	0.7±0.3	43±17	9±4	83±6
Benzoic acid	38	5.7±0.3	20±13	51±9[e]	7±2	87±4[e]
N,N-Diethyl-m-toluamide	103	21±6	14±4	38±10	5±1	83±3
Diethyl malonate[f]	24,900	40±10	10±3	30±10	2±1	85
Diisopropyl fluorophosphonate[f]	57,900	65±8	7±5	12±8	0.8±0.7	85

[a]Compounds were applied to fresh pig skin at a dose of 4 μg/cm².
[b]Unless otherwise indicated, values are for three replicates.
[c]Vapor pressures were taken from the literature: DDT (Spencer and Cliath, 1972); parathion and malathion (Guckel et al., 1973); lindane (Spencer and Cliath, 1970); benzoic acid (Davies and Jones, 1954); N,N-diethyl-m-toluamide (Blaine and Levy, 1974); diethyl malonate (Long and Wallace, 1981); and diisopropyl fluorophosphonate (Merck Index, 8th ed., 1968).
[d]Total recovery includes small percentages recovered from apparatus rinse.
[e]$n = 2$.
[f]Values were corrected for losses during application by adding the difference between actual and 85% assumed total recovery to trapped evaporation.

Source: Hawkins and Reifenrath (1984).

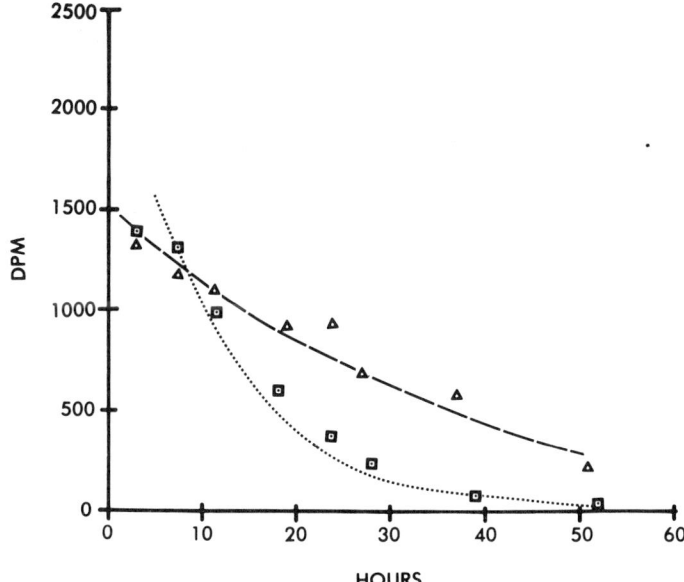

Figure 4 Evaporation (dpm) recovered from vapor traps) of N,N-diethyl-m-toluamide (320 $\mu g/cm^2$) versus time at air temperatures of 24°C (dashed curve) and 32°C (dotted curve). Specific activity, 345 dpm/μg. (From Hawkins and Reifenrath, 1984.)

identical to the 24°C plot shown.) At 32°C, penetration increased twofold over the value at 20°C and total evaporation was less than the value at 20°C.

The influence of air humidity on percutaneous penetration was examined by comparing the mean percent penetration for malathion, N,N-diethyl-m-toluamide, DDT, progesterone, testosterone, and caffeine at 0 and 75% relative humidity (Hawkins and Reifenrath, 1984). Adjustment of the relative humidity was achieved by conducting the experiments in an environmental chamber.

Increased relative humidity had the effect of increasing percutaneous penetration for relatively water-soluble compounds (N,N-diethyl-m-toluamide, caffeine, and malathion) whereas the penetration of more lipid-soluble compounds (progesterone, testosterone, and DDT) was unaffected (Fig. 6).

Dose and Vehicle

For the compounds testosterone, hydrocortisone, and benzoic acid, Wester and Maibach (1976) have demonstrated that the percentage of applied dose penetrating the skin of monkey and man increases as the applied dose decreases.

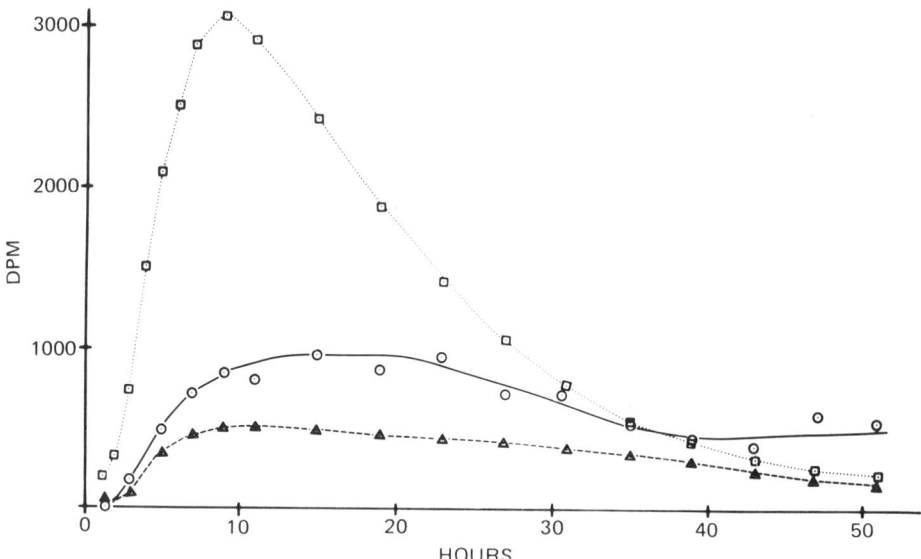

Figure 5 Percutaneous penetration (dpm outflow from the penetration cell) of N,N-diethyl-m-toluamide (320 μg/cm^2) versus time at air temperatures of 20°C (solid curve), 24°C (dashed curve), and 32°C (dotted curve). Specific activity, 345 dpm/μg. (From Hawkins and Reifenrath, 1984.)

Scheuplein and Ross (1974) reported a decrease in percentage percutaneous penetration of cortisone with increase in chemical dose on human skin in vitro. Of course, in both cases, the total amount absorbed through skin increased with increasing applied dose. In the case of the more volatile insect repellents, Reifenrath et al. (1981) found no significant increase in percentage penetration with decreasing dose for N,N-diethyl-m-toluamide, 2-ethyl-1,3-hexanediol, and 1-(butylsulfonyl)hexahydro-1H-azepine in in vivo studies using hairless dogs. When N,N-diethyl-m-toluamide was applied to pig skin in vitro, a higher evaporation rate was obtained at 320 μg/cm^2 compared to 4 μg/cm^2, while the percentage penetrating into the skin at the two doses was similar (Table 4).

The effect of dose and vehicle on skin disposition of volatile compounds was investigated using radiolabeled diethyl malonate (DEM) and radiolabeled diisopropyl fluorophosphonate (DFP). The compounds were uniformly applied to pig skin in vitro at chemical doses of 4 μg/cm^2 and 0.1 mg/cm^2 with ethanol as a vehicle and 0.1 mg/cm^2 without a vehicle (neat). Skin penetration was measured by the appearance of radioactivity in Tyrode's solution on the visceral side of the skin, and evaporation was measured by radioactivity recovered from vapor traps.

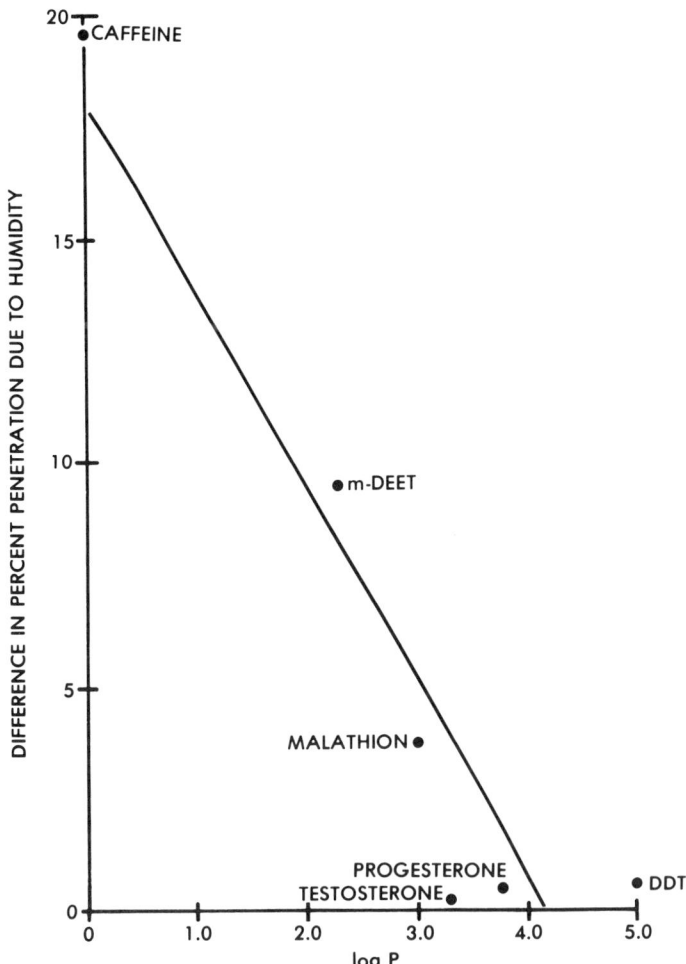

Figure 6 Plot of the difference in percent percutaneous penetration of six compounds (*m*-deet = *N,N*-diethyl-*m*-toluamide) when determinations were done with air flowing over the skin surface at high relative humidity (approximately 75%) and zero relative humidity versus log P, the logarithm of the octanol/water partition coefficient. (From Hawkins and Reifenrath, 1984.)

Table 4 The Effect of Chemical Dose on the Disposition of N,N-Diethyl-m-Toluamide from Pig Skin in Vitro

Dose ($\mu g/cm^2$)	Evaporation rate ($\mu g/0.8\ cm^2$/time interval)[a]						Skin surface[c]	Residue in skin[d]
	0-10 min	10-25 min	25-40 min	40-55 min	55-70 min	70-85 min		
4	0.05 ±0.01	0.09 ±0.01	0.07 ±0.01	0.07 ±0.01	0.06 ±0.01	0.06 ±0.01	24 ±4	53 ±4
320	0.54 ±0.08	1.3 ±0.5	1.2[b] ±0.3	1.3 ±0.2	1.2 ±0.4	1.2 ±0.2	29 ±3	52 ±2

[a] Mean ± standard deviation of microgram equivalents (μg Eq) of radioactivity recovered in the time intervals designated. Unless otherwise indicated, $n = 4$. Standard test conditions were employed, except that split-thickness pig skin (1 mm) was used, tissue culture media (RPMI, Gibco Laboratories, Santa Clara, Calif.) perfused the penetration cell and air was at ambient relative humidity (approximately 40%). Experiments were terminated at 85 min.
[b] $n = 3$.
[c] Percent of applied radioactive dose recovered from swabbing the skin surface with counting solution.
[d] Percent of applied radioactive dose recovered by oxidation of skin to liberate radioactivity as $[^{14}C]CO_2$.

Table 5 Disposition of Radioactivity After Topical Application of Radiolabeled Diethyl Malonate (DEM) and Diisopropyl fluorophosphonate (DFP) to Pig Skin in Vitro

Compound	Chemical dose	Solvent	Percent of applied radioactive dose (mean ± SD)[a]				
			Recovered evaporation	Penetration	Skin wash	Residue in skin	Total recovery
DEM	4 µg/cm^2	Ethanol	25±8	10±3	2±1	30±10	70±10
DEM	0.1 mg/cm^2	Ethanol	43±4	6±3	2±1	13±2	64±8
DEM	0.1 mg/cm^2	Neat	50±2	3±1	2.3±0.3	8.8±0.5	65±2
DFP	4 µg/cm^2	Ethanol	8±1	7±5	0.8±0.7	12±8	28±5
DFP	0.1 mg/cm^2	Ethanol	10±2	5±2	0.8±0.6	15±8	30±7
DFP	0.1 mg/cm^2	Neat	7±2	3±1	1.5±0.4	6±2	18±4

[a]Standard test conditions.
Source: Hawkins and Reifenrath (1984).

The disposition of radioactivity at the end of a 2-day period following topical application is given in Table 5. Overall recovery is low, particularly with DFP, considering that recoveries of at least 90% are routinely achievable with nonvolatile compounds or when volatile compounds are applied quickly. Time was taken to achieve a uniform application of compound, and the low recovery probably reflected evaporative loss during the application process. Considering this factor, skin evaporation was the major route of loss from the skin surface for these two compounds. Only 3% of the radioactive dose of DEM and DFP penetrated the skin when no vehicle was used. Greater penetration into the skin was observed when ethanol was used as a vehicle. On a percentage basis, greater penetration was obtained at 4 $\mu g/cm^2$ of DEM than at 100 $\mu g/cm^2$. On the other hand, DFP gave similar skin penetration percentages at the two dose levels.

PHARMACOLOGICAL SIGNIFICANCE OF EVAPORATION OF CHEMICALS FROM THE SKIN

Mosquito repellents are interesting examples of the importance of evaporative loss from the skin. By examination of homologous series of chemical structures that have repellent activity, optimal repellent activity was found to exist within a certain range of boiling point (Skinner and Johnson, 1980). These findings suggested that repellents are required to evaporate from the skin to be effective and that compounds with too high a vapor pressure dissipate too quickly from the skin and compounds with too low a vapor pressure don't emit enough vapor (Gabel et al., 1976). By measuring the evaporation rate from the application of a minimum effective dose (MED) of a compound to repel mosquitoes, it was possible to obtain a minimum effective evaporation rate (MEER). For N,N-diethyl-m-toluamide, the MED and MEER were found to be 25 and 1.2 ±0.3 $\mu g/cm^2 \cdot hr$, respectively (Reifenrath and Robinson, 1982).

Knowing the MEER, it is possible to approximate duration of repellent protection by determining the time required for the evaporation rate from a protective dose (300 $\mu g/cm^2$) to reach the MEER (Table 6). In vitro and in vivo duration increased in parallel fashion. Excluding sulfonamide, whose duration exceeded the test period for both in vivo and in vitro tests, a statistically significant correlation ($r = 0.97$, $p < 0.05$) existed between the values. Based on these results, the in vitro evaporation and penetration measurements have proven a useful tool for the screening of repellent formulations designed to extend the duration of repellent evaporation.

In a case of occupational cutaneous hazards, both evaporative loss from the skin surface and penetration are important processes when skin comes in contact with toxic compounds. In the case of the volatile, highly toxic organophosphorus anticholinergic compound soman, at least 60% of the compound evaporated from the skin surface during a 15-min period after a dose of 0.1

Table 6 Minimum Effective Evaporation Rate (MEER) and Duration of Protection for Five Mosquito Repellents

Compound	MEER[a] ($\mu g/cm^2 \cdot hr$, mean ± SD)[a]	Duration of protection (hr)	
		In vitro	In vivo (mean ± SD)[b]
N,N-Dicyclohexamethyleneurea	1.1±0.1	1	2.1±1.7
2-Ethyl-1,3-hexanediol	7.5±1.7	7	3.6±1.2
N,N-Diethyl-m-toluamide	1.2±0.3	12	5.7±1.8
N,N-Diethyl-p-toluamide	1.8±0.8	12	4.8±1.4
1-(Butylsulfonyl)hexahydro-$1H$-azepine	0.2±0.1	—	—

[a]Values for three replicates using full-thickness human skin (Reifenrath and Robinson, 1982).
[b]Values determined against *Aedes aegypti* mosquitoes in laboratory testing (Hill et al., 1979).

mg/cm^2 of the radiolabeled compound was spread over pig skin in vitro (Reifenrath et al., 1984b). Five percent of the radioactive dose was recovered from the skin surface, only 1% from within the skin tissue, and less than 0.1% from fluid beneath the skin. While evaporation in this case reduced the amount of compound available for penetration, the vapor creates the additional hazards of subsequent inhalation.

The surface area of skin exposing a compound can markedly influence disposition. When diethyl malonate, a compound with a vapor pressure similar to that of soman, was applied to the skin (mounted in evaporation/penetration chambers) in a single drop versus the same amount spread over a larger surface area, evaporative loss was reduced by half in the former case (Reifenrath, 1980). This factor, along with others, complicates the assessment of cutaneous hazards.

CONCLUSION

Evaporation is a major mode of loss from the skin surface for many substances, serving to cool the skin, to concentrate active ingredients in an emulsion at the surface, or to limit the amount of active material penetrating skin into the body. Wind, humidity, temperature, and vapor pressure play roles in evaporation from and penetration through skin and, thus, affect persistence on the skin surface where, in the case of mosquito repellents, volatile compounds repel mosquitoes. Other substances such as volatile toxic chemicals are readily removed from the surface by evaporation; however, they then constitute an inhalation hazard. For all chemicals coming in contact with the skin, evaporation must be considered, along with penetration and formation of skin reservoirs, as a potential factor in the pharmacological activity of topically applied materials.

ACKNOWLEDGMENTS

The authors wish to thank Christina Vancheri for the preparation of artwork and Patricia A. Cantrell for word processing.

REFERENCES

Bartek, M. J. and LaBudde, J. A. (1975). In *Animal Models in Dermatology*. Edited by H. I. Maibach. Churchill-Livingstone, New York, p. 103.
Blaine, R. L. and Levy, P. F. (1974). *Anal. Calorimetry 3*: 185.
Davies, M. and Jones, J. I. (1954). *Trans. Faraday Soc. 50*: 1042.
Feldmann, R. J. and Maibach, H. I. (1969). *J. Invest. Dermatol. 52*: 89.
Feldmann, R. J. and Maibach, H. I. (1970). *J. Invest. Dermatol. 54*: 399.
Gabel, M. L., Spencer, T. S., and Akers, W. A. (1976). *Mosquito News, J. Am. Mosquito Control Assoc. 36*: 141.
Guckel, W., Synnatschke, G., and Rittig, R. (1973). *Pestic. Sci. 4*: 137.
Hawkins, G. S. and Reifenrath, W. G. (1984). *Fundam. Appl. Toxicol. 4*: S133-S144.
Hill, J. A., Robinson, P. B., McVey, D. L., Akers, W. A., and Reifenrath, W. G. (1979). *Mosquito News, J. Am. Mosquito Control Assoc. 39*: 307.
Long, D. and Wallace, V. (1981). Technical Report No. T-180-A. U.S. Army Dugway Proving Ground, Dugway, Utah.
Merck Index, 8th ed. (1968). Edited by P. G. Stecher. Merck and Co., Rahway, N.J., p. 370.
Meyer, W., Schwarz, R., and Neurand, K. (1978). In *Current Problems in Dermatology*. Edited by G. A. Simon, Z. Paster, M. A. Klingberg, and M. Kaye. Karger, Basel, p. 39.
Reifenrath, W. G. (1980). Technical Report No. 86. Letterman Army Institute of Research, San Francisco.
Reifenrath, W. G. and Robinson, P. B. (1982). *J. Pharm. Sci. 71*: 1014.
Reifenrath, W. G., Robinson, P. B., Bolton, V., and Aliff, R. E. (1981). *Food Cosmet. Toxicol. 19*: 195.
Reifenrath, W. G., Chellquist, E. M., Shipwash, E. A., Jederberg, W. W., and Krueger, G. G. (1984a). *Br. J. Dermatol. III*, Supplement 27, 123-135.
Reifenrath, W. G., Mershon, M. M. Brinkley, F. B. Miura, G. A., Broomfield, C. A., and Cranford, H. B. (1984b). *J. Pharm. Sci. 73*: 1388.
Scheuplein, R. J. (1978). In *The Physiology and Pathophysiology of the Skin*. Edited by A. Jarrett. Academic, New York, p. 1731.
Scheuplein, R. J. and Ross, L. W. (1974). *J. Invest. Dermatol. 62*: 353.
Skinner, W. A. and Johnson, H. L. (1980). In *Drug Design*, Vol. 10. Edited by E. J. Ariens. Academic, New York, p. 277.

Spencer, T. S., Hill, J. A., Feldmann, R. J., and Maibach, H. I. (1979). *J. Invest. Dermatol.* 72: 317.
Spencer, W. F. and Cliath, M. M. (1970). *J. Agric. Food Chem.* 18: 529.
Spencer, W. F. and Cliath, M. M. (1972). *Agric. Food Chem.* 20: 645.
Wester, R. C. and Maibach, H. I. (1976). *J. Invest. Dermatol.* 67: 518.
Wester, R. C. and Maibach, H. I. (1977). In *Cutaneous Toxicity*. Edited by V. A. Drill and P. Lazar. Academic, New York, p. 111.

24
Dermal Decontamination and Percutaneous Absorption

Ronald C. Wester and Howard I. Maibach
University of California School of Medicine, San Francisco, California

Decontamination of chemical from the skin is commonly done by washing with soap and water. It has always been assumed that washing will remove chemical. However, recent evidence suggests that many times the skin and the body are unknowingly subjected to enhanced penetration and systemic absorption/toxicity because the decontamination procedure does not work or may actually enhance absorption.

EFFECTS OF OCCLUSION AND WASHING

Table 1 shows the effect of duration of occlusion on the rate of absorption of malathion (Feldmann and Maibach, 1974). What is important from this table is that 9.6% of the applied malathion was absorbed during a zero time duration. There was an immediate wash of the site of application with soap and water. However almost 10% of the applied dose was not washed off, but in fact persisted on the skin through the wash procedure and was later absorbed into the body.

Table 2 shows the effect of washing on the percutaneous absorption of hydrocortisone in a rhesus monkey. With a nonwashing sequence between dose applications, the percent dose absorbed was 0.55 ±0.06% of applied dose. When a post-24-hr wash procedure was introduced, the percent dose absorbed statistically ($p < 0.05$) increased to 0.72 ±0.06%. The post-24-hr wash was supposed to remove the excess materials and thus decrease absorption. However, the soap and water wash hydrated the skin and the rate of absorption of hydrocortisone increased.

Table 1 Effect of Duration of Occlusion on Percutaneous Absorption of Malathion in Man

Duration (hr)	Absorption (%)
0[a]	9.6
0.5	7.3
1	12.7
2	16.6
4	24.2
8	38.8
24	62.8

[a]Immediate wash with soap and water.
Source: Feldmann and Maibach (1974).

Table 3 shows dermal washing efficiency for polychlorinated biphenyls (PCBs) in the guinea pig. When 42% PCB was applied to guinea pig skin and immediately washed, only 58.9% of the applied dose could be removed. The rest of the material was available for subsequent percutaneous absorption. When 42% PCB was applied to guinea pig skin and 24 hr later the site of application was washed, only 0.9% of the applied dose was removed. Thus, all the applied PCB was available for absorption or had already been absorbed into the body. When 54% PCB was applied to guinea pig skin and washed 24 hr postapplication, 19.7% of the applied dose was removed. Thus, with 54% PCB, 80% of the applied dose could not be removed or had already been absorbed into the body.

Table 2 Effect of Washing on Percutaneous Absorption of Hydrocortisone in Rhesus Monkey

Treatment	Absorption (% ± SD)
No wash	0.55 ± 0.06
Post-24-hr wash[a]	0.72 ± 0.06 ($p < 0.05$)

[a]Soap and water wash.
Source: Wester et al. (1977).

Table 3 Dermal Wash Efficiency for Polychlorinated Biphenyls (PCBs) in Guinea Pig

PCB (%)	Wash time[a]	Dose removed (% ± SD)
42	Immediate	58.9 ± 7.5
42	Post-24-hr	0.9 ± 0.2
54	Post-24-hr	19.7 ± 5.5

[a]Wash procedure: twice with water, twice with acetone, twice with water.
Source: Wester et al. (1984).

Subsequent examination of the rate of absorption of PCB showed that most of the material was absorbed into the body. This study illustrates that the hypothesis that washing or bathing and any other applications of water will remove material from skin is wrong. Substantivity (the nonspecific absorption of material to skin) can be a strong force.

Figure 1 shows the percent dose absorbed per hour of a herbicide in the rhesus monkey (Wester and Maibach, 1983). At 24 hr postapplication time, the site of absorption was washed with water and acetone sequentially. The time curve shows a "washing-in effect" following the 24-hr postapplication wash. Thus, as we saw previously with hydrocortisone, there is definitely a washing-in effect. The application of water and acetone changed the barrier properties of skin and caused an increase in the rate of absorption of this herbicide.

It is generally assumed that pesticides and other chemicals can be easily removed from skin. Another series of experiments by Feldmann and Maibach (1974) was designed to determine just how effective the removal is in terms of decreasing percutaneous absorption. The experimental variable was the removal of applied pesticide in different groups of subjects at varying times. Decontamination was attempted by a 2-min wash with soap and hot water. Data are presented in Table 4. Absorption of azodrin at a concentration of 4 $\mu g/cm^2$ on the human forearm was 14.7% if the site was not washed for 24 hr. Washing after 4 hr decreased absorption to 8% of the dose. Washing after only 15 min decreased penetration, but still 2.3% of the dose was absorbed. With similar experimental variables, ethion washing in 15 min decreased the penetration from the 24-hr time period only from 3.3 to 1.6%. Malathion decrease from the 24-hr to 15-min wash was only 6.8 to 4.3%.

A similar relationship was maintained when the applied concentration was greatly increased. For instance, at a concentration of 4 $\mu g/cm^2$ of parathion, the penetration after washing at 24 hr was 8.6%, this only decreased by 1.9% by washing in 15 min.

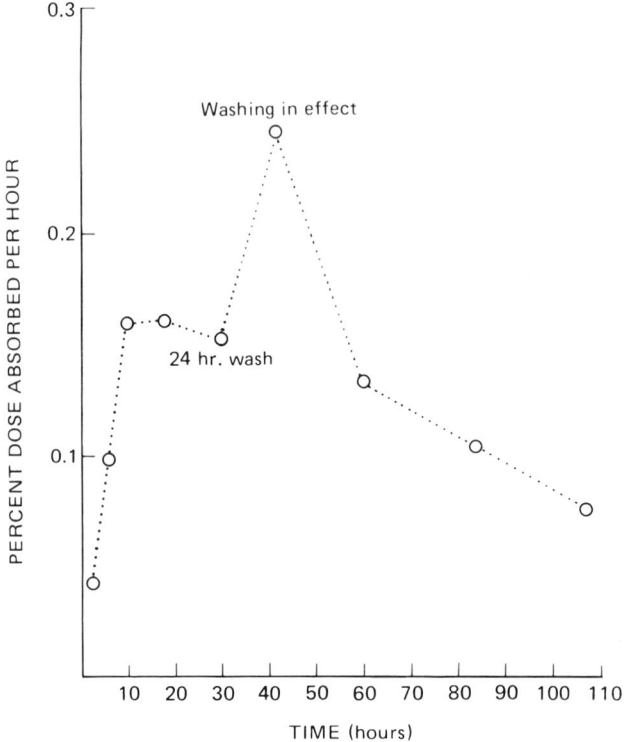

Figure 1 Washing-in effect of a 24-hr postapplication wash on the percutaneous absorption of a herbicide. (From Wester, 1983.)

The effect of the anatomic site was also studied. On the palm, the penetration of parathion was 11.8% with washing at 24 hr. There was no significant decrease in penetration washing in 15 min; in fact, there was a slight increase. Thus, the very potent pesticide parathion absorbs to skin despite washing, and is absorbed into the body.

Experiments with rubbing alcohol had similar results. When used with malathion, alcohol washing at 4 hr allowed 16.8% penetration and at 15 min, 17.7%. Penetration with parathion at 4 hr was 10.3%, and at 15 min, 8.2%. These data suggest that a careful examination be made of recommendations given to consumers and workers regarding when they can remove these substances from their skin and what materials should be used. It is obvious that protection from washing and bathing is not what had been predicted.

It is possible that attempts to remove pesticides with soap and water or rubbing alochol actually spread the material over the skin rather than removing it.

Table 4 Effect of Washing on Percent Penetration

Compound, dose (μg/cm², and site	Minutes				Hours				
	1	5	15	30	1	2	4	8	24
Soap and water									
Azodrin, 4, arm			2.3				8.6		14.7
Ethion, 4, arm			1.6				2.9		3.3
Guthion, 4, arm									
Malathion									
4, arm	1.3		4.3	4.5	6.1	8.3			
40, arm			4.7				6.8		
400, arm			1.4		2.0		4.7		6.8
Parathion									
4, arm	2.8		6.7		8.4		8.0	15.8	8.6
40, arm			3.1				6.9		9.5
400, arm			2.2		2.3		4.2		4.8
4, forehead	8.4		7.1	12.2	10.5	20.1	27.7		36.3
4, palm		6.2	13.6	13.3	11.7	9.4	7.7		11.8
Lindane, 4, arm		1.7	1.8	4.2	3.9	6.7	5.1		9.3
Baygou, 4, arm	1.2		4.7	4.5	4.7	11.8	15.5	11.3	19.6
2,4-D									
4, arm	0.5		0.7	1.8	1.2	3.7	3.7		5.8
40, arm			0.7				2.8		
Rubbing alcohol									
Malathion, 4, arm			17.7		5.8		16.8		
Parathion, 4, arm			8.2		7.0		10.3		

Source: Feldmann and Maibach (1974).

Table 5 Effect of Shower on Different Types of Removal at 4 hr

Compound	Absorption (%) after shower[a]		
	Arm	Forehead	Palm
Malathion	8.8	32.7	7.2
	(12.1)		
Parathion	16.5	41.9	13.4
	(8.0)	(27.7)	(7.7)
Baygon	9.9	20.5	8.7
	(15.5)		

[a]Values in parentheses: after washing.
Source: Feldmann and Maibach (1974).

It was questioned whether a whole body exposure to a solvent such as water might not be more effective at removing pesticides. For this reason a group of subjects were showered 4 hr after application instead of being washed locally with soap and water. The data for malathion, parathion, and baygon are in Table 5. The shower was no more effective and perhaps less effective than the local application of soap and water. Showering does not appear to be a solution to the problem.

CONCLUSION: SUBSTANTIVITY

"Substantivity" has been defined as the nonspecific adsorption of material from skin. It is obvious that the standard washing procedures do not readily remove materials from skin. How important is this in terms of occupational exposure? Kazen and co-workers (1974) did hexane hand rinsings on occupationally exposed people. They analyzed the rinsings by electron capture and flame photometric/gas-liquid chromatography for pesticide residues to determine whether these chemicals persisted on the skin long after exposure. Chlordane and dieldrin apparently persisted on the hands of a former pest control operator for at least 2 years. Methoxychlor, captan, and malathion persisted for at least 7 days on the hands of a fruit and vegetable grower. Parathion was found on the hands of one man 2 months after his last known contact with this pesticide. Endosulfan, DDD, kelthane, decthal, trithijon, imidan, and guthion have persisted on the hands of some exposed workers from less than a day to 112 days after exposure.

In conclusion, washing does *not* necessarily prevent penetration of some chemicals. Surely, the understanding of the mechanisms and the development of more efficient removal systems must be a high priority for research.

REFERENCES

Feldmann, R. J. and Maibach, H. I. (1974). Systemic absorption of pesticides through the skin of man. In Occupational Exposure to Pesticides: Report to the Federal Working Group on Pest Management from the Task Group on Occupational Exposure to Pesticides. Appendix B, pp. 120-127.

Kazen, C., Bloomer, A., Welch, R., Oudbier, A., and Price, H. (1974). Persistence of pesticides on the hands of some occupationally exposed people. *Arch. Environ. Health 29*: 315-318.

Wester, R. C. and Maibach, H. I. (1983). Advances in percutaneous absorption. In *Cutaneous Toxicity*. Edited by V. A. Drill and P. Lazar. Raven, New York, pp. 29-40.

Wester, R. C., Noonan, P. K., and Maibach, H. I. (1977). Frequency of application of percutaneous absorption of hydrocortisone. *Arch. Dermatol. 113*: 620-622.

Wester, R. C., Bucks, D. A. W., and Maibach, H. I. (1984). Polychlorinated biphenyls (PCBs): Dermal absorption, systemic elimination, and dermal wash efficiency. *J. Toxicol. Environ. Health*. In press.

25
Radial Transport in the Dermis

Richard H. Guy
University of California School of Pharmacy, San Francisco, California

Howard I. Maibach
University of California School of Medicine, San Francisco, California

Jonathan Hadgraft*
University of Nottingham, Nottingham, England

In percutaneous absorption, the ultimate step is generally considered to be uptake of penetrant by the cutaneous microcirculation and subsequent systemic dilution. In other words, the dermal capillaries are said to provide an effective "sink" for transcutaneously delivered molecules. The argument, on the whole, appears sensible: the stratum corneum (and the skin in general) is an excellent barrier to ingress of chemicals into the body; hence arrival of penetrant at the skin blood vessels may be expected to be slow and the concentration of substrate at this region will be low relative to the applied amount. These are the criteria characteristic of "sink" conditions. Hence, little attention has been focused on the intradermal behavior of molecules transported from the skin surface; their putative activity in this region has been confined to depletion by the blood supply.

However, review of the literature coupled with some simple observations of ourselves and others do indicate (albeit in a limited sense) that penetrant transport can take place within the dermis and can be quantified and interpreted. This chapter shows that the results can permit measurement of the radial movement of penetrant within the dermis, that the mechanism of such movement may involve the dermal capillaries, and that the uptake of penetrant into the systemic circulation is generally efficient.

EXPERIMENTAL OBSERVATIONS

It is not unusual to observe (Shuster, 1982), after the topical application of a chemical capable of producing local vasodilatation, (1) the appearance of

---
*Present affiliation: University of Wales Institute of Science and Technology, Cardiff, Wales

erythema at the contact site, (2) a progressive radial expansion in the visible area of redness, until (3) the attainment of maximum spread and intensity, followed by (4) gradual contraction and fading. These events are distinct from those typical of a classic axon reflex flare (DiSclafani and Wilkin, 1983) and are considered to reflect, therefore, concomitant transport and depletion of vasodilator within and from the dermis.

An early assessment of this phenomenon was provided by Fountain et al. (1969). They studied the rate of absorption and duration of action of four formulations of methyl nicotinate by measuring, in humans, the area and duration of erythema, which the chemical produced (Stoughton et al., 1960). Anatomic, temperature, concentration, and vehicle variables were investigated and each was shown to influence the time course and extent of the observations. The overall pattern, though, was essentially consistent and is exemplified by the data in Figure 1.

In a detailed investigation of the disposition of topically applied [^{3}H] escin in mice and rats (Lang, 1974), measurements were made of the activity residing in the skin beneath the application site and in several skin strips 0.5 cm wide at

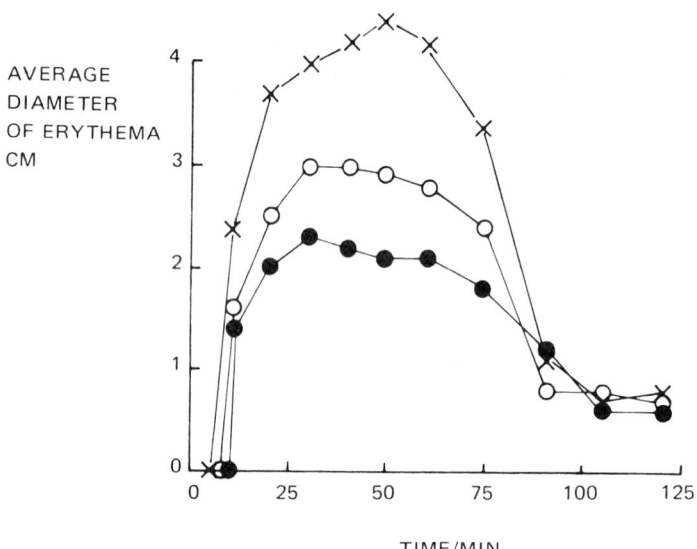

Figure 1 Lateral movement of methyl nicotinate in the skin as assessed by erythematous area. The drug was applied in aqueous solution at ambient temperature (25°C). Each data point is the average of five readings from various sites. Key: methyl nicotinate concentration (X) 1.0%; (●) 0.5%; (0) 0.25%. (Data from Fountain et al., 1969.)

Radial Transport in the Dermis

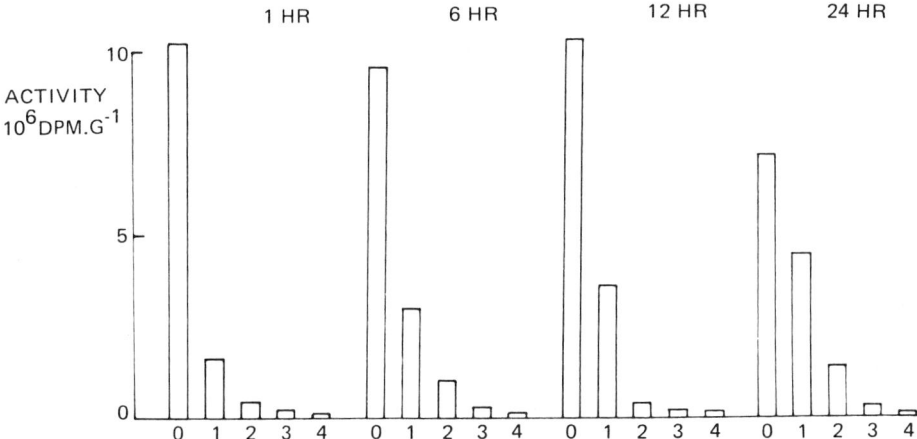

Figure 2 Radioactivity located in several skin areas at various times after cutaneous application of [^{3}H] escin to the mouse. Column 0 corresponds to skin directly under the application site. Columns 1, 2, 3, and 4 refer to skin strips at 0.5-cm intervals away from the contact zone. (Data from Lang 1974.)

distances of 1-5 cm from the center of the application zone. The results in Figure 2 for the mouse showed clearly that radial movement of drug within the skin was taking place.

Radial transport in the dermis as assessed by visual detection of a pharmacological effect is not confined to vasodilatation but has also been observed with the opposite effect (vasoconstriction) produced by corticosteroids (Osamura, 1982). In these experiments, blanching in human volunteers was visually assessed as a function of steroid and concentration applied. For hydrocortisone 17-butyrate-21-propionate, betamethasone-17-valerate and clobetasol-17-propionate, blanching beyond the applied area was regularly seen at concentrations greater than 0.025%.

However, it is further work with methyl nicotinate (Albery et al., 1983; Guy and Maibach, 1982) that has provided most insight and quantitation into the process of radial dermal movement. In this case, the radial increase in the erythematous area produced by topical application of the drug was measured (again, in man). The nicotinic acid ester was delivered to the skin in aqueous solution via circular absorbent test patches (two sizes were used). Erythematous contours were assessed at various times postapplication as functions of methyl nicotinate concentration and patch contact time. A typical set of experimental data is shown in Figure 3. The measured areas of redness (A) were converted to their corresponding radii (r), assuming circular erythema, and were normalized with

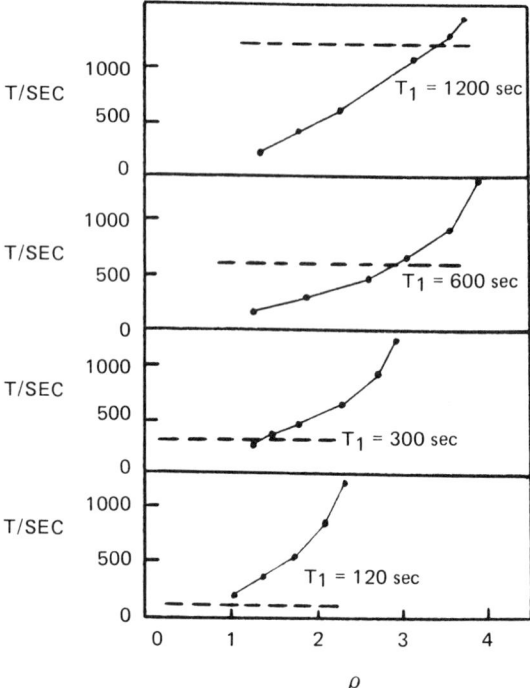

Figure 3 Radial spread of erythema caused by topical application of an aqueous 290 mM methyl nicotinate solution. Times of application (t_1) are shown. The area of application was 0.31 cm^2. (Data from Albery et al. 1983.)

respect to the radius of the application patch (r_0) to yield a radial distance parameter ρ:

$$\rho = \frac{r}{r_0} = \frac{1}{r_0}\left(\frac{A}{\pi}\right)^{1/2} \qquad (1)$$

The variation in ρ was followed until no further expansion in the observed erythema could be detected. Experiments were also conducted to determine the times of onset of erythema when the drug was continually delivered from the patch, and delivered as a pulse for a time (t_1) shorter than the erythema onset time for continuously delivered nicotinate at that concentration (Albery et al., 1983). In the following section, we discuss how the combined results of these studies were analyzed to permit calculation of (1) the rate of radial transport in the dermis and (2) the kinetics of uptake by the capillary system.

INTERPRETATION

The simple observations, such as those in Figure 3, make it plausible to characterize the behavior of methyl nicotinate in the dermis in terms of three basic processes:

1. The supply of drug from the epidermis (a function of the concentration applied and the duration of patch application).
2. The radial movement of nicotinate in the dermis (as shown by the increasing erythematous area).
3. The irreversible uptake of ester into the systemic circulation via the dermal microcirculation (indicated by the failure of vasodilatation to persist indefinitely).

Schematically, these events are illustrated by Figure 4, which shows that dermal radial movement is characterized by a transport coefficient D_D. The use of "diffusion coefficient" to describe the D_D process is avoided because of the

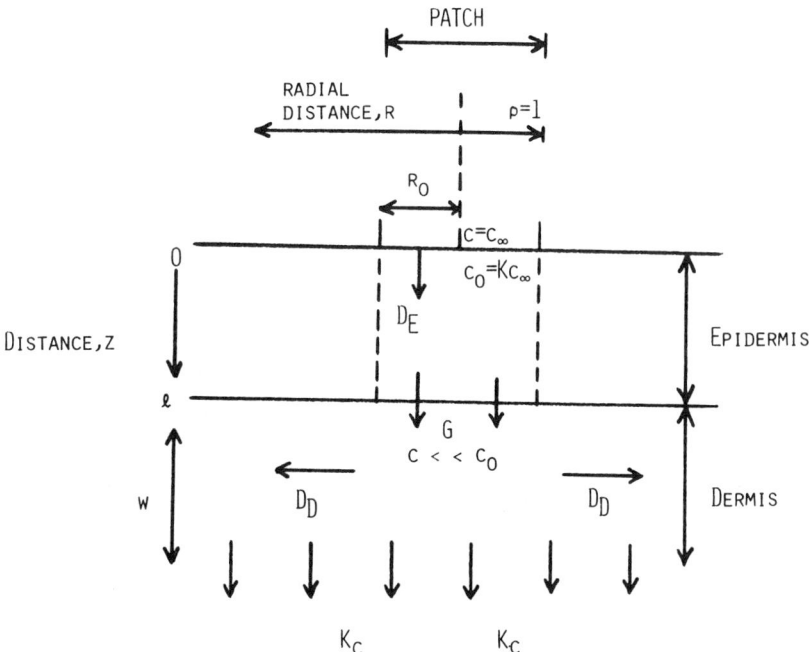

Figure 4 Schematic model (Albery et al., 1983) for transport from a circular patch through the epidermis with radial transport and depletion in the dermis.

following simple argument. The results in Figure 3 show that the rate of spread of erythema is such that the area of redness expands in diameter by 1 cm in about 10 min. This characteristic time corresponds to an *apparent* diffusion coefficient of approximately 10^{-3} cm^2/sec, a value 1000 times larger than that expected for an ordinary diffusion process (Scheuplein, 1976). No detailed mathematical analysis nor interpretive insight is required for this deduction. If the diffusion coefficient were a more reasonable 10^{-6} cm^2/sec, then the characteristic time τ to diffuse 1 cm would be:

$$\tau \simeq \frac{1 \text{ cm}^2}{2(10^{-6} \text{ cm}^2/\text{sec})} \simeq 6 \text{ days}$$

(Atkins, 1978), a value that plainly does not fit the experimental facts (Albery et al., 1983; Guy and Maibach, 1982). It follows that a much more efficient transport process is at work.

Elucidation of the mechanism involved first required a more detailed understanding of the complete transport process under consideration. Using the model shown in Figure 4, Albery et al. (1983) set out to solve the appropriate diffusion/transport equations for the system. Briefly, these can be summarized as follows:

Transport through the epidermis is described by Fick's second law of diffusion:

$$\frac{\partial c}{\partial t} = D_E \frac{\partial^2 c}{\partial z^2} \tag{2}$$

where c is the concentration of nicotinate and D_E is its diffusion coefficient in the epidermis. This equation holds for the region of skin under the patch ($r < r_0$). The boundary conditions for Equation (2) are:

1. On the skin surface, while the patch is applied,

$$c = c_0 = Kc_\infty \quad \text{at } z = 0 \text{ and } 0 < t < t_1 \tag{3}$$

   where K is the drug partition coefficient between the epidermis and water and c_∞ is the nicotinate concentration in the patch.

2. After the patch is removed,

$$\left(\frac{\partial c}{\partial z}\right)_0 = 0 \quad \text{at } z = 0 \text{ and } t > t_1 \tag{4}$$

3. At the epidermal-dermal junction,

$c \simeq 0 \quad \text{at } z = 1$ (5)

that is, it is assumed that removal by transport in the dermis and the circulatory system is rapid compared to transport across the epidermis. This assumption was confirmed experimentally by Katz and Poulsen (1971) and by the subsequent analysis.

4. At the start of the experiment for all values of z,

$c = 0 \quad \text{at } t = 0$ (6)

In the dermis, it is assumed that the distance (w) between the epidermal-dermal junction and the microcirculatory system is small enough for the concentration to be uniform. The processes occurring are therefore: supply of material from the patch, transport radially, and removal by the capillaries. The differential equation for the dermis is therefore:

$$\frac{\partial c}{\partial t} = D_D \left(\frac{\partial^2 c}{\partial r^2} + \frac{1}{r} \frac{\partial c}{\partial r} \right) + G - k_c \quad (7)$$

where D_D is the apparent drug diffusion coefficient in the dermis, k is a first-order rate constant describing removal by the microcirculation, and G describes the supply of material from the patch of radius r_0.

For $r < r_0$,

$$G = \frac{aD_E}{w} \left(-\frac{\partial c}{\partial z} \right)_{z=\ell} \quad (8)$$

and, for $r > r_0$

$G = 0$ (9)

The parameter a describes the fractional area of the interstitial channels through which the ester diffuses compared to the total area of the skin (Albery and Hadgraft, 1979a,b). The boundary conditions for Eq. (7) are:

$c = 0 \quad \text{at } t = 0$ (10)

$(\partial c/\partial r)_0 = 0 \quad \text{at } r = 0$ (11)

$c \to 0 \quad \text{as } r \to \infty$ (12)

The differential equations (2) and (7) are solved by the method of Laplace transformation and the results inverted using the convolution theorem. Equation (2) can be shown to reduce to the result:

$$\log(c_\infty t_E^{3/2}) = \log\left(\frac{n_E}{a\ell}\right) - \log\left\{\frac{4K}{\pi^{1/2}}\left(\frac{D_E}{\ell^2}\right)^{3/2}\right\} + \frac{\ell^2}{9.212 D_E t_E} \quad (13)$$

In this expression, t_E is the time of onset of erythema when the drug is continuously applied and n_E is the number of moles per square centimeter required to trigger erythema. Continuous application experiments (Albery et al., 1983) were performed for methyl nicotinate and it was found that:

$$D_E = 22 \times 10^{-8} \text{ cm}^2/\text{sec}$$

and

$$n_E = 9 \text{ pmol}/\text{cm}^2$$

These values were in good agreement with previous results (Albery and Hadgraft, 1979b; Stoughton et al., 1960) and with data from pulsed application studies. The D_E and n_E were evaluated first in this way because they were necessary parameters to reduce the number of unknowns in the complicated radial diffusion equation solution (Eq. (14)) to only two, namely, D_D and k:

$$\frac{n_E}{K\ell c_\infty} = \left(\frac{2r_0}{\pi r_E}\right)^{1/2}\left(\frac{D_E}{k\ell^2}\right)^{3/4}\{F1\}\exp\left\{-\left(\frac{2k\ell^2}{D_E}\right)^{1/2}\{F2\}\right\}$$

$$\cdot \text{erf}\left\{\left(\frac{\ell t_1}{2D_E^{1/2} t_E}\right)^{1/2}\{F2\}\right\} \quad (14)$$

where F1 and F2 are functions of D_D and k and of known or determined parameters. By choosing values of D_D, therefore, the corresponding value of k was calculated for each experimental point. It was found that there was a minimum value of D_D below which no fit to the data could be found. Above this value of D_D, reasonable fits could be found. As discussed below, it can be shown that the most plausible values for D_D and k are the smallest that will account for the data, namely,

$$D_D = 5 \times 10^{-4} \text{ cm}^2/\text{sec} \quad \text{and} \quad k = 5 \times 10^{-3} \text{ sec}^{-1}$$

The value of k is in good agreement with results from totally different types of experiment (DeSalva and Thompson, 1965; Helde and Seeberg, 1953; Hertzman and Randall, 1948; Tur et al., 1983), and it can be concluded that the lifetime of methyl nicotinate in the dermis is 3-10 min. This agreement between k values explains the choice of minimum results for D_D and k. Higher values would lead to implausible transport parameters.

The result for D_D is about 1000 times larger than the expected value for a dermal diffusion coefficient (Scheuplein, 1976). Because no fit to the data can be found with a significantly lower value of D_D, and because the simplistic argument with characteristic times (see above) shows that an ordinary diffusion mechanism is impossible, the very efficient process that transports the ester in a radial direction must involve the capillaries. To confirm this conclusion, Albery et al. (1983) presented a model in which the drug partitions into the capillaries, is carried radially outward, and then reenters the dermis. The model is shown in Figure 5: diffusion in the dermis is considered in only one dimension z, such that the basic differential equation for transport in the ith capillary becomes:

$$\frac{\partial c_i'}{\partial t} = k_c(c - c_i') - v_c \frac{\partial c_i'}{\partial x_i} \tag{15}$$

where c_i' is the concentration inside the capillary, c is the concentration in the adjoining dermis, v_c is the velocity of blood flow in the capillary, x_i describes the distance along the capillary from the point at which the drug entered the dermis,

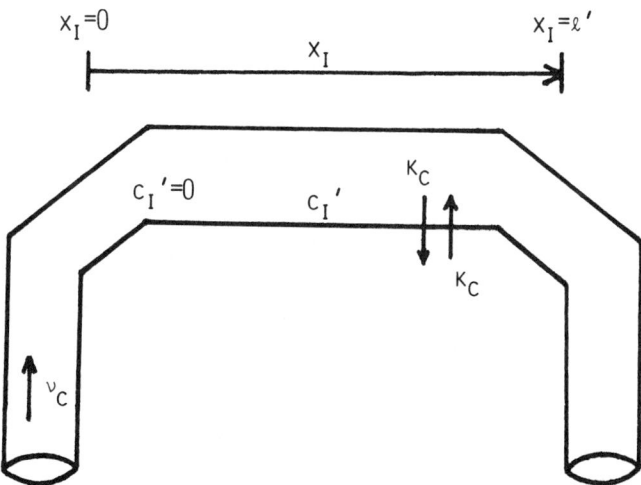

Figure 5 Capillary diffusion model illustrated for the *i*th capillary loop (Albery et al., 1983). The simulation assumes that the capillaries are randomly oriented in the dermis.

and k_c describes the rate of transfer between the dermis and the capillary (and assumes a dermis/blood partition coefficient for methyl nicotinate of unity). Equation (15) can be solved to give:

$$\frac{\partial c}{\partial t} = -kc + D_D \frac{\partial^2 c}{\partial z^2} \qquad (16)$$

where

$$k = \frac{\alpha v_c}{\ell'} [1 - \exp(-\ell'/\chi_c)] \qquad (17)$$

and

$$D_D = \frac{1}{2} \alpha v_c \chi_c \left\{ 1 - \frac{\chi_c}{\ell'} [1 - \exp(-\ell'/\chi_c)] \right\} \qquad (18)$$

Hence, the capillary diffusion model yields a kinetic diffusion equation (Eq. (16)) of the same form as Eq. (7), where now k and D_D are related to the geometry, kinetics, and flow rate of the capillary system. In Equations (17) and (18), α is the ratio of the area of the capillaries to that of the dermis, and $\chi_c = v_c/k_c$ and is the characteristic distance for the establishment of equilibrium in the capillaries. The ratio of distances χ_c/ℓ' is very important in this analysis. If χ_c is less than ℓ', then for most of the capillary's length in the dermis, the blood therein is equilibrated with the material in the dermis. On the other hand, if χ_c exceeds ℓ', equilibrium is not achieved.

Equations (17) and (18) can be approximated for the situations in which equilibrium is or is not reached. First, for $\chi_c > \ell'$ (nonequilibrated):

$$k = \alpha k_c \quad \text{and} \quad D_D = \frac{\alpha v_c \ell'}{4}$$

That is, k is given simply by the rate at which material transfers across the capillary wall from the dermis, and "diffusion" requires as large a value of ℓ' as possible to allow exchange. The approximations for the equilibrated case ($\chi_c < \ell'$) are:

$$k = \alpha v_c/\ell' \quad \text{and} \quad D_D = \frac{\alpha v_c \chi_c}{2}$$

For constant α, k decreases with increasing ℓ' because the larger ℓ' can be achieved only by having fewer capillaries. As each capillary is equilibrated, it is more efficient to have a larger number of shorter capillaries. In this case, D_D depends on χ_c; the larger χ_c, the more efficient the mixing process.

Comparison with the deductions from the experimental data showed that the model was in good agreement and that

$$\chi_c \simeq \ell' \simeq 0.6 \text{ cm}$$

The value of k_c corresponded to an interfacial transfer rate constant at the capillary wall of 2×10^{-4} cm/sec, a value about one order of magnitude less than that for the ester at an oil/water interface (Albery and Hadgraft, 1979c), hence entirely reasonable. The fact that $\chi_c \simeq \ell'$ is deduced from this study implies that each capillary is working at close to its maximum efficiency, such that the blood in each loop spends just enough time in the dermis for it to become equilibrated with its surroundings.

CONCLUSION

The investigations discussed in this chapter show that radial transport in the dermis represents a measurable pathway for drug movement after transepidermal penetration. The most detailed analysis indicates that the lateral transport is mediated via the capillaries of the cutaneous microcirculation via a mechanism very much more efficient than ordinary diffusion. For methyl nicotinate, the chemical that has been studied in greatest depth, the radial transport and capillary uptake parameters imply that the lifetime of ester within the dermis is very short (< 10 min) and that there appears to be an optimum arrangement of the geometry of the microcirculation for facilitating dermal movement.

ACKNOWLEDGMENTS

We thank the Wellcome Trust, the Burroughs Wellcome Fund, Alza Research, and Hoffman-LaRoche for support. We also wish to express our gratitude to Prof. John Albery, F.R.S. of Imperial College, London.

REFERENCES

Albery, W. J. and Hadgraft, J. (1979a). Percutaneous absorption: Theoretical description. *J. Pharm. Pharmacol. 31*: 129-139.
Albery, W. J. and Hadgraft, J. (1979b). Percutaneous absorption: In vivo experiments. *J. Pharm. Pharmacol. 31*: 140-147.
Albery, W. J. and Hadgraft, J. (1979c). Percutaneous absorption: Interfacial transfer kinetics. *J. Pharm. Pharmacol. 31*: 65-68.

Albery, W. J., Guy, R. H., and Hadgraft, J. (1983). Percutaneous absorption: Transport in the dermis. *Int. J. Pharm. 15*: 125-148.

Atkins, P. W. (1978). *Physical Chemistry.* Oxford University Press, Oxford, p. 842.

DeSalva, S. J. and Thompson, G. (1965). [^{22}Na]Cl skin clearance in humans and its relation to skin age. *J. Invest. Dermatol. 45*: 315-318.

DiSclafini, A. and Wilkin, J. K. (1983). The axon reflex flare. *Cutis 31*: 523-530.

Fountain, R. B., Baker, B. S., Hadgraft, J. W., and Sarkany, I. (1969). The rate of absorption and duration of action of four different solutions of methyl nicotinate. *Br. J. Dermatol. 81*: 202-206.

Guy, R. H. and Maibach, H. I. (1982). Rapid radial transport of methyl nicotinate in the dermis. *Arch. Dermatol. Res. 273*: 91-95.

Helde, M. and Seeberg, G. (1953). Cutaneous absorption studies using radiophosphorus. *Acta Dermatovenereol.* (Stockholm) *33*: 290-298.

Hertzman, A. B. and Randall, W. C. (1948). Regional differences in the basal and maximal rates of blood flow in the skin. *J. Appl. Physiol. 1*: 234-241.

Katz, M. and Poulsen, B. J. (1971). Absorption of drugs through the skin. In *Handbook of Experimental Pharmacology,* Vol. 28. Edited by B. B. Brodie and J. Gillette. Springer-Verlag, Berlin, pp. 103-174.

Lang, V. W. (1974). Untersuchungen zur perkutanen Absorption von [^{3}H] Aescin bei Maus und Ratte. *Arzneim.-Forsch. 24*: 71-76.

Osamura, H. (1982). Penetration of topical corticosteroids through human epidermis. *J. Dermatol. 9*: 45-58.

Scheuplein, R. J. (1976). Permeability of the skin: A review of major concepts and some new developments. *J. Invest. Dermatol. 67*: 672-676.

Shuster, S. (1982). The mechanism of UV erythema. *Br. J. Dermatol. 106*: 235-236.

Stoughton, R. B., Clendenning, W. B., and Kruse, D. (1960). Percutaneous absorption of nicotinic acid and derivatives. *J. Invest. Dermatol. 35*: 337-341.

Tur, E., Guy, R. H., Tur, M., and Maibach, H. I. (1983). Non-invasive assessment of local nicotinate pharmacodynamics by photoplethysmography. *J. Invest. Dermatol. 80*: 499-503.

26
Interrelationships in the Dose Response of Percutaneous Absorption

Ronald C. Wester and Howard I. Maibach
University of California School of Medicine, San Francisco, California

In most medical and toxicological specialties the administered dose is defined precisely. This has not always been the case in dermatoxicology and dermatopharmacology. This chapter defines our current, albeit far from perfect, understanding of the relation of applied dose to percutaneous absorption.

The interrelationships of dose response in dermal absorption are defined in terms of dose, surface area, frequency of application, and time of exposure. Dose is the concentration of applied chemical per unit of skin surface area. Surface area is usually defined in square centimeters of skin application or exposure. Frequency is either intermittent or chronic exposure. "Intermittent" can be one, two, and so on exposures per day. Chronic application is usually repetitive and on a continuing daily basis. Time of exposure is the duration of the period during which the skin is in contact with the chemical before washing. Such factors define skin exposure to a chemical and subsequent percutaneous absorption.

EFFECTS OF CONCENTRATION ON PERCUTANEOUS ABSORPTION

Maibach and Feldmann (1969) applied increased concentrations of testosterone, hydrocortisone, and benzoic acid from 4 $\mu g/cm^2$ in three steps to 2000 $\mu g/cm^2$ (4 $\mu g/cm^2$ is approximately equivalent to the amount applied in a 0.25% topical application; 2000 $\mu g/cm^2$ leaves a grossly visible deposit of chemical). Increasing the concentration of the chemical always increased total absorption. These data suggest that as much as gram amounts of some compounds can be absorbed through normal skin under therapeutic and environmental conditions.

Wester and Maibach (1976) further defined the relationship of topical dosing. Increasing concentrations of testosterone, hydrocortisone, and benzoic acid decreased the efficiency of percutaneous absorption (percent dose absorbed) in both the rhesus monkey and man (see Table 1), but the total amount of material absorbed through the skin always increased with increased concentration. Scheuplein and Ross (1974) also showed in vitro that the mass of material absorbed across skin increased when the applied dose was increased. The same relationship between dose applied and dose absorbed is also seen with the pesticides parathion and lindane in Table 2.

Wedig and co-workers (1977) compared the percutaneous penetration of different anatomic sites. A single dose of a ^{14}C-labeled magnesium sulfate adduct of dipyrithione at concentrations of 4, 12, or 40 $\mu g/cm^2$ per site was applied for an 8-hr contact time to the forearm, forehead, and scalp of human volunteers. The results again indicated that as the concentration increased, more was absorbed. Skin permeability for equivalent doses on different sites assumed the

Table 1 Percutaneous Absorption of Increased Topical Dose of Several Compounds in Rhesus Monkey and Man

Compound ($\mu g/cm^2$)	Totals for rhesus		Totals for man	
	Percent	Micrograms	Percent	Micrograms
Testosterone				
34	18.4	0.7	11.8	0.4
30	–	–	8.8	2.6
40	6.7	2.7	–	–
250	2.9	7.2	–	–
400	2.2	8.8	2.8	11.2
1600	2.9	46.4	–	–
4000	1.4	56.0	–	–
Hydrocortisone				
4	2.9	0.1	1.6	0.1
40	2.1	0.8	0.6	0.2
Benzoic acid				
3	–	–	37.0	1.1
4	59.2	2.4	–	–
40	33.6	134.4	25.7	102.8
2000	17.4	348.0	14.4	288.0

Sources: Maibach and Feldmann (1969); Wester and Maibach (1976).

Table 2 Effect of Applied Topical Concentration on Human Percutaneous Absorption

Compound (μg/cm^2)	Totals	
	Percent	Micrograms
Parathion		
4	8.6	0.3
40	9.5	3.8
400	4.8	19.2
2000	9.0	180.0
Lindane		
4	9.3	0.4
40	8.3	3.3
400	5.7	22.8
1000	3.4	34.0
2000	4.4	88.0

Source: Feldmann and Maibach (1974).

following order: forehead was equal to scalp, which was greater than forearm. The total amounts absorbed increased even when the percentage of dose excreted at two doses remained approximately the same. On the forehead proportionately more penetrated from the 40 than from the 4 and 12 μg/cm^2 doses. On the scalp the difference was even more striking, with almost twice as much proportionately penetrating from 40 than from 4 and 12 μg/cm^2. Thus, as the concentration of applied dose increased, the total amount of chemical penetrating the skin (and thus becoming systemically available) also increased for all the anatomic sites studied. Therefore, for exposure of many parts of the body, absorption can take place from all the sites. As the concentration of applied chemical and the total body exposure increase, the subsequent systemic availability will also increase.

Although the penetration at these doses varied between anatomic sites, the percent of the dose penetrating was similar at the three doses on the forearm and the forehead. However, on the occiput (of the scalp) there was an increasing percentage of penetration with increasing dosage. In other words, at the highest dose, the efficiency of penetration was the greatest.

This effect of concentration on percutaneous absorption also extends to the penetration of corticoids as measured by the vasoconstrictor assay. In this type of assay Maibach and Stoughton (1973) showed that in general, there is a dose-response relationship with increasing efficacy closely following increased dose. A severalfold difference in dose can override differences in potency between the halogenated analogs. If this applies for corticoids, it could also apply for other chemicals.

Reifenrath et al. (1981) determined the percutaneous penetration of mosquito repellents in hairless dogs. As the topical dose increased in concentration, the penetration in terms of percentage of applied dose was about the same (Table 3). However, the mean total amount of material absorbed increased dramatically. An application of 4 $\mu g/cm^2$ of N,N-diethyl-m-toluamide gave a 12.8% absorption resulting in a total absorption of 0.5 $\mu g/cm^2$. Increasing the dose to 320 $\mu g/cm^2$ decreased the percent absorbed to 9.4; however, the total amount of material absorbed was now up to 30.1 $\mu g/cm^2$, an increase of 60 times!

Roberts and Horlock (1978) examined the effects of concentration and repeated skin application on percutaneous absorption. Following single treatment application with 1, 5, and 10% ointments, the penetration fluxes for salicylic acid in hydrophilic ointment increased as the concentration increased (Table 4). With chronic application (on a daily basis) a change in flux was also observed. With chronic exposure the skin underwent a change and subsequently the penetration flux changed.

Wester (unpublished observations) looked at percutaneous absorption of nitroglycerin. The topical concentration of nitroglycerin was increased stepwise from 0.01 to 10 mg/cm^2. The percent dose absorbed remained basically the same between 0.01 and 1 mg/cm^2 (Table 5). But as this dose increased 10 times, the amount of material becoming systemically available also increased 10 times. At 10 mg/cm^2 the percent dose absorbed had markedly decreased. This suggests that the percent of absorption could become saturated at a high concentration.

Table 3   Percutaneous Penetration and Total Absorption of Repellents in Relation to Dose of Chemical Applied to Hairless Dog

Compound	Topical dose ($\mu g/cm^2$)	Penetration (% of applied dose)	Mean total absorbed ($\mu g/cm^2$)
Ethyl hexanediol	4	8.8	0.35
	320	10.3	33.0
N,N-Diethyl-m-toluamide	4	12.8	0.51
	320	9.4	30.1
Sulfonamide[a]	100	9.1	9.1
	320	7.5	24.0
	1000	5.4	54.0

[a]n-Butane sulfonamide cyclohexamethylene.
Source: Reifenrath et al. (1981).

Table 4 Mean Penetration Fluxes of Salicylic Acid in Hydrophilic Ointment Base Through Excised Rat Skin After Single Treatment

Salicyclic acid concentration (w/w)	Penetration flux of salicyclic acid (mg/cm^2·hr, ± SE)
1	0.014 ± 0.002
5	0.061 ± 0.003
10	0.078 ± 0.003

Source: Roberts and Horlock (1978).

Howes and Black (1975) determined the comparative percutaneous absorption of sodium and zinc pyrithione in shampoo, through rat skin. As the concentrations of material in shampoo increased from 0.1 to 2% the penetration also increased from 0.7 to 1 μg/cm^2 (Table 6).

Concentration and Newborns

Wester and co-workers (1977a) compared the percutaneous absorption in newborn versus adult rhesus monkeys. The total amount absorbed per square centimeter of skin again increased with increased applied dose and was further increased when the site of application was occluded. In the newborn the question of concentration may have special significance, since the ratio of surface area to body mass is greater than in the adult. Therefore, the systemic availability per kilogram of body weight can be increased by as much as threefold.

Table 5 Percutaneous Absorption of Nitroglycerin: Topical Concentration Versus Absorption for Neat Liquid Application

Topical nitroglycerin concentration (mg/cm^2)	Absorption	
	Percent	Total micrograms
0.01	41.8	0.004
0.1	43.5	0.04
1.0	36.6	0.4
7.0	26.6	1.9
10.0	7.8	0.8

Source: R. C. Wester, unpublished observations.

Table 6 The Effect of Concentration of Sodium Pyrithione in Shampoo on Absorption Through Rat Skin

Concentration in shampoo (% w/v)	Total absorption (%)
0.1	0.07
0.5	0.27
1.0	0.62
2.0	1.02

Source: Howes and Black (1975).

Concentration and Water Temperature

Cummings (1969) determined the effect of temperature on rate of penetration on n-octylamine through human skin. Increasing the temperature increased the rate of penetration as evidenced by octylamine-induced wheal formation and erythema. The increase in cutaneous blood flow mainly involved areas of the wheal. It was proposed that the effect of temperature on penetration involved epidermal factors. Therefore, increased temperature along with increased concentration will increase the percutaneous absorption.

Concentration and Duration of Contact

Howes and Black (1976) studied percutaneous absorption of trichlorcarban in rat and man. As the duration of contact increased, penetration increased.

Nakaue and Buhler (1976) examined the percutaneous absorption of hexachlorophene in adult and weanling male rats at exposure times from 1.5 to 24 hr and determined the plasma concentrations of hexachlorophene. The plasma concentrations of hexachlorophene increased with time from a low of just a few nanograms per milliliter of plasma up to 80+ ng/ml.

Duration of occlusion enhances percutaneous absorption. The significance of time in occlusion was shown by Feldmann and Maibach (1974), who concluded that the longer clothing occludes a pesticide, the greater the contamination potential becomes (Table 7).

Concentration, Duration of Contact, and Multiple Dose Application

Black and Howes (1979) studied the skin penetration of chemically related detergents (anionic surfactants) through rat skin and determined the absorption for multiple variables, mainly concentration of applied dose, duration of contact,

Table 7 Effect of Duration of Occlusion on Percutaneous Absorption of Malathion in Man

Duration (hr)	Absorption (%)
0[a]	9.6
0.5	7.3
1	12.7
2	16.6
4	24.2
8	38.8
24	62.8

[a]Immediate wash with soap and water.
Source: Feldmann and Maibach (1974).

Table 8 Concentration, Duration of Contact, and Multiple Application as Variables in Penetration of Anionic Surfactant Through Rat Skin

Variable	Penetration ($\mu g/cm^2$)
Concentration (% w/v)	
0.2	0.02
0.5	0.11
1.0	0.23
2.0	0.84
Duration of contact (min)	
1	0.25
5	0.47
10	0.69
20	0.97
Multiple application (× 5 min)	
1	0.14
2	0.25
4	0.36

Source: Black and Howes (1979).

and the effect of multiple dose applications. With alcohol sulfate and alcohol ether sulfate, as the concentration of applied dose increased and the duration of contact increased, penetration increased. With multiple applications there was also an increase in penetration (Table 8). Therefore, again the systemic availability and potential toxicity of a chemical depend on many variables. One of these, concentration, was discussed in the preceding paragraphs, other variables such as duration of contact and multiple application are also important.

Concentration and Surface Area

Sved and co-workers (1981) determined the role of surface area on percutaneous absorption of nitroglycerin. As the surface area of applied dose increased, the total amount of material absorbed and systemic availability of nitroglycerin increased. This was confirmed by the percutaneous absorption studies of Noonan and Wester (1980), but there was not a linear relationship between the size of the surface area and increase in absorption, but the same information held. The surface area of applied dose determines systemic availability of the chemical.

EFFECT OF APPLICATION FREQUENCY

Wester and co-workers (1977b) studied the effect of frequency of application on the percutaneous absorption of hydrocortisone. Material applied once or three times per day showed a statistical difference ($p < 0.05$) in the percutaneous absorption. One application per 24 hr of exposure gave a higher absorption than material applied at a lower concentration but more frequently, namely, three times a day. This study also showed that washing (effect of hydration) enhanced the percutaneous absorption of hydrocortisone. This relationship between frequency of application and percutaneous absorption is also seen with testosterone (1980a).

The studies noted above used intermittent application per single day of application. Another consideration is chronic versus acute administration and the subsequent effects on percutaneous absorption. Wester et al. (1980b) examined the percutaneous absorption of hydrocortisone with long-term administration. The work suggests that chronic exposure had some effect on the permeability parameters of skin and markedly increased percutaneous absorption.

With malathion, which apparently has no pharmacological effect on skin, the dermal absorption from day 1 was equivalent to day 8 application (Wester et al., 1983). Therefore, for malathion, the single-dose application data are relevant for predicting the toxic potential for longer term exposure.

APPLICATION FREQUENCY AND TOXICITY

There is a correlation between frequency of application, percutaneous absorption, and toxicity of applied chemocal. Wilson and Holland (1982) determined

Table 9 Incidence of Tumors After Application of Shale Oils

Shale oil	Dose and frequency	Total dose per week (mg)	Number animals with tumors
OCSO No. 6	10 mg, 4 times	40	2
	20 mg, 2 times	40	4
	40 mg, once	40	13
PCSO II	10 mg, 4 times	40	11
	20 mg, 2 times	40	17
	40 mg, once	40	19

Source: Wilson and Holland (1983).

the effect of application frequency in epidermal carcinogenic assays. Application of a single large dose of a highly complex mixture of petroleum or synthetic fuels to a skin site increased the carcinogenic potential of the chemical compared to smaller or more frequent applications (Table 9). This carcinogenic toxicity correlated well with the results of Wester et al. (1977b, 1980a), where a single applied dose increased the percutaneous absorption of the material compared to smaller or intermittent applications.

DISCUSSION

Many variables affect percutaneous absorption and subsequent dermal toxicity. Increased concentration of applied chemical on skin increases the body burden, as does increasing the surface area and the time of exposure. The opposite holds, namely, dilution of chemical will decrease the effects of applied concentration, provided other factors do not change (such as diluting chemical but spreading same total dose over larger surface area). The body burden is also dependent on the frequency of daily application and on possible effects due to chronic topical exposure.

The current data provide a skeleton of knowledge to use in the design and interpretation of toxicologic and pharmacologic studies, to increase their relevance to the most typical exposures for man. In essence, we have just begun to define the complexity of the interrelationships between percutaneous absorption and dermatoxicology (Table 10) (Wester and Maibach, 1982, 1983). Until an appropriate theoretical basis that has been experimentally verified becomes available, quantitating the various parameters listed here will greatly improve the usefulness of biologically oriented protocols utilizing the skin as a route of entry.

Table 10 Factors in the Dose-Response Interrelationships of Percutaneous Absorption

---
Concentration of applied dose ($\mu g/cm^2$)

Surface area of applied dose (cm^2)

Total dose

Application frequency

Duration of contact

Site of application

Temperature

Vehicle

Substantivity (nonpenetrating surface adsorption)

Wash-and-rub resistance

Volatility

Binding

Individual and species variations

Skin condition

Occlusion

Sources: Wester and Maibach (1983).

REFERENCES

Black, J. G. and Howes, D. (1979). Skin penetration of chemically related detergents. *J. Soc. Cosmet. Chem. 30*: 157-165.

Cummings, E. G. (1969). Temperature and concentration effects on penetration of *N*-octylamine through human skin in situ. *J. Invest. Dermatol. 53*(1): 64-79.

Feldmann, R. J. and Maibach, H. I. (1979). Systemic absorption of pesticides through the skin of man. In *Occupational Exposure to Pesticides: Report to the Federal Working Group on Pest Management from the Task Group on Occupation Exposure to Pesticides*. Appendix B, pp. 120-127.

Howes, D. and Black, J. G. (1975). Comparative percutaneous absorption of pyrithiones. *Toxicology 5*: 209-220.

Howes, D. and Black, J. G. (1976). Percutaneous absorption of trichlorocarban in rat and man. *Toxicology 6*: 67-76.

Maibach, H. I. and Feldmann, R. J. (1969). Effect of applied concentration on percutaneous absorption in man. *J. Invest. Dermatol. 52*: 382.

Maibach, H. I. and Stoughton, R. B. (1973). Topical corticosteroids. *Med. Clin. North Am. 57*(5): 1253-1264.

Nakaue, H. S. and Buhler, D. R. (1976). Percutaneous absorption of hexachlorophene in the rat. *Toxicol. Appl. Pharmacol. 35*: 381-391.

Noonan, P. K. and Wester, R. C. (1980). Percutaneous absorption of nitroglycerin. *J. Pharm. Sci. 69*(3): 385.

Reifenrath, W. G., Robinson, P. B., Bolton, V. D., and Aliff, R. E. (1981). Percutaneous penetration of mosquito repellents in the hairless dog: Effect of dose on percentage penetration. *Food Cosmet. Toxicol. 19*: 195-199.

Roberts, M. S. and Horlock, E. (1978). Effect of repeated skin application on percutaneous absorption of salicylic acid. *J. Pharm. Sci. 67*(12):1685-1687.

Scheuplein, R. J. and Ross, L. W. (1974). Mechanism of percutaneous absorption. V. Percutaneous absorption of solvent-deposited solids. *J. Invest. Dermatol. 62*: 353-360.

Sved, S., McLean, W. M., and McGilveray, I. J. (1981). Influence of the method of application on pharmacokinetics of nitroglycerin from ointment in humans. *J. Pharm. Sci. 70*(12): 1368-1369.

Wedig, J. H., Feldmann, R. J., and Maibach, H. I. (1977). Percutaneous penetration of the magnesium sulfate adduct of dipyrithione in man. *Toxicol. Appl. Pharmacol. 41*: 1-6.

Wester, R. C. and Maibach, H. I. (1976). Relationship of topical dose and percutaneous absorption in rhesus monkey and man. *J. Invest. Dermatol. 67*: 518-520.

Wester, R. C. and Maibach, H. I. (1982). In vivo percutaneous absorption. In *Dermatotoxicology,* 2nd ed. Edited by F. Marzulli and H. I. Maibach. Hemisphere, Washington, D.C., pp. 131-146.

Wester, R. C. and Maibach, H. I. (1983). Cutaneous pharmacokinetics: 10 steps to percutaneous absorption. *Drug Metab. Rev. 14*: 169-205.

Wester, R. C., Noonan, P. K., Cole, M. P., and Maibach, H. I. (1977a). Percutaneous absorption of testosterone in the newborn rhesus monkey: Comparison to the adult. *Pediatr. Res. 11*: 737-739.

Wester, R. C., Noonan, P. K., and Maibach, H. I. (1977b). Frequency of application on percutaneous absorption of hydrocortisone. *Arch. Dermatol. Res. 113*: 620-622.

Wester, R. C., Noonan, P. K., and Maibach, H. I. (1980a). Variations in percutaneous absorption of testosterone in the rhesus monkey due to anatomic site of application and frequency of application. *Arch. Dermatol. Res. 267*: 299-235.

Wester, R. C., Noonan, P. K., and Maibach, H. I. (1980b). Percutaneous absorption of hydrocortisone increases with long-term administration. *Arch. Dermatol Res. 116*: 186-188.

Wester, R. C., Maibach, H. I., Bucks, D. A. W., and Guy, R. H. (1983). Malathion percutaneous absorption following repeated administration to man. *Toxicol. Appl. Pharmacol.* In press.

Wilson, J. S. and Holland, L. M. (1982). The effect of application frequency on epidermal carcinogenesis assays. *Toxicology 24*: 45-54.

27
Does Rubbing Enhance In Vivo Dermal Absorption?

James McMaster, Howard I. Maibach, Ronald C. Wester, and Daniel A. W. Bucks
University of California School of Medicine, San Francisco, California

Tradition suggests that rubbing topical medicaments enhances dermal absorption. We examined this by applying [^{14}C] cortisone cream (4 µg/cm^2) to the naked retroauricular area of the guinea pig and the abdomen of the rhesus monkey in a crossover experiment (nonrubbed versus rubbed). In the guinea pig 20.1 ±4.3% of the applied nonrubbed dose was absorbed compared to 20.0 ±3.7% of the rubbed dose ($p > 0.05$), while in the rhesus monkey 5.3 ±3.3% of the applied nonrubbed dose was absorbed compared to 6.2 ±2.7% of the nonrubbed dose ($p > 0.05$). Therefore, the tradition of rubbing a medicament, at least for cortisone cream, probably does not enhance delivery into the skin.

INTRODUCTION

Traditional wisdom states that when topically applying a drug in ointment or cream, absorption is enhanced by rubbing the formulation into the skin. There have not been studies to confirm or deny this assumption. Percutaneous absorption has been studied in the guinea pig (Andersen et al., 1980) and in the rhesus monkey (Wester and Maibach, 1975) as animal models for man. Results suggest that the rhesus monkey provides a suitable model for percutaneous absorption studies. Cortisone, a low penetrant in man and rhesus monkey, was used here to determine the absorption effect of rubbing a compound into the skin.

METHODS

The method used was the procedures of Anjo et al. (1980) and Wester and Maibach (1975) where absorption is quantified on the basis of percent of radioactivity excreted in the urine following applications to the skin of a known amount of the labeled compound. To correct for excretion by other routes and for retention of radioactivity in the body, urinary excretion data obtained after dermal application of the compound are adjusted in accordance with urinary excretion after parenteral administration (intramuscular administration in this study).

Six guinea pigs and six male rhesus monkeys (trained for metabolic studies) were used. For the intramuscular administrations cortisone was mixed with propylene glycol and injected into the thigh. The amount given was half the topical dose, 0.5 μCi/dose. The dose was topically applied by either rubbing or spreading cortisone ointment: 1 μCi of [^{14}C] cortisone in 4 μl of hydrophilic ointment was applied to a 2-cm^2 retroauricular skin area in the guinea pig and on the abdomen in the rhesus. In the first group the dose was rubbed into the area with 100 strokes using a metal spatula. In the second, the dose and application were identical, only the method of application differed. The dose was evenly spread with a spatula, but not rubbed. After 24 hr the skin site of application was washed with soap and water. Urine aliquots (1.0 ml) from the guinea pig urine samples were diluted with 4.0 ml of distilled water and mixed with 14 ml of PCS scintillation cocktail (Amersham). A 5.0-ml aliquot from the monkey urine samples was mixed with PCS scintillation cocktail. Total radioactivity was determined by scintillation spectrometry using the internal standards method of quench correction.

Table 1 Effect of Rubbing and Spreading on Dermal Absorption of Cortisone

Time (days)	Percent dose excreted			
	Rhesus monkey		Guinea pig	
	Rub	Spread	Rub	Spread
1	2.2 ±1.7	1.2 ±1.0	15.7 ±4.3	15.6 ±5.0
2	1.9 ±0.9	1.7 ±1.5	2.0 ±0.6	2.1 ±0.4
3	0.8 ±0.3	0.9 ±0.5	0.8 ±0.2	0.9 ±0.2
4	0.4 ±0.2	0.6 ±0.2	0.5 ±0.2	0.5 ±0.2
5	0.2 ±0.1	0.4 ±0.0	0.3 ±0.1	0.4 ±0.1
6	0.3 ±0.0	0.3 ±0.1	0.4 ±0.2	0.4 ±0.1
7	0.4 ±0.3	0.2 ±0.0	0.4 ±0.2	0.3 ±0.1
Total	6.2 ±2.7	5.3 ±3.3	20.0 ±3.7	20.1 ±4.3

RESULTS

In the guinea pig 67.1 ±2.3 and in the rhesus 96.6 ±3.3% of the parenteral doses was excreted in urine over 7 days. These numbers were used as the parenteral correction.

Table 1 gives the dermal absorption of topically applied (rubbed and nonrubbed) cortisone in the guinea pig and rhesus monkey. Means and standard deviations for the individual time periods and 7-day total excretion are given. In both animal models there was no difference ($p > 0.05$) in absorption between application by rubbing versus nonrubbing. There was a three- to fourfold increase in the amount of absorption in the guinea pig studies compared to the rhesus monkey studies. This difference could be due to species differences, difference in site of application, or both (Wester and Maibach, 1983).

DISCUSSION

This study suggests that application by rubbing compared to simply spreading an ointment had no obvious effect on the dermal absorption. Clinically, this may have bearing on topical drug administration. Treatment of patients with damaged skin might be more efficacious if the less traumatic application by spreading were employed instead of rubbing. This initial experiment, although conclusive for this chemical and these species, cannot yet be extrapolated to be a general rule.

REFERENCES

Andersen, K. E., Maibach, H. I., and Anjo, M. D. (1980). The guinea pig: An animal model for human skin absorption of hydrocortisone, testosterone and benzoic acid. *Br. J. Dermatol. 102*: 447.

Wester, R. C. and Maibach, H. I. (1975). Percutaneous absorption in the rhesus monkey compared to man. *Toxicol. Appl. Pharmacol. 32*: 394.

Wester, R. C. and Maibach, H. I. (1983). Cutaneous pharmacokinetics: 10 steps to percutaneous absorption. *Drug. Metab. Rev. 14*: 169.

28
Polychlorinated Biphenyls
Dermal Absorption, Systemic Elimination, and Dermal Wash Efficiency

Ronald C. Wester, Daniel A. W. Bucks, and Howard I. Maibach
University of California School of Medicine, San Francisco, California

John H. Anderson
California Primate Research Center, University of California, Davis, California

This study determines the dermal absorption, systemic elimination, and dermal wash efficiency for polychlorinated biphenyls (PCBs). Radiolabeled PCBs containing 42 and 54% chlorine ([^{14}C] 42% PCB and [^{14}C] 54% PCB) were topically and parenterally administered to rhesus monkeys and guinea pigs. Dermal absorption, determined by ^{14}C urinary excretion, was extensive. Absorption in guinea pigs was 33.2% ±6.3% (SD of the applied [^{14}C] 42% PCB dose (4.6 μg/cm^2) and 55.6 ±2.6% of the [^{14}C] 54% PCB dose (5.2 μg/cm^2). A topical dose of 4.1 μg/cm^2 [^{14}C] 42% PCB was 17.3 and 33.9% absorbed by two rhesus monkeys. The topical concentration was increased 4.5-fold to 19.3 μg/cm^2 and absorption was 15.2 and 19.4% for the respective animals. This represents a 3.3-fold increase in actual mass (micrograms) transferred across the skin when the concentration was increased.

The [^{14}C] 42% PCB applied to guinea pig skin was immediately washed with water and acetone. Only 58.9 ±7.5% of the applied dose was removed from the skin. A post-24-hr washing removed only 0.7 ±0.2% of applied [^{14}C] 42% PCB and 19.7 ±5.5% of applied [^{14}C] 54% PCB. Postcontamination washing cannot be assumed to remove all contaminated PCB from skin.

The body elimination of ^{14}C was continuous and slow, with elimination half-lives on the order of days. Only 50-65% of an intramuscular dose could be accounted for in urine and feces for up to 28 days excretion. The elimination half-lives following topical administration were not much greater than that following intramuscular administration. This suggests that PCBs are rapidly and extensively

---

Reprinted from *J. Toxicol Environ. Health 12:* 511-519, 1983 with permission of the publisher.

absorbed through the skin, that they are probably generally distributed throughout the body, and then slowly eliminated.

INTRODUCTION

The polychlorinated biphenyls (PCBs) have been used extensively for industrial purposes for 50 years. Their properties made them ideal for use in adhesives, paints, varnishes, and printing inks, and as general fillers. Since they do not conduct electricity, they found widespread use in electrical equipment such as transformers (Allen, 1975). This widespread use, coupled with their resistance to degradation in the environment, resulted in extensive PCB contamination of animal foods (Kolbye, 1972) and people. Detectable levels of PCBs are present in over 30% of randomly sampled inhabitants of the United States (Yobs, 1972). During the past 15 years the health significance of these compounds has been brought to public attention. Common symptoms observed include chloracne and disorders of the peripheral nervous system (Garmon, 1982).

The most obvious route of human contamination is thought of as oral consumption of PCBs through the food chain. However, with such extensive use, dermal exposure to PCBs seems obvious. The skin is a primary body contact with the environment and the route by which many chemicals enter the body. Some chemicals applied to the skin have proved to be toxic (Wester and Maibach, 1982). Therefore, our objectives were to determine the dermal absorption, systemic elimination, and dermal wash efficiency for PCBs. The animals chosen for this study were the rhesus monkey and the guinea pig, both of which have been shown to have some relevance to man as models for percutaneous absorption (Andersen et al., 1980; Wester and Noonan, 1980).

MATERIALS AND METHODS

Dermal absorption was determined by the methods of Feldmann and Maibach (1965, 1970) and Wester and Maibach (1975, 1976) using the following relationship:

$$\frac{\text{Percent dose absorbed}}{} = \frac{\text{total }^{14}\text{C urinary excretion after topical administration}}{\text{total}^{14}\text{C urinary excretion after parenteral administration}} \times 100$$

The percent dose absorbed, as determined by urinary excretion, is actually that percentage when compared to a parenteral route of administration, where 100% absorption is assumed. The parenteral dose is often referred to as the correction factor.

Dermal Absorption of PCBs

The [^{14}C] 42% PCB (24.4 mCi/mmol; molecular weight 257.6) and [^{14}C] 54% PCB (31.3 mCi/mmol; molecular weight 326.5) used were obtained from New England Nuclear Corp., Boston. The PCBs contained 42 and 54% chlorine, respectively.

Adult female rhesus monkeys were placed in metabolic chairs for the first 24 hr, the time of topical drug application. Each chair had thoracic arm restrainers (which separated the site of application, the abdomen, from the animal's mouth, hands, and feet), as well as a belly plate below the application site (to separate the site from the animal's feet). Any topical drug that fell from the skin by exfoliation landed on the belly plate, not in the urine. Thus, the site of application was isolated from contaminating the urine and feces. After 24 hr the application site was washed three times with soap and water, and the animals were placed in metabolism cages for continuing urine and feces collection.

Four rhesus monkeys were topically dosed with either 5.0 (two animals) or 23.8 (two animals) μCi of [^{14}C] 42% PCB as a 50-μl solution (benzene/hexane 1:1 v/v) spread over 13 cm^2 of abdominal skin (4.1 or 19.3 μg/cm^2) after light clipping of hair with an Oster clipper. Light clipping of hair does not affect percutaneous absorption (Wester and Maibach, 1975). After a 1-month washout period, each of the same animals received a single 50-μl dose of 5.0 μCi of [^{14}C] 42% PCB by intramuscular injection into the thigh. Daily urine samples were collected for 28 days following both topical and parenteral administration; fecal samples were collected following parenteral administration only, daily for 28 days.

Adult guinea pigs were used. Urine and feces were collected in metabolism cages. For topical application, the animals were dosed and placed in a restrictive metal cylinder open on each end. The cylinder plus guinea pig was then placed in the metabolism cage. The head portion of the cylinder was raised relative to the butt end. The animal could not or would not move in the cylinder to disrupt the topical application. Urine and feces, due to cylinder tilt, fell directly into the metabolism cage. The animals were hand fed and watered during this period. After 24 hr each animal was removed from its cylinder, the application site washed, and the animal replaced in the metabolism cage for continual urine and fecal sample collection.

Three guinea pigs each received a single 50-μl dose of 5.3 μCi of [^{14}C] 54% PCB by intramuscular injection into the thigh. Daily urine samples were collected for 16 days. Fecal samples were collected daily and pooled for ^{14}C analysis. Fifty microliters of the [^{14}C] 54% PCB solution containing 5.2 μCi was spread over 10.1 cm^2 of postauricular (in back of ear) skin (5.2 μg/cm^2), lightly clipped of hair using an Oster clipper. After 24 hr, the application site was washed two times with distilled water then two times with acetone. This procedure was repeated once again for a total of eight individual washings per application site. The wash solvent was applied to a cotton ball attached to a pair of curved, blunt forceps. The application site was wiped with the solvent-laden cotton ball. The amount of ^{14}C from the wash was determined by liquid scintillation spectroscopy of the cotton ball. Daily urine and fecal (parenteral dose only) samples were collected for 12 days, then once again after 4 days' accumulation. Urine samples were assayed individually and fecal samples pooled for assay.

Three guinea pigs each received a single dose of 5.0 µCi of [^{14}C] 42% PCB injected into the thigh musculature. Daily urine and fecal samples were collected. Fifty microliters of [^{14}C] 42% PCB solution containing 5.0 µCi was applied over 11.4 cm^2 (4.6 µg/cm^2) of skin on the back of the ears. After 24 hr the application site was washed twice with a fine spray of acetone, then two more times with water. The wash solutions were collected for assay. Daily urine samples were collected for 15 days.

Three other guinea pigs each received a single dose of 5 µCi of [^{14}C] 42% PCB in 50-µl solution spread over 11.4 cm^2 of skin on the back of the ears (4.6 µg/cm^2). The site of application was then washed immediately with the method used for 42% PCB.

A 1- or 2-ml aliquot of guinea pig urine or pooled washing solution was mixed with 4 or 5 ml of distilled water and 14 ml of PCS scintillation fluid (Amersham). Then five ml of monkey urine was mixed directly with 14 ml of PCS. The ^{14}C content was determined by liquid scintillation spectrometry. A ^{14}C internal standard was added to a triplicate vial of each sample to determine the extent of quench.

Total fecal sample collections were blended in distilled water and the total volume adjusted to 1 liter. One 0.5-ml aliquot of each fecal preparation was analyzed using the wet ashing method of Bucks and Maibach (1981).

A σ- analysis was performed to determine the ^{14}C elimination half-life. The differences between the total percent dose excreted over all the collection intervals and the percent dose excreted up to the end of each collection interval are equivalent to the amount of the compound not yet excreted to the ends of the collection intervals. A semilog arithmic plot of these differences versus time yields a straight line with a slope proportional to the elimination half-life (Wagner, 1975).

RESULTS

Table 1 gives the disposition of radioactivity by rhesus monkeys following parenteral administration of [^{14}C] 42% PCB. For the 30-day collection period, 43.4% (± 3.3% SD) was excreted in the urine and 22.4 ±2.1% was excreted in the feces, totaling 65.8% of the administered dose. Radioactivity elimination was not markedly great for any particular time period, but was characterized more as a steady, continual elimination, slightly faster in the first days.

Table 1 Disposition of Radioactivity After Parenteral Administration to Four Rhesus Monkeys of [^{14}C] 42% PCB

Day	Percent dose excreted (mean ±SD)	
	Urine	Feces
1	5.0 ±1.0	3.9 ±3.2
2	6.8 ±1.8	1.8 ±0.4
3	5.0 ±3.1	1.7 ±0.4
4	5.8 ±0.6	1.8 ±0.5
5	3.2 ±1.1	0.8 ±0.2
6-10	9.8 ±2.4	6.1 ±1.2
11-20	6.0 ±2.5	3.3 ±0.3
21-30	1.6 ±0.7	2.9 ±0.3
Total	43.4 ±3.3	22.4 ±2.1
Total urine + feces	65.8	

Table 2 gives the disposition of radioactivity following parenteral administration of [^{14}C] 42% PCB and [^{14}C] 54% PCB to guinea pigs. With [^{14}C] 42% PCB, 32.3 ±3.0% of the administered dose was excreted in the urine and 20.0 ±3.6% was excreted in the feces, totaling 52.3% elimination for the 16-day collection period. In contrast, with [^{14}C] 54% PCB the larger portion (46.6 ±3.6%) of the administered dose was excreted in the feces, and 14.9 ±1.9% was excreted in the urine, totaling 61.5% elimination for the 16-day collection period. The elimination rate was similar to that in the rhesus, characterized as steady, continual elimination, slightly faster in the first days.

Table 3 shows the dermal absorption of [^{14}C] 42% PCB in rhesus monkey. At a topical concentration of 4.1 μg/cm^2, the absorption was 17.3 and 33.9% of applied dose for two animals. Increasing the topical dose 4.7-fold, the absorption was 15.2 and 19.4% for two animals. With the 4.7-fold increase in dose the average percentage of absorption decreased just slightly (25.5 to 17.3%); however, the average mass absorbed (as micrograms per square centimeter) increased threefold. Thus the body burden can be increased dramatically with increased topical concentration.

Table 4 gives the dermal absorption of PCBs in guinea pigs. An average 33.2 ±6.3% of the topical 4.6-μg/cm^2 [^{14}C] 42% PCB dose was absorbed and 55.6 ±2.6% of the 5.2-μg/cm^2 [^{14}C] 54% PCB dose was absorbed. Thus PCB dermal

Table 2 Disposition of Radioactivity After Parenteral Administration to Three Guinea Pigs of PCB

	Percent dose excreted (mean ±SD)			
	[^{14}C] 42% PCB		[^{14}C] 54% PCB	
Day	Urine	Feces	Urine	Feces
1	5.3 ±1.5		1.3 ±0.5	
2	8.0 ±1.1		2.7 ±1.1	
3	5.7 ±1.7		2.4 ±0.4	
4	4.2 ±0.6		2.2 ±0.4	
5	2.4 ±0.4		1.5 ±0.3	
6–10	5.3 ±1.1		3.4 ±0.5	
11–16	1.6 ±0.2		1.2 ±0.5	
Total	32.3 ±3.0	20.0 ±3.6	14.9 ±1.9	46.6 ±3.6
Total urine + feces	52.3		61.5	

Table 3 Dermal Absorption of [^{14}C] 42% PCB in Four Rhesus Monkeys

	Percent dose excreted			
	4.1 µg/cm² dose		19.3 µg/cm² dose	
	Animal number		Animal number	
Day	1	2	3	4
1	4.7	9.5	2.4	6.0
2	2.9	4.0	[a]	2.0
3	2.3	2.9	1.6	1.9
4	1.2	1.8	1.3	1.4
5	1.1	0.9	0.4	0.4
6–10	2.0	4.1	4.0	3.0
11–20	2.4	6.2	3.6	2.9
21–28	0.7	4.5	1.9	1.8
Total	17.3	33.9	15.2	19.4
Average percent	25.6		17.3	
Average mass (µg/cm²)	1.0		3.3	

[a] Sample lost.

Table 4 Dermal Absorption of PCBs in Three Guinea Pigs

Day	Percent dose excreted (mean ±SD)	
	[^{14}C] 42% PCB, 4.6 μg/cm^2	[^{14}C] 54% PCB, 5.2 μg/cm^2
1	12.7 ±2.7	14.1 ±0.1
2	5.7 ±0.2	14.2 ±1.8
3	4.2 ±1.4	7.1 ±1.7
4	2.7 ±1.1	4.3 ±0.6
5	2.0 ±0.7	3.2 ±0.3
6–10	4.0 ±0.7	8.1 ±0.6
11–16[a]	1.8 ±0.3	4.6 ±0.2
Total	33.2 ±6.3	55.6 ±2.6

[a]Days 11–15 for [^{14}C] 42% PCB.

absorption in guinea pigs is high, that of the more highly chlorinated PCB is greater than the 42% PCB.

Dermal absorption of 42% PCB was studied in both guinea pig and rhesus monkey. The topical concentration for two of the monkeys was the same as in guinea pigs; therefore the two species can be compared. Absorption in the guinea pig was just slightly higher than the rhesus monkey, and therefore might be considered to be a reasonable model.

Table 5 gives the radioactivity elimination half-lives following intramuscular and topical administration of [^{14}C] 42% and [^{14}C] 54% PCB to monkey and

Table 5 Radioactivity Elimination Half-life After Administration of [^{14}C] PCB

Animal	Chlorine in PCB (%)	Route of administration	Half-life (days)
Monkey	42	Intramuscular	4.3
Monkey	42	Topical	6.9
Guinea pig	42	Intramuscular	2.2
Guinea pig	42	Topical	1.9/12.6[a]
Guinea pig	54	Intramuscular	2.5
Guinea pig	54	Topical	2.9

[a]Elimination biphasic 1.9 is for day 0–10 interval, 12.6 is for day 10–15 interval.

Table 6 Dermal Wash Efficiency for PCBs in Three Guinea Pigs

Chlorine in PCB (%)	Wash time	Dose removed (% ±SD)
42	Immediate	58.9 ± 7.5
42	Post-24 hr	0.7 ± 0.2
54	Post-24 hr	19.7 ± 5.5

guinea pig. All the half-lives were linear for the duration of urinary collection, except for 42% PCB in the guinea pig, and all the half-lives are of long duration (days). This is suggestive of a slow but continual body elimination. The half-lives following topical administration are only slightly longer than those following intramuscular administration. This suggests that the long half-life is due to body elimination, not absorption. PCBs are thus probably rapidly absorbed (as suggested by the high absorption percentage) and slowly eliminated from the body.

Table 6 shows the dermal wash efficiency for PCBs in the guinea pig. When topically applied and immediately washed with water and acetone, only about half (58.9 ±7.5%) of the [^{14}C] 42% PCB could be recovered. When left in place for 24 hr, none of the 42% PCB and only 19.7 ±5.5% of the 54% PCB could be removed from the skin.

DISCUSSION

The dermal absorption of PCBs was extensive, ranging from about 20% of applied dose in the rhesus monkey to above 50% for 54% PCB in the guinea pig. Additionally, when the topical dose in the rhesus moniey was increased 4.5-fold, the dermal absorption also increased 3.3-fold. Therefore, the potential for large quantities entering the systemic circulation via the dermal route is high. Many factors determine the toxic potential of a topically applied chemical. The most obvious is that the chemical must be inherently toxic. The systemic availability is then determined by rate of dermal absorption, concentration of applied dose, surface area covered, and length of exposure. Other factors such as occlusion (such as plastic protective clothing) and anatomic sites exposed will also affect the absorption (Wester and Maibach, 1982, 1983a,b). PCBs are inherently toxic, and their potential for dermal absorption is great.

With the use of any industrial chemical, appropriate warnings recommend immediate washing upon skin contamination. It is assumed that washing will remove the chemical. An extensive washing procedure immediately after dermal application of 42% PCB removed only about 60%. The other 40% remained available for systemic absorption. A post-24-hr wash failed to remove any PCB. Presumably, all the PCB had been absorbed or was irreversibly bound to the stratum corneum. Topically applied compounds exhibit substantivity (nonpenetrating surface absorption) and rub-and-wash resistance (Wester and Maibach, 1983). The key lesson of PCBs is that postcontamination washing cannot be assumed to remove all contaminated chemical from skin. This is not unique for PCBs. Surface washing not only will fail to remove skin contaminated chemical, but it can also alter the percutaneous absorption of the chemical (Maibach and Feldmann, 1974; Wester and Maibach, 1983). It is possible that more efficient systems for removing PCB from skin can be developed.

Allen (1975) reported on the disposition of PCBs in adult rhesus monkeys. Only 10% of a single oral dose of Arochlor 1248 was detected in excreta within 14 days. With tritiated tetrachlorobiphenyl (TCB), less than 5% of the tritium was eliminated in the excreta within 72 hr. Over 95% of the TCB in the body was in an unmetabolized form, primarily associated with tissue protein and nucleic acids and serum albumin of the blood. Allen suggested that PCBs, not their metabolites, are responsible for the acute toxic effects. In our study, the disposition of radioactivity from the animals was also slow, and at best only 50-60% of the administered dose was recovered in the excreta. The elimination half-lives were on the order of days, and were not much greater following topical application. This suggests that PCBs can be rapidly and excessively absorbed through the skin, are distributed throughout the entire body, and then slowly eliminated.

ACKNOWLEDGMENTS

This chapter was supported in part by the National Institutes of Health, Division of Research Resources, Grant No. RR00169, and a grant from Pacific Gas and Electric of California.

REFERENCES

Allen, J. R. (1975). Response of the nonhuman primate to polychlorinated biphenyl exposure. *Fed. Proc. 34*: 1675-1679.

Andersen, K. E., Maibach, H. I., and Anjo, M. D. (1980). The guinea pig: An animal model for human skin absorption of hydrocortisone, testosterone and benzoic acid? *Br. J. Dermatol. 102*: 447-453.

Bucks, D. and Maibach, H. (1981). Measurement of low level carbon-14 in biologic specimens by wet ashing. *Arch. Dermatol. Res. 271*: 241-242.

Feldmann, R. J. and Maibach, H. I. (1965). Penetration of [^{14}C] hydrocortisone through normal skin. *Arch. Dermatol. 91*: 661-666.

Feldmann, R. J. and Maibach, H. I. (1970). Absorption of some organic compounds through the skin in man. *J. Invest. Dermatol. 54*: 399-404.

Feldmann, R. J. and Maibach, H. I. (1974). Percutaneous penetration of some pesticides and herbicides in man. *Toxicol. Appl. Pharmacol. 28*: 126-132.

Garmon, L. (1982). Puzzled over PCBs. *Sci. News 121*: 361-363.

Kolbye, A. C. (1972). Food exposure to polychlorinated biphenyls. *Environ. Health Perspect. 1*: 85-93.

Maibach, H. I. and Feldmann, R. J. (1974). Systemic absorption of pesticides through the skin of man. In Occupational Exposure to Pesticides. Report to the Federal Working on Pest Management from the Task Group on Occupational Exposure to Pesticides. Appendix B, pp. 120-127.

Wagner, J. G. (1975). *Fundamentals of Clinical Pharmacokinetics.* Drug Intelligence Publications, Hamilton, Ill., p. 77.

Wester, R. C. and Maibach, H. I. (1975). Percutaneous absorption in the rhesus monkey compared to man. *Toxicol. Appl. Pharmacol. 32*: 394-398.

Wester, R. C. and Maibach, H. I. (1976). Relationship of topical dose and percutaneous absorption in rhesus monkey and man. *J. Invest. Dermatol. 67*: 518-520.

Wester, R. C. and Maibach, H. I. (1982). In vivo percutaneous absorption. In *Dermatotoxicology,* 2nd ed. Edited by F. N. Marzulli and H. I. Maibach. Hemisphere, Washington, D.C., pp. 131-146.

Wester, R. C. and Maibach, H. I. (1983a). Cutaneous pharmacokinetics: 10 steps to percutaneous absorption. *Drug Metab. Rev. 14*: 169-205.

Wester, R. C. and Maibach, H. I. (1983b). Advances in percutaneous absorption. In *Cutaneous Toxicity.* Edited by V. Drill and P. Lazar. Raven, New York.

Wester, R. C. and Noonan, P. K. (1980). Relevance of animal models for percutaneous absorption. *Int. J. Pharm. 7*: 99-110.

Yobs, A. R. (1972). Food exposure to polychlorinated biphenyls. *Environ. Health Perspect. 1*: 79-84.

29
Artificial Membranes and Skin Permeability

Sergio Nacht and David Yeung
Richardson-Vicks, Inc., Shelton, Connecticut

The percutaneous absorption of topically applied chemicals has been a subject of scientific interest for many years (Makee et al., 1945; Scheuplein et al., 1969; Stoughton et al., 1960; Trekerne, 1956) and studies on the permeability of the skin have been thoroughly reviewed (Franz, 1975, 1983; Idson, 1975; Scheuplein and Blank, 1971).

Skin permeation studies conducted primarily with excised human skin specimens obtained at autopsy have demonstrated that the stratum corneum is the rate-limiting membrane, which behaves mainly like a passive diffusion barrier (Scheuplein and Blank, 1971). Recently, Franz (1975) has shown good correlation between results obtained with excised human skin in diffusion cells and those obtained in vivo, supporting the use of excised human skin in vitro as a model to predict percutaneous absorption in vivo. However, this tissue is not readily available and, when obtained, it has a limited viability (Galey et al., (1976).

The use of animal skin as a human model has been considered (Bartek et al., 1972; Wester and Maibach, 1975). The skin of the rhesus monkeys and miniature swine most closely resembles the permeability characteristics of human skin, at least for those compounds tested (Bartek et al., 1972).

Synthetic membrane models have been used to study drug diffusion kinetics. Early studies using dimethyl polysiloxane membranes were pioneered by Garrett and Chemburkar (1968). Barry et al. (Barry and Brace, 1977; Barry and ElEini, 1976) used a cellulose acetate membrane to study the influence of temperature and nonionic surfactants on the permeation rate of various steroids. However, although the use of synthetic membranes in studying drug diffusion kinetics has

Table 1 Permeants Used to Evaluate Artificial Membrane Systems

Polarity	Compound	Water solubility (mg/ml)
Polar	Water	∞
↓	Salicylic acid	2.0
Nonpolar	Hydrocortisone	0.53

not been unusual (Herzog and Swarbrick, 1971; Levy and Mroszczak, 1968), no correlation has yet been established between the permeability characteristics of such membranes and that of human skin.

Obviously, there are significant differences between a structurally simple synthetic membrane and the highly complex human skin. Even if we focus just on the stratum corneum, since this is the effective permeability barrier of the skin, we have a multilayered membrane of considerably greater complexity than a single membrane. Electron microscope studies conducted by Lavker (1976) and Elias (1981) have shown that the stratum corneum layers are held together by multilaminar sheets of lipids exquisitely organized as a sequence of hydrophobic and hydrophilic regions to form a water barrier, as well as to provide cellular adhesion. Thus, it seems logical that multilaminated membranes consisting of alternate hydrophilic and hydrophobic polymeric materials could provide a permeation model that would resemble the properties of human skin more closely than any of the individual materials per se.

To explore the use of synthetic membranes as a model for the study of drug permeation through human skin, we used as model permeants the materials listed in Table 1.

These compounds have been widely studied in terms of skin permeability, they cover a reasonably wide range of polarity, and measurements of their relative permeability through the various membranes considered, compared to that through excised human skin, can be helpful in the design of a suitable model to mimic the permeability characteristics of human skin.

MATERIALS AND METHODS

Human Skin Samples

Excised human skin was obtained at autopsy either from the abdomen or from the inner aspect of the thigh with an electric keratome (Padgett Electro Dermatome, model B, Kansas City Assemblage Co., Kansas City, Mo.) set at maximum depth. The skin was obtained in strips of 700-800 μm thick, 10 cm wide, and 15-20 cm long. When freshly excised skin samples were not used immediately, they were stored at 4°C in a sterile skin bank fluid as described by Galey et al. (1976). For diffusion studies, discs of skin 4.3 cm in diameter were punched out and equilibrated with a pH 7.2 phosphate-buffered Ringer's solution for 12-20 hr. Streptomycin (0.1 mg/ml) and penicillin (0.061 mg/ml) were added to the buffer solution to prevent bacterial growth.

Synthetic Membranes

A dimethyl polysiloxane nonreinforced sheeting (Silastic medical grade dimethyl polysiloxane, Dow Corning Corp., Medical Products Division, Midland, Mich.) 0.005 in. thick was used.

Cellulose acetate membranes annealed at different temperatures with a wet thickness of 0.0086 in. were supplied by Dr. H. K. Lonsdale (Bend Research, Inc., Bend, Ore.) and UOP, Inc. (Fluid Systems Division, San Diego, Calif.). Diaflo ultrafiltration membranes type 10 PM10, 43 mm in diameter, were purchased from Amicon Corp. (Lexington, Mass.).

Circular discs 4.3 cm in diameter of all synthetic membranes were punched out and equilibrated at room temperature in physiological phosphate-buffered Ringer's solution, pH 7.2, for 20 hr before use in drug permeation studies.

Diffusion Cells

The diffusion cell design used in all skin permeation studies (Fig. 1) has been previously described (Nacht et al., 1981). The cell is composed of two compartments, the lower chamber is made of Plexiglass and the top is made of either Teflon or Delrin. The skin membrane is mounted with the stratum corneum side exposed to the air and held on to the Teflon top with a rubber O-ring; a perfect seal between the two compartments is achieved by tightening the set screws. The cell has an effective diffusional area of 5.08 cm^2 and the dermis side of the skin is constantly bathed by filling the receptor compartment with 40 ml of a physiological saline buffer, pH 7.2. Adequate mixing of the receptor solution is accomplished with a Teflon-coated magnetic bar moved by a 120-rpm electric synchronous motor located below the cell bath. The whole diffusion cell assembly is immersed in a water bath maintained at 30 ±0.4°C by an immersion thermostatic pump (Thermomix 1440, B; Braun Melsungen).

Figure 2 shows the design of the diffusion cells used in all the synthetic membranes permeation studies. These cells are similar to those used in skin permeation studies except that the Teflon top is cylindrical instead of conical and fits snugly into the receptor compartment. A flat rubber O ring is placed on top of the membrane, and a perfect seal between the two compartments is achieved by tightening the set screws in the top. These diffusion cells have a larger effective diffusion area (8.03 cm^2) and a receptor volume of 45 ml. Other experimental conditions for the synthetic membranes permeation studies are similar to those described above for human skin.

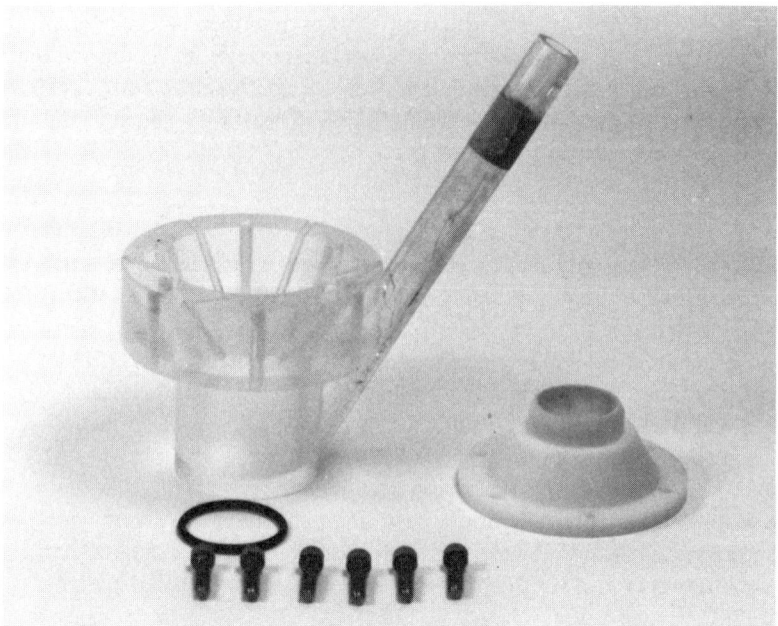

Figure 1 Diffusion cell for skin permeation studies.

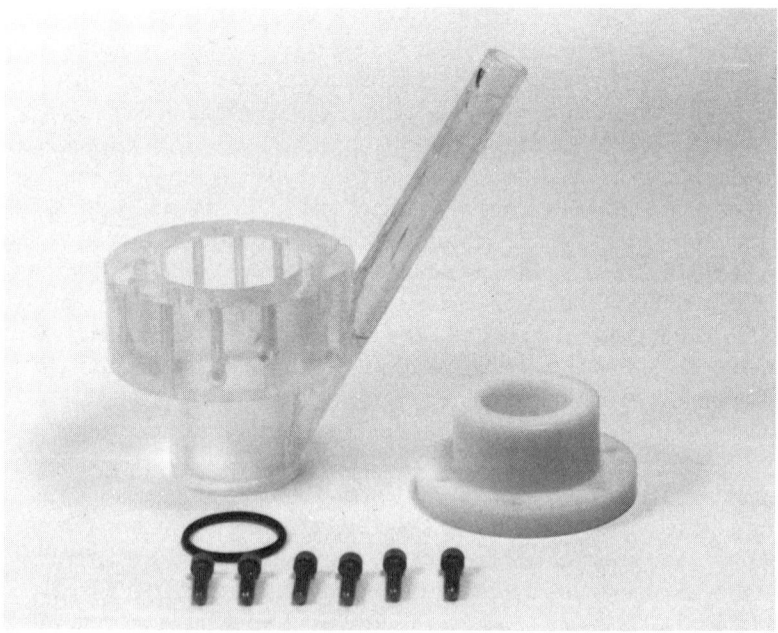

Figure 2 Diffusion cell used with synthetic membranes.

Experimental Procedure

Once the membrane has been mounted between the two cell compartments, Ringer's phosphate buffer, pH 7.2, is added to the receptor side and the cell is equilibrated in the water bath at 30 ±0.5°C for 20 min. Then 2 ml of the donor solution containing a radioactive tracer is accurately measured and applied to the membrane surface. The cell is stoppered with a glass stopper to prevent fluid evaporation and to maintain steady-state conditions. At selected time intervals, an aliquot of the receptor buffer is withdrawn through the side arm of the lower compartment and analyzed for radioactive content by liquid scintillation counting. All experiments were run in triplicate and the results were averaged. If any of the cell provided results higher than the other two by more than 20%, that run was considered invalid due possibly to pinholes, and was repeated.

Radioactive Materials and Chemicals

All radioactive labeled compounds were obtained from New England Nuclear Corp. in Boston, as either ^{14}Carbon or tritium-labeled species. High specific activity [^{3}H] hydrocortisone (80.6 Ci/mM) had to be used to obtain adequate counting rates because of its low rate of penetration. Nonradiolabeled hydrocortisone was purchased from Organon Inc. U.S. Pharmacopoeia grade salicylic acid was obtained from McKesson Chemical Co. All organic solvents used were spectra grade obtained from J. T. Baker Chemical Co., Phillipsburg, New Jersey.

Measurement of Drug Transfer

The specific activities of the radiolabeled materials in the test solutions were determined by liquid scintillation counting of an aliquot of known concentration in a Nuclear Chicago Mark II scintillation counter (Searle Analytic, Inc., Des Plaines, Ill.). The samples were prepared for counting by adding 15 ml of ACS aqueous counting scintillant (Amersham) to up to 2 ml of the sample. The samples were thoroughly shaken and each was counted for at least 10 min or 10,000 counts. The radioactivity counts were corrected for quenching by the external standard channel ratio method (Nuclear-Chicago Technical Bulletin) and converted to amounts of drug transferred using the previously determined specific activities. The cumulative transfer of the drug was computed with a Hewlett-Packard HP-25 programmable calculator, using suitably developed programs.

Concentration of salicylic acid and hydrocortisone in the donor solutions was determined by measuring the peak UV absorbance of diluted solutions in an ultraviolet scanning spectrophotometer (Beckman model 25 UV-V).

Specific activities of various donors were calculated as follows:

$$\text{specific activity (dpm/}\mu\text{g)} = \frac{\text{dpm/ml of donor solution}}{\text{concentration of drug (}\mu\text{g/ml) in donor solution}}$$

Calculations

The flux (J_s) of solute was calculated by determining the amount of drug transferred per unit time, expressed as micrograms per square centimeter per hour. The apparent permeability coefficient (P_s) was calculated with the integrated form of Fick's law for steady-state diffusion:

$$J_s = \frac{DK}{A} \Delta C = P_s \Delta C = P_s C_d \quad \text{or} \quad P_s = \frac{J_s}{\Delta C} = \frac{J_s}{C_d} \quad \text{if } C_r = 0$$

where

J_s = flux of solute
D = solute diffusion coefficient in the membrane
K = partition coefficient of the solute in the membrane
ΔC = solute concentration gradient across the membrane
A = effective diffusional area of the membrane (5.08 and 8.03 cm^2 for the skin diffusion cells and artificial membrane cells, respectively)
P_s = K × D = permeability coefficient of the solute (cm/hr)
C_d = solute concentration in the donor solution
C_r = solute concentration in the receptor solution

Care was taken to prevent buildup of solute in the receptor buffer during the experiment; under these conditions, ΔC is practically equal to the solute concentration in the donor solution (C_d).

RESULTS

Table 2 summarizes the steady-state fluxes and permeability coefficients measured for different membranes with a saturated solution of salicylic acid in a 50% alcohol/water vehicle on the donor side. Of the various synthetic membranes tested, no single polymeric membrane was found to mimic the permeability of human skin. The Silastic surgical sheet yielded an average flux of 703 µg/cm^2·hr, closer to that of excised human skin than other membranes tested. Its permeability coefficient was thus the closest to that of excised human skin, albeit somewhat larger. Cellulose acetate membranes annealed at different temperatures showed notably higher fluxes than the other membranes tested: Silastic sheeting, Diaflo ultrafiltration membrane, and excised human skin. However, the annealing temperature had little or no effect on the permeability characteristics of the membranes, since all three cellulose acetate membranes, annealed at 60, 70, and 90°C, resulted in similar steady-state diffusion rates for salicylic acid. On the other hand, a very slow steady-state diffusion rate (48 µg/cm^2·hr) acid was observed for salicylic acid with the non-

Table 2 Steady-state Flux of Salicylic Acid Through Various Membranes[a]

Membrane	Average flux ($\mu g/cm^2/hr$)	Permeability coefficient, P_s (cm/hr)[b]
Cellulose acetate at annealing temperatures		
60°C	1124	1.83×10^{-2}
70°C	1132	1.84×10^{-2}
90°C	1079	1.76×10^{-2}
Diaflo-ultrafiltration	48	7.80×10^{-4}
Silastic surgical sheet	703	1.14×10^{-2}
Trilaminar cellulose acetate	321	5.21×10^{-3}
Trilaminar Silastic surgical sheet	167	2.72×10^{-3}
Multimembrane system (cellulose acetate/Silastic/cellulose acetate)	402	6.38×10^{-3}
Excised human skin	409	6.36×10^{-3}

[a]Vehicle used was ethanol/water (50/50). In all cases, the donor was a saturated solution of salicylic acid in this vehicle.
[b]Standardized flux.

cellulose microporous Diaflo ultrafiltration membrane, probably due to its superfine pore size.

When either three Silastic or cellulose acetate membranes (annealed at 60°C) were stacked together to form trilaminar membrane systems, the steady-state fluxes of salicylic acid through these trilaminar membranes were lower than through the single membranes, as expected.

When both types of membrane were combined to form a multimembrane with the Silastic membrane sandwiched between two cellulose acetate membranes (CSC), the values obtained for the flux (402 $\mu g/cm^2 \cdot hr$) and permeability coefficient (6.38×10^{-3} cm/hr) were almost identical to those obtained with excised human skin (409 $\mu g/cm^2 \cdot hr$ and 6.36×10^{-3} cm/hr).

Hydrocortisone, a much slower permeating species, was used for the evaluation of permeability characteristics of different membranes. Table 3 presents the steady-state fluxes and permeability coefficients of hydrocortisone from a 50% ethanol/water vehicle through each of two single artificial membranes and through the composite.

Cellulose acetate membrane alone was found to be extremely permeable to hydrocortisone, with steady-state fluxes about 1000 times larger than those measured with excised human skin. The flux through Silastic sheeting is only 2.5 times faster than through the composite membrane but about 8 times faster than through excised human skin.

Table 3 Steady-state Flux of Hydorcortisone Through Various Membranes[a]

Membrane	Average flux (μg/cm^2/hr)	Permeability coefficient, P_s (cm/hr)[b]
Cellulose acetate[c]	73	6.4×10^{-3}
Silastic surgical sheet	0.61	5.3×10^{-5}
Multimembrane system (cellulose acetate/Silastic/cellulose acetate)	0.25	2.3×10^{-5}
Excised human skin	0.07	7.0×10^{-6}

[a]The donor was a saturated solution of hydrocortisone in ethanol/water (50/50).
[b]Standardized flux.
[c]Annealing temperature, 60°C.

Again, the multimembrane sandwich system (CSC) yielded the closest steady-state flux (0.25 μg/cm^2·hr) and permeability coefficient (2.3 × 10^{-5} cm/hr) to those of excised skin (0.07 μg/cm^2·hr and 7.0 × 10^{-6} cm/hr, respectively).

Water permeation was measured through various model membrane systems and excised human skin. As results summarized in Table 4 indicate, while the water fluxes and permeability coefficients through the trilaminated cellulose acetate or Silastic surgical sheet are quite different from excised human skin, the CSC membrane system behaves very similarly, with permeability coefficient only 1.5 times greater than that of human skin.

To further test the validity of the CSC model in the evaluation of drug release from different vehicles and to better correlate the diffusion characteristics of this membrane system with those of human skin, the permeation of salicylic acid from saturated solutions in different hydroalcoholic vehicles was assessed. The steady-state flux of salicylic acid from each vehicle was determined for both membranes and the apparent permeability coefficients were calculated; the

Table 4 Water Permeation Through Multimembrane Systems and Excised Human Skin

Membrane	Average flux (mg/cm^2/hr)	Permeability coefficient, P_s (cm/hr)[a]
Trilaminated cellulose acetate	26	2.6×10^{-2}
Trilaminated Silastic surgical sheet	0.08	8.0×10^{-5}
Multimembrane (cellulose acetate/Silastic/cellulose acetate)	0.62	6.2×10^{-4}
Excised Human Skin	0.42	4.2×10^{-4}

[a]Standardized flux.

Table 5 Effect of Vehicle Composition on Salicylic Acid Permeation: Multimembrane System Versus Human Skin[a]

Vehicle	CSC[b] Multimembrane		Excised human skin		P_m/P_s
	Flux (μg/cm^2/hr)	P_m^c (cm/hr)	Flux (μg/cm^2/hr)	P_s^d (cm/hr)	
Deionized water	43	2.40×10^{-2}	28	1.32×10^{-2}	1.8
30% Ethanol	136	1.04×10^{-2}	92	6.13×10^{-3}	1.7
50% Ethanol	402	6.38×10^{-3}	409	6.36×10^{-3}	1.0
70% Ethanol	642	3.96×10^{-3}	532	2.55×10^{-3}	1.6
Ethanol	1571	2.68×10^{-3}	638	1.55×10^{-3}	1.7

[a]In all cases, the donor is a saturated solution of salicylic acid in the specified vehicle.
[b]Cellulose acetate/Silastic/cellulose acetate.
[c]P_m = permeability coefficient for multimembrane system (standardized flux).
[d]P_s = permeability coefficient for excised human skin (standardized flux).

Table 6 Effect of Vehicle Composition on Hydrocortisone Permeation: Multimembrane System Versus Human Skin

Vehicle	CSC[a] Multimembrane		Excised human skin		P_m/P_s
	Flux ($\mu g/cm^2/hr$)	$P_m{}^b$ (cm/hr)	Flux ($\mu g/cm^2/hr$)	$P_s{}^c$ (cm/hr)	
Saturated in saline	1.56×10^{-2}	2.97×10^{-5}	6.90×10^{-3}	1.31×10^{-5}	2.3
1% in a hydroalcoholic vehicle[d]	1.46×10^{-1}	1.42×10^{-5}	6.13×10^{-2}	5.96×10^{-6}	2.4
0.5% in a polymer vehicle[e]	2.65×10^{-2}	4.65×10^{-6}	8.99×10^{-3}	1.58×10^{-6}	2.9

[a]Cellulose acetate/Silastic/cellulose acetate.
[b]P_m = permeability coefficient for multimembrane system (standardized flux).
[c]P_s = permeability coefficient for excised human skin (standardized flux).
[d]Ethanol/water (50/50).
[e]Contained 5% hydroxyethyl methacrylate polymer in ethanol/water (50/50).

results are summarized in Table 5. The ratio of the permeability coefficients obtained with the CSC membrane (P_m) to that obtained with human skin (P_s) was found to be fairly constant, ranging from 1.0 to 1.8. Thus, in most cases salicylic acid penetrated the artificial membrane system approximately 1.6 times faster than human skin. Table 6 summarizes the steady-state permeation rates of hydrocortisone from different vehicles through the CSC membrane and through excised human skin. The P_m/P_s ratio was computed and found rather constant, ranging from 2.3 to 2.9.

DISCUSSION

The epidermis is the protecting epithelial membrane of the body and it is limited by an aggregate lamellae of cornified cells composed mainly of keratin. These keratinized layers of cells (the stratum corneum) are held together by lipids, which constitute the effective water barrier of the skin. These lipids can be pictured as a multilaminate of alternate hydrophilic and lipophilic regions. Therefore, a multilayered membrane with both hydrophilic and lipophilic properties can be rationalized a priori as mimicking the critical permeation paths of the stratum corneum.

The compounds selected as model permeants in this investigation, salicylic acid and hydrocortisone, are of interest in topical pharmacology and, although both are capable of permeating into human skin, they do so at significantly different rates. Water was also used, since it probably can be considered to be the standard for human skin permeability studies.

In the present investigation, the type of membrane employed in the initial screening had been previously used by other researchers to study drug diffusion kinetics (Barry and Brace, 1977; Barry and El Eini, 1976; Garrett and Chemburkar, 1968; Herzog and Swarbrick, 1971). Confirming the previous findings of Garrett and Chemburkar (1968), the diffusion and permeation characteristics of salicylic acid and hydrocortisone through Silastic medical grade sheeting indicate that this membrane acts as a lipidlike barrier and that the diffusion kinetics through this membrane are in accordance with Fick's law.

Conversely, the different types of cellulose acetate membrane tested behaved as a hydrophilic barrier, but the annealing temperature of the cellulose acetate did not alter the permeability characteristic of the membranes.

The Diaflo ultrafiltration membrane used is a noncellulosic, synthetic, microporous membrane with an apparent pore radius of 20 Å and is hydrophobic; therefore, it should be very permeable to salicylic acid. The low fluxes observed may have resulted from the incomplete wetting of the pores of the membrane; otherwise, we would have expected the fluxes through the Diaflo membranes to be substantially higher than through the other membranes tested.

Of the three types of membranes tested, the cellulose acetate and the Silastic surgical sheet showed permeability characteristics closest to those of excised human skin. However, these membranes are either hydrophilic or lipophilic, and thus they are suitable for screening only hydrophilic or lipophilic compounds. The concurrent use of both types of membrane could provide the capability of screening a wider range of compounds for their permeability characteristics, offering distinct advantages over a single-membrane system.

From the systems studied both with salicylic acid and with hydrocortisone as model drugs, the CSC multimembrane yielded the fluxes and permeability coefficients closest to those of full-thickness excised human skin, even though, in general, skin was found to be somewhat more permeable. Perhaps values even closer to those of human skin could be obtained with a multilaminated membrane composed of more than three layers or with a combination of different hydrophilic and lipophilic membranes. However, from a practical point of view, this would make the experimental setup more cumbersome while, probably, it would not significantly increase the relative validity of the data obtained, compared to real-life situations.

Further support for the potential usefulness of this multimembrane system as a model for excised human skin is provided by the comparison of the permeability coefficients of water through the two membrane models. The remarkably close permeability coefficients for water found with the two membrane systems indicate that they are of very similar permeability characteristics. We also compared the permeability coefficients of salicylic acid in the CSC multimembrane and in excised human skin, using simple alcohol/water donors with different ethanol concentrations. As predicted by the theory, the flux of salicylic acid through either membrane system increases with the increase in ethanol concentration (and drug concentration) in the donor solutions. This further extends the observation that the permeation through the CSC membrane is Fickian. Moreover, the relatively constant ratio obtained between the respective permeability coefficients of salicylic acid and hydrocortisone through the two membrane systems over a wide range of ethanol concentrations demonstrates the similarity in the permeability characteristics of human skin and those of the artificial multimembrane model. Thus, the rank orders of drug permeation through the CSC membrane and through excised human skin were the same.

To provide predictable information, a useful membrane model system should exhibit permeabilities for different drugs similar to those of excised human skin. In addition, the ratio of these permeabilities should be relatively constant; the observed 1.6 and 2.5 times higher permeabilities determined for salicylic acid and hydrocortisone, respectively, represent an acceptable multiple. Since the same multiple was obtained with drug permeability coefficients that ranged from 10^{-3} to 10^{-5} cm/hr, it is reasonable to expect that a 2–3 times higher flux will be obtained with the CSC membrane for other drugs or delivery systems. Additionally, the small discrepancy in fluxes between human skin and the multimembrane model might eventually be corrected by using a somewhat thicker or more complex multimembrane system.

In conclusion, the results reported here substantiate that the CSC multimembrane system is a suitable permeability model for excised human skin and that this model may be useful in the preliminary screening of drug release from different vehicles and formulations.

REFERENCES

Barry, B. W. and Brace, A. R. (1977). Permeation of oestrone, oestradiol, oesteriol and dexamethasone across cellulose acetate membrane. *J. Pharm. Pharmacol. 29*: 394-400.

Barry, B. W. and El Eini, D. I. D. (1976). Influence of nonionic surfactants on permeation of hydrocortisone, dexamethasone, testosterone and progesterone across cellulose acetate membrane. *J. Pharm. Pharmacol. 28*: 219-227.

Bartek, M. J., LaBudde, J. A., and Maibach, H. I. (1972). Skin permeability in vivo: Comparison in rat, rabbit, pig and man. *J. Invest. Dermatol. 58*: 114-123.

Elias, P. M. (1981). Epidermal lipids, membranes, and keratinization. *Int. J. Dermatol. 20*(1): 1-17.

Franz, T. J. (1975). Percutaneous absorption. On the relevance of in vitro data. *J. Invest. Dermatol. 64*: 190-195.

Franz, T. J. (1983). Kinetics of cutaneous drug penetration. *Int. J. Dermatol. 22*(9): 499-505.

Galey, W. R., Lonsdale, H. K., and Nacht, S. (1976). The in vitro permeability of skin and buccal mucosa to selected drugs and tritiated water. *J. Invest. Dermatol. 67*: 713-717.

Garrett, E. R. and Chemburkar, P. B. (1968). Evaluation, control, and prediction of drug diffusion through polymeric membranes. *J. Pharm. Sci. 57*(6): 944-959.

Herzog, K. A. and Swarbrick, J. (1971). Drug permeation through thin-model membranes. III. *J. Pharm. Sci. 60*(11): 1666-1668.

Idson, B. (1975). Percutaneous absorption. *J. Pharm. Sci. 64*: 901.

Lavker, R. S. (1976). Membrane coating granules: The fate of the discharged lamellae. *J. Ultrastruct. Res. 55*: 79.

Levy, G. and Mroszczak, E. J. (1968). Effect of complex formation on drug absorption VI. Drug permeation through an artificial lipid barrier. *J. Pharm. Sci. 57*(2): 235-239.

Makee, G., Sulzberger, M., Herrman, F., and Baer, R. (1945). Histological studies on percutaneous penetration with special reference to the effect of vehicles. *J. Invest. Dermatol. 6*: 43-59.

Nacht, S., Yeung, D., Beasley, J. N., Anjo, M. D., and Maibach, H. I. (1981). Benzoyl peroxide: Percutaneous penetration and metabolic disposition. *J. Am. Acad. Dermatol. 4*(1): 31-37.

Nuclear-Chicago Technical Bulletin No. 13. How to determine efficiency automatically in liquid scintillation counting.

Scheuplein, R. J. and Blank, I. H. (1971). Permeability of the skin. *Physiol. Rev. 51*(4): 702-747.

Scheuplein, R. J., Blank, I. H., Brauner, G. J., and MacFarlane, D. J. (1969). Percutaneous absorption of steroids. *J. Invest. Dermatol. 52*: 63-70.

Stoughton, R. B., Clendenning, W. E., and Kruse, D. (1960). Percutaneous absorption of nicotinic acid and derivatives. *J. Invest. Dermatol. 35*: 337.

Treherne, J. E. (1956). The permeability of skin to some nonelectrolytes. *J. Physiol. 133*: 171.

Wester, R. C. and Maibach, H. I. (1975). Percutaneous absorption in the rhesus monkey compared to man. *Toxicol. Appl. Pharmacol. 32*: 394-398.

30
Receptor Fluid Penetrant Interactions and the In Vitro Cutaneous Penetration of Chemicals

Ronald T. Riley and Barbara W. Kemppainen*
R. B. Russell Research Center, U.S. Department of Agriculture, Agricultural Research Service, Athens, Georgia

The in vivo elimination from the body of chemicals that have partitioned into the skin is rate limited by processes that occur within the skin (Guy et al., 1982). While the stratum corneum is the primary barrier, there are other factors that can alter the rate of penetration. One is the subcutaneous blood flow. According to Scheuplein (1980), if the subcutaneous blood flow is not sufficient to maintain a low concentration of penetrant in the viable epidermis, the blood flow will become the limiting factor for penetration. Increased perfusion rate in vitro has been shown to increase dermal penetration of compounds (Crutcher and Maibach, 1969). Anjo et al. (1980) demonstrated, in vitro, that perfusion rate can limit penetration of parathion.

When using simple static diffusion cells to model in vivo penetration, the receptor fluid is analogous to the blood. If the penetrant is not metabolized and the receptor compartment volume is small, the concentration gradient at the interface will decrease rapidly until equilibrium is approached. The equilibrium concentration is dependent on the relative affinity of the penetrant for the skin and receptor fluid. If the receptor compartment is large, the time to approach equilibrium should be great. In the static system, the total quantity of penetrant that can accumulate in the receptor compartment is determined by its affinity for the receptor fluid and the volume of the receptor compartment. This assumes that the penetrant is not metabolized and that the relative affinity for the skin and receptor fluid is constant. Taken together, the relative affinity and receptor volume define the "holding capacity" of the static receptor compartment. In a perfused in vitro system, the receptor compartment becomes theoretically large as the perfusion rate is increased. In a static system, the receptor

---

Present affiliation: Auburn University School of Pharmacy, Auburn, Alabama

volume is fixed. Assuming negligible metabolism, the holding capacity can be increased only by changing the relative affinity of the penetrant for the receptor fluid.

This chapter shows that the chemical composition of the receptor fluid can affect the rate of penetration in vitro. The effect may be due to increased affinity of the penetrant for the receptor fluid or alterations in the skin itself.

METHODS

Test System

Penetration of test agents through isolated epidermis (stratum corneum plus underlying epidermis) was estimated using static diffusion cells (Riley, 1983). Pig skin was obtained from the abdominal area of suckling pigs, and nonselected human skin was obtained either at autopsy or from amputations. Pig skin was stored in sterile banking fluid at 4°C and human skin was treated and stored as described by Franz (1975). Epidermal sheets of pig skin and human skin were obtained by the method of Scheuplein and Blank (1973).

Test Agents

[^{35}S]Parathion was custom synthesized by Amersham Corp. (Arlington Heights, Ill.) and [G-^{14}C]aflatoxin B_1 (AFB_1) was obtained from Moravek Biochemicals, Inc. (Brea, Calif.). The radiochemical purities were determined by thin-layer chromatography (TLC) to be 95 and 93% for parathion and AFB_1, respectively. Doses were prepared in methanol or as adsorbed formulations on attapulgus clay particles (20-30 mesh). After application, the methanol carrier was evaporated. Adsorbed formulations were applied by weight ($\sim$ 5 mg).

Experimental

These experiments determine whether the use of different receptor fluids affects the rate of penetration of parathion and AFB_1. The control receptor fluids were phosphate-buffered saline with penicillin and streptomycin (PBSA) and filtrates resulting from the ultrafiltration of serum using Diaflo ultrafilters (Amicon, Lexington, Mass.). Antibiotics were also added to filtrates. Six diffusion cells (three controls and three treated) were used in each experiment. Samples of receptor fluid (50 μl) were removed at predetermined intervals and radioactivity was determined by standard liquid scintillation counting techniques. Penetration of test agents using PBSA was compared to penetration using serum or serum fractions (in PBSA), 5% Triton X100 (in PBSA) or 1% sodium lauryl sulfate (in PBSA). The radiochemical purity of penetrants was determined by TLC after extraction from the receptor fluids. The solubility of parathion in

PBSA and swine serum and solubility of AFB_1 in PBSA, serum, Triton $\times 100$, and sodium lauryl sulfate (SDS) was determined by the method of Cadwallader and Madan (1981).

RESULTS AND DISCUSSION

The total quantity of $[^{35}S]$ parathion that penetrated pig skin was always greater whenever swine serum or the fraction of swine serum having a molecular weight greater than 500 was compared to penetration using PBSA or 500-MW filtrate, respectively (Fig. 1A). The differences between PBSA and serum were apparent regardless of whether the dose was applied in methanol or as the adsorbed formulation. Parathion penetration across human skin was significantly greater with human serum as the receptor fluid (Fig. 1B). The solubilities of parathion in PBSA and whole serum were 220 ±58 and 3426 ±379 nmol/ml, respectively. Gel filtration (Bio Gel P2, BioRad, Richmond, Calif.) of the swine serum/parathion mixture revealed that the increased affinity of parathion for the serum may have been partially a result of interactions of parathion with specific constituents of the serum (11%); however, most of the parathion in the serum (89%) was not tightly bound but was associated with a rapidly reversible binding to serum proteins (Riley and Wallner, 1983). An increased affinity of parathion for serum proteins, relative to PBSA, could ultimately result in an increased holding capacity of the receptor compartment and thus an increased penetration of parathion relative to PBSA.

The total penetration of $[^{14}C]$ AFB_1 was not increased when human serum was used as the receptor fluid, however, both 5% Triton $\times 100$ and 1% SDS significantly increased the total penetration relative to PBSA (Table 1). The solubility of AFB_1 is much greater in serum, Triton $\times 100$, and SDS than in PBSA (Table 2). However, serum and Triton are equally effective solvents for AFB_1. With AFB_1, increased affinity for the serum did not result in increased penetration. Recently, Bronaugh and Stewart (1983) have shown that rabbit serum, 3% bovine serum albumin, organic solvents, and nonionic surfactants enhanced the in vitro penetration of cinnamyl anthranilate and acetylethyl tetramethyl tetralin. Both Triton and SDS are strong surfactants capable of solubilizing nonpolar chemicals. The lipid components of the stratum corneum are essential to its barrier function (Grayson and Elias, 1982). Solubilization of the lipid-enriched intercellular "mortar" by these surfactants could enhance the penetration of AFB_1 by altering the permeability characteristics of the stratum corneum or by providing intercellular channels down which AFB_1 could diffuse.

Regardless of the mechanisms, the results of this study indicate that the chemical composition of the receptor fluid can affect the kinetics of penetration and therefore should be considered when designing in vitro systems to assess percutaneous absorption.

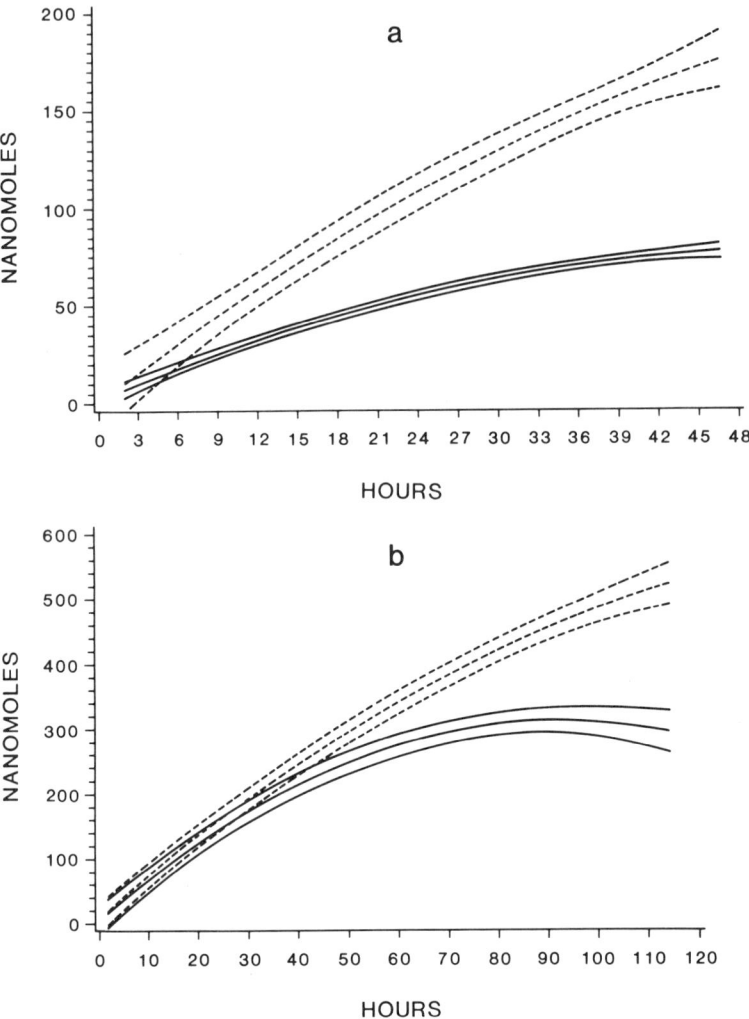

Figure 1 (a) Penetration of [^{35}S] parathion across isolated pig epidermis under conditions of occlusion of the donor chamber at 24°C. Upper and lower 95% confidence limits and least-squares fit of the data are given. The appplied dose was 0.89 μmol. Solid lines are penetration with 500-MW filtrate as the receptor fluid [r^2 = 0.97, degree of freedom (df) = 23] and dotted lines are the 500-MW dialysate of whole swine serum (r^2 = 0.94, df = 23). (b) Penetration of [^{35}S]-parathion across isolated human epidermis under conditions of occlusion at 25°C. The applied dose was 7.62 μmol. Solid lines are penetration with PBSA (r^2 = 0.97, df = 26) and dotted lines are whole human serum (r^2 = 0.94, df = 26).

Table 1 Penetration of $[^{14}C]AFB_1$ Through Human Skin Using Different Receptor Fluids[a]

Fluid	Penetration of PBSA controls (% ±SD)[a]
Human serum (47 hr)	82.3± 4.0
5% Triton X100 (50 hr)	146.1±43.2[b]
1% SDS (24 hr)	322.9±81.9[b]

[a]Values are relative to matched PBSA controls after period of time given in parentheses; $n = 3$.
[b]Significantly greater than PBSA controls, $P < 0.05$.

Table 2 Solubility of AFB_1 in Receptor Fluids

Receptor fluid	Solubility (nmol/ml, mean ±SD)[a]
PBSA	49.8± 0.9
Whole serum	209.5±20.0
5% Triton X100	220.0± 4.8
5% SDS	3254.7±89.7

[a]Values at equilibrium (~ 48 hr); $n = 3$.

REFERENCES

Anjo, D. M., Feldmann, R. J., and Maibach, H. I. (1980). Methods of predicting percutaneous penetration in man. In *Percutaneous Absorption of Steroids*. Edited by P. Mauvais-Jarvis, C. F. H. Vickers, and J. Wepierre. Academic, New York, pp. 31–51.

Bronaugh, R. L. and Stewart, R. F. (1983). Hydrophobic compounds—A potential problem for in vitro percutaneous absorption studies. *J. Invest. Dermatol. 80*: 347 (Abstr.).

Cadwallader, D. E. and Madan, D. K. (1981). Effect of macromolecules on aqueous solubility of cholesterol and hormone drugs. *J. Pharm. Sci. 70*: 442–446.

Crutcher, W. and Maibach, H. I. (1969). The effect of perfusion rate on in vitro percutaneous penetration. *J. Invest. Dermatol. 53*: 264.

Franz, T. J. (1975). Percutaneous absorption. On the relevance of in vitro data. *J. Invest. Dermatol. 64*: 190–195.

Grayson, S. and Elias, P. M. (1982). Isolation and lipid biochemical characterization of stratum corneum membrane complexes: Implications for the cutaneous permeability barrier. *J. Invest. Dermatol. 78*: 128–135.

Guy, R. H., Hadgraft, J., and Maibach, H. I. (1982). A pharmacokinetic model for percutaneous absorption. *Int. J. Pharm. 11*: 119-129.

Riley, R. T. (1983). Starch-xanthate encapsulated pesticides: A preliminary toxicological evaluation. *J. Agric. Food Chem. 31*: 202-206.

Riley, R. T. and Wallner, B. M. (1983). Cutaneous penetration of lipophilic toxicants through swine skin: Serum concentration rate limiting in in vitro system. *J. Animal Sci. 57*: 34 (Abstr.).

Scheuplein, R. J. (1980). Percutaneous absorption: Theoretical aspects. In *Percutaneous Absorption of Steroids*. Edited by P. Mauvais-Jarvis, C. F. H. Vickers, and J. Wepierre. Academic, New York, pp. 1-17.

Scheuplein, R. J. and Blank, I. H. (1973). Mechanism of percutaneous absorption. IV. Penetration of nonelectrolytes (alcohols) from aqueous solutions and from pure liquids. *J. Invest. Dermatol. 60*: 286-296.

31
Blood Flow Studies and Percutaneous Absorption

Richard H. Guy
University of California School of Pharmacy, San Francisco, California

Ethel Tur,* Ronald C. Wester, and Howard I. Maibach
University of California School of Medicine, San Francisco, California

Various approaches are currently available to study the kinetics and extent of percutaneous absorption. The suitability of the different techniques (e.g., human in vivo, animal models, in vitro) depends on the question being asked of the experiment and on the philosophy of the investigator. Debate on the relevance of model studies (animal or in vitro) to human skin penetration has been and will continue to be conducted vigorously, and examples of this discussion can be found in this volume. One point of agreement that may be accepted is that absorption through the skin of man is best considered by performing penetration studies in live human subjects. The work described in this chapter summarizes new procedures for following, in vivo in man, the time course of drug behavior at and within the region of topical application. It will be shown that information is collected with negligible perturbation to the skin and with excellent subject compliance. Observations and measurements are thus made of *local*, in vivo, absorption, a sequence of events (of much clinical and toxicological relevance) that has previously been accessible to study only through somewhat indirect means.

We have employed the noninvasive optical procedures of laser Doppler velocimetry and photopulse plethysmography, which are sensitive to changes in skin blood flow (number of erythrocytes times velocity) and volume, respectively, to monitor the percutaneous penetration of vasodilative chemicals. Hence,

---

**Present affiliation*: Ichilov Medical Center, Tel Aviv, Israel

the objective of this work has been to collect and interpret pharmacodynamic effects on the cutaneous microcirculation elicited by topical vasodilators with the purpose of deducing the local kinetics of skin absorption and elimination.

EXPERIMENTAL TECHNIQUES

Laser Doppler Velocimetry

The laser Doppler velocimetry (LDV; see Fig. 1) technique has been described in detail (Bonner et al., 1981; Holloway and Watkins, 1977; Nilsson et al., 1980a,b; Stern et al., 1977; Watkins and Holloway, 1978). Briefly, light at 632.9 nm from a 5-mW helium-neon laser is directed into the skin. The radiation is multiply scattered and reflected by both stationary tissue components and mobile red blood cells. The former backscatter radiation at the incident frequency, the latter reflect light that has been frequency (or Doppler) shifted by an amount proportional to the product of their number multiplied by their velocity. The devices employed (either the LD5000 capillary perfusion monitor of Medpacific, Seattle, or the Periflux LD flowmeter of Perimed, Sweden) separate the frequency-shifted component, amplify the signal, and display the result as a fluctuating voltage. Laser light is transmitted to the skin from the velocimeters, and the reflected radiation is returned, along identical optical fibers. Physical support to the fibers at the point where they interface with the skin is provided by a small cylindrical probe, which is attached to the application site using a double-sided adhesive disc.

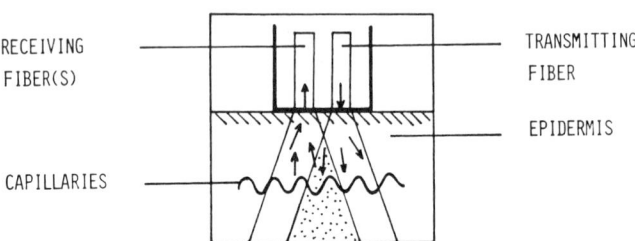

Figure 1 Laser Doppler velocimetry (LDV). Light from a helium-neon laser (λ = 632.9 nm) is transmitted to the skin via an optical fiber. The backscattered light consists of radiation at the same frequency as the incident source (reflected from nonmoving tissue) and radiation that has been Doppler shifted as a result of reflection from mobile red blood cells. The LDV extracts the frequency-shifted signal and derives an output proportional to the flux (number times velocity) of erythrocytes in the observed cutaneous microcirculation.

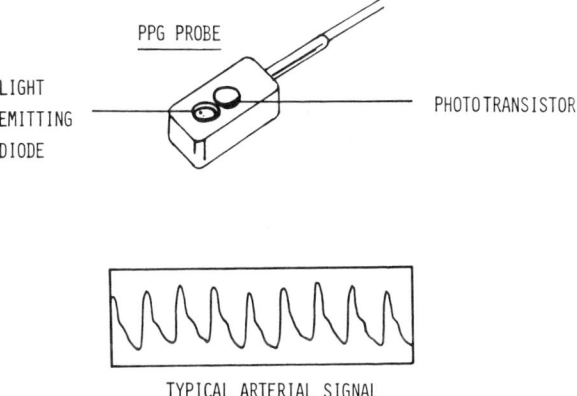

Figure 2 Photopulse plethysmography (PPG). This method utilizes a diode emitting infrared light and determines changes in blood volume passing through the dermal capillaries by the percentage of incident radiation absorbed. The output appears as a series of pulsations on which, at high sensitivity, the dicrotic notch may be seen.

Photopulse Plethysmography

Descriptions of the procedure for photopulse plethysmography (PPG; see Fig. 2) have appeared previously (Challoner, 1979; Guy et al., 1983). An infrared light-emitting diode directs radiation into the skin. The wavelength range of the source (800-940 nm) spans a region for which the tissue is transparent; on the other hand, hemoglobin absorbs measurably in this part of the spectrum. Hence the reflected radiation, which is measured with a phototransistor, contains information about the volume of blood in the skin site under observation. As with LDV, PPG is believed to monitor the microcirculation to a depth of 1-2 mm (Guy et al., 1983; Tur et al., 1983). Again, radiation is transmitted to the skin and received back via a small probe (housing the diode and phototransistor) held in position by double-sided adhesive tape. The blood volume fluctuations are processed by a photoplethysmograph (Medasonics, Mountain View, Calif.). Increases in perfusion are registered by an enhancement of the control output oscillations (Challoner, 1979; Guy et al., 1983; Tur et al., 1983).

RESULTS

LDV and PPG are suitable techniques to consider changes in skin blood flow caused by the local delivery of vasoactive agents. Indeed, application of PPG in this way has been reported for both vasodilators (Cummings, 1969; Hertzman and Randall, 1948) and vasoconstrictors (Ramsay, 1969; Thune, 1971).

Recently, in our laboratories, we have begun to consider systematically the local pharmacodynamic response to topically applied vasodilators. We have considered nicotinic acid esters, in particular the methyl ester, nitroglycerin, and minoxidil. The overall objective of these studies has been to attempt to follow the penetration, residence, and elimination of the drug into, within, and from the local region of skin at the application site, and to increase our understanding of percutaneous absorption kinetics in vivo in man.

Initial work focused on the beginning of the erythemal reaction and correlation of instrumentally detected response with visual observation (Guy et al., 1983). A typical LDV response curve is shown in Figure 3. Here hexyl nicotinate at 200 mM in a propylene glycol/isopropanol vehicle was applied via an absorbent disc (1 cm diameter) for 15 sec. The drug solution was then removed and the LDV probe placed with its center coincident with that of the application area. Similar experiments using both LDV and PPG with methyl nicotinate in aqueous solution have been carried out over a 100-fold concentration range. The data are summarized in Table 1. Figure 4 shows the pattern of changes detected locally

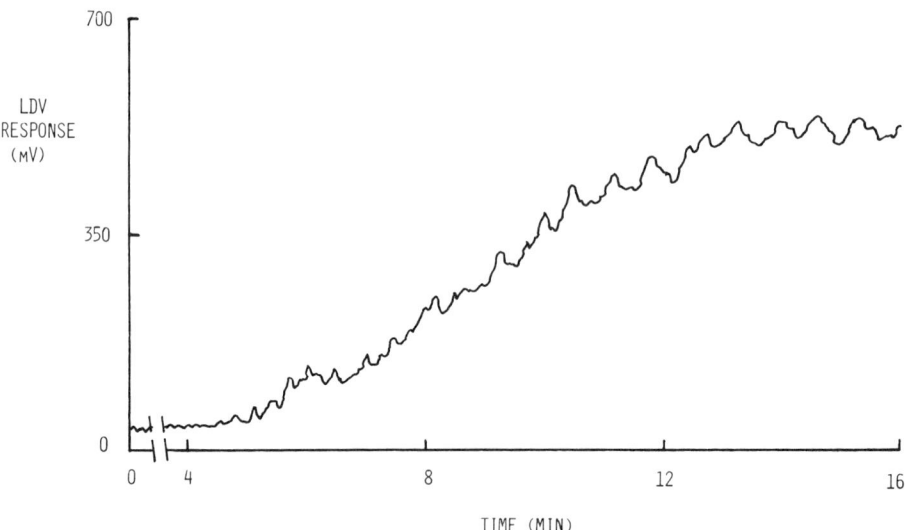

Figure 3 Early time portion of a characteristic LDV response curve. The vasodilator was hexyl nicotinate (200 mM) in a propylene glycol/isopropanol vehicle. The application site was the human ventral forearm. Time of application was 15 sec; area of application was 0.785 cm^2.

Table 1 LDV and PPG Experimental Results[a] After 15-sec Topical Applications of Aqueous Methyl Nicotinate Solutions to Flexor Aspect of Human Forearm

Methyl nicotinate concentration (mM)	Onset of LDV response (sec)	Onset of PPG response (sec)	Observed onset of erythema (sec)	Decay time of response[b] postapplication (min)
Subject 1				
150	120	125	125	40–60
15	160	180	165	20–35
1.5	250	270	260	15–25
Subject 2				
150	135	150	180	40–60
15	300	325	370	30–50
1.5	615	635	645	20–35

[a] All data represent the average of duplicate or triplicate experiments (±10%).
[b] Approximate time ranges covering the period between the start of the response decay and the return to baseline LDV or PPG output.
Source: Guy et al. (1983).

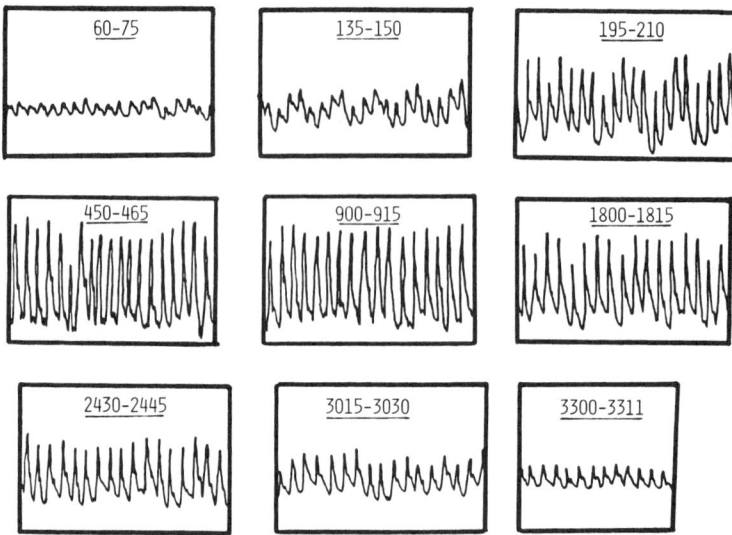

Figure 4 A representative time sequence (t in seconds) of the PPG output following a 15-sec topical application of 150 mM methyl nicotinate to human forearm skin (area = 0.785 cm^2).

by PPG during one such experiment. The optical techniques' responses provide simply quantifiable profiles of the pharmacodynamic changes elicited by these compounds without the subjectivity common to visual assessment of a reaction.

Different application sites have also been considered to probe the sensitivity of various anatomic regions of skin to a similar stimulus. Using the PPG only, Tur et al. (1983) followed the effect of aqueous methyl nicotinate (1000 mM, applied to a 1-cm diameter area for 15 sec) at five body positions. The results are summarized in Table 2 and results from the upper back and shin are compared in Figure 5. Overall, it could be shown that no statistical difference, in terms of the *relative* change from baseline perfusion, existed between the sites.

Dose-response behavior to aqueous methyl nicotinate application has been further investigated (Guy et al., 1984). Typical sets of LDV and PPG response curves are shown in Figure 6 and data from four subjects are summarized in Table 3. With increasing drug concentration, the response is saturable such that the duration of the effect, rather than the magnitude, is enlarged. Because the goal of these experiments was to learn more about the kinetics of percutaneous absorption, a simple model (Fig. 7) was formulated and hypothesized as a description of the results. We assume that input (In) of drug during the application period (15 sec) is constant and that delivery of nicotinate to and its elimination

Table 2 PPG Data[a] After 15-sec Topical Application of Aqueous Methyl Nicotinate (1000 mM) to Various Sites

Site	Time to maximum PWA[b] (min)	Time to decay (min)	$\ln \dfrac{\text{max PWA}}{\text{baseline PWA}}$
Upper forearm	7.5 ±2.2	75.2 ±7.1	1.99 ±0.3
Lower forearm	5.7 ±0.8	70.0 ±8.8	1.76 ±0.3
Upper back	6.4 ±2.5	67.5 ±12	1.85 ±0.2
Lower back	7.0 ±0.5	80.0 ±5.1	1.64 ±0.4
Shin	9.2 ±3.3	80.0 ±6.1	1.46 ±0.2

[a]Data (means ±SD) are from three volunteers: quadruplicate readings from one, duplicates from the other two. In each column, analysis of variance indicates no statistical difference between the results from different sites ($p < 0.05$).
[b]PWA = pulse wave amplitude of PPG response (see Fig. 2).
Source: Tur et al. (1983).

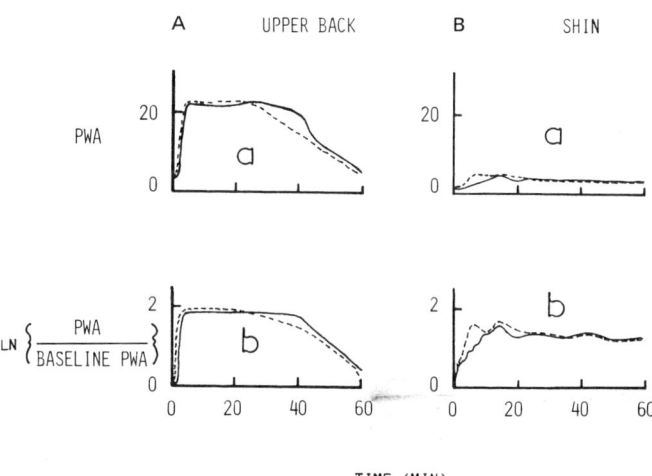

Figure 5 (A) Time dependence of the PPG pulse wave amplitude (PWA) following a 15-sec topical administration of aqueous methyl nicotinate (1000 mM) applied to (A) the upper back and (B) the shin. Curves (a) show the direct reading from the recorder output; curves (b) show the natural logarithm of the ratio PWA/baseline PWA. Solid line: left side. Dashed line: right side.

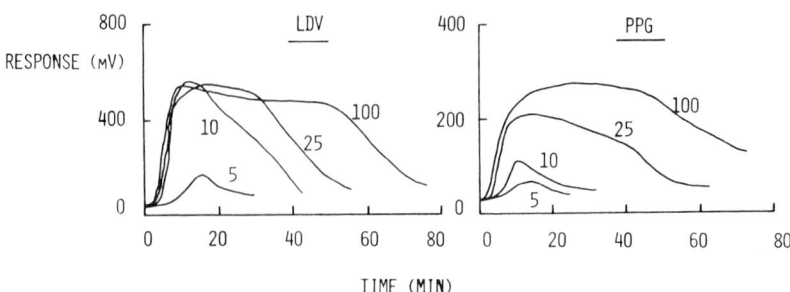

Figure 6 LDV and PPG response curves obtained in one subject following a 15-sec topical application of four aqueous solutions of methyl nicotinate of different concentrations (mM). Each curve is the mean of at least three separate determinations.

Table 3 Summary of Dose-Response Data (mean ±SE) to Methyl Nicotinate from Four Subjects[a]

Methyl nicotinate concentration (mM)[b]	Maximum instrument response (mV)		Area under response-time curve (mV·hr)		Time (min) for response to decay to 75% of maximum value	
	LDV	PPG	LDV	PPG	LDV	PPG
100	536 ± 23	173 ± 30	385 ± 52	124 ± 44	59 ± 7	56 ± 11
25	507 ± 39	135 ± 26	252 ± 30	70 ± 22	44 ± 3	41 ± 7
10	421 ± 78	66 ± 11	163 ± 20	23 ± 7	36 ± 8	31 ± 5
5	131 ± 52	48 ± 14	32 ± 13	12 ± 5	21 ± 4	20 ± 2

[a]Results have been normalized to eliminate differences in control (i.e., pre-drug-application) perfusion levels.
[b]Methyl nicotinate was applied in aqueous solution for 15 sec over an area 1 cm in diameter.
Source: Guy et al. (1984).

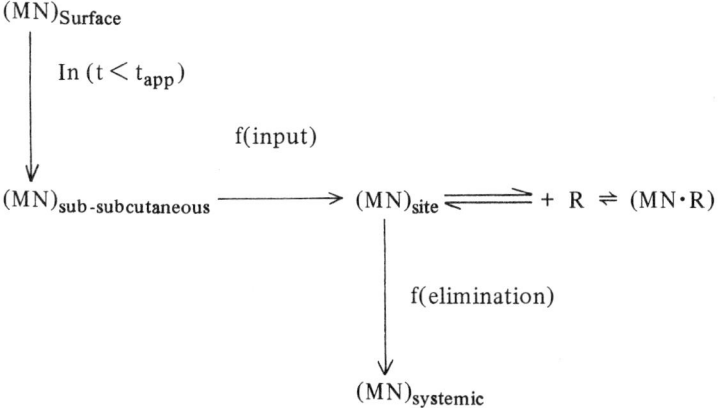

Figure 7 Pharmacokinetic/pharmacodynamic model for the determination of methyl nicotinate percutaneous absorption kinetics.

from the receptor site is first order with rate constants k_i and k_e, respectively. Binding at the receptor is assumed to obey the generalized Hill equation (Tallarida and Jacob, 1979):

$$(E - E_0) = \frac{E_{max} C^N}{C_{50}^N + C^N} \quad (1)$$

where C is concentration at the receptor, E is measured response, E_0 is the baseline response (i.e., perfusion level), E_{max} is the maximum response, C_{50} is the concentration producing 50% of E_{max}, and N is a parameter affecting the steepness of the E versus C curve. To interpret our observations with the model, therefore, requires that a relationship between E, C, and time be established. This is possible (Guy et al., 1984) and yields the result:

$$E - E_0 = \frac{E_{max} R^N}{R^N + C_{SS,50}^N} \quad (2)$$

where

$$R = k \cdot C_{APP} \cdot t_{APP} \cdot u \quad (3)$$

and C_{APP} is applied nicotinate concentration and t_{APP} is time of application. Results analysis shows that k_i and k_e are very close and not distinguishable by the regression techniques employed; thus $k = k_i = k_e$. The parameter u is a normalized concentration:

$$u = \frac{CV}{Q} = kt' \exp(-kt') \tag{4}$$

where V is the local volume of distribution, Q is the amount of drug delivered into the skin in a time equal to t_{APP}, and t' is time corrected for the lag period between drug application and response onset. The final parameter in Eq. (2) is $C_{SS,50}$ which is the hypothetical steady-state applied nicotinate concentration that would be necessary to maintain half the maximum possible increase in skin blood flow that the chemical can produce (assuming no tolerance). Thus, $C_{SS,50}$ may be considered to be a sensitivity measure of the cutaneous microcirculation to drug-induced vasodilatation. Fitting the data to Equation 2 produced the results in Table 4. Inter- and intrasubject variability is indicated, and the excellent agreement between LDV and PPG is manifest. The $C_{SS,50}$ values show that it should be possible to induce vasodilatation using very low steady-state applied levels of nicotinate (much lower than those concentrations used in this study). Preliminary results imply that this prediction is correct (Guy et al., unpublished data). The values of k show that the half-lives for drug delivery to and elimination from the site of action span a range of 4-15 min (mean = *8* min). Hence, we show that input to the site is rapid and measurable and that drug removal is equally fast and quantifiable. The former observation is consistent with what one sees using this chemical; the latter agrees with other determinations of this parameter for methyl nicotinate (e.g., Albery et al., 1983). Further work is proposed to extend the analysis of pharmacodynamic profiles in this way to provide quantitiative assessments of often inaccessible aspects of transcutaneous kinetics in vivo.

In more limited studies, we have considered local penetration of two other potent vasodilators, nitroglycerin (GTN) and minoxidil (Wester et al., 1984). The response to GTN was followed primarily after application of a commercial 2% ointment (Nitrobid, Marion Laboratories, Kansas City, Mo.). As an example of the type of behavior seen, Figure 8 shows the LDV response after 50 μl of ointment was applied over a 2-cm diameter area for 10 min, under occlusion. Residual ointment was removed before the probe was positioned to record the effect. Measurements were also taken through a transparent occlusive dressing; that is, the ointment was not at any point removed from the application site. A typical curve is shown in Figure 9. Observations of this type are of relevance to the transdermal delivery of GTN, and we have initiated work to monitor blood flow through specially prepared transdermal systems.

Minoxidil is an orally effective peripheral vasodilator that occasionally produces hair growth as a side effect. A hypothesis for this action is that the micro-

Table 4 Results of Nonlinear Least-Squares Regression Analysis (average values ±SE) of Data Sets of Type Illustrated in Figure 6[a]

Subject	k (min^{-1})		$C_{SS,50}$ (mM)		E_{max} (mV)		N	
	LDV	PPG	LDV	PPG	LDV	PPG	LDV	PPG
1	0.063	0.046	0.19	0.15	524	313	2.78	3.31
	±0.007	±0.001	±0.01	±0.06	±38	±39	±0.39	±0.68
2	0.117	0.143	0.18	0.04	441	110	2.24	1.38
	±0.010	±0.026	±0.10	±0.01	±65	±3	±0.34	±0.44
3	0.082	0.075	0.09	0.12	517	262	2.51	1.75
	±0.008	±0.010	±0.01	±0.03	±44	±15	±0.43	±0.16
4	0.167	0.086	0.09	0.08	642	503	1.19	3.05
	±0.010	±0.006	±0.02	±0.05	±82	±664	±0.19	±0.88
Population	0.106	0.079	0.12	0.08	521	224	2.10	1.94
	±0.020	±0.010	±0.03	±0.02	±25	±50	±0.33	±0.25

[a]Equation 2 based on the pharmacokinetic/pharmacodynamic model in Figure 7 was employed. The population averages were obtained using appropriately weighted individual subject parameters.
Source: Guy et al. (1984).

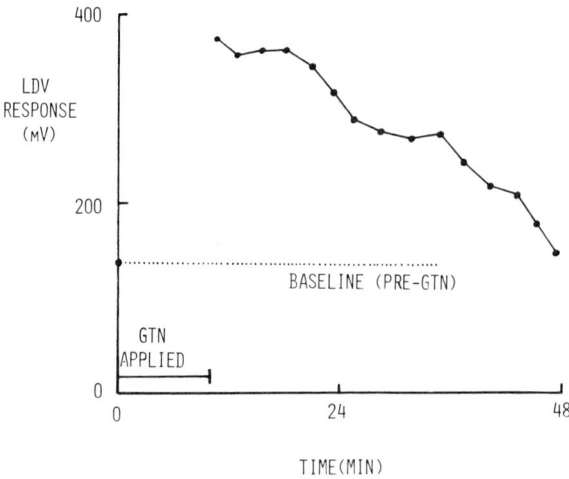

Figure 8 LDV monitoring of cutaneous vasodilatation in man induced by topical nitroglycerin application: 50 μl of Nitrobid ointment was applied over 3.14 cm² of forearm skin under occlusion for 10 min and was then removed. Perfusion was followed thereafter for the period shown.

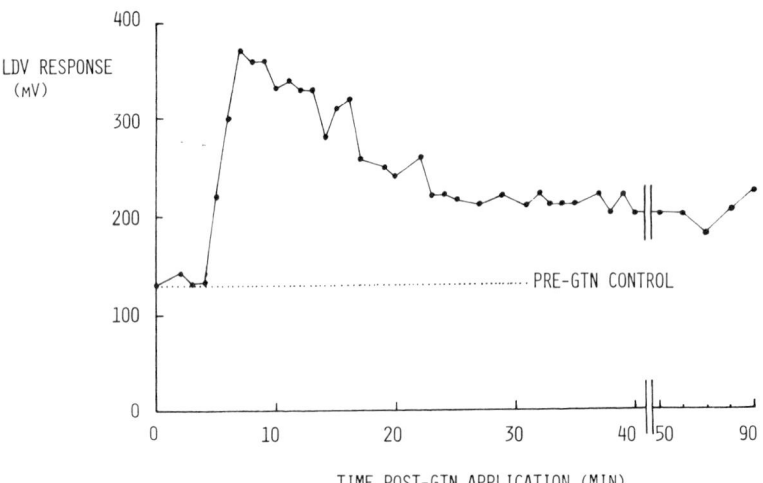

Figure 9 LDV monitoring of cutaneous vasodilatation in man induced by topical application of nitroglycerin. Excess ointment (Nitrobid) was gently massaged into a 5-cm² area of forearm skin and the site was occluded with Saran wrap. The laser probe was then attached to the plastic film and blood flow alterations were measured directly in situ through the occlusive dressing while drug was continuously delivered from the ointment.

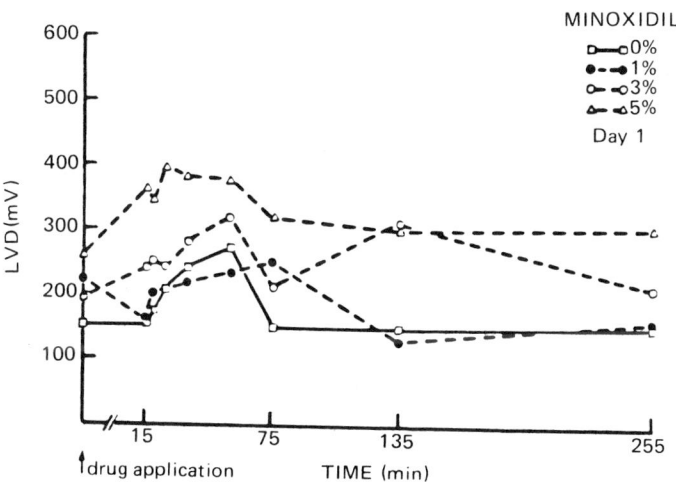

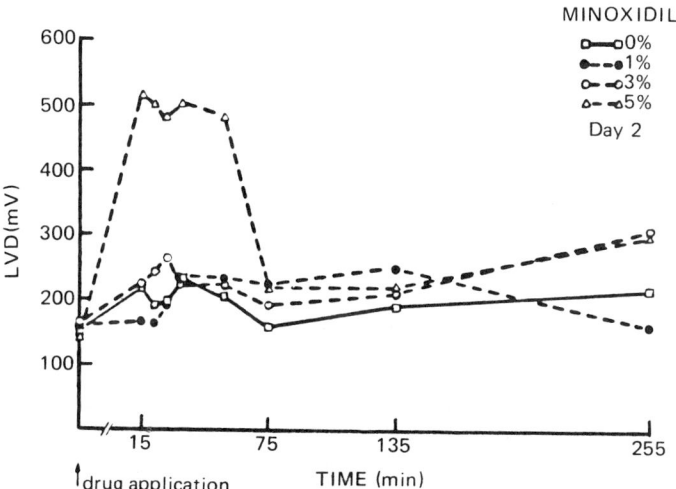

Figure 10 LDV responses to various minoxidil topical solutions applied twice over 2 consecutive days; 250 µl of each solution was applied over 100 cm^2 of bald human scalp (results shown are the means from four subjects).

circulation around hair follicles is stimulated, leading to hypertrichosis. Topical solutions of minoxidil (0, 1, 3, and 5% in propylene glycol/ethanol/water) were therefore tested with LDV and PPG for their ability to increase skin blood perfusion to the scalps of balding human volunteers. In a double-blind study (Wester et al., 1984) that involved drug application on two consecutive days (one dose per day), 250 μl was applied over 100 cm^2. LDV results, which showed the largest effect (Fig. 10) imply that minoxidil, at least at the highest concentration, is vasodilative under the conditions of this study. The significance of the observations, however, remains to be determined.

CONCLUSIONS

We believe that the research described in this chapter has started to attain its stated objectives. The noninvasive methodology does appear to be capable of elucidating kinetic and dynamic information pertinent to our understanding of in vivo percutaneous absorption in man. The data are collected easily, and the perturbation induced to living skin with the LDV and PPG techniques is minimal. Of course, there are limitations; for example, the penetrant under study must alter blood flow in some way if its progress through the skin is to be monitored optically. Furthermore, it has not yet been established whether the procedures are sufficiently sensitive to adequately assess a vasoconstrictive response (see, e.g., Amantea et al., 1983). However, the results to date are exciting and offer many fruitful avenues for further investigation. Determination of optimal vehicle formulations and evaluation of chemical-induced irritancy are just two large areas in which application of LDV and PPG may prove invaluable. It appears to us very likely that we shall hear more of these techniques in the not too distant future.

ACKNOWLEDGMENTS

We thank Medasonics, Medpacific, and Perimed (Sweden) for instrumental assistance and advice. We are also grateful to the following for their interpretive and experimental aid: Moshe Tur, Ph.D., Lewis B. Sheiner, M.D., Larry Schall, M.D., Constantine Gean, M.D., Sharif Elamir, M.D., Caroline Gaebel, Barry Bugatto, Michael Amantea, Kim Bergstrom, and Brad Roter. Support for this work was provided in part by Alza Research, Hoffman-La Roche, and the Thompson Medical Company.

REFERENCES

Albery, W. J., Guy, R. H., and Hadgraft, J. (1983). Percutaneous absorption: Transport in the dermis. *Int. J. Pharm. 15*: 125-148.

Amantea, M., Tur, E., Maibach, H. I., and Guy, R. H. (1983). Preliminary skin blood flow measurements appear unsuccessful for assessing topical corticosteroid effect. *Arch. Dermatol. Res. 275*: 419-420.

Bonner, R. F., Clem, T. R., Bowen, P. D., and Bowman, R. L. (1981). Laser Doppler continuous real-time monitor of pulsatile and mean blood flow in tissue microcirculation. In *Scattering Techniques Applied to Supramolecular and Non-Equilibrium Systems,* NATO, ASI Series B. Vol. 73. Edited by S. H. Chen, B. Chu, and R. Nossal. Plenum, New York, pp. 685-702.

Challoner, A. V. J. (1979). Photoelectric plethysmography for estimating cutaneous blood flow. In *Non-Invasive Physiological Measurements,* Vol. I. Edited by P. Rolfe. Academic, London, pp. 125-151.

Cummings, E. G. (1969). Temperature and concentration effects on penetration of n-octylamine through human skin in situ. *J. Invest. Dermatol. 53*: 64-70.

Guy, R. H., Wester, R. C., Tur, E., and Maibach, H. I. (1983). Noninvasive assessments of the percutaneous absorption of methyl nicotinate in humans. *J. Pharm. Sci. 72*: 1077-1079.

Guy, R. H., Tur, E., Bugatto, B., Gaebel, C., Sheiner, L., and Maibach, H. I. (1984). Pharmacodynamic measurements of methyl nicotinate percutaneous absorption. *Pharm. Res. 1*: 76-81.

Hertzman, A. B. and Randall, W. C. (1948). Regional differences in the basal and maximal rates of blood flow in the skin. *J. Appl. Physiol. 1*: 234-241.

Holloway, G. A. and Watkins, D. W. (1977). Laser Doppler measurement of cutaneous blood flow. *J. Invest. Dermatol. 69*: 306-309.

Nilsson, G. E., Tenland, T., and Öberg, P. A. (1980a). A new instrument for continuous measurement of tissue blood flow by light beating spectroscopy. *IEEE Trans. Biomed. Eng. BME-27*: 12-19.

Nilsson, G. E., Tenland, T., and Öberg, P. A. (1980b). Evaluation of a laser Doppler flowmeter for measurement of tissue blood flow. *IEEE Trans. Biomed. Eng. BME-27*: 597-604.

Ramsay, C. (1969). Vascular changes accompanying white dermographism and delayed blanch in atopic dermatitis. *Br. J. Dermatol. 81*: 37-43.

Stern, M. D., Lappe, D. L., Bowen, P. D., Chimosky, J. E., Holloway, G. A., Keiser, H. R., and Bowman, R. L. (1977). Continuous measurement of tissue blood flow by laser-Doppler spectroscopy. *Am. J. Physiol. 232*: H441-H448.

Tallarida, R. J. and Jacob, L. S. (1979). *The Dose-Response Relationship in Pharmacology.* Springer-Verlag, New York, pp. 1-17.

Thune, P. (1971). Plethysmographic recordings of skin pulses. IV. The vasoconstrictive effect of steroids in normal and stripped skin. *Acta Dermatovenereol.* (Stockholm) *51*: 261-267.

Tur, E., Guy, R. H., Tur, M., and Maibach, H. I. (1983). Noninvasive assessment of local nicotinate pharmacodynamics by photoplethysmography. *J. Invest. Dermatol. 80*: 499-503.

Watkins, D. W. and Holloway, G. A. (1978). An instrument to measure cutaneous blood flow using the Doppler shift of laser light. *IEEE Trans. Biomed. Eng. BME-25*: 28-33.

Wester, R. C., Maibach, H. I., Guy, R. H., and Novak, E. (1984). Minoxidil stimulates cutaneous blood flow in human balding scalps. *J. Invest. Dermatol. 82*: 515-517.

32
Hair Dye Penetration in Monkey and Man

Leszek J. Wolfram
Clairol, Inc., Stamford, Connecticut

Hair dyes have been in use for decades, yet even recent studies of their skin penetration potential have been restricted primarily to their evaluation in rats and dogs (Frenkel and Brody, 1973; Howes and Black, 1983; Hruby, 1977; Hruby et al., 1979; Nakao and Takeda, 1979; Tsomi and Kalopissis, 1982). Although undoubtedly useful, the results of these experiments are difficult to extrapolate to man and to relate to the percutaneous absorption that occurs under conditions of practical usage of fully formulated products. Sporadic attempts have been made to single out individual ingredients for studies in man (Kiese and Rauscher, 1968; Maibach et al., 1975), but these could not be readily quantitated.

A thorough study by Wester et al. (1979), comparing the percutaneous absorption in man and different animal species while pointing to the experimental advantages of using animal models, stresses the need for frequent checks at each stage of the penetration process. The authors conclude that both in vivo and in vitro studies of the skin of the rhesus monkey approximate the permeability characteristics of human skin.

We recently initiated (Maibach and Wolfram, 1981) a comprehensive evaluation of skin penetration potential of hair dyes from both permanent and semipermanent color categories. This chapter summarizes our results. The investigation focuses on man, although in most cases a comparison study also has been carried out using rhesus monkey as the animal model. The methodology is, in general, patterned after the procedure developed by Feldmann and Maibach (1970) for measurement of percutaneous absorption in man. This method involves quantifying absorption on the basis of the percentage of radioactivity excreted in the urine following application of a known amount of the labeled compound.

EXPERIMENTAL

Hair Dyes

Commercially available hair dye products, representatives of permanent and semipermanent hair color categories (Nice 'n Easy and Loving Care formulations, respectively) were individually labeled with radioactive materials. The radioactively labeled dyes together with their urinary recoveries following parenteral (P) or oral (O) administration are listed in Table 1.

Dyeing Procedure

Process instructions, specific for each hair color product, were followed. Net weights of single-application hair coloring products vary between 3 (semipermanent dyes) and a 4 fl. oz. (oxidative, permanent dyes). While this is sufficient to color up to 120 g of hair, the average weight of female scalp hair 4 in. long is about 60 g. The ratio of lotion to hair commonly operative during hair coloring is thus 1.5–2.0, and the latter value was chosen to arrive at the quantity of the dye mixture that was used in the studies with rhesus monkey.

Human Volunteers

The coloring was performed with one subject at a time. The subject was seated in a chair having his head rested on a specially constructed sink support for comfort and easy collection of rinse water. The dye mixture was applied to dry hair and worked gently into the hair mass over a period of 5–8 min and left on the hair for an additional 20 (permanent color) or 30 (semipermanent color) min. In the latter case, a plastic turban was wrapped around the hair for the dyeing period. The dyed hair was thoroughly rinsed, towel blotted, dried, and either clipped with an electric clipper or left on (see below).

Rhesus Monkeys

Animals were tranquilized with 0.2 ml of ketamine and placed comfortably in a supine position on a laboratory bench top. The head of each monkey was rested on a specially designed sink support to facilitate the coloring process and to assure quantitative collection of the rinse water. The dye lotion (total of 5 g, in the case of oxidative dyes consisting of 2.5 g of the dye solution and 2.5 g of 6% aqueous hydrogen peroxide) was worked into the dry scalp hair until all the dye mixture was used ($\sim$ 3 min). The operator wore vinyl disposable gloves. Twenty minutes was allowed for the dyeing process to proceed (30 min in the case of semipermanent dye, where a plastic turban was also used). After dyeing, the hair was rinsed with a microshower until the rinsing water was free of color. The

Table 1 Dyes Studied in this Work

Dye structure	Dye	Species and yield of urinary recovery from parenteral (P) or oral (O) administration
1,4-diaminobenzene	p-Phenylenediamine (PPD)	Man, 72% (P)
1,3-dihydroxybenzene	Resorcinol	Rhesus monkey, 79% (P)
2-methyl-5-amino-phenol (OH, CH₃, NH₂)	4-Amino-2-hydroxytoluene	Man, 94% (O)
2-methoxy-1,4-diaminobenzene (OCH₃, NH₂, NH₂)	2,4-Diaminoanisole (DAA)	Rhesus monkey, 61% (P)
2-nitro-1,4-diaminobenzene (NH₂, NO₂, NH₂)	2-Nitro-PPD	Rhesus monkey, 56% (P)
2-nitro-4-aminophenol (OH, NO₂, NH₂)	2-Nitro-4-aminophenol	Rhesus monkey, 68% (P)
HNCH₃, NO₂, N(CH₂CH₂OH)₂	HC Blue No. 1	Man, 94% (O)
NHCH₂CH₂OH, NO₂, N(CH₂CH₂OH)₂	HC Blue No. 2	Man, 51% (O)

excess water remaining on the hair was blotted with a paper towel and dyed hair was cut off with electric clippers.

Urine Collection

Human Volunteers

The subjects were given plastic urine containers for each time period: 0-4, 4-8, 8-12, and 12-24 hr and then for every 24-hr period for as long as required.

Rhesus Monkeys

After the dyeing procedure was completed, all the monkeys were restrained in ophthalmological chairs, thus preventing the animals from touching the scalp area. Urine samples were collected at 6, 12, and 24 hr and from then on at 24-hr intervals for 7 days. For both species and for each time period, total urine weights were recorded and an aliquot removed for analysis.

Radioactivity Determination in Urine

All urine samples were filtered and assayed in PPD/Triton/toluene with a liquid scintillation spectrometer. A $[^{14}C]$ toluene internal standard (100,000 cpm) was added to each counting vial to determine the extent of quenching. The counting cocktail was 81% efficient and the background was 22 cpm. Most specimens were also counted by the wet ashing method (Feldmann and Maibach, 1970). The assay values listed in the tables have been corrected for incomplete excretion from internal application. For the latter, see Table 1.

Radioactivity Determination in Dyed Hair and Stratum Corneum

Samples of hair or of the horny layer were digested overnight in counting vials, each containing 1 ml of Unisol. The digested samples were decolorized by the addition of 50% hydrogen peroxide and each was diluted with 15 ml of Unisol complement. Clear samples were equilibrated in the counting chamber at 4°C before counting on a Packard Tricarb liquid scintillation spectrometer. Three samples were analyzed for each hair lot and one of the stratum corneum, with three radioactivity determinations for each sample.

RESULTS

Two methodological approaches (denoted "Application Only" and "Application and Wear"), reflecting different experimental objectives, have been developed in the course of this study. In the first one, the hair was removed immediately following the completion of the coloring procedure; in the other, the hair was left on. The first approach allowed us to evaluate the extent of skin penetration by hair dyes resulting from the hair coloring procedure alone. The second approach recognized that (1) people color their hair to wear it as such, and (2) the dyed hair represents a reservoir of dye moieties that through a variety of routes, may become bioavailable.

Application Only

The data on total excretion of radiolabeled dye ingredients are given in Table 2. In most cases, they reflect the counts obtained over 144 hr following application of the dye; occasionally a time span of 96 hr was used if the counts at longer times were at the background level.

Two entries of Table 2, namely $T_{1/2}$ and Total dose excretion, should be clarified. It was found that the urinary excretion followed satisfactory first-order kinetics and thus, time required for 50% excretion ($T_{1/2}$) was employed as an additional quantifying parameter. Regarding the dose, bear in mind that in the process of hair coloring, the product is usually applied in the form of a viscous lotion and uniformly distributed within the hair mass. Clearly, only the product that is in contact with the scalp serves as a dye reservoir available for skin penetration. The quantity available depends on the retention of the product by hair, which in turn is a function of total surface area of the hair mass and the viscosity of the product. Unless the product is applied sparingly (product/hair ratio much less than 1—a situation that is unlikely to be encountered in hair dyeing), the thickness of the product film present on the scalp is at least 5-10 times that of the horny layer of the scalp; and under such conditions, the quantity of the absorbed dye reaches a limiting value and is independent of the quantity of lotion used (Tsomi and Kalopissis, 1982). Throughout this work, every attempt was made to maintain a constant ratio of product to hair weight ($\sim$2) and thus to make the dose excretion values intercomparable.

From the five dyes that were concurrently evaluated on both man and the rhesus monkey, three of them (DAA, PPD, and HC Blue No. 1) show striking equivalence in cutaneous absorption between these two species. This parallels the earlier finding of Wester et al. (1979) and Bartek and LaBudde (1975), who noted a similar pattern for absorption of benzoic acid, testosterone, and hydrocortisone. Two remaining dyes (2-nitro-PPD and resorcinol), representing the semipermanent and permanent categories, respectively, do not follow this pattern. Both dyes show greater absorption for rhesus monkey than man, although the $T_{1/2}$ values are identical in both species.

The results also indicate that except for DAA, the dyes appear to penetrate the skin to a similar extent. This is in spite of substantial differences in the chemical structure of the dyes, in the nature of the dye bases, and in the reaction pathways responsible for color formation. The observed effect is, however, somewhat fortuitous because the various dyes are present in their respective

Table 2 Parameters of Percutaneous Absorption of Hair Dyes

Hair color category	Labeled ingredient	Species	Number of subjects	Total dose excretion [% (±SD)]	$T_{1/2}$ of urinary excretion (hr)
Permanent (oxidative)	2,4-Diaminoanisole (DAA)	Man	3	0.022 (0.01)	18
		Rhesus monkey	2	0.032	20
	Resorcinol	Man	3	0.076 (0.03)	31
		Rhesus monkey	3	0.177 (0.03)	31
	4-Amino-2-hydroxytoluene	Man	3	0.20 (0.10)	24
	p-Phenylenediamine (PPD)	Man	5	0.190 (0.06)	16
		Rhesus monkey	3	0.182 (0.06)	22
Semipermanent	2-Nitro-PPD	Man	3	0.143 (0.04)	24
		Rhesus monkey	3	0.551 (0.10)	24
	4-Amino-2-nitrophenol	Man	3	0.235 (0.08)	10
	HC Blue No. 1	Man	5	0.151 (0.12)	18
		Rhesus monkey	3	0.127 (0.03)	40

Table 3 Flux of Hair Dyes Through Human Scalp

Dye	Flux (mol/cm² hr)
DAA	9.2×10^{-11}
Resorcinol	2.2×10^{-10}
4-Amino-2-hydroxytoluene	4.5×10^{-10}
2-Nitro-PPD	4.7×10^{-10}
HC Blue No. 1	4.9×10^{-10}
PPD	6.3×10^{-10}
4-Amino-2-nitrophenol	8.3×10^{-10}

formulations at different concentrations. A better perception of their penetration potential can be deduced from the flux values, which were calculated for individual dyes from the 24-hr excretion data, normalizing the quantity applied in each case to 10 $\mu M/cm^2$ (Table 3).

There is approximately a 10-fold spread in the flux, with DAA being at the low end of the scale and 4-amino-2-nitrophenol exhibiting the highest potential. No apparent correlation to either molecular weight or the chemical structure is evident, but the spread in molecular weight is relatively small (it varies between 100 and 250), and all the dyes are unchanged under dyeing conditions. It is also interesting that the flux ranking of dyes is not reciprocated by their solubility characteristics. The membrane/vehicle partition coefficients (which reflect the solubility properties of materials in media of differing polarities) are considered to be important factors in determining the flux of materials through the stratum corneum but, surprisingly, their utility in this case is minimal (Table 4).

The octanol/water partition coefficients seem to be at odds as well with those determined for stratum corneum/water with no evidence of a pattern that could be persuasively interpreted. The data all but imply that the lipid domains in the horny layer are the unlikely sites for retention of lipophilic dyes. That the distribution of dyes in the stratum corneum is highly complex is further evidenced by the fact that the delipidization of stratum corneum by chloroform/methanol increases the values of partition coefficients of dyes irrespective of whether they are hydrophilic or prefer a nonpolar environment. Clearly, the removal of the lipids augments the reservoir capacity of the horny layer. It would be presumptuous, however, to assume that such an increase would simply translate into faster or more extensive diffusion, since the latter is likely to be critically dependent on the binding of the dyes to the stratum corneum and there is no information about how delipidization affects the binding characteristics.

An additional and useful insight into the mechanism of scalp penetration by hair dyes can be gained from the $T_{1/2}$ values of urinary excretions. The results

Table 4 Partition Coefficients of Hair Dyes Between Octanol/Water and Guinea Pig Stratum Corneum/Water

Dye	Partition coefficients		
	Octanol/ water	Intact stratum corneum/ water	Delipidized stratum corneum/ water
DAA	0.7	—	—
Resorcinol	7.0	3.6	7.7
4-Amino-2-hydroxytoluene	25.4	8.0	21.1
2-Nitro-PPD	3.6	13.2	28.9
HC Blue No. 1	10.8	2.8	7.3
PPD	0.2	4.0	7.3
4-Amino-2-nitrophenol	10.1	5.0	9.1

of monitoring the urinary recoveries of dyes administered by parenteral injection or orally show that elimination of those materials from the organisms of either rhesus monkey or man is rapid, yielding $T_{1/2}$ values of 4 hr or less. That is clearly not the case with the urinary dye recoveries following hair dyeing, where $T_{1/2}$ values vary from 10 to 40 hr, suggesting that only trivial amounts of dye penetrate the stratum corneum during the actual process of hair coloring. It follows that the bulk of the urine-recovered dye must have been taken up into the horny layer and then slowly released into the circulation. Some penetration of hair follicles and/or sweat ducts might also have occurred, but this shunt mechanism—judging again by high $T_{1/2}$ values—seems to be of less importance. A direct experimental support for the magnitude of the horny layer reservoir has been obtained by applying a measured quantity of dye formulation to forearms of human volunteers, mimicking the dyeing procedure, and then removing sequential layers of stratum corneum all the way to the glistening layer by stripping with adhesive tape. The application areas were large enough to allow for stripping adjacent regions 16 or 18 hr after the color application. Figures 1 and 2 illustrate the results obtained in the case of PPD and HC Blue No. 1, respectively. The change in the concentration profiles of both dyes with time is a dramatic demonstration of their mobility in the horny layer and serves as an independent confirmation of the observed kinetics of scalp penetration. It is worth adding that the calculations based on the reservoir potential in both cases strongly suggest that the urinary excretion values, which are the measure of the extent of dye penetration, can be satisfactorily accounted for by the dye absorbed within the stratum corneum.

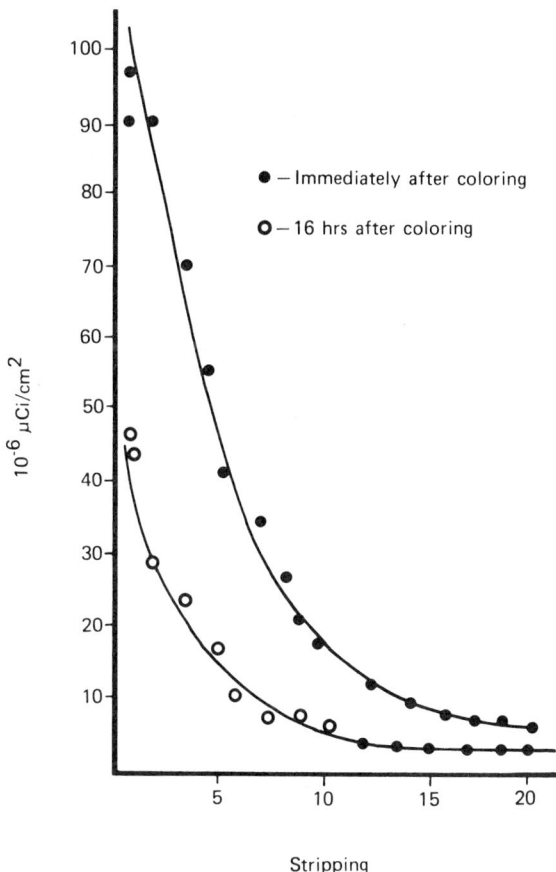

Figure 1 Distribution of radioactive PPD in the horny layer.

Application and Wear

The hair coloring procedures employed in this study were identical to those described earlier, however, the collections of urine and their radioactive assays continued for as long as 30 days following the dye application. The results of the assays, both total and interim, are given in Table 5. The half-times ($T_{1/2}$) of urinary excretions are also included as informative guides.

The results fall into a pattern that one would anticipate from the mechanism of hair coloring that is characteristic for a given class of dyes. In the case of oxidative (permanent) dyes (based on PPD and its couplers), the color-forming reactions convert the small, mobile, and colorless molecules into much bulkier dye

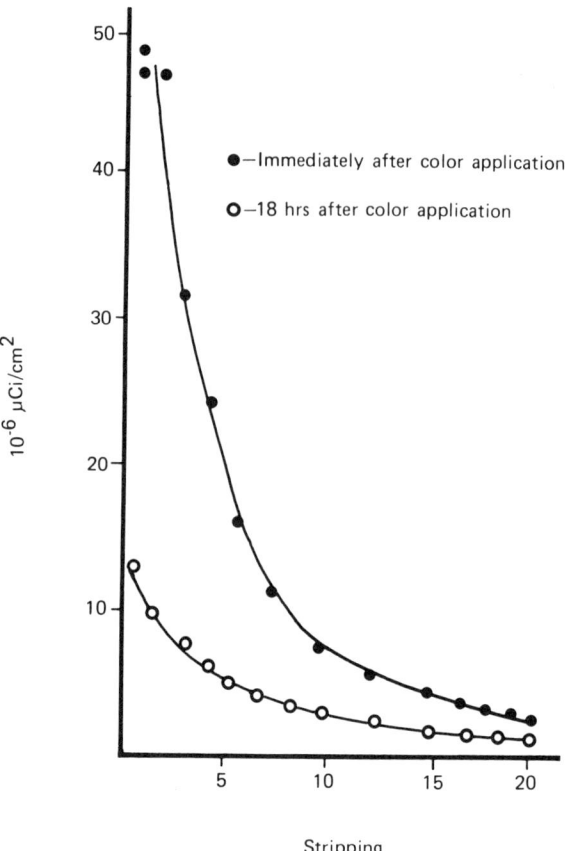

Figure 2 Distribution of radioactive HC Blue No. 1 in the horny layer.

Table 5 Dose Absorption of Hair Dyes in Man Under Conditions of Use (application + 30 days wear)

Dye	Number of subjects	Cumulative dose absorption (%)					$T_{1/2}$ (hr)
		1st day	10th day	20th day	30th day	(±SD)	
PPD	3	0.19	0.31	0.34	0.34	(0.12)	26
2-Nitro-PPD	4	0.19	0.42	0.62	0.75	(0.30)	150
HC Blue No. 1	4	0.15	0.28	0.30	0.50	(0.15)	138
HC Blue No. 2	4	0.01	0.07	0.094	0.094	(0.02)	52

moieties trapped within the structure of the hair. There is little chance for these materials to diffuse out of the hair, even when it becomes fully swollen during shampooing. On the other hand, the semipermanent dyes do not undergo any changes in size upon their deposition in the fiber, and they retain a high degree of mobility, which translates into a potential for outward diffusion. Thus, while the hair acts as a repository for both types of dye, their bioavailabilities are clearly different. The latter finds its experimental verification in the urinary excretion data. There is only a marginal increase in the dosage absorption of PPD when compared to the "Application Only" values, with most of the increase generated within 2 days of color application. HC Blue No. 1 and 2-nitro-PPD, on the other hand, register a four- to fivefold increase with measurable absorption values spread over several weeks. This trend is also reflected in the $T_{1/2}$ values of urinary excretion—a trivial change for PPD, but a substantial increase for both HC Blue No. 1 and 2-nitro-PPD.

The excretion data of Table 5 reflect not only scalp penetration but also include dye that has become bioavailable through other ports of entry (dermal as well as oral)—a real-life situation. In this sense, the $T_{1/2}$ values do not have the same meaning as those of Table 2, where they referred exclusively to scalp permeation.

The higher mobility of semipermanent dyes when compared to their oxidative counterparts implies faster depletion of the hair "reservoir." This is fully attested to by the results of the radioactive assays of the dyed hair. Over the 30-day wear period, the hair colored with permanent dyes lost approximately 10% of its original dye content, while losses of well over 60% were recorded for hair dyed with semipermanent dyes.

Table 5 contains one entry (HC Blue No. 2) that appears to be at odds with the remainder of the data. This dye is strikingly similar in its chemical structure to HC Blue No. 1, it remains unaltered during the dye-out, yet in its skin permeation characteristics it does not behave like a semipermanent. The octanol/water partition coefficient for HC Blue No. 2, at 1.6, is much lower than that of HC Blue No. 1, and the dye partitions poorly into the stratum corneum from water. A clue to the unusual behavior of this dye was furnished by the skin stripping experiments. Figures 3 and 4 are the dye content profiles of human stratum corneum stripped from the forearms dyed with components containing either HC Blue No. 1 or No. 2. The stripping was done immediately upon dyeing and again 6 hours later. The radioactivities of the dye lotions were almost identical, and so were the assays of stratum corneum strips harvested right after dyeing (29.7×10^{-4} μCi for HC Blue No. 1, and 30.3×10^{-4} μCi for HC Blue No. 2). Obviously, both dyes were diffusing at comparative rates while the dye lotions were on. The assays of the 6-hr strips revealed, however, that while the activity of the skin dyed with HC Blue No. 1 decreased to 24.5×10^{-4} μCi (16% loss),

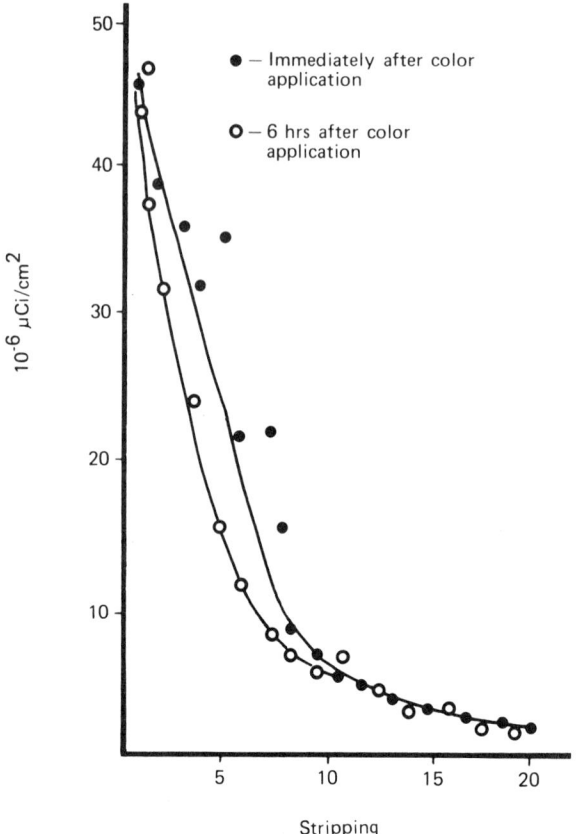

Figure 3 Distribution of radioactive HC Blue No. 1 in the horny layer.

that of tissue dyed with HC Blue No. 2 remained unchanged. The HC Blue No. 2 is thus obviously bound much more strongly to the stratum corneum than HC Blue No. 1, yet such a conclusion would hardly be arrived at on the basis of its partition coefficient.

There is little doubt that an increase in the tenacity of binding is inversely related to the dye mobility within the horny layer and thus adversely affects the diffusion of the dye into viable epidermis. With the diffusion process markedly slowed down, the natural process of desquamation attains an important role. The bulk of the dye reservoir is located in a few uppermost layers of the stratum corneum, and their loss by desquamation can lead to a rapid and precipitous drop in the quantity of the bioavailable dye, hence in the total extent of skin penetration. It appears from the results presented here that HC Blue No. 2 exemplifies such a behavior.

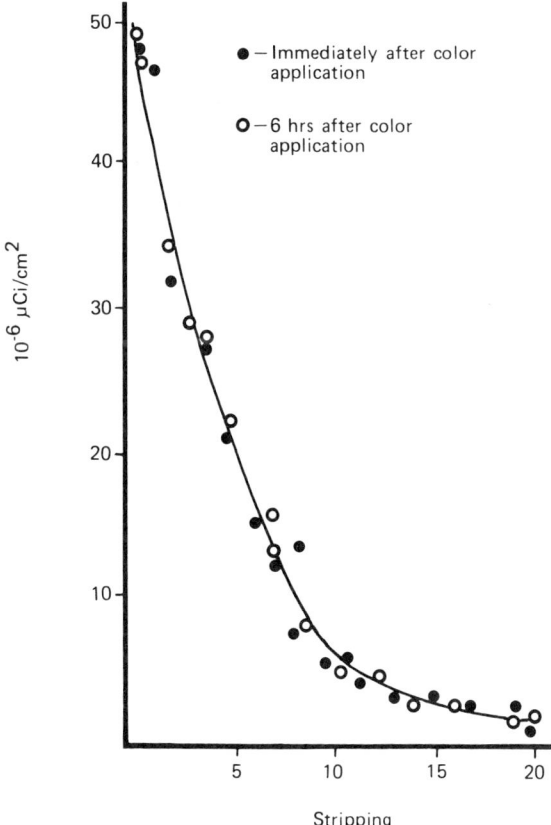

Figure 4 Distribution of radioactive HC Blue No. 2 in the horny layer.

REFERENCES

Bartek, M. J. and LaBudde, J. A. (1975). *Animal Models in Dermatology: Relevance to Human Dermatopharmacology and Dermatotoxicology.* Edited by H. I. Maibach. Churchill-Livingstone, London, pp. 103-120.

Feldmann, R. J. and Maibach, H. I. (1970). Absorption of some organic compounds through the skin of man. *J. Invest. Dermatol.* 54: 399-404.

Frenkel, E. P. and Brody, F. (1973). Percutaneous absorption and elimination of an aromatic hair dye. *Arch. Envir. Health* 27: 401-404.

Howes, D. and Black, J. G. (1983). Percutaneous penetration of 2-nitro-*p*-phenylenediamine. *Int. J. Cosmet. Sci.* 5: 215-226.

Hruby, E. (1977). The absorption of *p*-toluenediamine by the skin of rats and dogs. *Cosmet. Toxicol.* 15: 595-599.

Hruby, E. (1979). Cutaneous resorption of 2,4-diaminoanisole in the rat and dog. SGAE Report A0037, March.

Kiese, M. and Rauscher, M. (1968). The absorption of *p*-toluenediamine through human skin in hair dyeing. *Toxicol. Appl. Pharmacol. 13*: 325-331.

Maibach, H. I. and Wolfram, L. J. (1981). Percutaneous penetration of hair dyes. *J. Soc. Cosmet. Chem. 32*: 223-229.

Maibach, H. I., Leaffer, M. A., and Skinner, W. A. (1975). Percutaneous penetration following use of hair dyes. *Arch. Dermatol. 111*: 1444-1445.

Nakao, M. and Takeda, Y. (1979). Body distribution, excretion and metabolism of *p*-phenylenediamine in rats. *J. Pharm. Soc. Japan 99*: 1149-1153.

Tsomi, V. and Kalopissis, G. (1982). Cutaneous penetration of some hair dyes in the hairless rat. *Toxicol. Eur. Res. 4*: 119-127.

Wester, R. C., Noonan, P., and Maibach, H. I. (1979). Recent advances in percutaneous absorption using the rhesus monkey model. *J. Soc. Cosmet Chem. 30*: 297-307.

33
Penetration of Mycotoxins Through Excised Human Skin

Barbara Kemppainen* and Ronald T. Riley
R. B. Russell Research Center, U.S. Department of Agriculture, Agricultural Research Service, Athens, Georgia

Judith G. Pace
U.S. Army Medical Research Institute of Infectious Diseases, Fort Detrick, Frederick, Maryland

Mycotoxins are common contaminants of agricultural products. T-2 toxin (T-2), a potent cytotoxic agent, is a contaminant of corn in the midwestern United States. T-2 concentrations in corn have been reported as high as 2 ppm (Mirocha et al., 1977). Aflatoxin B_1 (AFB_1), one of the most potent carcinogens known, is a common contaminant of corn in the southern United States. Airborne dust samples collected during corn harvesting in Georgia contained 15-382 ppb AFB_1 (Burg et al., 1982). Dust samples collected from grain elevators in Georgia contained 29-543 ppb aflatoxin B_1 and B_2 (Burg et al., 1982). Agricultural workers dermally exposed to mycotoxin-contaminated corn may absorb these toxins through the skin. Bamburg and Strong (1971) found that a single cutaneous dose of T-2 (8 mg/kg) was fatal to rats, however, they did not report the use of measures to prevent inadvertent ingestion of the toxin. Previous studies on the dermal absorption of AFB_1 have resulted in conflicting results. Cutaneous application of AFB_1 caused liver lesions within 48 hr of dosing conscious rabbits (Ungar and Joffe, 1969) and rats (Wei et al., 1970). When AFB_1 was applied to the skin of conscious and unconscious rats, it was absorbed by the conscious rats only (Purchase and Steyn, 1973). Purchase and Steyn concluded that the absorption of AFB_1 by conscious rats was due to ingestion of toxin present on the hind foot pads as a result of grooming, and they suggested that the same phenomenon may have occurred in the other experiments where liver necrosis was reported after dermal exposure to AFB_1.

The views of the author do not purport to reflect the positions of the Department of the Army or the Department of Defense. (para. 4-3, AR 360-5).
Present affiliation: Auburn University School of Pharmacy, Auburn, Alabama

This chapter summarizes recent findings on the cutaneous penetration of mycotoxins through excised human skin. Penetration studies of mycotoxins adsorbed to corn dust required high specific activity [^{3}H]T-2 and [^{3}H]AFB$_1$. Unfortunately, the [^{3}H]AFB$_1$ underwent extensive tritium exchange. This was not the case with [^{3}H]T-2. Therefore, aflatoxin penetration was studied with [^{14}C]AFB$_1$ dissolved in methanol.

METHODS

The relevance of our in vitro test system (Riley, 1983) to in vivo percutaneous penetration was validated by measuring the rate of penetration of [^{14}C]urea and [^{14}C]benzoic acid through excised human skin (Table 1). The methods used were similar to the techniques used by Franz (1975) so that the results could be compared to previous in vitro (Franz, 1975) and in vivo (Feldmann and Maibach, 1970) percutaneous penetration studies. Unselected human skin from amputations was stored at $-20°C$. In each experiment skin from one specimen was mounted on six diffusion cells. Whole skin was obtained by the method of Franz (1975) and epidermal sheets by the method of Scheuplein (1965). The dermal side of the skin was bathed by receptor fluid, which consisted of phosphate-buffered saline with 157 mg/liter of penicillin and 250 mg/liter of streptomycin (PBSA). The epidermal surface was exposed to room air. Each penetration experiment was conducted at room temperature (22-25°C). Radioactivity in the receptor fluid was analyzed by standard liquid scintillation counting (LSC) procedures.

Table 1 Relevance of the In Vitro Test System (using excised human skin) to In Vivo Penetration in Humans

	Total penetration (% of applied dose, mean ±SD)	
	[^{14}C]Urea	[^{14}C]Benzoic acid
In vivo		
Feldmann and Maibach (1970)	6.0±1.9 [4][a]	42.6±16.5 [6][a]
In vitro		
Whole skin		
Franz (1975)	11.1 (5.2, 29)[b] [22]	44.9 (29, 53)[b] [18]
Kemppainen et al.	7.9±5.7 [3][c]	47.6±11.5 [3][c]
Epidermis		
Kemppainen et al.	3.8±0.7 [3][c]	18.5±7.9 [3][c]

[a]Number of subjects studied.
[b]Median (95% confidence interval).
[c]Number of diffusion cells used in each experiment.

Penetration of T-2 Through Excised Human Skin

The [^{3}H] T-2 (11.65 Ci/mmol) was custom synthesized by Amersham Corp. The crude [^{3}H] T-2 preparation was purified by preparative thin-layer chromatography (TLC). The radiochemical purity was determined to be greater than 99%.

Corn dust (120 mesh) was prepared by grinding kernels of corn first with a Wiley mill and then with a mortar and pestle. The corn dust was slurried in chloroform for 5 min before the [^{3}H] T-2 was added. After mixing the corn, the chloroform was evaporated. The [^{3}H] T-2 concentration in the corn dust was 18.2 ±2.0 ppm (mean ±SD).

[^{3}H] T-2 penetration through human whole skin was compared to penetration through human epidermal sheets. After the skin was mounted on three diffusion cells, 3.27 to 4.75 mg of 18.2-ppm [^{3}H] T-2 corn dust was applied to each epidermal surface. [^{3}H] T-2 metabolites in the receptor fluid were identified by thin-layer radiochromatography. In each experiment two skins from each treatment group were digested with Soluene (Amersham) and the radioactivity measured by LSC techniques to determine how much of the applied dose was recovered. Penetration of [^{3}H] T-2 through whole human skin was replicated four times; penetration through human epidermis was replicated five times.

Curve fitting was accomplished by linear regression analysis (Barr et al., 1979). Except where indicated differently, all values given in the text are the mean plus or minus standard deviation. The number of independent samples (n) is in parentheses following each value.

Penetration of AFB$_1$ Through Excised Human Skin

The chemical purity of the AFB$_1$ standard was determined by its UV spectra in methanol (Cole and Cox, 1981) and mobility on silica gel G TLC plates. The radiolabeled AFB$_1$, [G-^{14}C] AFB$_1$ (50 mCi/mmol), was obtained from Moravek Biochemical Inc. (Brea, Calif.). The radiochemical purity of [^{14}C] AFB$_1$ was determined by TLC to be 93%. No attempt was made to remove the two radiolabeled fluorescent contaminants (7% of the radioactivity) in the [^{14}C] AFB$_1$.

Three separate experiments were conducted with a total of eight diffusion cells. Human epidermal sheets were used in all the [^{14}C] AFB$_1$ experiments. Between 7.5 and 9.3 μg of [^{14}C] AFB$_1$ in methanol was applied to each epidermal surface. The methanol was evaporated and the experiment conducted under subdued light. At the end of each experiment with AFB$_1$ the receptor fluids from each treatment group were pooled, chloroform extracted, and radioactive penetrants identified by thin-layer radiochromatography.

RESULTS AND DISCUSSION

Analysis of the receptor fluid bathing human whole skin revealed that 69% of the radioactivity was associated with T-2 and 25% was associated with the metabolite HT-2. The identification of T-2 and HT-2 in the receptor fluid demonstrated that T-2 can penetrate through excised human skin that has been exposed to [^{3}H] T-2 adsorbed onto corn dust. This is consistent with previous observations that T-2, HT-2, and diacetoxyscirpenol penetrate through intact rat skin (Bamburg and Strong, 1971). The HT-2 in the receptor fluid was probably formed as a result of hydrolytic reactions carried out by the skin. In vitro studies have demonstrated that esterases in the intestine (Yoshizawa et al., 1980) and liver (Ellison and Kotsonis, 1974) are capable of selectively removing the C_4 acetyl group of T-2, resulting in the formation of HT-2. It is improbable that the HT-2 was formed as a result of hydrolysis in the receptor fluid because trichothecenes are stable to a variety of environmental conditions (Smalley and Strong, 1974). Excised rat, guinea pig, and human skin carry out several hydrolytic reactions (Pannatier et al., 1978). We (unpublished data) identified both T-2 and HT-2 in the receptor fluid bathing excised guinea pig skin that had been dosed with [^{3}H] T-2 in 1% sodium lauryl sulfate. The transformation of T-2 into HT-2 by guinea pig skin may not be a detoxification reaction, because HT-2 is more toxic than T-2 in the guinea pig (Mirocha, 1983).

After 26 hr [^{3}H] T-2 penetration was greater through epidermis than through whole skin (Fig. 1). The slopes of the lines representing the rate of [^{3}H] T-2 penetration under occluded conditions were greater than the slopes under nonoccluded conditions. Recovery of the applied dose was 88.7 ±13.4% (n = 12) and 91.4 ±12.1% (n = 15) for the whole skin and epidermis, respectively. The low coefficients of determination for the whole skin (r^2 = 0.36) and for the epidermis (r^2 = 0.25) indicate that there was a great deal of variability between replicated experiments not explained by the linear regression. Differences in age, state of health of the donor, race, and anatomic location of the human skin specimens could contribute.

Since the stratum corneum is the main barrier to diffusion through the skin, the tendency toward greater accumulation of [^{3}H] T-2 in the receptor fluid bathing the epidermis is consistent with the hypothesis that the dermis may act as a reservoir for T-2 toxin. Dermal exposure to small amounts of T-2 causes cutaneous lesions (Hayes and Schiefer, 1979). The following sequence of gross and histopathological changes occurs in the rat after a single cutaneous dose of 0.24 μg of T-2: nonspecific acute dermal inflammatory reaction, characterized by hyperemia, edema, and neutrophil exudation, with necrosis (Hayes and Schiefer, 1979).

The results of the [^{14}C] AFB_1 penetration experiments indicated that aflatoxin can penetrate the stratum corneum (Fig. 2). Once the steady-state rate of AFB_1 penetration had been reached under nonoccluded conditions, the total penetration of AFB_1 in 48 hr was 0.030 ±0.034 nmol (n = 8), which represented 0.12 ±0.14% of the applied dose. The major radioactive compound in the receptor fluid was AFB_1. The two fluorescent radioactive contaminants present in

Penetration of Mycotoxins

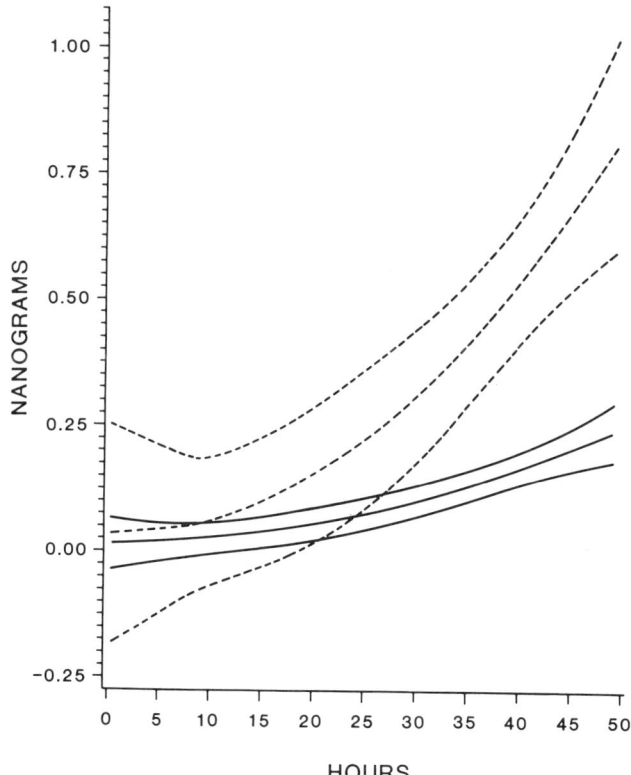

Figure 1 Penetration of [^{3}H] T-2 through excised human skin. The epidermal surfaces were nonoccluded during the first 24 hr and then occluded for an additional 24 hr. Upper and lower 95% confidence limits and least-squares fit of the data are given. The applied dose was 78.8±10.2 ng of T-2 (n = 27) adsorbed on corn dust. Solid curves are penetration through whole skin [r^2 = 0.36, degrees of freedom (df) = 83] and dashed curves are for epidermis (r^2 = 0.25, df = 104).

the dose also penetrated the skin. Total recovery expressed as a percentage of the applied radioactivity was 98.0 ±6.4% (n = 10).

These studies support the hypothesis that dermal exposure to T-2 and AFB$_1$ could pose a potential risk of contact dermatitis. The degree of risk to those occupationally exposed is impossible to assess from the current studies. One way that humans have received doses of pure T-2 or AFB$_1$ as surface deposits on the skin has been accidental exposure in research laboratories (Bamburg and Strong, 1971; Bamburg et al., 1968; Deger, 1976). Agricultural workers are routinely ex-

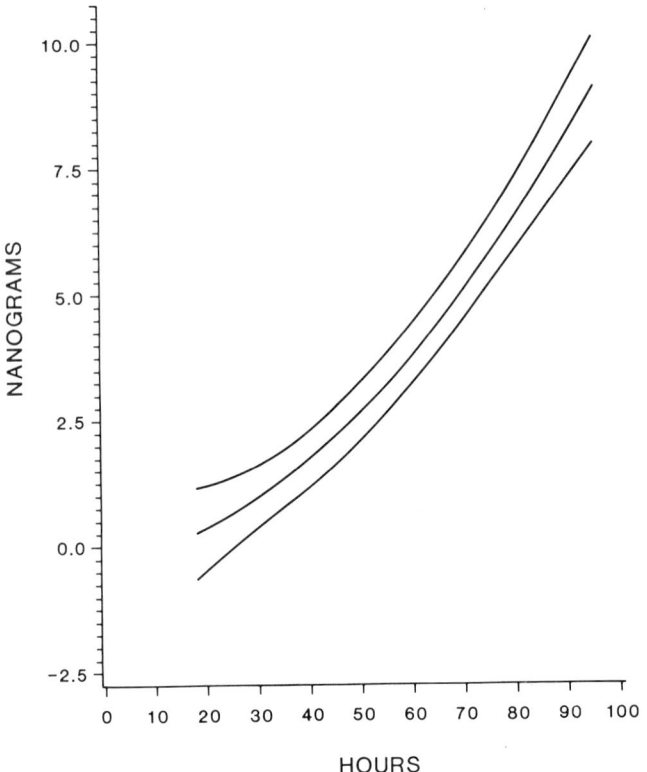

Figure 2 Penetration of [^{14}C]AFB$_1$ through excised human epidermis under conditions of exposure to ambient humidity. Upper and lower 95% confidence limits and least-squares fit of the data are given ($r^2 = 0.92$, df = 21). The applied dose was 9.3±0.6 μg (n = 3) as a surface deposit.

posed to dusts contaminated with high levels of aflatoxins (Burg et al., 1982). It is likely that aflatoxins and T-2 adsorbed on dust can partition into and penetrate human epidermis in vivo. The extent of risk can be assessed only if valid kinetic data can be obtained.

REFERENCES

Bamburg, J. R. and Strong, F. M. (1971). 12,13-Epoxytrichothecenes. In *Microbial Toxins, Vol. VII. Algal and Fungal Toxins.* Edited by S. Kadis, A. Ciegler, and S. Ajl. Academic, New York, pp. 207-292.

Bamburg, J. R., Marasas, W. F., Riggs, N. V., Smalley, E. B., and Strong, F. M.

(1968). Toxic spiroepoxy compounds from *Fusaria* and other hyphomycetes. *Biotechnol. Bioeng. 10*: 445-455.

Barr, A. J., Goodnight, J. H., Sall, J. P., Blair, W. H., and Chilko, D. M. (1979). *A User's Guide to SAS*. SAS Institute, Raleigh, N.C.

Burg, W. R., Shotwell, O. L., and Saltzman, B. E. (1982). Measurements of airborne aflatoxins during the handling of 1979 contaminated corn. *Am. Ind. Hyg. Assoc. J. 43*: 580-586.

Cole, R. J. and Cox, R. H. (1981). *Handbook of Toxic Fungal Metabolites*. Academic, New York.

Deger, G. E. (1976). Aflatoxin—Human colon carcinogenesis. *Ann. Intern. Med. 85*: 204.

Ellison, R. A. and Kotsonis, F. N. (1974). In vitro metabolism of T-2 toxin. *Appl. Microbiol. 27*: 423-424.

Feldmann, R. J. and Maibach, H. I. (1970). Absorption of some organic compounds through the skin of man. *J. Invest. Dermatol. 54*: 399-404.

Franz, T. J. (1975). Percutaneous absorption. On the relevance of in vitro data. *J. Invest. Dermatol. 64*: 190-195.

Hayes, M. A. and Schiefer, H. B. (1979). Quantitative and morphological aspects of cutaneous irritation by trichothecene mycotoxins. *Food Cosmet. Toxicol. 17*: 611-621.

Mirocha, C. J. (1983). Effect of trichothecene mycotoxins on farm animals. In *Trichothecenes—Chemical, Biological, and Toxicological Aspects*. Edited by Y. Ueno. Elsevier, New York, pp. 177-194.

Mirocha, C. J., Pathre, S. V., and Christensen, C. M. (1977). Chemistry of *Fusarium* and *Stachybotrys* mycotoxins. In *Mycotoxic Fungi Mycotoxins, and Mycotoxicosis: An Encyclopedic Handbook*. Edited by T. D. Wyllie and L. C. Morehouse. Dekker, New York, pp. 365-420.

Pannatier, A., Jenner, P., Testa, B., and Etter, J. C. (1978). The skin as a drug-metabolizing organ. *Drug Metab. Rev. 8*: 319-343.

Purchase, I. F. H. and Steyn, M. (1973). Absence of percutaneous absorption of aflatoxin. *Toxicol. Appl. Pharmacol. 24*: 162-164.

Riley, R. T. (1983). Starch-xanthate-encapsulated pesticides: A preliminary toxicologic evaluation. *J. Agric. Food Chem. 31*: 202-206.

Scheuplein, R. J. (1965). Mechanism of percutaneous absorption. I. Routes of penetration and the influence of solubility. *J. Invest. Dermatol. 45*: 334-346.

Smalley, E. B. and Strong, F. M. (1974). Toxic trichothecenes. In *Mycotoxins*. Edited by I. G. F. Purchase. Elsevier, Amsterdam, pp. 199-227.

Ungar, H. and Joffe, A. Z. (1969). Acute liver lesions resulting from percutaneous absorption of aflatoxins. *Pathol. Microbiol. 33*: 65-76.

Wei, R. D., Liu, G. X., and Lee, S. S. (1970). Uptake of aflatoxin B_1 by the skin of rats. *Experientia 26*: 82-83.

Yoshizawa, T., Swanson, S. P., and Mirocha, C. J. (1980). In vitro metabolism of T-2 in rats. *Appl. Environ. Microbiol. 39*: 1172-1177.

34
In Vitro Methods Used to Study Dermal Delivery and Percutaneous Absorption

Boyd J. Poulsen
*Institute of Pharmaceutical Sciences, Syntex,
Palo Alto, California*

Gordon L. Flynn
University of Michigan College of Pharmacy, Ann Arbor, Michigan

Earlier reviews include: Johnson and Lee (1943), Gemmell and Morrison (1957), Blank (1960), Ainsworth (1960), Katz and Poulsen (1971), Grasso and Lansdown (1972), Nugent and Wood (1980), and De Kay (1962).

What might be gained through in vitro study of the events surrounding diffusive penetration of the skin? Theorists use such investigations to shed light on the nature of the barrier properties within the skin and amplify our understanding of the mechanism of percutaneous absorption, so that we are in a more favorable position to select compounds or to chemically modify compounds for the purpose of dermal delivery. As the mechanistic elements involved in diffusion are made clearer, we can consider what might be done to the skin to make it more permeable to those drugs for which it has great diffusional resistance. These provide a means to clarify skin-vehicle interactions and physical and biological interactions of permeants within the skin's strata.

There often is an implicit assumption that the processes being followed in vitro mirror in crucial ways the actual drug delivery events. When this assumption is invalid, in vitro initiatives are not helpful and are actually wasteful of time and effort. Thus, the experimenter must have a good grasp of the thermodynamic and kinetic possibilities involved in the real situation, at least to the point that a qualitative assessment of the parallelism of the in vitro work to the in vivo case can be made, thereby permitting an estimate of the degree to which the data obtained can be reasonably extrapolated. The in vitro design must be examined side by side with the mechanism of the in vivo response and differences between these two different situations weighed critically with respect to the interpretations to which the in vitro data may be put.

IN VITRO DIFFUSION STUDIES: NO MEMBRANE

Gemmell and Morrison (1957) state that "in vitro methods are of limited value but they are a means of assessing the ability of a vehicle or base to liberate medicament under the conditions of the test." This statement can accurately be applied to membraneless systems of investigation. The usual assumption is that the release of a drug from a solvent or vehicle into a second medium is similar to the release of the drug in the clinical situation. Application of this approach to the investigation of release of a given chemical entity from vehicles systematically varied in their solvency or other properties has contributed positively to our understanding of dermal delivery systems. Enormous potential differences between in vivo and in vitro situations exist, and thus the consequence of unjustified extrapolation may be most severe. Figure 1 represents schematically two traditional membraneless in vitro diffusion systems applicable to many past investigations. Both utilize simple passive diffusion into an agar gel to assess drug and/or vehicle effects. The first frames of the drawings beneath the sketches of two representative experimental configurations illustrate the effective concentration (thermodynamic activity) profiles that develop after a drug-containing vehicle and a receptor phase have been brought into contact. In one case the drug is all in solution and, in the second, the drug is formulated as a suspension. The arrows indicate the interface between the two phases. The second and third frames illustrate how the activity gradients can be expected to develop when neither donor phase (vehicle) nor receptor phase is stirred. In these circumstances, significant gradients in activity of the drug can form on either side of the interface. This is especially true when the application is thickly applied, a significant departure from the usual realities of use. On occasion, the formulation has been layered over the receptor phase to depths measured in whole centimeters. Almost without exception, the receptor phase has been a thick slab. Thus for either the solution or suspension case, release rates may be governed by one or both of the media found on either side of the interface. Eventually recession of the gradients from the interface may cause the more diffusionally resistant medium to assume rate control. Overall, the release is a receding boundary phenomenon and will, at least roughly, follow a square root of time relationship. The conditions are such that the kinetics reflect the mixed features of diffusion from a semi-infinite medium and diffusion into a semi-infinite medium. If the vehicle is the most diffusionally resistant of the media involved, it becomes the principal determinant of the mass transfer rate. Then what is learned may be directly applicable to the system's performance in vivo, depending on the nature of the system and how it is clinically used. On the other hand, if the rate-controlling phase is the reservoir and the reservoir bears no resemblance to the skin, little that is useful may have been learned. Unfortunately, it is next to impossible to ascertain from zones of inhibition, or other such endpoints, much about the mechanism and even the rates of the processes involved.

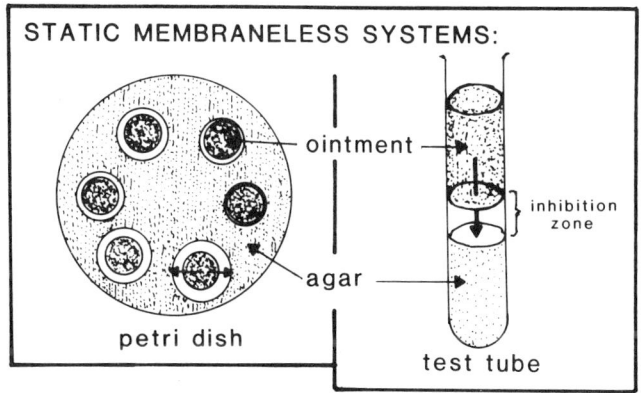

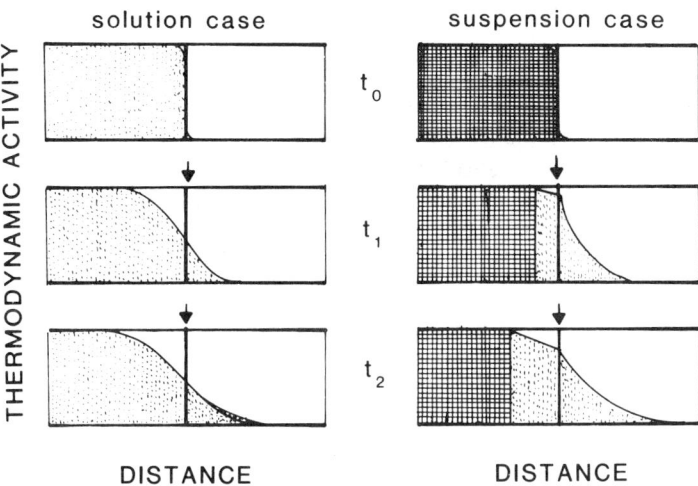

Figure 1 Static membraneless systems and diffusion profiles for solution case and suspension case as a function of time, t.

This is especially true of such studies that have relied on assay at but one point in time, as for instance has been done with zones of inhibition of antibiotics released into a microorganism-seeded agar. In such cases, extrapolations to clinical behavior are especially weak.

Because of the obvious differences between the physicochemical characteristics of the skin's surface layers and watery gels such as agar and gelatin used as a receptor phase, much work has been called into question (Poulsen et al., 1968). The past objectives need not be restated. It is clear that experiments involving release from a thick application layer under closed conditions, which prevent the normal compositional adjustments that occur on the skin from taking place, may yield results totally unrelated to release under the clinical conditions of system use. A related concern is that the receptor phase of the in vitro system can selectively absorb components of the donor phase other than the drug, with alterations in system composition sufficient to cause drift away from the desired usage simulation. This factor limits the choice of the reservoir phase by placing a requirement on the reservoir that it not be able to solubilize much of the vehicle used for the drug.

Despite such limitations, some important conceptual work has been done utilizing membraneless systems (Poulsen, 1970). In studies at Syntex (Ostrenga et al., 1971a,b), the release of fluocinolone acetonide and of fluocinolone acetonide acetate from propylene glycol/water gel systems was followed in each case into stirred isopropyl myristate, a light oil that was in sufficient volume to act as a diffusional sink. Carbopol was the gelling agent, and at the concentration used, had a negligible effect on drug diffusion. The total concentrations of each of the steroids in the gel vehicles corresponded to those suitable for clinical efficacy. These concentrations greatly exceeded the solubility of the steroids in pure water but were well below saturation solubilities of the agents in the pure glycol. Since the gel composition could range from one pure solvent to the other, a full spectrum of compositions (and solubilization capacities) existed between these two extremes. As the percentage of propylene glycol was increased, the drug-containing media thus changed from suspensions to highly unsaturated solutions for a given drug concentration, in the course passing through the singular binary solvent composition simultaneously yielding full solution and saturation. The glycol/water composition at which saturation occurred depended, of course, on each steroid's unique solubility and on the total concentration of steroid present.

Figure 2 shows the gel, contained in a petri dish, submerged in the oil. Isopropyl myristate, which has good solvency for the two steroids, was stirred, thus limiting its influence on the release process to that of a nominal hydrodynamic layer. Therefore, while the release of the drug might momentarily be zero order and controlled by the boundary layer, as suggested in the first set of activity accompanying the sketch of the system, it must change to a square root of time dependency as the gradient recedes into the gel, an unavoidable event represented by the latter frames of Figure 2. As seen by comparison of the two sets of profiles in Figure 3, a maximum in the release profiles was observed at essentially the same place on the profile when the release was from 0.025% systems for a given steroid irrespective of whether the assay point in time was 2, 6, or 12 hr. This fact alone signifies that the mechanism was for practical purposes invariant over the 12-hr period and thereby rules out a zero-order period of significant duration. However, the glycol/water composition required to produce this maximum was different for each steroid when formulated at 0.025% concentration

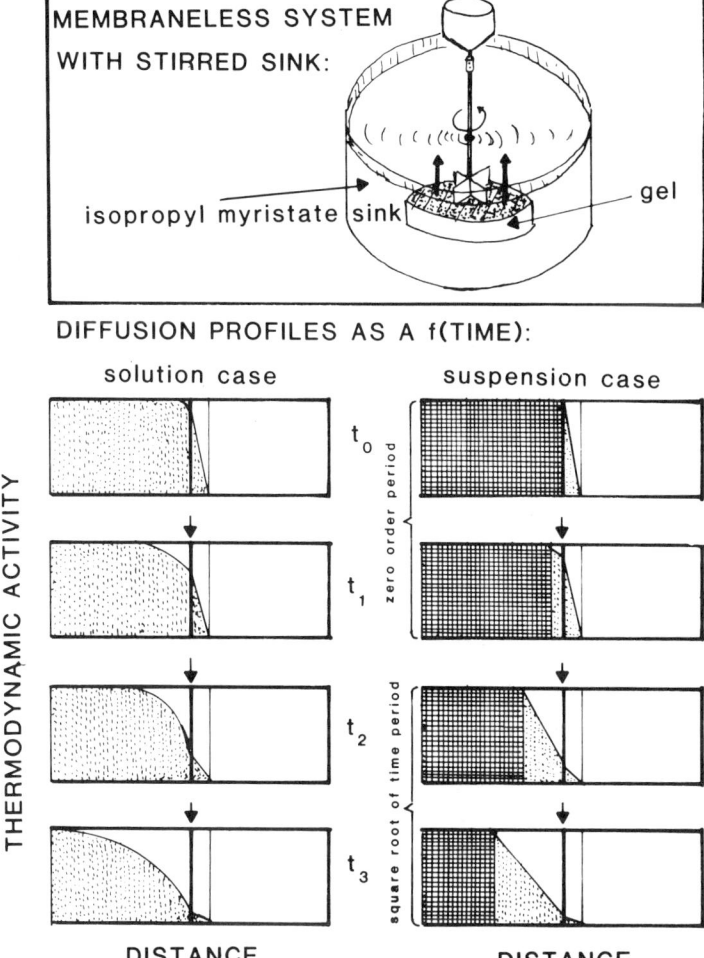

Figure 2 Membraneless system with stirred sink and diffusion profiles for solution case and suspension case as a function of time, t.

and (Fig. 4), was also different for fluocinolone acetonide at each of three different initial concentrations, 0.01, 0.025, and 0.1%. Independent solubility studies proved the position of these maxima to lie consistently near the binary solvent composition, yielding a totally solubilized, saturated system for a given concentration, irrespective of the steroid involved. Thus, the studies suggested that the optimum formulation composition for topical corticosteroids would fall at or

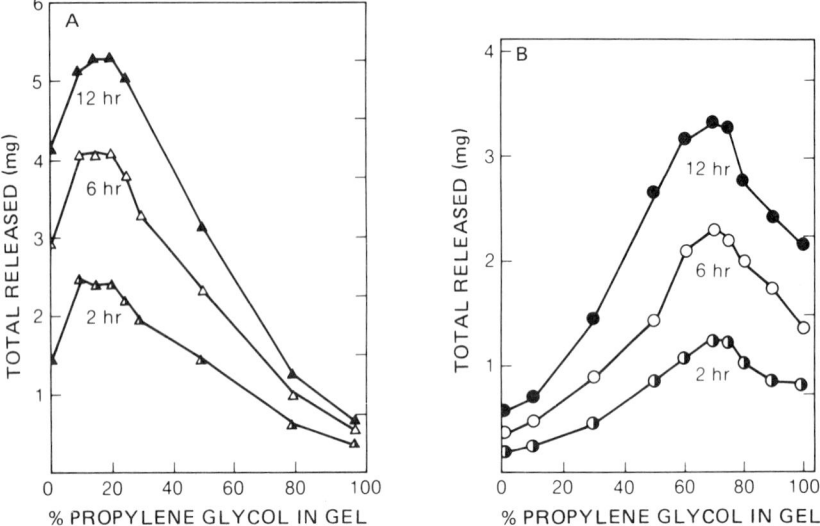

Figure 3 Effect of propylene glycol concentration on the release of (A) 0.025% fluocinonide acetonide and (B) its 21-acetate ester fluocinonide from propylene glycol/water gels at 37°C: release as a function of time.

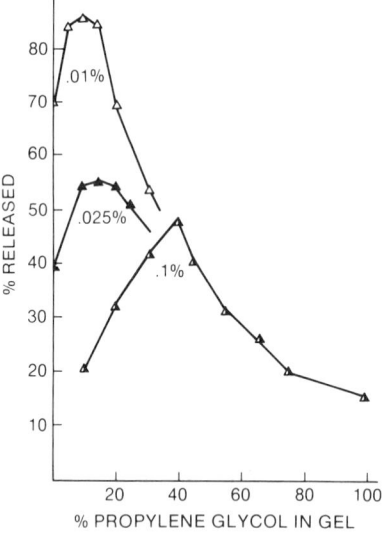

Figure 4 Comparison of release of 0.01, 0.025, and 0.1% fluocinolone acetonide from propylene glycol/water gels after 6 hr at 37°C.

near the position of total solubilization and concurrent saturation. Although in the suspension region of the profile all systems were initially of isothermodynamic activity with respect to the drug (the activity established by the solid), other factors, especially the development of the depleted zone in the gels, were obviously able to kinetically override simple thermodynamic control of drug release, and release diminished as the fraction of dissolved drug was reduced. Later studies (Ostrenga et al., 1971a) showed that similar behavior is to be expected for creams; that is, release is greatest when the drug is 100% solubilized in the formulation as long as the drug is saturated or nearly so (Fig. 5). If parallels exist in the in vivo delivery of drugs, these studies suggest some general direction for the formulation of topical drugs. Therefore it is of great importance that the studies have been given credibility through independent experiments that (1) have shown that topical corticosteroids of this type are absorbed through the skin via a lipid pathway (Scheuplein et al., 1969), making the choice of the reservoir phase (isopropyl myristate) somewhat relevant, and (2) have demonstrated rank-order correlation between physiological responses measured in vivo with the well-known vasoconstrictor assay and the in vitro release characteristics of both gels (Haleblian et al., 1977) and creams (Ostrenga et al., 1971a).

These investigations and concepts were a logical extension of theoretical analyses and speculations by T. Higuchi regarding the mechanism of release from

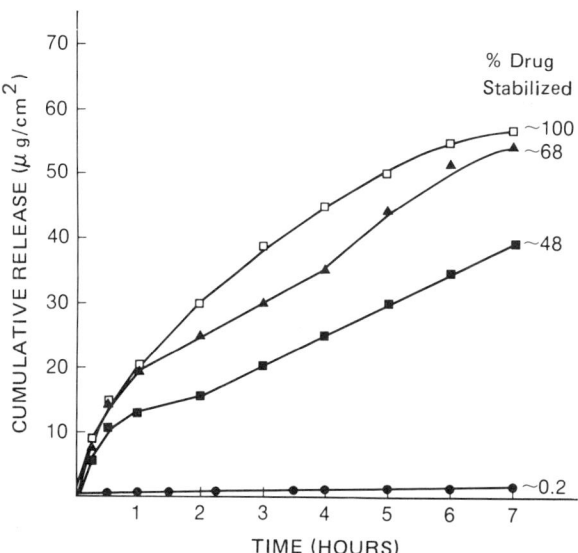

Figure 5 Fluocinonide release into isopropyl myristate at 25°C from o/w creams with varying degrees of solubilizing capability for the drug.

topical systems (Higuchi, 1960, 1961). For release from solutions through a planar surface and into a diffusional sink he formulated the following equation:

$$Q = AhC_0 \left[1 - \frac{8}{\pi^2} \sum_{m=0}^{\infty} \frac{1}{(2m+1)^2} \exp\left(-\frac{D(2m+1)^2 \pi^2 t}{4h^2} \right) \right]$$

where Q is the quantity of drug released over an interface of area A, h is the thickness of the receding boundary layer, C_0 is the initial drug concentration, and D is the diffusion coefficient of the drug in the vehicle, t stands for time, and m represents the set of integers with values from zero to infinity. It was pointed out that for the first 30% or so of release:

$$Q = 2AC_0 \left(\frac{Dt}{\pi} \right)^{1/2}$$

It might be noted that these equations are written assuming no significant boundary layer influence. A square root of time dependency to 30% of the total amount released is evident.

Equations for the situation of the drug being in suspension were also derived by T. Higuchi (1960) with the same overall assumptions (no significant boundary layer, release over a planar surface, and a receiver reservoir acting as a sink) with the following results:

$$Q = A(2W - C_s) \left[\frac{Dt}{1 + 2(W - C_s)/C_s} \right]^{1/2}$$

In this equation W is the total amount of drug suspended and in solution in the vehicle and C_s is the solubility of the drug. It follows that:

$$\frac{dQ}{dt} = \frac{1}{2} A(2W - C_s) \left(\frac{1 + 2(W - C_s)t}{C_s} \right)^{1/2}$$

and when $W \gg C_s$:

$$Q = \sqrt{2WDC_s t}$$

and:

$$\frac{dQ}{dt} = \left(\frac{WDC_s}{2t} \right)^{1/2}$$

It is seen that this situation also results in the release being proportional to the square root of time. In this instance there is no condition on the fraction of drug released.

STUDIES INVOLVING MEMBRANES OTHER THAN THE SKIN

Other living membranes such as frog skin (Bracho et al., 1971), the membrane encasing the chick embryo (Hunter and Smith, 1952; Ruggiero and Skauen, 1962a,b), manmade membranes like hydrated dialysis membranes (Howze and Billups, 1966), porous cellulosic membranes with lipid-filled interstices (Guy and Fleming, 1979), and silicone rubber films (Flynn and Roseman, 1971) have been utilized as skin substitutes. Unfortunately, none bears an exact resemblance to skin; all studies must be questioned in the same way membraneless system of study have been questioned. That is, until a parallelism has been shown with appropriate experiments, conclusions must be considered suspect. In some well-defined instances, qualitative effects of system design on bioavailability may be deciphered. To make such judgments, it is minimally necessary that the mechanism of permeation of the nonskin membrane to the compound or compounds in question be similar to the mechanism of skin permeation. Specifically, for compounds that breach the skin principally by way of the lipid fraction of the stratum corneum, a hydrophobic membrane structure may properly sort out relative permeation behaviors. On the other hand, if the permeants in question are so hydrophobic that their access to the deeper tissues and systemic circulation is regulated by their passage across the living, cellular layers of the epidermis and the thin wedge of dermis lying just above the local capillary bed, a functionally aqueous diffusional stratum from all that can be told, then diffusion through something like a dialysis membrane may take on meaning.

One factor to be considered here is that we generally do not know enough about percutaneous absorption to assess a priori the mechanism for unknown substances. Since it is generally possible to use excised skin in lieu of a synthetic or a nonskin biological membrane, reliance on a membrane other than a skin section for such investigations should be carefully weighed. With this caveat in mind, an examination of what has been accomplished with this approach can be made.

Jurist (1953) introduced a method of studying the release of water-soluble materials from ointment bases that involved the use of a dialysis membrane separating the ointment system and the aqueous phase used as the receptor phase. Essentially the membrane minimized cross-contamination of the phases. This procedure (Billups and Sager, 1965; Howe and Billups, 1966; Multimer et al., 1956a,b; Wood et al., 1962) has been used with slight modifications. Usually the aqueous phase is stirred but may even be continuously perfused past the membrane. The factors setting this system apart from systems where the diffusion is from an ointment into a gel matrix are the membrane itself and the fact that stirring sets a limit on the resistance of the watery regions, namely, the summed resistances found on the hydrous membrane and in the effective hydrodynamic layer external to the membrane.

The system operation is like that described for release of drug from aqueous or glycol/water gels into isopropyl myristate except that the roles of the aqueous and oily phases are reverse. The initial release will be at a constant rate. As time elapses, the amount being released should become proportional to the square root of time. How long it is until the transition in mechanism takes place depends on the physicochemical characteristics of the ointment and membrane, on the membrane's thickness, and on the vigor of the stirring (the latter determines the net influence of the boundary layer). The initial zero-order phase of release from this system depends on partitioning of the drug from the oily vehicle to the hydrated phase of the membrane, with diffusion through the membrane and across the boundary layer of the receiver setting the rate. If the partition from oil to water is difficult for a drug, the rate of its appearance in the aqueous external medium will be slow relative to another compound for which water has a high affinity. All other factors being equal, the duration of the zero-order phase of release will be longer, the more hydrophobic a compound is, because the rate of recession of the front of the depletion zone in the vehicle will be slowed by increasingly shallow gradients initially formed across the membrane and boundary layer. A comprehensive model of the operation of this system must account for two distinctly different dependencies of release.

Roseman and W. Higuchi (1970) developed equations describing this overall behavior, applying them to the release of steroids suspended in silicone rubber matrices. Again using W as the total drug load per unit volume of the releasing system and C_s as the solubility, and beginning with the assumption that $W \gg C_s$, then Q, the quantity released over the operating area A, would be:

$$Q = AWL$$

The receding boundary's thickness L is related to time through:

$$L^2 + \frac{2DhKL}{D_{BL}} = \frac{2DC_s t}{W}$$

where D and t are as defined previously and D(BL) is the diffusivity in the boundary layer, h is the thickness of the boundary layer, and K is the matrix/external medium partition coefficient. Initially $2DhK/D(BL) \gg L$ and therefore:

$$Q \simeq \frac{AD_{BL}C_s t}{Kh}$$

and:

$$\frac{dQ}{dt} \simeq A \frac{D_{BL}C_s}{Kh}$$

In time, however, $L \gg 2DhK/D(BL)$ and:

$$Q \simeq A\sqrt{2WDC_s t}$$

and:

$$\frac{dQ}{dt} = A\left(\frac{WDC_s}{2t}\right)^{1/2}$$

For drugs finely suspended in a semisolid oily vehicle and released across a dialysis membrane, the only qualitative difference between the ointment system and the model silicone rubber system is the presence of the dialysis membrane, which accentuates the effect of the watery region external to the releasing system, further delaying the onset of square root of time kinetics. Two phases of release can be expected when the drug is in solution in the vehicle, since this situation also begins with rate control by the membrane but leads to a receding boundary of rate-controlling proportions in time.

What place do these systems have in topical drug delivery system development? One possibility would be release under an application into a moist region, as would occur over badly broken skin. Others could include release over skin burned even momentarily at temperatures much higher than 80°C and over moist mucosal surfaces such as the buccal cavity's lining and the lining of the vaginal vault. The physical features of tissue uptake are reasonably approximated by the combined membrane and boundary layer, and the results of in vitro initiatives may serve qualitatively to guide the course of product development. If percutaneous absorption of intact, horny skin is a critical step in the activity cascade, then extrapolations may give false directions. This is expected because the cornified structure of skin acts as a lipid matrix to the permeation of many agents of interest. Even when such is not the case, most substances and especially polar substances find the stratum corneum's resistance far greater in magnitude than the resistance of the in vitro membrane and boundary layer together; therefore the initial absorption by the skin will necessarily be very much slower than suggested by in vitro release kinetics. Moreover, the interposition of a high-resistance element as the stratum corneum as a dominating element of the barrier will either delay or preclude the onset of square root of time control. Thus, there can be failings of approximation of a qualitative as well as a quantitative nature, in which the in vitro system is plainly a deceptive or misleading model.

In the hydrophobic extreme, drugs tend not to be restricted in permeation by the stratum corneum but by the cellular and fibrous tissues beneath, which, as stated, are functionally aqueous, and thus the substrata of the skin can play the same role played in vitro by the dialysis membrane and its hydrodynamic layer.

Thus, this is another possible circumstance in which reasonable in vivo-in vitro agreement might be obtained, but the precondition represented is uncommon and the chance of this dependency developing, rare. Perhaps the real issue here is not that under some foreseeable circumstances the behaviors of ointments tested on the lab bench will coincide with their actual drug delivery capabilities, but that even the most experienced development scientist is unable to confidently predict when such agreement is to be expected. In more cases than not the extent of in vivo-in vitro parallelism will be unsatisfactory. This latter generalization is over and above considerations of differences with respect to thicknesses of application and other obvious departures of the in vitro experiments from the manner in which topical drug delivery systems are actually used clinically. Limitations of the type discussed under membraneless systems apply equally here.

On occasion, hydrophobic membranes have been used in the development of fundamental data and understandings concerning topical dosage forms. In some early work of theoretical significance Lueck et al. (1957) studied the diffusion of substrates across thin slabs of white petrolatum and polyethylene jelled mineral oil, obtaining the first quantitative information on diffusion through these media. The classic paper of T. Higuchi (1960) concerned with the release of medicaments from ointment bases, which introduced the idea of a receding boundary into the pharmaceutical literature, was an outgrowth of this work. W. Higuchi (1962) demonstrated the applicability of the theory, showing that the amount of iodine released from a petroleum jelly medium (data of Patel et al., 1961) was, as predicted, proportional to the square root of time. He deduced the diffusion coefficient of iodine from the square root dependency, possibly the first such application of the derived equations. Spang-Brunner and Speiser (1976) expanded on this use of the theory, gathering fundamental diffusion data on a number of important pharmaceutical semisolids. Table 1 summarizes diffusion coefficients obtained in this fashion. Diffusion is up to 100 times faster in hydrogels than in ointmentlike media, where a typical diffusion coefficient is on the order of 1.5×10^{-8}. These not only suggest the mechanisms of the release processes but provide magnitudes of the parameters needed for modeling of the systems. That the real drug delivery situation is complex and not totally described by these relationships is proven when the simple release concepts are put to test in clinical research. Ostrenga et al. (1971a) entertained the idea of using square root of time kinetics to evaluate vasoconstriction responses of variously formulated fluocinolone acetonide creams but were able to show rank-order agreement between the theoretical expectations and the blanching index only.

Table 1 Vehicle Diffusion Coefficients

Permeant	Vehicle	D (cm^2/sec)
Sodium iodide	Ointment bases	0.43 to 3.6 × 10^{-6}
Resorcinol	Polyacrylate gels	3.4 × 10^{-6}
Resorcinol	Carboxymethyl cellulose gels	2.4 × 10^{-6}
Resorcinol	Starch gels	1.7 × 10^{-6}
Resorcinol	Lipo gels	1.9 to 7.8 × 10^{-8}
Resorcinol	Labrafils (hydrogenated palm oils)	0.42 to 1.3 × 10^{-7}

Many studies with artificial membranes having hydrophobic character have sharpened our understanding of the relationship between chemical structure and the physicochemical behavior of organic molecules that determine their relative abilities to diffusionally pass through lipid membranes. Such relationships are integral to our understanding of the functioning of biomembranes as biologic barriers, including the skin. Firm structure-partitioning, structure-diffusivity, and structure-solubility relationships are essential to the deciphering of the mechanism of percutaneous absorption from permeation data and are cornerstones of the construction of functional models of the skin. In this sense basic physicochemical works form a body of relevant in vitro studies. Flynn et al. (1974) summarized these findings through the early 1970s.

On occasion manmade lipid membranes have been used as actual facsimiles of the skin. This carries too far the notion that the skin acts diffusionally as a "partitioning membrane," a phrase intended to convey that a compound's oil/water (o/w) distribution coefficient is the principal determinant of its gradient across the horny structure of the skin and therefore of its rate. A watery vehicle is, of course, the reference vehicle. To an extent, the relative ability to partition to oil from water does govern the permeation of many compounds, but surprising exceptions exist that make reliance on this simple lipid picture of the skin barrier very risky. The only reliable membrane for study of the mechanism of percutaneous absorption is a suitable skin preparation. This admonition is not intended to rule out the use of synthetic membranes when the purpose of the artificial membrane is to contrast specific behavior of the skin to that of a prototype hydrophobic or watery barrier (Behl et al., 1983b; Durrheim et al., 1980) or to build-upon the basic concepts governing all permeation.

IN VITRO STUDIES IN WHICH SKIN IS THE MEMBRANE

There are two distinctly separable research strategies that involve the use of skin membrane preparations. The first involves mass transfer studies under circumstances of a steady state or quasi-steady state being obtained during the course of an experiment. This allows reduction or the rate of permeation to a mass transfer coefficient that characterizes the permeation of the compound in a way unique to the compound, the skin membrane preparation, and the vehicle of application.

A second type involves the application to excised skin of a small quantity of a substance, either in its neat state or as a solution or suspension in a prototype vehicle, to ascertain how much of the substance permeates the tissue in a given amount of time. The procedure has become known as the finite-dose technique, and the experimental conditions usually preclude the reduction of the data to precise mass transfer coefficients. Nevertheless this approach to skin permeability is particularly useful because a drug can be applied to the skin surface in a manner relatively faithful to the way that the drug is applied clinically. Such studies provide the best means of gauging the potential for systemic absorption of topically applied substances short of actual live animal or human trials.

Before elaborating on these two strategies, we consider the choice of the skin membrane. Whatever a skin's source, it is tacitly assumed that the excised tissue retains its barrier functions. The assumption that the stratum corneum's barrier properties are locked into an essentially dead and metabolically inactive tissue is by all accounts reasonable. But this is not the sole source of diffusional resistance within skin and not even the main source for some hydrophobic compounds, and the overall thickness of the skin membrane preparation may influence the mass transfer rates. In the living human the diffusion process terminates at the point of systemic entry, which can be within the region immediately beneath the epidermis if the local capillaries are well perfused with blood. The outermost reach of the skin's microvasculature is within 200 μm of the skin's surface over most of the body area. Therefore, thick slabs of skin, especially human cadaver skin, as are occasionally used in in vitro studies, may fail to fairly represent the living situation. For large, polar compounds having the greatest difficulty of passage through the stratum corneum, it generally matters little how thick the skin section is, but for nonpolar substances the relative roles of the skin's strata in the natural state might be obfuscated when the skin is too thick. Investigators have developed techniques to isolate the epidermis itself to better approximate the functioning thicknesses of the skin's barrier-bearing elements. Chemical and physical vesication of the skin of living man and animals has been one means of isolation, with the tops of the blisters removed for study. Others have taken whole excised skin and treated it mildly with heat (60°C for 60 sec) to effect separation at the epidermal-dermal junction. Another technique has been to simply dermatome the skin as thinly as possible. In this case an indeterminate layer of dermis becomes part of the membrane.

Even sunburn peelings and callus have been used. Some argue that skin membranes for in vitro work should be prepared from human skin; otherwise the test material will lack critical properties that set human skin apart from that of other creatures in the animal kingdom. Others have relied heavily on animal skins. Either choice can be alarmingly inadequate if done without thought. Irrespective of their manner of preparation, almost all membranes from human sources have been stored in a chilled, frozen, or dessicated state for long periods because the working samples of skin are obtained intermittently in batches. Since the skins of different human cadavers vary, it is common for investigators to use the same source for a set of experiments, providing another reason for the protracted storage of skin samples. The variability seen with human skin samples is to be expected, since normally no control can be exercised over the characteristics (age, health, sex, race, skin care habits, etc.) of the donors, usually cadavers. Considering all the manipulation of human skin samples involved in their preparation as membranes and recognizing the often protracted and varied means of storage, some misgivings should exist concerning the use of excised human skin, as are invariably raised over the use of animal skins.

The alternative to using human skins as the source of the membranes of study is to prepare membranes from the skin of another living animals. This choice suffers the general criticism that all animal integuments differ structurally and functionally from human skin and therefore lack representativeness. However, to dismiss all sources of animal skin on this basis is shortsighted, considering the above-mentioned genuine concerns over the uniformity of human skin preparations. Therefore, it seems that a better approach to the question of use of animal tissue involves considering the properties of skin that give it its essential barrier features and then determining whether there are animal skins that have these critical properties in the proper balance to make them suitable substitutes for percutaneous absorption and drug delivery investigations. Every land-dwelling creature has developed some form of protection against the dessicating influences of the nonaquatic environment. The horny layer of human skin plays this protective role. Unlike many furry animals, man does not derive moisture loss protection from a thick coat of hair for, with the usual exception of the scalp, man's hair distribution is too sparse. Mammals that share with man the attribute of having little or no hair of necessity also have skins overlayered with a thin but relatively moisture-impervious cornified tissue. Histologic evidence indicates that these skins and human skin are anatomically constructed in a fashion similar. Physicochemical studies, including permeability work, indicate comparably important similarities of general physical function. It is reasonable to expect that skins as close to man's as these will function as a diffusional barrier approximating that of human skin to a satisfactory degree. Animals such as the hairless varieties of mice are sufficiently inexpensive that it is possible to sacrifice them as skin is needed and do all work with fresh membranes. Animals such as the pig, although generally too costly to sacrifice, are large enough for bioavailability studies and can be used to test delivery concepts first developed in in vitro studies. Either type of animal can be kept in a regulated environment and the variables of age, sex, and health controlled. Certainly much can be learned about the diffusional behavior of skin and of topical drug delivery systems from these animal models. It is absolutely certain that these skins make more representative models of human skin than the synthetic structures sometimes pressed into action as skin facsimiles.

Having dealt with the issue of choice of membrane for in vitro work, we can consider in some further detail the strategies that have been used to elucidate the mechanism of percutaneous absorption. Diffusion equations that can be readily applied have proved to be the most useful for characterization of human skin as a barrier to penetrants, including drugs. These experimental approaches embrace the first research strategy using skin as a membrane referred to at the beginning of this topic.

In the typical experiment involving steady-state kinetics, a stirred drug solution is placed on the stratum corneum. Drug concentration is measured over time in a second stirred phase on the opposite (dermal) side of the skin membrane. Conditions are adjusted so that the concentration difference across the skin is held constant, or nearly so. Furthermore, buildup of drug on the dermal side is controlled so that "sink" conditions prevail. The transport process is followed well into the period where the rate of diffusion dQ/dt is steady. The mass transfer coefficient, the critical experimental parameter being sought, is computed from the simple equation:

$$\frac{dQ}{dt} = PA\Delta C$$

The parameter P is the mass transfer coefficient or, as it is more usually referred to, the permeability coefficient. It is the reciprocal of the total diffusional resistance that a diffusing species encounters in traversing the membrane system, including all boundary layers. In the same equation, A is the diffusional area involved, ΔC is the difference in concentration expressed across the membrane as measured in the external phases to the membrane, and dQ/dt is the experimentally measured mass transfer rate in terms of the quantity penetration of time. As defined, the mass transfer coefficient has the units distance divided by time and it can be viewed as the average velocity of the molecules of the diffusing species in the barrier field. This rate is affected by diffusivity of the permeant in all phases of the membrane, by partitioning of the permeant into and between all phases of the membrane, and by the thicknesses and configurations of the phases of the barrier. The permeability coefficient may reflect events taking place throughout the barrier, or it may be determined by only a thin section of the membrane that is particularly impervious. The latter appears to be true when it comes to the skin, because the intact stratum corneum, which is only about 10 μm thick, usually sets the mass transfer rate for skin preparations fully 10-100 times as thick.

Permeability coefficients from one permeant to another change in predictable ways based on chemical structure. Since physical parameters underlying the permeability coefficient to like diffusivities and o/w partition coefficients have predictable structural dependencies, one can begin to place the mass transfer data for a given membrane into a self-consistent picture and construct a working model of the barrier using these known physicochemical tendencies. Such studies have provided the most definitive insights into the mechanism of percutaneous absorption and, as the data bank of mass transfer coefficients expands, we are coming closer to the day when it will be possible to predict the percutaneous absorption rates of novel, untested compounds.

While there are older works of some relevance, work begun by Blank (1964, 1969) and theoretically amplified soon after by his close research collaborator Scheuplein (1965, 1967, 1975, 1976) is regarded by many as the beginning of modern, systematic characterization of the skin's barrier properties. The members of a simple homologous series, the n-alkanols, were the permeants of human epidermal sheets prepared by the standard scalding technique. Separate partitioning studies showed that the o/w partition coefficients of these solutes increased exponentially using an organic liquid as the oil phase but that partitioning into the skin is a more complex phenomenon, with only the higher homologs exhibiting the exponentially increasing behavior. The permeability coefficients of the series grow exponentially over the greater part of the series, a sign that the skin is discriminating the alkanols on the basis of their partitioning properties. Deviations from the simple lipid membrane pattern at C_9 and C_{10} were caused by the increasing importance of the underlying cellular (aqueous) resistance. The behaviors of methanol and ethanol appeared anomalous, since these species permeated the skin sections at nearly the same rate as water. The dermis was unable to discriminate the compounds on the basis of their relative hydrophobicities, suggesting that it acts as an aqueous resistance in series in the intact skin. These studies demonstrated that, for alkanols at least, the skin acts principally as a lipid membrane. Studies with a diverse group of steroids showed this to be true for larger structures (Michaels et al., 1975; Scheuplein et al., 1969). The work with the steroids led to the speculation that parallel pathways must exist through the skin. This conclusion was necessary to rationalize the clinical effectiveness of topical corticosteroids when many days were required to obtain the steady-state current in vitro. The first anatomically rigorous physical modeling of the skin evolved from this work.

Flynn and co-workers have worked with the alkanols using hairless mouse skin and, through direct comparison with Scheuplein's data, have shown the animal skin to exhibit striking parallels in barrier attributes to its human counterpart (Behl et al., 1980a, 1982, 1983a; Durrheim et al., 1980; Flynn et al.,

1981a,b). This skin can be separated into its dermal and epidermal elements either by scalding or by soaking it in saline for periods approaching a full day. The stratum corneum can be stripped away as well by use of well-established tape-stripping procedures. It has thus proved possible to independently define its constituent diffusional resistances; these are similar in magnitude to human skin (Table 2). Figure 6 illustrates that the stratum corneum of hairless mouse skin has the same chemical sensitivity to phenol as human stratum corneum; it takes phenol concentrations in excess of 2% to chemically denature the structure and open it to perfuse permeation (Behl et al., 1983b). Heat denatures at the same temperature as the human stratum corneum, maintaining the bulk of its barrier integrity to about 80°C and then deteriorating rapidly with further increases in temperature as seen in Figure 7 (Behl et al., 1980b, 1981). Hairless mouse skin functions as an essentially lipid barrier to corticosteroids (Fig. 8), in which permeability coefficients of some ester homologs of hydrocortisone increase exponentially.

The following examples illustrate the manner of carrying out permeation studies and their possibilities. Figure 9 presents the essence of the two-compartment diffusion cell. A membrane is placed between the cell halves and, once assembled, the compartments are filled with suitable media. The figure also depicts the gradual buildup of penetrant with time in the membrane, eventually establishing a quasi-steady state with respect to diffusion. Normally, physiologic saline or similar medium is used in both compartments, the only difference being that the medium in touch with the stratum corneum surface is charged with a permeant species. But in some studies other solvents have been employed, either diluted with water, or in an essentially neat state and on either side of the skin

Table 2 Comparison of Permeability Constants: Human and Mouse Skin Membranes

Compound	P (cm/hr $\times 10^3$)	
	Man	Mouse[a]
Water	0.5	1.6
Methanol	0.5	2.1
Ethanol	0.8	2.1
Butanol	2.5	5.3
Hexanol	13	19.4
Heptanol	32	65.9
Octanol	52	78.2

[a]Data for fresh mouse skin.

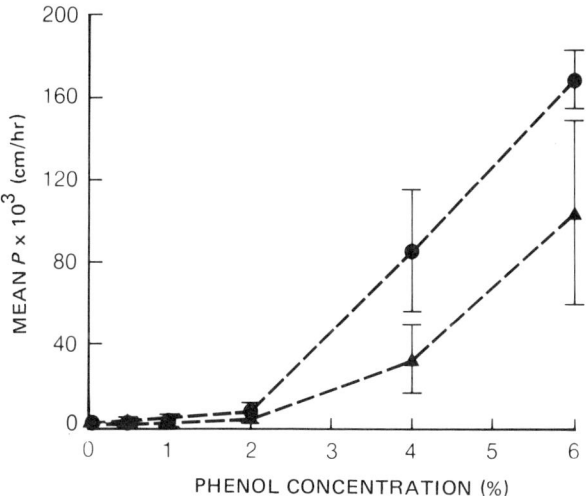

Figure 6 Plots of the mean permeability coefficients P of methanol obtained in concentration-effect (●) and reversibility (▲) experiments. Bars represent standard deviation for each mean value.

membrane. While the diffusion process can in principle be characterized by following either the appearance of drug in the receiver side or the disappearance of drug from the donor side, the former technique is generally a more satisfactory experimental procedure, and it is used except under special circumstances that make donor depletion methods more convenient. The raw data are usually obtained as the penetrant concentration in the receptor phase as a function of time, a quantity readily converted to the amount penetrated as a function of time. From the steady-state rate dQ/dt and the cell's dimensions, the permeability coefficient is calculated as mentioned previously. In investigations with corticosteroids, Franz (1978) found two distinct phases of permeation to the profiles and two steady-state rates. For hydrocortisone, the rate of the second phase was about 30 times that of the initial phase (Fig. 10). This suggested that parallel pathways were operating, with one possibility being that these pathways were part of the natural makeup of the stratum corneum and another that the long soaking of the skin in saline eventually brought about an extreme degree of horny layer hydration.

There are a number of examples of studies involving finite dose methodology that have provided useful and sometimes surprising insight into the diffusional and kinetic processes involved during topical drug application. Figure 11 illustrates the essential elements of a finite dose system. As indicated, a finite dose (layer) of formulation is applied to the surface of the membrane. Ordinarily, the

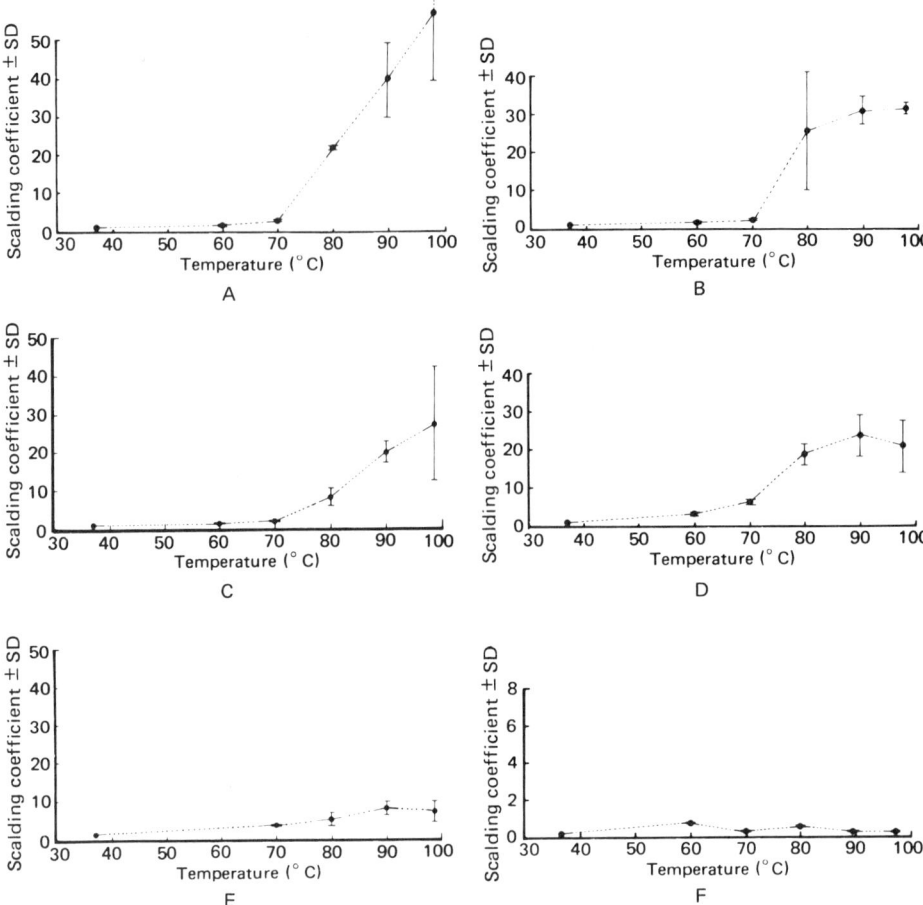

Figure 7 Plots of scalding coefficients as a function of temperature of burn for (a) water, (b) methanol, (c) ethanol, (d) butanol, (e) hexanol, and (f) octanol. Burning time = 60 sec.

top of the reservoir is left open to permit loss of volatile vehicle components, as would occur during clinical use conditions. Establishment of classical steady-state kinetics is not the objective in this method. [*Note*: This is possible, however, if the diffusional resistance to drug is exceptionally high and drug depletion from the donor phase is negligible during the experiment.] This methodology more closely parallels actual clinical conditions of drug usage and application and, for this reason, can provide information particularly pertinent to the vehicle used to deliver a drug to the skin surface.

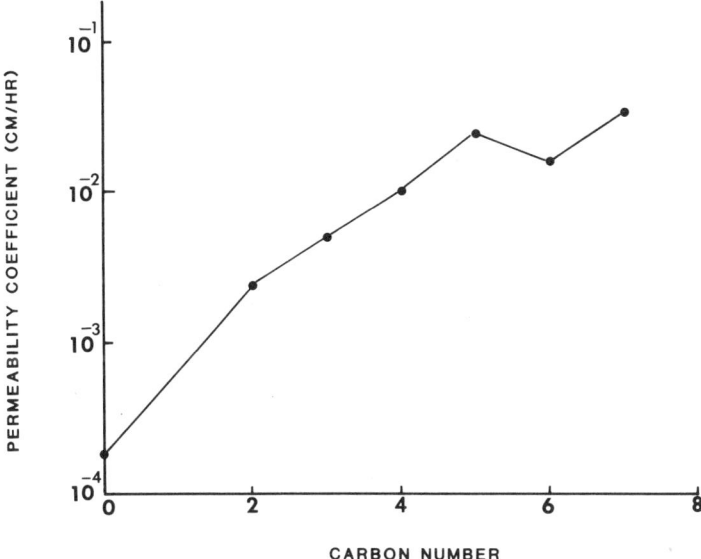

Figure 8 Effect of 21-*n*-alkyl chain length (number carbon atoms) on permeability coefficients of ester homologs of hydrocortisone.

Too little experimental attention has been given to what might be termed "vehicle dynamics" following application of a drug-vehicle combination to the skin. Finite-dosage studies, in which a layer of vehicle comparable to that used in clinical circumstances is used, provide a means for examining this aspect of topical drug delivery. It is intuitively obvious that the vehicle begins a dynamic and often dramatic change immediately after application to the skin. This could involve loss of volatile components, influx of skin components, emulsion inversion, precipitation of drug on other components, and a myriad of other significant changes in the physical state of the drug-vehicle system. It is utterly predictable that these changes can significantly affect drug delivery and efficacy. One must be aware that many in vitro experimental systems *exclude* these, to reduce variability in the experiment or to intentionally fix certain parameters. These procedures are normally logical and traditional. It is, however; essential that differences between laboratory necessity and clinical reality be recognized and understood.

The potential for postapplication changes in vehicle composition was clearly demonstrated in studies done with vehicles containing mixtures of (relatively) volatile and nonvolatile solvents (Coldman et al., 1969). It was shown that in vitro drug delivery will be radically effected by solubility effects induced by loss of the volatile component following application to the skin. Representative

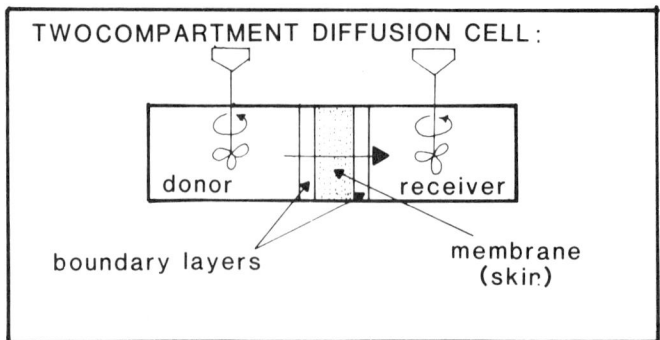

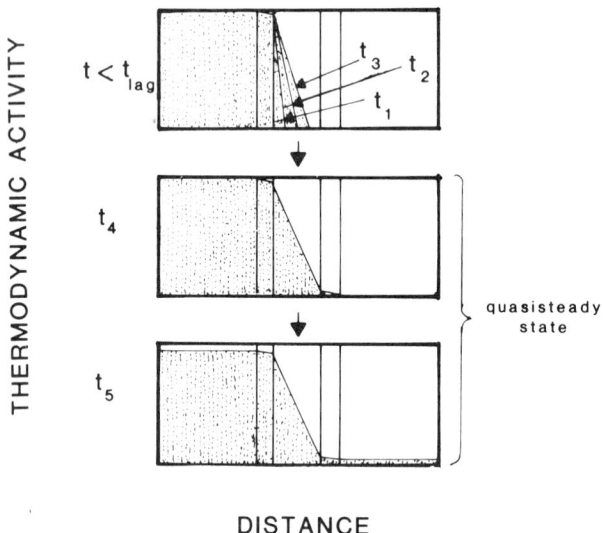

Figure 9 Typical two-compartment diffusion cell and diffusion profiles as a function of time, t.

results are shown in Figure 12, which indicates that a remarkable increase in the amount of fluocinonide acetonide penetrating excised human skin from isopropanol-propylene glycol mixtures is obtained by appropriate adjustment of solvent proportions. For 0.025% fluocinonide acetonide solutions, vehicles containing appropriately 10% of the nonvolatile component (propylene glycol) produced penetration rates many times greater than those achieved with nonoptimal solvent mixtures or with the optimal system when it was occluded to prevent loss

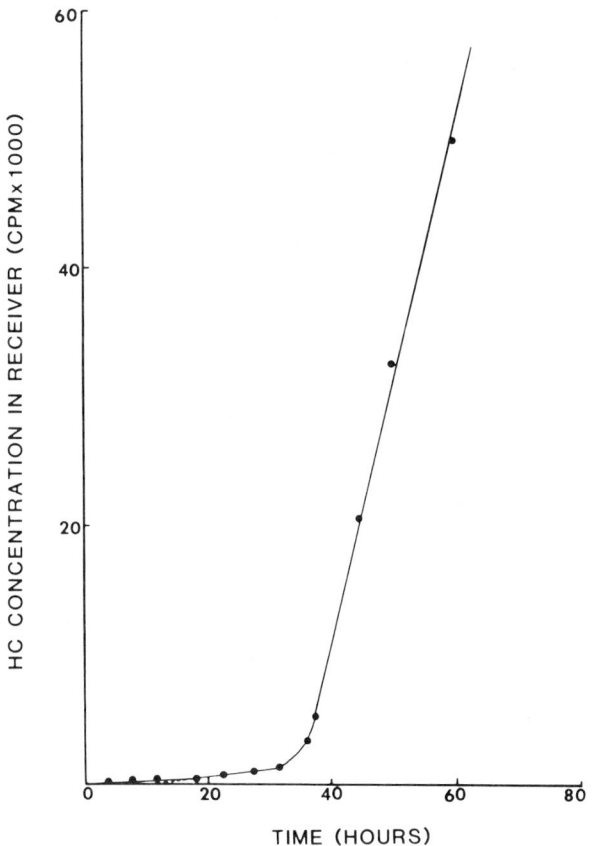

Figure 10 Biphasic diffusion profile of hydrocortisone (HC) penetrating hairless mouse skin.

of solvent by volatilization. The volatile-nonvolatile systems behaved predictably in these in vitro experiments. Accordingly, the composition of the optimal vehicle was a function of drug solubility and of initial concentration.

The importance of finite-dose techniques was also illustrated in a study (Coldman et al., 1971) in which unexpected dose-volume effects with dimethyl sulfoxide (DMSO) were found. In these experiments, it was found that the in vitro penetration of the corticosteroid fluocinonide was inversely proportional to the volume of drug-containing DMSO applied to human abdominal skin in vitro. Thus, application of more drug actually reduced percutaneous absorption. This paradoxical effect was rationalized as due to effects produced by water flux

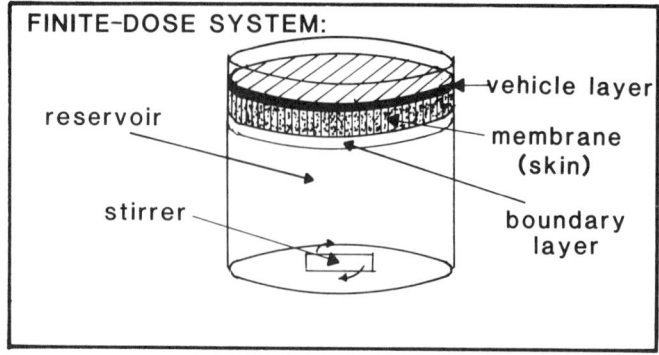
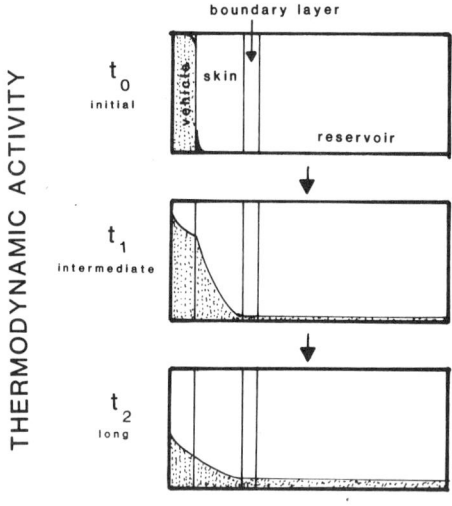

Figure 11 Schematic representation of a finite-dose system and diffusion profiles as a function of time, t.

from the skin specimen and/or receptor phase into the DMSO donor phase. It was shown a large increase in thermodynamic activity of fluocinonide occurred with small volume applications of DMSO. Since this increase in diffusional driving force would be larger for relatively thin films of applied vehicle, it was possible to reduce in vitro drug penetration by increasing the total amount of DMSO-corticosteroid applied to the skin surface. It is likely that numerous parallels, involving postapplication changes in vehicle composition, exist with products

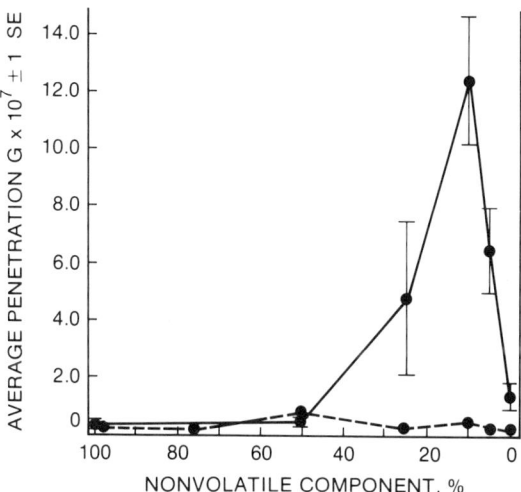

Figure 12 Penetration of fluocinolone acetonide through human skin from 0.05 ml, 0.025% solution in isopropanol/propylene glycol after 16 hr at 37°C. Solid curve, test site not occluded; dashed curve, test site occluded.

currently in clinical use. Their presence can best be detected and rationalized by the use of finite-dose methodology designed to closely simulate actual use conditions.

SUMMARY

Proper use of in vitro diffusion methodology can be an extremely useful technique for the design and development of dosage forms for both new and old topical drugs. A substantial theoretical and experimental base exists to guide undertakings in this area (Flynn and Smith, 1972; Flynn et al., 1974; Poulsen, 1972, 1973; Scheuplein, 1976b). Considering the available options, there are strong advantages to pursuit of experiments using actual excised skin as the diffusional barrier. This approach greatly increases confidence that properly designed and executed experiments will yield data with acceptable relevance. It is possible that use of excised human or animal skin may actually reduce the number of experiments required because at the conclusion of the study there will be fewer questions regarding the pertinence of the in vitro model. Finally, in the best of circumstances, the physicochemical parameters derived, and other observations made during such studies gradually enhance and expand our understanding of the complicated interactions between drug, vehicle, and skin.

REFERENCES

Ainsworth, M. (1960). Methods for measuring percutaneous absorption. *J. Soc. Cosmet. Chem. 11*: 69–78.

Behl, C. R., Flynn, G. L., Kurihara, T., Harper, N., Smith, W., Higuchi, W. I., Ho, N. F. H., and Pierson, C. L. (1980a). Hydration and percutaneous absorption. I. Influence of hydration on alkanol permeation through hairless mouse skin. *J. Invest. Dermatol. 75*: 346–352.

Behl, C. R., Flynn, G. L., Kurihara, T., Smith, W., Gatmaitan, O., Higuchi, W. I., Ho, N. F. H., and Pierson, C. L. (1980b). Permeability of thermally damaged skin. I. Immediate influences of 60°C scalding on hairless mouse skin. *J. Invest. Dermatol. 75*: 340–345.

Behl, C. R., Flynn, G. L., Barrett, M., Walters, K. A., Linn, E. E., Mohamed, Z., Kurihara, T., Ho, N. F. H., Higuchi, W. I., and Pierson, C. L. (1981). Permeability of thermally damaged skin. II. Immediate influences of branding at 60°C on hairless mouse skin permeability. *Burns, 7*: 389–399.

Behl, C. R., Barrett, M., Flynn, G. L., Kurihara, T., Walters, K. A., Gatmaitan, O. G., Harper, N., Higuchi, W. I., Ho, N. F. H., and Pierson, C. L. (1982). Hydration and percutaneous absorption. III. Influences of stripping and scalding on hydration alteration of the permeability of hairless mouse skin to water and *n*-alkanols. *J. Pharm. Sci. 71*: 229–234.

Behl, C. R., El-Sayed, A. A., and Flynn, G. L. (1983a). Hydration and percutaneous absorption. IV. Influence of hydration on *n*-alkanol permeation through rat skin; Comparison with hairless mouse skin. *J. Pharm. Sci. 72*: 79–82.

Behl, C. R., Linn, E. E., Flynn, G. L., Pierson, C. L., Higuchi, W. I., and Ho, N. F. H. (1983b). Permeation of skin and eschar by antiseptics. I. Baseline studies with phenol. *J. Pharm. Sci. 72*: 391–397.

Billups, N. F. and Sager, R. W. (1965). Microbiological and diffusion methods for determining drug release characteristics from ointment bases. *Am. J. Pharm. 137*: 57–68.

Blank, I. H. (1960). Percutaneous absorption. Statement of problem and critical review of past methods. *J. Soc. Cosmet. Chem. 11*: 59–68.

Blank, I. H. (1964). Penetration of low-molecular-weight alcohols into skin. I. Effect of concentration of alcohol and type of vehicle. *J. Invest. Dermatol. 43*: 415–420.

Blank, I. H. (1969). Transport across the stratum corneum. *Toxicol. Appl. Pharmacol. Suppl. 3*: 23–29.

Bracho, H., Erlij, D., and Martinez-Palomo, A. (1971). The site of the permeability barriers in frog skin epithelium. *J. Physiol. 213*: 50p–51p.

Coldman, M. F., Poulsen, B. J., and Higuchi, T. (1969). Enhancement of percutaneous absorption by the use of volatile: nonvolatile systems as vehicles. *J. Pharm. Sci. 58*: 1098–1102.

Coldman, M. F., Kalinovsky, T., and Poulsen, B. J. (1971). The in vitro penetration of fluocinonide through human skin from different volumes of DMSO. *Br. J. Dermatol. 85*: 457–461.

DeKay, H. G. (1962). The release of medication from an emulsified ointment base. *Am. Perfum. Cosmet. 77*: 109-115.

Durrheim, H. H., Flynn, G. L., Higuchi, W. I., and Behl, C. R. (1980). Permeation of hairless mouse skin. I. Experimental methods and comparison with human epidermal permeation by alkanols. *J. Pharm. Sci. 69*: 781-786.

Flynn, G. H. and Roseman, T. J. (1971). Membrane diffusion. II. Influence of physical adsorption on molecular flux through heterogeneous dimethyl polysiloxane barriers. *J. Pharm. Sci. 60*: 1788-1793.

Flynn, G. J. and Smith, R. W. (1972). Membrane diffusion. III. Influence of solvent composition and permeant solubility on membrane transport. *J. Pharm. Sci. 61*: 61-66.

Flynn, G. L., Yalkowsky, J. H., and Roseman, T. J. (1974). Mass transport phenomena and models: Theoretical concepts. *J. Pharm. Sci. 63*: 479-510.

Flynn, G. L., Behl, C. R., Walters, K., Gatmaitan, O., Wittkowsky, A., Kurihara, T., Ho, N. F. H., Higuchi, W. I., and Pierson, C. L. (1981a). Permeability of thermally damaged skin. III. Influence of scalding temperature on mass transfer of water and *n*-alkanols across hairless mouse skin. *Burns 8*: 47-58.

Flynn, G. L., Durrheim, H. H., and Higuchi, W. I. (1981b). Permeation of hairless mouse skin. II. Membrane sectioning techniques and influences on alkanol permeabilities. *J. Pharm. Sci. 70*: 52-56.

Franz, J. (1978). The finite dose technique as a valid in vitro model for the study of percutaneous absorption in man. *Curr. Probl. Dermatol. 7*: 58-68.

Gemmell, D. H. O. and Morrison, J. C. (1957). The release of medicinal substances from topical applications and their passage through the skin. *J. Pharm. Pharmacol. 9*: 641-656.

Grasso, P. and Lansdown, A. B. G. (1972). Methods of measuring, and factors affecting, percutaneous absorption. *J. Soc. Cosmet. Chem. 23*: 481-521.

Guy, R. H. and Fleming, F. (1979). A novel method to study the permeability of a phospholipid barrier. *J. Chem. Soc., Chem. Commun.* 729-730.

Haleblian, J. K., Poulsen, B. J., and Burdick, K. H. (1977). Development of fluocinonide gel: Correlation of in vitro assays, in vivo bioassays and clinical trials. *Curr. Ther. Res. 22*: 713-721.

Higuchi, T. (1960). Physical chemical analysis of percutaneous absorption process from creams and ointments. *J. Soc. Cosmet. Chem. 11*: 85-97.

Higuchi, T. (1961). Rate of release of medicaments from ointment bases containing drugs in suspension. *J. Pharm. Sci. 50*: 874-875.

Higuchi, W. I. (1962). Analysis of data on the medicament release from ointments. *J. Pharm. Sci. 51*: 802-804.

Howze, J. M. and Billups, N. F. (1966). Drug release from ointment bases: Characteristics, measurement and evaluation. III. Dialysis cell method. *Am. J. Pharm. 138*: 193-203.

Johnson, G. W. and Lee, C. O. (1943). A radioactive method of testing absorption from ointment bases. *J. Am. Pharm. Assoc., Sci. Ed. 32*: 278-280.

Hunter, M. C. and Smith, F. J. (1952). Determination of certain properties of ointment bases by use of chick embryos. *J. Am. Pharm. Assoc., Sci. Ed. 41*: 125-130.

Jurist, A. E. (1953). A rapid qualitative method for measuring the ion exchanging activity of dermatologic preparations containing an ion exchange resin. *J. Invest. Dermatol. 20*: 331–332.

Katz, M. and Poulsen, B. J. (1971). Absorption of drugs through the skin. In *Handbook of Experimental Pharmacology*, New Series, Vol. 28. Edited by B. B. Brodie and J. Gillette, Springer-Verlag, Heidelberg, pp. 103–174.

Lueck, L. M., Wurster, D. E., Higuchi, T., Lemberger, A. P., and Busse, L. W. (1957). Investigation and development of protective ointments. I. Developments of a method for measuring permeation of mechanical barriers. *J. Am. Pharm. Assoc., Sci. Ed. 46*: 694–698.

Michaels, A. S., Chandrasekaran, S. K., and Shaw, J. E. (1975). Drug permeation through human skin: Theory and in vitro experimental measurement. *AIChE J. 21*: 985–996.

Multimer, M. N., Riffkin, C., Hill, J. A., and Cyr, G. N. (1956a). Modern ointment base technology. I. Properties of hydrocarbon gels. *J. Am. Pharm. Assoc., Sci. Ed. 45*: 101–105.

Multimer, M. N., Riffkin, C., Hill, J. A., Glickman, M. E. and Cyr, G. N. (1956b). Modern ointment base technology. II. Comparative evaluation of bases. *J. Am. Pharm. Assoc., Sci. Ed. 45*: 212–218.

Nugent, F. J. and Wood, J. A. (1980). Methods for the study of percutaneous absorption. *Can. J. Pharm. 15*: 1–7.

Ostrenga, J., Haleblian, J., Poulsen, B., Ferrell, B., Mueller, N., and Shastri, S. (1971a). Vehicle design for a new topical steroid, fluocinonide. *J. Invest. Dermatol. 56*: 392–399.

Ostrenga, J., Steinmetz, C., and Poulsen, B. (1971b). Significance of vehicle composition. I. Relationship between topical vehicle composition, skin penetrability, and clinical efficacy. *J. Pharm. Sci. 60*: 1175–1179.

Patel, K. C., Banker, G. S., and DeKay, H. G. (1961). Study of anionic and cationic surfactants in a hydrophilic ointment base. II. The effect of the surfactant and its concentration on medicament release. *J. Pharm. Sci. 50*: 300–305.

Poulsen, B. J. (1970). The use of models in estimating vehicle effects on the activity of topical corticosteroid formulations. *Br. J. Dermatol. 82* (Suppl 6): 49–52.

Poulsen, B. J. (1973). Design of topical drugs products: Biopharmaceutics. In *Drug Design*, Vol. 4. Edited by Ariens. Academic, New York, pp. 149–192.

Poulsen, B. J. (1972). Diffusion of drugs from topical vehicles: An analysis of vehicle effects. In *Pharmacology and the Skin*, Vol. XII, *Advances in Biology of Skin*. Edited by W. Montagna, R. B. Stoughton, and E. J. Van Scott. Appleton-Century-Crofts, New York, pp. 495–509.

Poulsen, B. J., Young, E., Coquilla, V., and Katz, M. (1968). Effect of topical vehicle composition on the in vitro release of fluocinolone acetonide and its acetate ester. *J. Pharm. Sci. 57*: 928–933.

Roseman, T. J. and Higuchi, W. I. (1970). Release of medroxyprogesterone acetate from a silicone polymer. *J. Pharm Sci. 59*: 353–357.

Ruggiero, J. S. and Skauen, D. M. (1962a). Chick embryo technique for the evaluation of absorption of radioactive sodium iodide from ointment bases. *J. Pharm. Sci. 51*: 233-235.

Ruggiero, J. S. and Skauen, D. M. (1962b). Evaluation of the absorption of radioactive sodium iodide from various ointment bases by means of a chick embryo technique. *J. Pharm. Sci. 51*: 235-237.

Scheuplein, R. J. (1965). Mechanism of percutaneous absorption. I. Routes of penetration and the influence of solubility. *J. Invest. Dermatol. 45*: 334-345.

Scheuplein, R. J. (1967). Mechanism of percutaneous absorption. II. Transient diffusion and the relative importance of various routes of skin penetration. *J. Invest. Dermatol. 48*: 79-88.

Scheuplein, R. (1975). Skin permeation. In *The Physiology and Pathophysiology of the Skin*. Edited by A. Jarrett. Academic, New York, pp. 1693-1739.

Scheuplein, R. J. (1976a). Percutaneous absorption after twenty-five years; or old wine in new wineskins. *J. Invest. Dermatol. 67*: 31-38.

Scheuplein, R. J. (1976b). Permeability of the skin: A review of major concepts and some new developments. *J. Invest. Dermatol. 67*: 672-676.

Scheuplein, R. J., Blank, I. H., Brauner, G. J., and MacFarlane, D. J. (1969). Percutaneous absorption of steroids. *J. Invest. Dermatol. 52*: 63-70.

Spang-Brunner, B. H. and Speiser, P. P. (1976). Release of a drug from homogeneous ointments containing the drug in solution. *J. Pharm. Pharmacol. 28*: 23-28.

Wood, J. A., Rising, L. W., and Hall, N. A. (1962). Diffusion of sodium salicylate and salicylic acid within hydrophilic ointments. Measurement with a new diffusion cell. *J. Pharm. Sci. 51*: 668-671.

35
Calculations of Body Exposure from Percutaneous Absorption Data

Richard H. Guy
University of California School of Pharmacy, San Francisco, California

Howard I. Maibach
University of California School of Medicine, San Francisco, California

It is probably reasonable to say that most measurements of percutaneous absorption in vivo in humans use the forearm as the penetrant application site. It is apparent from the literature, however, that obvious differences exist in skin absorption resistance as a function of anatomic site (see Wester et al., Chap. 16, this volume). These two facts assume significance when it is recognized that where toxic effects result from dermal exposure, the forearm may not be the skin contact site or may be only a small fraction of the total exposed area. In this chapter we compare total body exposure evaluated using percutaneous absorption data obtained at different anatomic sites with that predicted on the basis of forearm penetration results alone. We make the same comparison for limited dermal exposure to specific body regions, namely, the face and hands. Because of the scarcity of regional absorption data, it must be stressed that our treatment is illustrative rather than definitive; nevertheless, we believe that the approach is relevant to any analysis of risk following the dermal exposure of man to harmful chemicals.

CALCULATIONS

We divide the body into five regions: genitals, arms, legs, trunk, and head, having surface areas A_G, A_A, A_L, A_T and A_H cm^2, respectively. To each region we assign a penetration index P_i (i = G, A, L, T, or H) defined as follows:

$$P_i = \frac{\text{amount of chemical penetrating 1 cm}^2 \text{ of skin at site } i \text{ in time } t}{\text{amount of chemical penetrating 1 cm}^2 \text{ of forearm skin in time } t}$$

Therefore, if experiment shows that N μg of chemical penetrate 1 cm² of forearm skin in time t, we may predict potential total body exposure (TBE) using Equation 1:

$$TBE = N(A_G P_G + A_A P_A + A_L P_L + A_T P_T + A_H P_H) \, \mu g \tag{1}$$

Conversely, if we assume that forearm penetration is representative of the whole body surface, then the "forearm" total body exposure (FTBE) prediction is:

$$FTBE = NP_A \, A_{TOT} \, \mu g \tag{2}$$

where A_{TOT} (= $A_G + A_A + A_L + A_T + A_H$) is the total body surface area. Furthermore, since most penetration measurements have been made using the forearm application site, P_A is invariably 1.

Only two comprehensive studies have been reported in the literature for which the five P_i values have been evaluated: for hydrocortisone (Feldmann and Maibach, 1967), and for malathion and parathion (Maibach et al., 1971); see Table 1.

To exemplify TBE and FTBE calculations, two sample "human" subjects (adult and neonate) are considered. Their height, weight, and body surface area characteristics are given in Table 2. This information, together with that in Table

Table 1 Penetration Indices for Five Anatomic Sites Assessed Using Hydrocortisone Skin Penetration Data and Pesticide (malathion and parathion) Absorption Results

Site	Penetration index based on:	
	Hydrocortisone data (Feldmann and Maibach, 1967)	Pesticide data (Maibach et al., 1971)
Genitals	40	12[a]
Arms	1	1
Legs	0.5[b]	1[c]
Trunk	2.5[d]	3[e]
Head	5[f]	4[g]

[a] Parathion value; P_G was not determined for malathion.
[b] Estimated on the basis of a value for the ankle.
[c] Estimated value using results from ball of foot.
[d] Assigned value using results for back and axilla.
[e] Assigned from data for abdomen and axilla.
[f] Evaluated from scalp, jaw angle, and forehead penetration indices and relative surface areas.
[g] Rounded average of scalp, jaw angle, and forehead data.

Table 2 Body Surface Areas Distributed Over Five Anatomic Regions for Adult and Neonate[a]

Anatomic region	Adult[b]		Neonate[c]	
	Percent of body area	Area (cm^2)	Percent of body area	Area (cm^2)
Genitals	1	190	1	19
Arms	18	3,420	19	365
Legs	36	6,840	30	576
Trunk	36	6,840	31	595
Head	9	1,710		365
Totals		19,000		1920

[a] For the adult, surface area percentages were assigned by the "rules of nine" (Wallace, 1951). Total body area was determined using the classic nomogram of Du Bois and Du Bois (1916) and agrees with a more recent and rigorous evaluation (Gehan and George, 1970). Distribution of body surface area in the neonate was assessed by the method of Lund and Browder (1944) together with published age-height-weight relationships (Blank, 1956; Heimendinger 1964a,b; Talbot et al., 1953, 1955) and the Du Bois and Du Bois (1916) child nomogram.
[b] Weight, 70 kg; height, 1.83 m.
[c] Weight, 3 kg; height, 0.49 m.

1, can now be applied, using Equations (1) and (2) to calculate TBE and FTBE values for the adult and neonate. The results, based on P_i data for both hydrocortisone and the pesticides, are given in Table 3.

We may evaluate predicted *limited* exposures in a similar fashion. For example, consider the realistic possibility of exposure to the head and hands. Assuming again that N μg of penetrant are absorbed through 1 cm^2 of forearm skin in time t, the amount transporting across the skin of the hands and face (N_{HH}) in a similar period is:

$$N_{HH} = N(A_H P_H + 0.25 A_A P_A) \, \mu g \tag{3}$$

where we have assumed that the surface area of the skin of the hands is 0.25 A_A. The amount (FN_{HH}) predicted by forearm penetration, however, is given by:

$$FN_{HH} = NP_A (A_H + 0.25 A_A) \tag{4}$$

Results for N_{HH} and FN_{HH}, again based on both hydrocortisone and pesticide P_i values, are presented in Table 4 for the model "adult" subject.

Table 3 Total Body Exposure (TBE) and "Forearm" Total Body Exposure (FTBE) Calculated Using Equations 1 and 2, Respectively, from Both Sets of Penetration Indices in Table 1 and the Two Groups of Body Surface Areas in Table 2

Exposure[a]	Adult	Neonate
TBE (10^4 N μg)[b]	4.01	0.473
FTBE (10^4 N μg)[b]	1.90	0.192
TBE/FTBE	2.11	2.46
TBE (10^4 N μg)[c]	3.99	0.441
FTBE (10^4 N μg)[c]	1.90	0.192
TBE/FTBE	2.10	2.30

[a]N = micrograms of penetrant absorbed across 1 cm² of forearm skin in time t.
[b]Values determined using penetration indices based on hydrocortisone absorption data (Feldmann and Maibach, 1967).
[c]Values determined using penetration indices based on pesticide absorption data (Maibach et al., 1971).

Table 4 Adult Exposure Estimates to the Head and Hands as Assessed by Equations 3 and 4

Exposure[a]	For hydrocortisone[b]	For pesticide[c]
N_{HH} (N μg)	9405	7695
FN_{HH} (N μg)	2565	2565
N_{HH}/FN_{HH}	3.67	3.00

[a]N = micrograms of penetrant absorbed across 1 cm² of forearm skin in time t.
[b]Values determined using penetration indices based on absorption data of Feldmann and Maibach (1967).
[c]Values determined using penetration indices based on absorption data of Maibach et al. (1971).

CONCLUSIONS

The results in Tables 3 and 4 essentially speak for themselves and show the possible inaccuracies that may result when one assumes that forearm percutaneous penetration is indicative of absorption at all body sites. TBE exceeds FTBE by approximately a factor of 2, while N_{HH}/FN_{HH} (the ratio for the limited exposure example) is about 3. Agreement between estimates based on hydrocortisone and pesticide P_i values is good for all the example exposure situations considered.

We may conclude, therefore, that a dermal exposure toxicity hazard depends on the anatomic sites contacted and that forearm percutaneous absorption data may provide an underestimate of risk. Other variables, of course, impinge on percutaneous absorption; this chapter has addressed the fact that an inherent physiological variable is provided by the anatomic region(s) at which skin penetration occurs. Again, we emphasize the limited data base on which our calculations depend, and we must accept (and can show) that there will very probably be instances when forearm absorption is a reliable predictor of certain exposure situations (Guy and Maibach, 1984). Overall, though, this chapter suggests that: (1) forearm penetration does not always reliably predict absorption at all anatomic sites and may significantly underestimate potential toxicity resulting from dermal exposure, and (2) there is much need for skin absorption to be measured as a function of anatomic site for a range of chemicals of different physicochemical characteristics.

ACKNOWLEDGMENT

This work was supported in part by grants OH-01830-01 and 1-KO1-OH-00017 from the National Institute of Occupational Safety and Health (RHG). A detailed description of this work appeared in the *Journal of Applied Toxicology*, 1984.

REFERENCES

Blank, J. H. (1956). *Clinical Recognition and Management of Disturbances of Body Fluids.* Saunders, Philadelphia.

Du Bois, D. and Du Bois, E. F. (1916). A formula to estimate the approximate surface area if height and weight be known. *Arch. Intern. Med. 17*:863-871.

Feldmann, R. J. and Maibach, H. I. (1967). Regional variation in percutaneous penetration of [^{14}C] cortisol in man. *J. Invest. Dermatol. 48*:181-183.

Gehan, E. A. and George, S. L. (1970). Estimation of human body surface area from height and weight. *Cancer Chemother. Rep. Part I 54*:225-235.

Guy, R. H. and Maibach, H. I. (1984). Correction factors for determining body exposure from forearm percutaneous absorption data. *J. Appl. Toxicol. 4*: 26-28.

Heimendinger, J. (1964a). Gemischt longitudinale Messungen von Körperlänge, Gewicht, oberem Segment, Thoraxumfang und Kopfumfang bei 1-24 Monate alten Säuglingen. *Helv. Paediatr. Acta 19*:406-436.

Heimendinger, J. (1964b). Die Ergebnisse von Körpermessungen an 5000 Basler Kindern von 2-18 Jahren. *Helv. Paediatr. Acta 19*: Suppl. 13.

Lund, C. C. and Browder, N. C. (1944). The estimation of areas of burns. *Surg. Gynecol. Obstet. 79*:352-358.

Maibach, H. I., Feldmann, R. J., Milby, T. H., and Serat, W. F. (1971). Regional variation in percutaneous penetration in man. *Arch. Environ. Health 23*: 208-211.

Talbot, N. B., Crawford, J. D., and Butler, A. M. (1953). Homeostatic limits to safe parenteral fluid therapy. *New Engl. J. Med. 248*:1100-1108.

Talbot, N. B., Kerrigan, G. A., Crawford, J. D., Cochran, W., and Terry, M. (1955). Application of homeostatic principles to the practice of parenteral fluid therapy. *New Engl. J. Med. 252*:856-862.

Wallace, A. B. (1951). The exposure treatment of burns. *Lancet 1*:501-504.

DRUG DELIVERY

36
Percutaneous Penetration as a Method of Delivery to Muscle and Other Tissues

Jean-Paul Marty
Université de Picardie, Amiens, France

Richard H. Guy
University of California School of Pharmacy, San Francisco, California

Howard I. Maibach
University of California School of Medicine, San Francisco, California

This chapter reviews the literature that demonstrates that significant drug delivery can be achieved to local subcutaneous structures following topical administration. The results discussed illustrate that the cutaneous microcirculation does not always act as a perfect "sink" and that lower tissue (e.g., the muscle beneath the subcutaneous fat) can be reached in significant amount via the transdermal route (Fig. 1).

EXPERIMENTAL RESULTS

Steroids

The most extensive studies of local subcutaneous delivery of chemicals have been performed in France by Marty, Wepierre, and co-workers. The approach involved is application of radiolabeled penetrant in a suitable vehicle to a defined skin site of a mouse or rat. Contact zones are protected for the experimental duration (up to 24 hr), after which the animal is sacrificed and dissected for tissue analysis. Radioactivity levels are determined by liquid scintillation counting and the results may then be converted to amounts of penetrant present in nanograms per gram of tissue. In some cases, similar data following oral dosing have been derived for comparative purposes.

The disposition of tritiated dexamethasone has been studied in mice and rats after both topical and oral administration of the drug (James et al., 1975, 1976). Tables 1 and 2 summarize the results. The conclusions from the data are self-evident and support the earlier results of these workers (James et al., 1974). For example, in mice, under the area of topical application, the levels of radioactivity

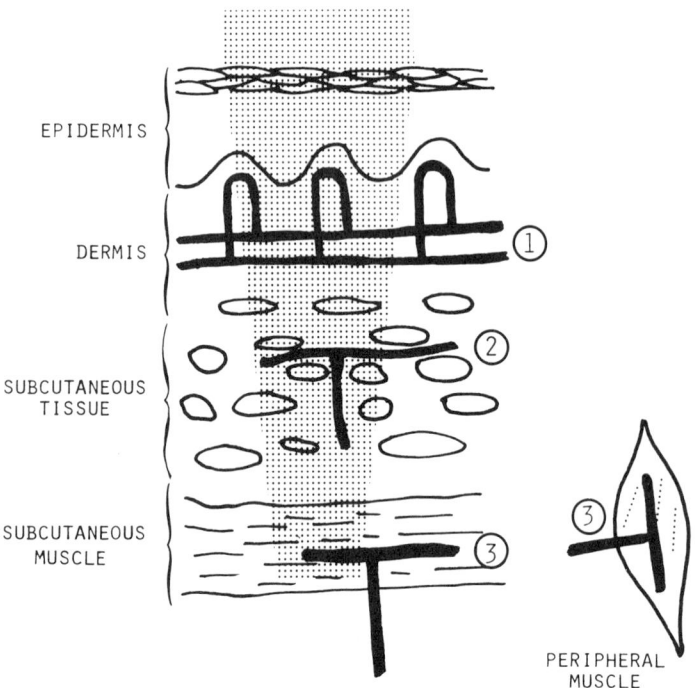

Figure 1 Schematization of several steps involved in the percutaneous delivery of drug to subcutaneous and muscle tissues located beneath the application area: 1, cutaneous vessels; 2, subcutaneous vessels; 3, muscle vessels (systemic circulation); shaded area, drug flux through the skin tissues.

Table 1 Percutaneous Absorption of 19-μg/cm^2 Doses of [^{3}H]Dexamethasone in Mice

Application duration (hr)[a]	Tissue concentration (ng/g)		Concentration in homogenized mouse (ng/g)
	Subcutaneous tissue[b]	Abdominal muscle	
1	49±19	4.1±1.3[b]	0.90±0.14
2	69±10	12±3.5[b]	2.6±1.7
4	97±30	29±13[c]	3.3±1.0

[a]N = 5 at 1 hr, N = 6 at 2 and 4 hr.
[b]Significance of difference between tissue and homogenized mouse, $p < 0.05$.
[c]Significance of difference, $p < 0.01$.
Source: James et al. (1975, 1976).

Table 2 Tissue Concentrations (ng/g) of [^{3}H] Dexamethasone After Topical (19 μg/cm^2) and Oral (40 μg/kg) Administration to Rats

Time (hr)[a],[b]	Plasma	Subcutaneous tissue	Abdominal muscle	Leg muscle	Liver	Kidneys
			Topical administration			
2	0.19±0.06	8.1±2.1[c]	0.77±0.14[c]	0.27±0.08	1.05±0.30	0.65±0.14
4	0.19±0.03	5.2±0.9[c]	0.68±0.30[d]	0.25±0.04	1.52±0.30	0.67±0.20
6	0.34±0.10	4.9±0.5[c]	1.6±0.6[c]	0.43±0.15	0.99±0.10	1.44±0.50
			Oral administration			
1	22±1	13±2	11.5±1.3	11.6±1.7	145±9	44±6
4	19±0.5	8.1±1.6	8.9±0.4	9.5±0.7	168±27	36±3
24	2.7±0.4	1.6±0.5	1.50±0.35	1.5±0.3	11±1.6	3.6±0.6

[a]Time = duration of application for topical dose and survival time for oral dose.
[b]$N = 5$ for all times except $t = 2$ hr (topical) for which $N = 12$.
[c]Significance of difference between tissue and plasma, $p < 0.05$.
[d]Significance of difference, $p < 0.01$.
Source: James et al. (1975, 1976).

in subcutaneous tissue and in the lower muscle were 30 and 10 times higher, respectively, than in other tissues. Levels and distribution were quite different following oral administration; the plasma concentration was higher, and large amounts were located in liver and kidney. Such a pattern of behavior (topical vs. oral) was intimated to be of potential importance in terms of the metabolic inactivation of the administered chemical.

For estradiol and progesterone (Marty et al., 1980) (Fig. 2, Tables 3 and 4), accumulation was again found in the connective tissue of the abdominal muscle in the region under application. The effect was not seen after subcutaneous administration (Table 4). As before, the authors argued that the results demonstrate slow exchanges between blood and tissue such that the steroids are not removed efficiently as they diffuse in the intercellular fluids. Their observations were emphasized to be distinct from the classic "reservoir" effect noted for this class of compound, but it was suggested that the latter would mean that the likelihood of deeper penetration was increased. It was concluded that the data constitute pharmacokinetic proof contributing to the confirmation of local subcutaneous pharmacological effects of topically administered hormones.

Pesticides

The fixation of topically applied materials in the superficial structures of the skin, and its relevance to problems of decontamination and bioavailability, has been reported (Marty, 1976; Marty et al., 1980). The materials studied were diisopropyl fluorophosphate (DFP), malathion, and parathion. Experiments were conducted in the mouse and rat using procedures comparable to those employed in the steroid investigations. The results are collected in Tables 5-7. In the mouse, approximately 28% (105 μg) of the total quantity of DFP absorbed was found in the abdominal muscle under the application region. Malathion gave similar results, with 36% of the absorbed chemical being located in subcutaneous tissue at or near to the application zone. The subjacent tissue contained a malathion concentration on the order of 1000 μg/g compared with the animal carcass level of less than 5 μg/g. Parathion data closely paralleled those for malathion.

An analogous pattern of behavior was found in the rat (Table 7) and it seems clear, therefore, that the organophosphorus pesticides represent another category of chemicals for which deep subcutaneous penetration is common.

Nonsteroidal Anti-Inflammatory Drugs

Panse et al. (1974) reported on the cutaneous absorption of anti-inflammatory agents. In rats treated topically with flufenamic acid, a significantly elevated level of drug was found in the tissues beneath the application site. The concentrations achieved were double those produced in the same region when the animal was given *six* times the drug dose administered orally. Representative data are shown in Figure 3.

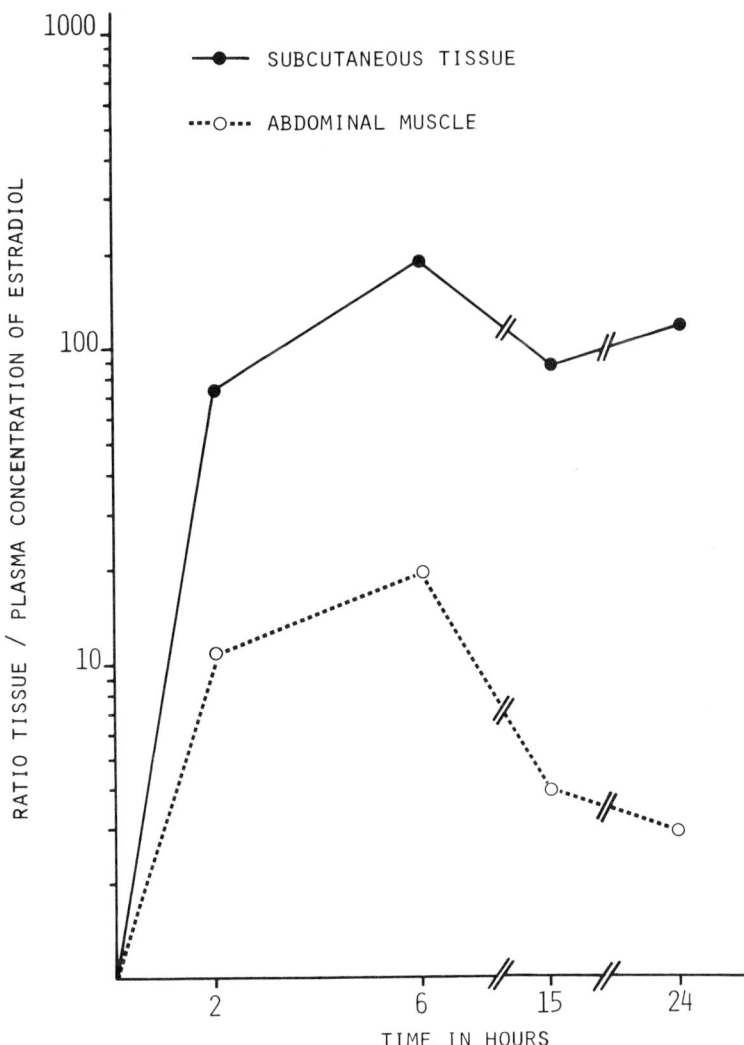

Figure 2 Ratio of tissue/plasma concentrations of estradiol in subcutaneous tissue and in muscle under application zone as a function of time after cutaneous administration to the rat. (From Marty et al., 1980.)

Table 3 Skin Absorption of Estradiol and Progesterone in Mice

Steroid	Concentration of steroid (µg/g)	Concentration in tissue under application zone (ng/g)			Concentration in whole crushed mouse (ng/g)
		Subcutaneous tissue	Muscle tissue		
Estradiol	600	1695±350	804±191		43±8
Progesterone	5000	43,600±1100	9350±2900		342±52

Source: Marty et al. (1980).

Table 4 Local Concentrations of Steroids in Subcutaneous Tissue Beneath the Application Zone on the Skin After 2 hr

Animal	Steroid and concentration (%)	Reference concentration of steroid, S (ng/g)[a]	Ratio of tissue to S	
			Subcutaneous	Muscle
Mouse	Estradiol (0.06)	43±8	39	19
Rat[b]	Estradiol (0.06)	1.93±0.18	75	11
Mouse	Progesterone (0.5)	342±52	125	27
Rat	Progesterone (0.5)	15.1±1.1	200	19

[a]The reference concentration for mouse is that in the whole crushed carcass after local excision; for the rat, the reference is plasma concentration.
[b]After subcutaneous injection (10 μg/kg), S = 0.88±0.05 and tissue/S = 2 (subcutaneous) and 0.75 (muscle).
Source: Marty et al. (1980).

Table 5 Percutaneous Absorption of [^{3}H]Diisopropyl Fluorophosphate (DFP), [^{35}S]Malathion, and [^{35}S]Parathion in Mice[a]

Penetrant[b]	Quantities of 10-μl applied dose found in tissues						
	Muscle under and circumscribed at application area		Mouse carcass		Overall absorption		
	μg	%	μg	%	μg	%	
DFP	105±10	1.05±0.10	250±60	2.5±0.6	355±70	3.5±0.7	
Malathion	60±10	0.50±0.08	110±25	0.9±0.2	170±40	1.4±0.3	
Parathion	50±8	0.40±0.06	130±25	1.0±0.2	180±20	1.4±0.2	

[a]Dose was applied over a surface area of 1 cm² for 1 hr.
[b]N = 6 for DFP and parathion, N = 7 for malathion.
Source: Marty (1976).

Table 6 Tissue Concentrations (μg/g) of Diisopropyl Fluorophosphate (DFP), Malathion, and Parathion After Absorption in Mice[a]

Penetrant[b]	Muscle under application area, M_1	Circumscribed muscle, M_2	Carcass, B	M_1/B	M_2/B
DFP	3920±520	1610±610[c]	11±3.5	355	145
Malathion	1880±570	650±200[d]	3.4±0.8	550	190
Parathion	2140±730	530±180[e]	4.0±0.7	535	130

[a] A 10-μl dose was applied over a surface area of 1 cm² for 1 hr.
[b] $N = 6$ for DFP and parathion, $N = 7$ for malathion.
[c] Significance of the difference between M_1 and M_2 (by paired series method), $p < 0.001$.
[d] Significance, $p < 0.02$.
[e] Significance, $p < 0.05$.
Source: Marty (1976).

Table 7 Distribution of Diisopropyl Fluorophosphate (DFP), Malathion, and Parathion in Rat Tissues After Percutaneous Application[a]

Penetrant[b]	Concentration in tissue ($\mu g/g$)		
	DFP	Malathion	Parathion
Subcutaneous tissue	130±25[c]	145±20[c]	155±60[c]
Muscle beneath zone	14±2[c]	2.5±0.6	1.45±0.45[d]
Paw muscle	4.0±1.5	1.7±0.6	Not detectable
Blood	1.3±0.3	3.6±0.6	0.4±0.1
Liver	4.1±0.5[c]	1.4±0.2	0.10±0.02[d]
Plasma	2.3±0.7	Not detectable	Not detectable
Kidney	8.9±1.5[c]	2.3±0.7	0.20±0.03

[a] A 100-μl dose was applied over a surface area of 5 cm² for 3 hr.
[b] N = 7 for DFP and N = 8 for malathion and parathion.
[c] Significance of the difference between blood and tissue concentrations, $p < 0.01$.
[d] Significance, $p < 0.05$.
Source: Marty (1976).

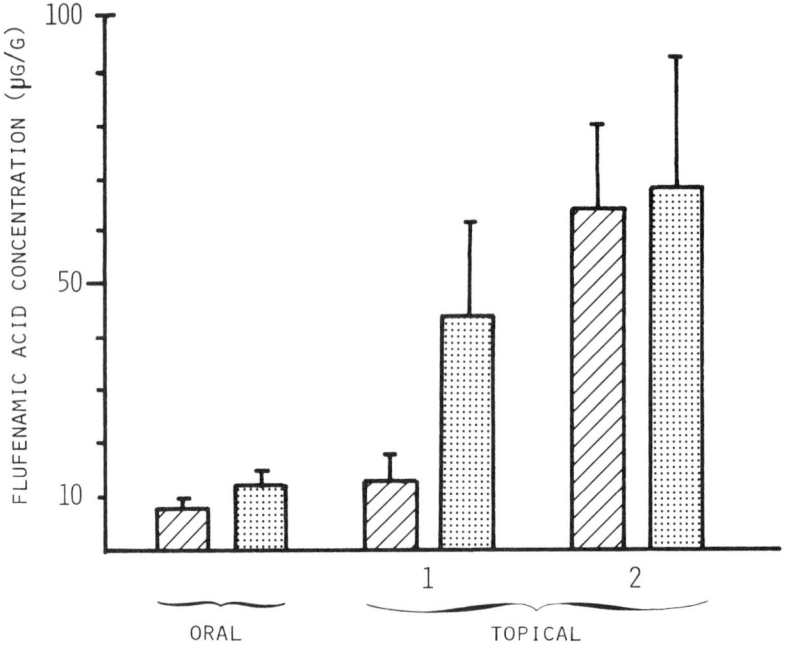

Figure 3 Flufenamic acid distribution in rat tissues 180 min after oral administration and after percutaneous application. ▤, Subcutaneous tissue; ▨, subcutaneous muscle. 1, tissues located around the application area; 2, tissues located beneath the application area (oral dose = 100 mg; topical dose = 16.5 mg/20 cm²). (From Panse et al. 1974.)

Ishihama et al. (1979) reported that indomethacin (ID) penetrated percutaneously into guinea pig skin and muscles after topical application of a gel containing 1% drug. ID was applied on the back once every 12 hr; the tissue distribution was evaluated after 1 to 20 dosings. The radioactivity was measured in the skin and the muscles beneath the application area, which was divided into two parts: a shallow part (2-4 mm in depth from the skin surface) and a deep part (4-6 mm). After five applications, the ID concentration in the skin reached a constant level of about 400 µg/g. During the same period the concentration of ID reached a constant level of about 0.7 µg/g in the shallow part of the muscle. In the deep part of the muscle the average detected amount of ID was 0.2 µg/g after 10 applications of the ointment (i.e., after 5 days). However, the concentration of ID in the skin and muscle of nonapplied portion was negligible. These results show that topically applied ID penetrates through the skin and reaches the muscle as deep as 5 mm from the surface without appreciable systemic distribution. Furthermore, the ID concentration in the muscle increased to a constant level after multiple applications.

Wada et al. (1981) then studied percutaneous absorption and distribution of ID in rats. The right hind paws of the animals were treated under occlusion with 100 mg of an ointment containing 1% of the [^{14}C]ID. Two hours postapplication the ointment was removed and a carrageenan solution injected subcutaneously in both hind paws. Three hours later the rats were sacrificed and the radioactivity measured in blood and in total exudate and muscle from inflamed tissues of both paws. The measured ID concentrations are in Table 8. The radioactivity levels in the exudate and muscle of the treated paw were, respectively, 72 and 7 times higher than in the blood. Likewise, the amounts detected in the contralateral paw were 36 and 10 times lower.

Under the same conditions of time and treatment, the edema volume of both hind paws was measured using a plethysmometer. ID significantly inhibited inflammation in the treated paw only; it had no influence on the edema of the

Table 8 Distribution of Radioactivity in the Carrageenan-Induced Paw Edema of Rats After Topical Application of 1% [^{14}C]Indomethacin Ointment

	Concentration in tissues (µg/g)			E/B	M/B
	Exudate, E	Muscle, M	Blood, B		
Applied foot, F_A	60.4±15.5	6.09±1.47	0.84±0.13	72	7
Nonapplied foot, F_N	1.68±0.23	0.61±0.08		2	0.7
F_A/F_N	36	10	–	–	–

Source: Wada et al. (1981).

nonapplied paw. The authors concluded that topically applied ID accumulates in the inflammatory site to produce local pharmacological effects in rats. These effects did not extend to the contralateral paw tissues, where the ID concentrations are close to the blood level.

In a recent paper, Rabinowitz et al. (1982) studied the local, articular, and systemic absorption of oral and topical salicylates in dogs and man using radioisotope techniques. Specifically, tissue disposition following oral [^{14}C] aspirin was compared to that after topical administration of triethanolamine [^{14}C] salicylate. In the canine part of the study, one group of five beagles received per os a 500-mg capsule of [^{14}C] aspirin; a second group had administered to the shaved right knee 10 g of labeled triethanolamine salicylate cream. Urine and blood samples were taken at 30 and 60 min and the animals were then sacrificed and various tissue samples taken for salicylate disposition analysis (see Table 9). In the human experiments, six subjects with seropositive adult-onset rheumatoid arthritis and active knee synovitis were studied. Each subject was dosed, on separate occasions, with an oral [^{14}C] aspirin capsule and topically with 10 g of triethanolamine [^{14}C] salicylate cream to one knee; 2-6 weeks elapsed between the two administrations. Blood and urine samples were taken pretreatment and 60 and 120 min postdosing. At 120 min a synovial fluid aspiration was performed, taking care to avoid sample contamination from the application site.

Table 9 Canine Study: Average Concentration of [^{14}C] Salicylate (± SEM) in Tissue After Oral and Topical Salicylate Administration

Tissue	Concentration in tissue (μg/g)	
	Oral	Topical
Blood (30 min)	34.80±2.33	2.60±0.02
Blood (60 min)	30.60±0.24	0.22±0.02
Urine	12.57±5.16	0.16±0.09
Skin	0.64±0.09	312.20±40.80
Muscle	1.76±0.16	38.20±5.16
Fascia	1.04±0.28	16.40±1.96
Fat pad	1.00±0.10	5.60±1.20
Tendon	0.20±0.03	3.00±0.44
Ligament	0.50±0.16	2.00±0.20
Cartilage	0.43±0.03	1.62±0.49
Synovial fluid	1.00±0.10	0.80±0.12
Synovium	0.62±0.10	0.74±0.12

Source: Rabinowitz et al. (1982).

Patients were also asked to rate their subjective pain relief after the two medications.

As Table 9 indicates, canine blood levels achieved after topical dosing were 10-100 times lower than those after oral administration of an equimolecular quantity of salicylate. However, the topical route resulted in higher local salicylate levels: the skin was, expectedly, highest but superior levels were seen in all local deeper tissues (ligament, tendon, cartilage, fascia, fat). The adjacent muscle showed 20 times more radioactivity posttopical than postoral.

The human results are given in Table 10. Despite blood level differences spanning orders of magnitude (oral ≫ topical), topical dosing produced 60% of the salicylate level in synovial fluid found after oral aspirin. Subjective improvement was reported by two-thirds of the study group for both salicylate administration routes. Hence, once again, topical delivery is seen to produce high local subcutaneous levels of drug despite appreciably reduced blood concentrations. Direct deep penetration is thus the mechanism implicated. The authors of this study concluded that the lipid solubility of triethanolamine salicylate permits it to remain localized and to be slowly absorbed into the blood. This suggested a desirable feature for providing pain relief of local discomfort without systemic side effects.

Parenthetically, a study performed by A. Fujii, L. G. Nutine and E. S. Cook (personal communication, 1982) in the rabbit using two commercial preparations of triethanolamine salicylate found as much salicylate in the muscle beneath the application site as in the same tissue following oral dosing of aspirin. Also, a double-blind investigation carried out by Golden (1978) using similar salicylate preparations on 40 patients again indicated that equally effective subjective pain relief could be attained using topical triethanolamine salicylate as with oral aspirin. The topical delivery route was suggested to offer a superior alternative in the alleviation of certain rheumatic conditions.

Finally, Areh (1982) prepared and studied percutaneous absorption of five salicylate derivatives: diethylamine salicylate, triethanolamine salicylate, glycol

Table 10 Human Study. Average Concentration of [^{14}C] Salicylate (± SEM) in Tissue 1 and 2 hr After Oral and Topical Salicylate Administration

Tissue	Concentration in tissue (μg/ml)			
	Oral, 1 hr: $N = 6$	Oral, 2 hr: $N = 4$	Topical, 1 hr: $N = 6$	Topical, 2 hr: $N = 4$
Blood	10.27±1.04	10.33±1.06	0.03±0.00	0.08±0.01
Urine	0.64±0.13	1.45±0.27	0.02±0.01	0.18±0.06
Synovial fluid	0.29±0.03	0.40±0.08	0.16±0.02	0.25±0.04

Source: Rabinowitz et al. (1982).

monosalicylate, methyl salicylate, and sodium salicylate. From a polyethylene glycol 400 vehicle, the diffusion through full-thickness rabbit skin in vitro followed the order: glycol monosalicylate > triethanolamine salicylate > diethylamine salicylate > methyl salicylate > sodium salicylate. The results correlated with the compounds' physicochemical properties. A cream and a clear gel were formulated with diethylamine salicylate and applied to the femoral skin areas of rabbits. Two hours later blood, skin, and muscle under the application area were sampled and total salicylate determined. The values obtained for blood, muscle, and skin were, respectively, 0.25, 2.03, and 13.5 mg% for the cream and 0.94, 3.44, and 19 mg% for the gel. These two dosage forms are capable of providing therapeutic salicylate levels in local muscle tissue after transdermal delivery.

Miscellaneous

In the late 1960s Gorog and Kovacs (1968) studied the anti-inflammatory properties of dimethyl sulfoxide (DMSO) in rats. It was found that carrageenan-induced rat paw edema was improved by both oral and topical DMSO therapy. Furthermore, and of greater relevance, arthritis induced by *Mycobacterium* adjuvant was significantly more inhibited by topical, as opposed to oral DMSO administration. In the same way, DMSO applied to the skin of rats with experimental arthritis produced by 6-sulfanilamidazole was also powerfully inhibitory. These early data, therefore, argue strongly for local deep penetration of the solvent.

A more detailed investigation on the disposition of topically applied ^{3}H-labeled escin was performed in mice and rats by Lang (1974). The radioactive compound was applied to the animals' backs, and tissue distribution was subsequently evaluated at various times by organ dissection after sacrifice. The tissues monitored were the back muscles, blood, liver, kidney, heart, lungs, spleen, testes, brain, leg muscle, femur, and stomach lining. In the mouse the amount of activity detected in the back muscle beneath the skin application site exceeded by 20-100 times that amount detected in any of the other regions. A similar pattern of behavior, though less pronounced (10-30 times more in the back muscle) was observed in the rat.

The time course of disposition to the back muscle in the two animals is shown in Figure 4. It is apparent that significant levels of escin are present in the deeper local tissue over prolonged periods of time. A further observation reported in Lang's paper (and elsewhere) implies that all material penetrating the upper skin layers is not immediately subjected to a sink condition. Measurements were made of activity residing in the skin beneath the application site and in several skin strips 0.5 cm wide at distances of 1-5 cm from the center of the application zone. The data for the mouse clearly showed that radial movement of drug within the skin is an additional transport pathway to the expected capillary uptake

Delivery to Muscle and Other Tissue

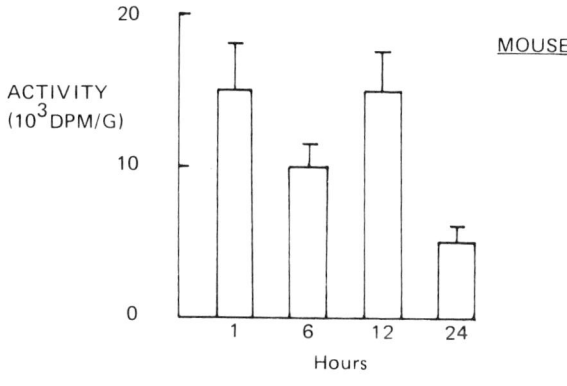

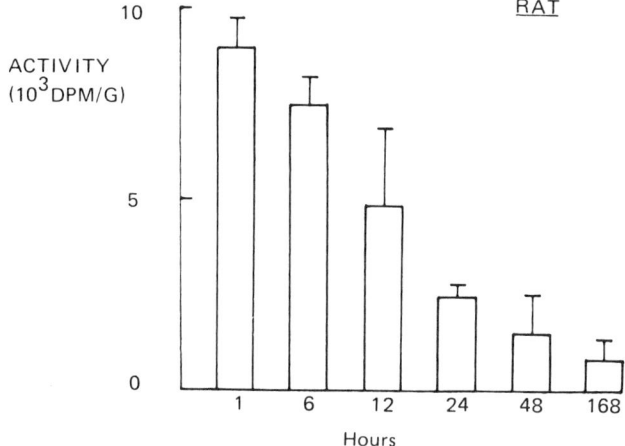

Figure 4 Radioactivity in mouse and rat back muscles at various times after cutaneous application of [^{3}H]escin. (Adapted from Lang, 1974.)

process. It should be pointed out that implied radial movement within the skin has been reported on other occasions (see Guy et al., Chap. 25, this volume).

The study of local subcutaneous delivery of thyroid hormones (thyroxine and triiodothyronine) has been performed by James et al. (1976) in an attempt to explain the localized and deep therapeutic effect of certain dermatologic preparations. The authors demonstrated that percutaneous absorption was accompanied by diffusion and retention in the connective and muscle tissues located beneath the administration area.

Radiolabeled compounds were applied in alcoholic solution to the shorn abdomen or back of Sprague-Dawley rats. The contact zones were protected and covered for periods of 0.5-2 hr. At the end of the test the rat was killed and blood was drawn from the carotid artery. The skin site of application was dissected and fragments of subcutaneous tissue, muscle, and brown interscapular fat were removed from below the contact area. Samples of liver, kidneys, and part of the muscle from a rear paw were also collected and weighed. Liquid scintillation counting was used to determine the radioactive concentrations in the various organs; the results were converted to amounts of drug equivalent present in nanograms per gram of tissue. For thyroxine (Fig. 5) after 1 hr, the levels in plasma, liver, kidneys, and skeletal muscle were not significantly different. Beneath the application area, the radioactive concentration was 100 times greater in the subcutaneous tissue than in the plasma. The subjacent muscle showed the same phenomenon though of less intensity. The ratio of concentra-

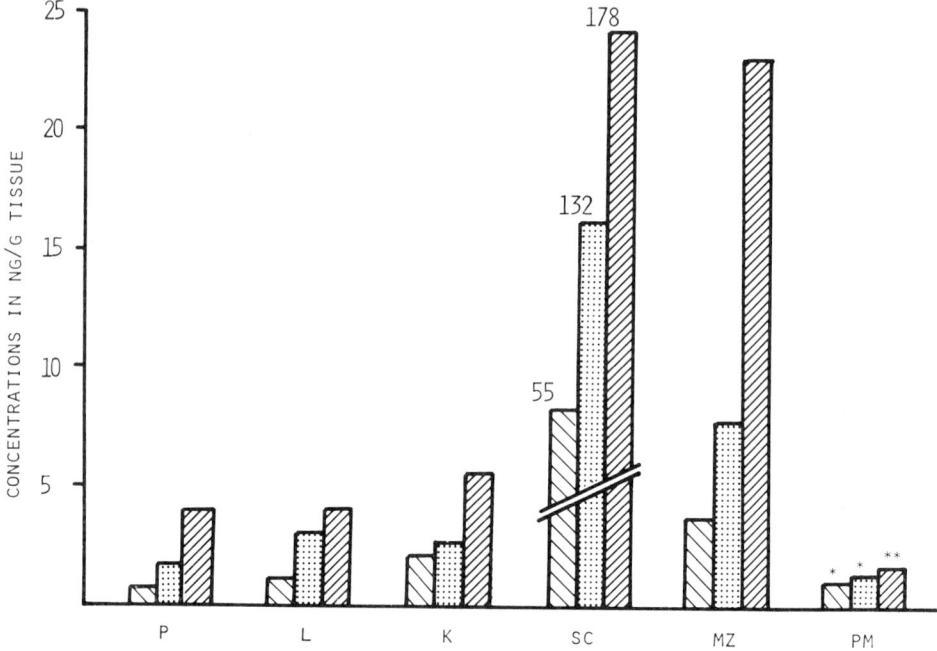

Figure 5 Distribution of [^{125}I] thyroxine in different tissues in the rat after application to the skin: P = plasma, L = liver, K = kidneys, SC = subcutaneous tissue, MZ = muscle under application zone, PM = paw muscle. Significance of difference between MZ and PM: *p < 0.05, **p < 0.01. Experiment duration: ▨ 2 hours, ▧ 0.5 hour, ▦ 1 hour. (Adapted from James et al. 1974.)

Delivery to Muscle and Other Tissue

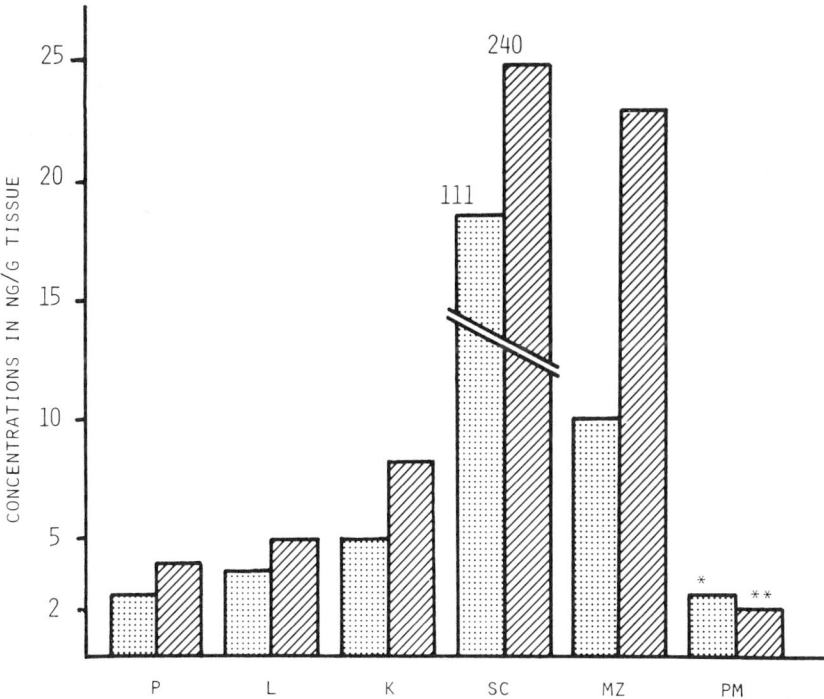

Figure 6 Distribution of [^{125}I] triiodothyronine in different tissues in the rat after application to the skin: P = plasma, L = liver, K = kidneys, SC = subcutaneous tissue, MZ = muscle under application zone, PM = paw muscle. Significance of difference between MZ and PM: *$p < 0.05$, **$p < 0.01$. Experiment duration: ▨ 1 hour, ▨ 2 hours.

tion in muscle below application zone to concentration in paw muscle increased substantially as time increased (4.2 at 30 min, 8.6 at 60 min, and 14.3 at 2 hr). Triiodothyronine (Fig. 6) gave similar results, with much retention in the subcutaneous tissue and deeper muscle. Liver and kidney levels matched the plasma concentration.

CONCLUSIONS

The research summarized in this chapter establishes that the subcutaneous delivery of topically applied chemicals is possible and that the cutaneous microcirculation is not always a perfect "sink" for penetrating molecules. The kinetics and absolute quantification of the phenomenon await further study, however, to determine the significance of the observations discussed in terms of body load and drug delivery. As far as the latter is concerned, a clear clinical advantage appears possible; namely, a concentration of active compound in local muscular tissue in excess of that which may be achieved with practical alternative administration routes. Thus, improved therapy is attainable with fewer potential side effects (i.e., much lower systemic drug levels). The pharmacological and pharmacokinetic ramifications of the experimental work presented, therefore, will no doubt be studied extensively in the not too distant future.

ACKNOWLEDGMENTS

This work was supported in part by National Institutes of Health grant (RHG) 1-R01-OH01830-01. An initial account of the literature reviewed here was reported by R. H. Guy and H. I. Maibach: "Drug delivery to local subcutaneous structures following topical administration," *Journal of Pharmaceutical Sciences*, 72 (1983) 1375-1380.

REFERENCES

Areh, O. M. (1982). Ph.D. thesis. Massachusetts College of Pharmacy and Allied Health Science, Boston.

Golden, E. L. (1978). A double-blind comparison of orally ingested aspirin and a topically applied salicylate cream in the relief of rheumatic pain. *Curr. Ther. Res.* 24:524-529.

Gorog, P. and Kovacs, I. B. (1968). Effect of dimethyl sulphoxide (DMSO) on various experimental inflammations. *Curr. Ther. Res.* 10:486-492.

Ishihama, H., Kimata, H., and Mizushima, Y. (1979). Percutaneous penetration of indomethacin. *Experientia* 35:798-799.

James, M., Marty, J.-P., and Wepierre, J. (1974). Diffusion localisée des substances absorbées par voie percutanée. *C.R. Hebd. Séances Acad. Sci. Ser. D* 278:2063-2066.

James, M., Marty, J.-P., and Wepierre, J. (1975). Comparison de l'absorption et de la distribution de la dexaméthasone ^{3}H après administration par voie percutanée ou orale chez la souris et le rat. *C.R. Hebd. Séances Acad. Sci. Ser. D 281*:1525-1528.

James, M., Marty, J.-P., and Wepierre, J. (1976). Percutaneous absorption of dexamethasone-^{3}H in rats and mice: Comparative study with oral administration. *Eur. J. Drug Metab. Pharmacokinet.* 2:69-72.

Lang, V. W. (1974). Untersuchungen zur perkutanen Absorption von ^{3}H-Aescin bei Maus und Ratte. *Arzneim.-Forsch.* 24:71-76.

Marty, J.-P. (1976). Ph.D. thesis. Université de Paris-Sud.

Marty, J.-P., James, M., Hajo, N., and Wepierre, J. (1980). Percutaneous absorption of estradiol and progesterone: Pharmacokinetic studies. In *Percutaneous Penetration of Steroids*. Edited by P. Mauvais-Jarvis, C. F. H. Vickers, and J. Wepierre. Academic, New York, pp. 205-218.

Panse, V. P., Zeiller, P., and Sensch, K. H. (1974). Zur perkutanen Resorption von antiphlogistisch wirksamen Substanzen. *Arzneim.-Forsch.* 24:1298-1301.

Rabinowitz, J. L., Feldman, E. S., Weinberger, A., and Schumacher, H. R. (1982). Comparative tissue absorption of oral [^{14}C] aspirin and topical triethanolamine [^{14}C] salicylate in human and canine knee joints. *J. Clin. Pharmacol.* 22:42-48.

Wada, Y., Etoh, Y., Ohira, A., Kimata, H. Koide, T., Ishihama, H., and Mizushima, Y. (1982). Percutaneous absorption and anti-inflammatory activity of indomethacin in ointment. *J. Pharm. Pharmacol.* 34:467-468.

37
Optimizing Percutaneous Absorption

Brian W. Barry
University of Bradford, Bradford, West Yorkshire, England

How to optimize topical formulations so that they provide controlled bioavailability of the incorporated drug is an important quest in modern therapy. Dermatologists prescribe traditional preparations, such as creams or ointments, with the usual intention of treating a skin disease by direct application; however, general physicians may also use ointments or transdermal devices to deliver drugs through the integument so as to achieve a systemic effect (e.g., with scopolamine, nitroglycerin, clonidine, or estradiol). For both approaches, the product may control the rate and extent of drug delivery to the biophase—the bioavailability—in two main ways, which may be used singly or combined (Barry, 1983). In the first scheme, the medicament exhibits its maximum chemical potential, and thus its maximum thermodynamic activity, within the vehicle. Thus, the formulator designs the preparation or device without deliberately modifying the barrier properties of the stratum corneum, but arranges for the drug to have a maximum tendency to leave the system and partition into the skin. This escaping tendency is quantified by the chemical potential μ. In general, the potential of a component is the same in all the phases of a system at equilibrium and at a fixed temperature and pressure, and it relates to the activity a by:

$$\mu = \mu^0 + RT \ln a \tag{1}$$

where μ^0 is the standard potential, R is the gas constant, and T is the absolute temperature.

The second method of approach deliberately decreases the barrier resistance of the stratum corneum, dynamically and reversibly, by inserting penetration enhancers into the tissue.

This chapter illustrates these concepts by discussing some of the work performed at Bradford University and Portsmouth Polytechnic, under two categories: cadaver skin experiments (in vitro approach) and vasoconstrictor assays (in vivo procedure). Each division examines some thermodynamic control methods and the value of penetration enhancers.

CADAVER SKIN EXPERIMENTS: IN VITRO METHODS

Thermodynamic Control

When we consider how vehicle formulation may control drug flux through the skin (under conditions in which the tissue remains unmodified), the permeation model incorporates certain assumptions (Poulsen, 1972). In its most restrictive form this model assumes that the skin is a homogeneous, intact membrane without shunt routes, with the stratum corneum providing the rate-limiting step during release and absorption of the drug. Noninteracting, nonionic diffusing species behave ideally, being unaffected by pH changes in the vehicle. Only the drug diffuses out of the formulation—other compounds do not leave (by evaporation or permeation), and skin secretions do not enter the product. The diffusion coefficient is invariant with time or position in the vehicle or horny layer; the viable tissues provide sink conditions. The donor phase does not deplete nor the skin change its permeability; the drug remains unaltered (e.g., no degradation or metabolism). An expression for flux estimates at steady state, as deduced from the diffusional model for simple zero-order flux under Fickian conditions (Crank, 1975) is:

$$J = \frac{KCD}{h} \tag{2}$$

where J is the steady-state flux of penetrant per unit area of the skin; K is the partition coefficient between the stratum corneum and the formulation; C is the dissolved, *effective* concentration of the drug in the vehicle; D is the diffusion coefficient of the penetrant within the stratum corneum; and h is the horny layer thickness.

Workers often use Equation (2) to develop topical products; but flux measurements require multiple, lengthy diffusion experiments with limited supplies of variable human skin. They could simply optimize K and C, assuming that D and h are constant; however, difficulties still remain in determining K for human skin and in measuring C in the vehicle (bearing in mind that C represents the concentration of drug freely available for diffusion within the vehicle and for partitioning into the skin). Thus, it would be valuable to be able to relate some simple physicochemical property of a drug in its vehicle, however complex the vehicle, to the flux developed through the skin. This could lead, in principle, to the prospect of predicting, controlling, and optimizing the bioavailability of a drug while using only the minimum number of diffusion experiments to confirm theoretical estimates.

Now, rewriting Equation (2) produces:

$$J = \frac{aD}{\gamma h} \tag{3}$$

where a is the thermodynamic activity of a drug in its vehicle and γ is the effective activity coefficient of the molecule within the skin barrier. As T. Higuchi (1960) indicated, Equation (3) predicts that under ideal conditions (as defined previously) the drug flux through the skin should be directly proportional to drug activity in the vehicle, provided D, γ, and h remain constant. One direct corollary of Equation (3) is that for maximum flux, the penetrant should exhibit its highest activity in the vehicle. The limiting value for this activity at equilibrium is that of the pure form of the substance at the environmental temperature and pressure (we will not concern ourselves with high-energy polymorphs or supersaturated solutions). Now all vehicles that contain the drug as a finely ground suspension also exist as saturated solutions of the drug. The thermodynamic activity of this dissolved drug is also maximal, being equal to that of the solid drug with which it is in equilibrium, and thus all such vehicles should produce the same maximum penetration rate. (This treatment assumes that the composition or structure of the crystal phase is identical in each vehicle. We can also note that the chemical potential and the thermodynamic activity must remain the same in all saturated vehicles, if we refer all measurements to the same standard state of the solute—Eq. (1).) We need to reemphasize that Equation (3) applies to *ideal* conditions, including the special requirements here that the different vehicles do not themselves affect the skin's properties and the particles must dissolve fast enough to maintain a constant donor concentration in the vehicle; that is, dissolution must not become rate limiting during the permeation process.

To test the hypothesis that the drug flux should relate directly to the thermodynamic activity (under ideal conditions), we chose as a model penetrant benzyl alcohol and used a variety of simple liquids as vehicles: butan-1-ol, butyl acetate, toluene, isopropyl myristate, *n*-heptane, propylene carbonate, and isophorone (Harrison et al., 1982; Barry et al., 1985a). To measure thermodynamic activity, we used headspace analysis by gas chromatography, with the GC response to pure benzyl alcohol vapor representing unit activity. We then related the activity of the benzyl alcohol to its mole fraction in each vehicle. (A useful way of thinking about thermodynamic activity is that it represents the "escaping" tendency of a molecule from a vehicle or system; headspace analysis measures the actual equilibrium amount of material—per unit volume—that is released by a vehicle,

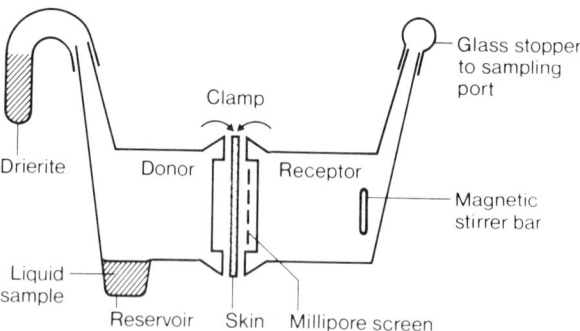

Figure 1 Glass cell for measuring vapor diffusion through skin: D, donor compartment; R, receptor compartment; M, skin membrane; P, sampling port; BM, bar magnet; SS, stainless steel support; W, well; Dr, drierite.

and this concentration, expressed as a ratio of the vapor concentration provided by the pure compound, provides a measure of the activity.)

Using binary mixtures of benzyl alcohol in the various solvents (at 0.5 mole fraction), we determined the benzyl alcohol vapor flux through dermatomed human abdominal skin mounted in a diffusion cell at 30°C (Fig. 1). The receptor solution (equal parts of ethanol and water) was sampled and analyzed by GC. As predicted by Equation (3), the steady-state vapor fluxes increased linearly with activity as found by headspace analysis, provided the solvent did not damage the skin (Fig. 2). It thus seems that this approach could be useful for preliminary experiments aimed at optimizing the bioavailability of a topical formulation. However, further work showed that fluxes developed from the liquid state (i.e., when the vehicle contacted the stratum corneum directly) were higher than vapor fluxes (Harrison et al., 1983; Barry et al., 1985b). This suggests that interfacial effects are important in a comparison of vapor rates with liquid rates and that vapor analyses may reveal only *trends*, not absolute values, relative to clinical fluxes.

Penetration Enhancers

Nontoxic substances that temporarily diminish the impermeability of the stratum corneum may promote drug penetration for local and for systemic effects. Such materials may be called accelerants, sorption promoters, or penetration enhancers (Allenby et al., 1969; Ritschel, 1969; for a review, see Barry, 1983). We are interested here in compounds that significantly enhance drug penetration through the horny layer without irritating or damaging the viable tissues; our definition implies a reversible change in the specific barrier properties of the surface layer. Katz and Poulsen (1971) detailed a spectrum of properties the ideal penetration enhancer should possess; although no candidate employed

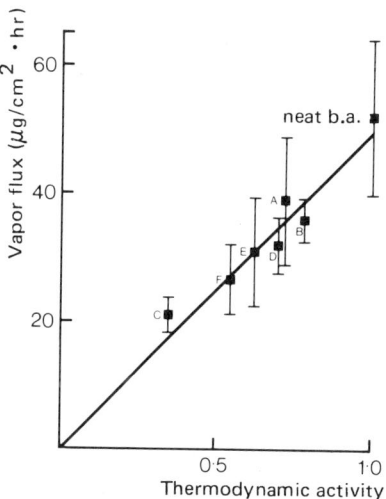

Figure 2 Benzyl alcohol vapor diffusion through human skin and its dependence on thermodynamic activity in the vehicle as measured by headspace analysis; benzyl alcohol presented neat and as 0.5 mole fraction binary mixtures with designated solvents: A, isopropyl myristate; B, toluene; C, isophorone; D, propylene carbonate; E, butan-1-ol; F, butyl acetate; b.a., benzyl alcohol. (From Harrison et al., 1982.)

so far exhibits all these attributes, some substances have shown sufficient promise for limited clinical use. However, a more cautious approach now tempers the initial excessive enthusiasm for some enhancers.

In the past, the most widely used penetration enhancers were the aprotic solvents—dimethyl sulfoxide, dimethylformamide, and dimethylacetamide (Fig. 3). They accelerate the permeation of many drugs, including antifungal agents, antibiotics, barbiturates, steroids, and local anesthetics, and they enhance stratum corneum reservoirs (e.g., for griseofulvin and corticosteroids). However, initial optimism for these solvents has been reduced because of irritancy, toxicity, and odor (dimethylsulfide, a metabolite of dimethyl sulfoxide, produces a foul breath). The pyrrolidones also promote skin penetration and establish drug reservoirs in the horny layer and in the nails (Resh and Stoughton, 1976; Southwell and Barry, 1983). Azone (Fig. 4), a relative newcomer to the clinic, is being actively promoted for use with antifungals, antibacterials, steroids, and so on, as well as compounds in development (Stoughton, 1981, 1982; Stoughton and McClure, 1983).

Surfactants may promote absorption via the appendages by lowering interfacial tensions; anionics in particular may also reduce horny layer resistance by altering keratin helices and interacting with binding sites. Long-chain derivatives

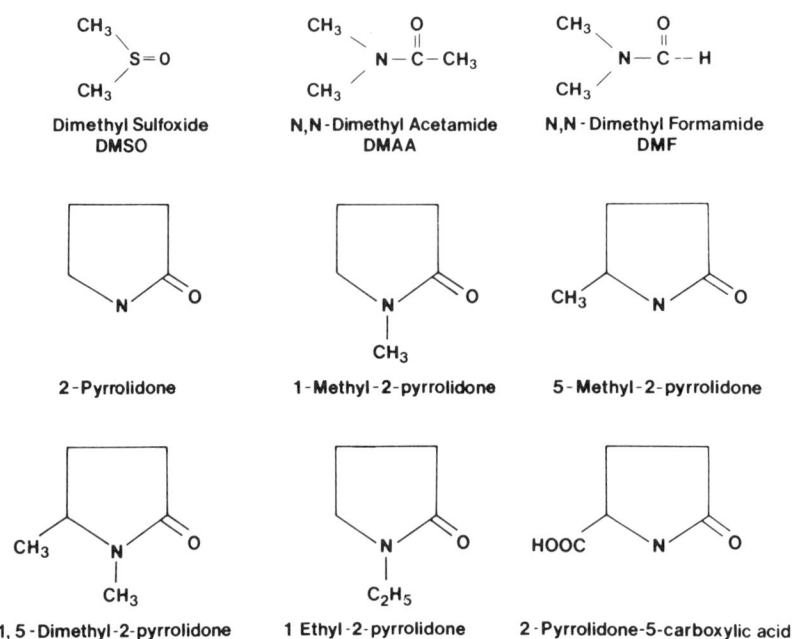

Figure 3 Examples of suggested penetration enhancers: aprotic solvents and pyrrolidone derivatives.

of sulfoxides may act similarly and thus also promote polar route penetration. Combinations of oleic acid (or other long-chain compounds with cis double bonds or a bulky chain), dissolved in a solvent such as propylene glycol, may boost nonpolar penetration (Cooper, 1984). Other candidates include phosphine oxides, sugar esters, tetrahydrofurfuryl alcohol, urea, diethyl-*m*-toluamide, and any material that raises the water content in the stratum corneum.

We investigated many possible penetration enhancers, using pseudo-steady-state experiments and in vivo mimic designs. In our mimic arrangement, the

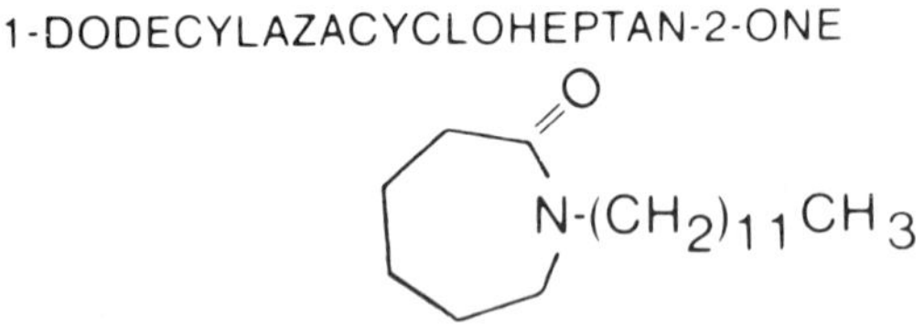

Figure 4 Azone, the latest penetration enhancer.

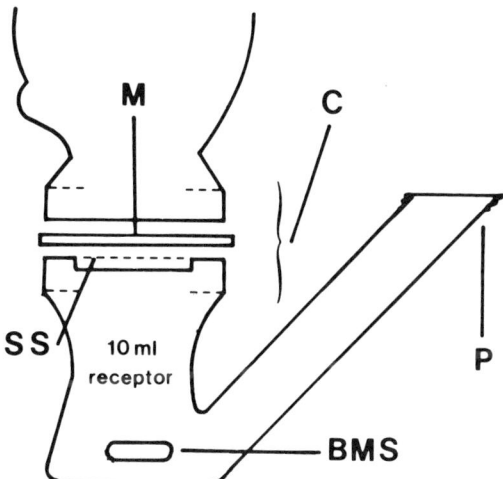

Figure 5 Glass cell for measuring diffusion under simulated in vivo conditions: C, clamp; M, skin membrane; SS, stainless steel support; P, sampling port; BMS, bar magnet stirrer.

horny layer is in contact with controlled environmental conditions (e.g., 22°C and 60% relative humidity) and the receptor solution is at body temperature (Fig. 5). The drug may be applied in a volatile or nonvolatile solvent, in a semisolid preparation, or in a drug device. Water and temperature gradients develop across the skin, similar to those operating in vivo. The investigator may control skin hydration, observe the effects of dose size variation, multiple application, and washing procedures, and monitor the action of penetration enhancers. We can therefore study the absorption of compounds in a form and dose most applicable to their in vivo use (Franz, 1978).

As an example of work with penetration enhancers, Figure 6 illustrates penetration data for Ibuprofen (a nonsteroidal anti-inflammatory agent) after deposition from acetone onto dermatomed skin clamped in an open cell. The plots show the cumulative amount of drug penetrated M and the derived flux J, and the effects of acetone deposition, occlusion, and the addition of the enhancer N-methyl-2-pyrrolidone. A clear rate maximum arises from drug partitioning from the solvent and subsequent permeation; this peak falls as the dissolution rate of drug crystals on the skin surface becomes the rate-limiting step in percutaneous absorption. Occlusion does not increase the dissolution rate, and therefore it does not affect the flux. Addition of the pyrrolidone redissolves the Ibuprofen and accelerates its penetration through the skin, producing a marked increase in the flux profile (Akhter and Barry, 1985; Akhter et al., 1982).

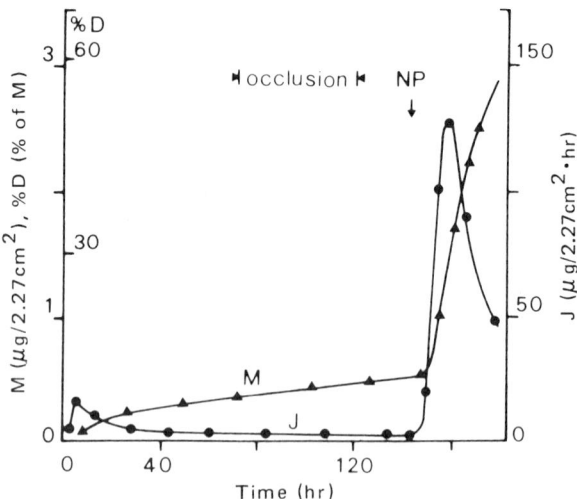

Figure 6 The absorption through human skin of Ibuprofen under in vivo mimic conditions and the effects of occlusion and the addition of N-methyl-2-pyrrolidone (NP); M is the cumulative amount penetrated, %D is the percent of dose applied, and J is the derived flux.

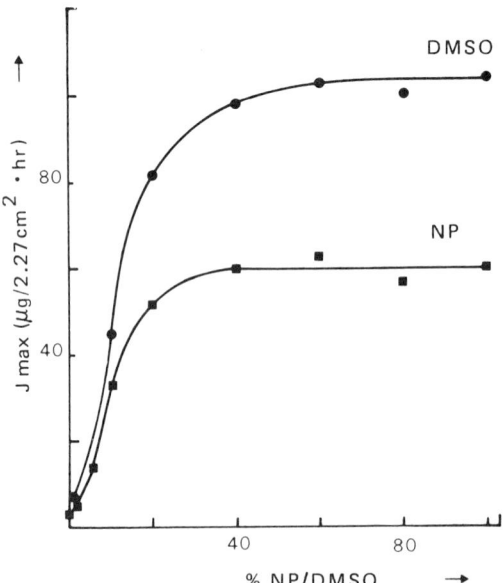

Figure 7 The penetration of Flurbiprofen through human skin under in vivo mimic conditions and the effect of dimethyl sulfoxide (DMSO) and N-methyl-2-pyrrolidone (NP) aqueous solutions on the maximum flux, J_{max}. (From Akhter and Barry, 1983.)

Akhter and Barry (1983) used a similar agent, Flurbiprofen, to investigate the enhancer activities of the pyrrolidone and dimethyl sulfoxide, as functions of concentration (Fig. 7). The in vivo mimic approach showed that these accelerants operated at relatively low initial concentrations and that the effect leveled off at about 40% enhancer concentration.

We now consider some results obtained in healthy volunteers.

VASOCONSTRICTOR ASSAY: IN VIVO METHOD

The vasoconstrictor bioassay for topical steroids is an excellent procedure for assessing the combination of intrinsic activity at a receptor site and skin penetrability of a topical corticosteroid. The assay can assess factors that modify drug bioavailability by scoring the skin pallor induced in volunteers. We can screen novel synthetic steroids for clinical efficacy, develop topical formulations, test marketed preparations and rank them in terms of clinical efficacy, perform fundamental studies on percutaneous absorption, and generate dosage regimens for topical steroids (Barry, 1983). The term "bioavailability" in this context means the relative absorption efficiency for a medicament as illustrated by steroid release from the formulation and subsequent penetration through the stratum corneum and viable tissues to initiate the characteristic blanching response (Barry, 1976). Thus, the intensity and duration of steroid-induced pallor assesses both corticosteroid activity and bioavailability from different vehicles via a pharmacological response (Barry and Woodford, 1978).

Our modification of the *occluded* vasoconstrictor assay uses a panel of 10 volunteers selected to provide a balance of good, medium, and poor responders. We apply 5 ± 1 mg (or μl) of each formulation to the washed flexor surface of both forearms, using as application sites paired 7×7 mm^2 areas punched out from double-sided adhesive Blenderm polyethylene tape. The sites are occluded with Melinex film for 6 hr; we then wash the regions with soap and water at body temperature, dry, and assess the pallor 10 min later using a 0-4 scale with half-point ratings. Subsequent readings provide data points for skin blanching over 5 days. A full blanching profile may be drawn from the average results of 10 volunteers (20 replicates of each formulation).

Our *nonoccluded* bioassay is similar, except that after applying samples to the skin, we remove the Blenderm tapes and use a protective perforated plastic secreen for 6 hr instead of the Melinex film.

Thermodynamic Control

We used the occluded vasoconstrictor assay to test the bioavailability of mechlorisone dibutyrate at 0.2% concentration in six experimental solutions (Woodford and Barry, 1982). These solutions were blended from various polar solvents (hexylene glycol, propylene glycol, propylene carbonate, polyethylene glycol 400, and water). Within each solution, the solvent composition was adjusted so that the steroid was at 90% saturation (i.e., ideally at the same chemical potential and thermodynamic activity). This assumption is a simplification, because the potential in a real system depends on concentration in different ways for diverse nonideal systems. However, the assumption that all formulations were initially at the same potential provides us with a starting point to examine any deviations from theory.

Figure 8 illustrates blanching curves derived by plotting the percent total possible score (a measure of the blanching response) against time. Table 1 com-

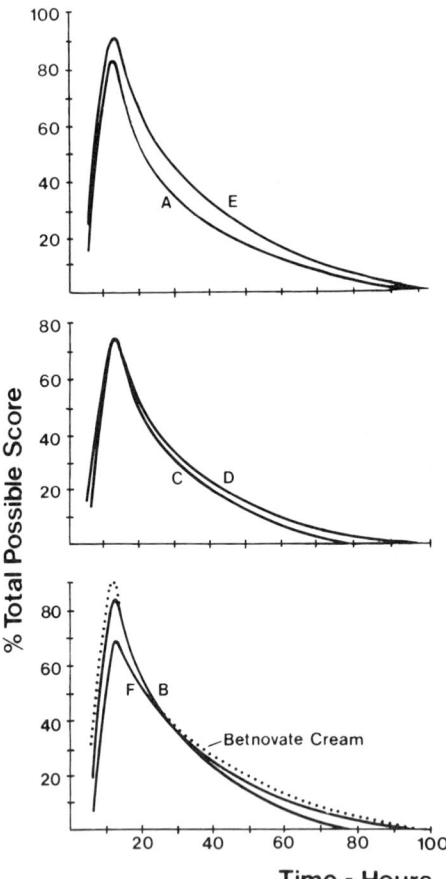

Figure 8 Blanching curves for 0.2% steroid solutions and for control preparation, Betnovate Cream; thermodynamic control experiments.

Table 1 Blanching Responses to 0.2% Steroid Solutions, Arranged in Rank Order of Area Under the Curve Values

Solution	Area under the curve (% × h)	Summed % total possible score	$T_m/10$ mean value[a]	Bioavailability[b] (i)	Bioavailability[b] (ii)
E	2650	413	5.72	1.00	1.00
A	2140	345	5.23	0.81	0.84
B	2080	339	5.18	0.79	0.82
D	1910	305	4.92	0.72	0.74
F	1780	265	4.59	0.67	0.64
C	1720	282	4.73	0.65	0.68

[a]The minimum significant range value k = 0.28 (p = 0.05). That is, if the $T_m/10$ values of the two preparations differ by more than 0.28, there is a significant difference between these preparations.
[b]Defined by the relationships:

$$\frac{\text{"area under the curve" for preparation}}{\text{"area under the curve" for most active preparation}} \quad (i)$$

$$\frac{\text{summed \% total possible score for preparation}}{\text{summed \% total possible score for most active preparation}} \quad (ii)$$

Source: Modified from Woodford and Barry (1982).

pares the different steroid solutions using three parameters: the summed percent total possible score, the square root transformation of the sum of scores divided by the number of volunteers $T_m/10$ (this parameter allows the solutions to be ranked statistically), and the area-under-curve values. The table also includes two ways for assessing steroid bioavailability.

Our data reveal that there *were* statistically significant differences between the solutions (Table 1); this may have been because the solvent compounds were not truly inert. (This is not surprising; topical vehicle components are seldom entirely inactive—see Barry, 1983.) For example, individual solvents could have acted as penetration enhancers, skin irritants, or dehydrating agents, or they could have complexed with the steroid and thus reduced its thermodynamic activity.

If the test had compared only pairs of similar solvent systems, many of these complications would be common to members of each pair and the situation would be clearer. Therefore a second series of formulations used the same solvents (but in slightly different ratios within any one pair) to maintain constant the thermodynamic activity of the steroid while its overall concentration was either 0.1 or 0.2% (both still at 90% saturation). The results in Figure 9 and Table 2 show that within any solvent system, there was no significant difference between gels containing different *concentrations* of steroid (p = 0.05). This finding accords with thermodynamic predictions on the basis that the complicating effects mentioned previously would be approximately constant within any one pair of formulations. However it is interesting to note that there may be a concentration effect in that the lower strengths of steroid always provided a diminished response (within each pair), although the differences were not statistically significant.

Penetration Enhancers

An extension of our work on the bioavailability optimization of steroids moved on from the thermodynamic approach to use the alternative strategy of incorporating penetration enhancers in the formulation. The first trial assessed the bioavailability of 0.1% betamethasone-17-benzoate presented in several potential enhancers, using the standard occluded vasoconstrictor assay. As candidates we selected some pyrrolidones, 2-pyrrolidone (2-P), N-methyl-2-pyrrolidone (NMP), 1-ethyl-2-pyrrolidone (EP), the aprotic solvent dimethylformamide (DMF), diethyl-m-toluamide (DEET, a compound recently investigated as an enhancer), and propylene glycol (PG, a popular solvent in dermatological formulations). Since DEET is a skin irritant, we also used a 75% solution in ethanol (DEET 75%) to reduce the possibility of erythema. Acetone (AC) provided an example of a volatile solvent that would rapidly evaporate and precipitate steroid crystals on the skin; dimethylisosorbide (DMI) served as a baseline vehicle with which to

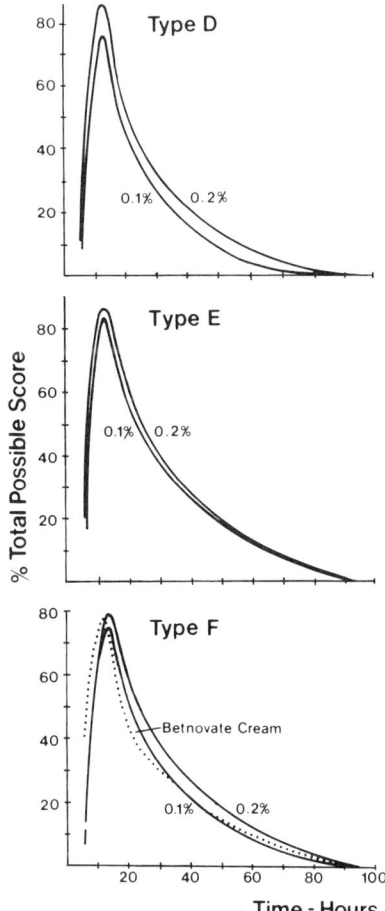

Figure 9 Blanching curves for 0.1 and 0.2% steroid gels and for control preparation, Betnovate Cream; thermodynamic control experiments.

compare the other materials. This trial looked simply for dramatic effects, and so the test solutions were not adjusted to the same thermodynamic activity of the steroid, nor did we allow for different partition coefficients—stratum corneum to solvent (Barry et al., 1984).

The type of analysis detailed in the preceding section indicated that only NMP increased the steroid bioavailability compared with DMI; acetone, DMF, 2-P, and EP were equal to DMI, while PG, DEET, and DEET 75% were poorer. Figure 10 illustrates these results in the form of a histogram of the bioavailabilities,

Table 2 Blanching Responses to Steroid Gels

Gel	Area under the curve (% × h)	Summed % total possible score	$T_m/10$ mean value[a]	Bioavailability[b]	
				(i)	(ii)
E 0.2%	2430	412	5.68	1.00	1.00
E 0.1%	2240	380	5.48	0.92	0.92
F 0.2%	2220	331	5.10	1.00	1.00
F 0.1%	1890	304	4.90	0.85	0.92
D 0.2%	2020	336	5.14	1.00	1.00
D 0.1%	1590	281	4.71	0.79	0.84

[a]The minimum significant range value $k = 0.58$. See note a, Table 1, for definition of T_m.
[b]As defined in Table 1, note b.
Source: Modified from Woodford and Barry (1982).

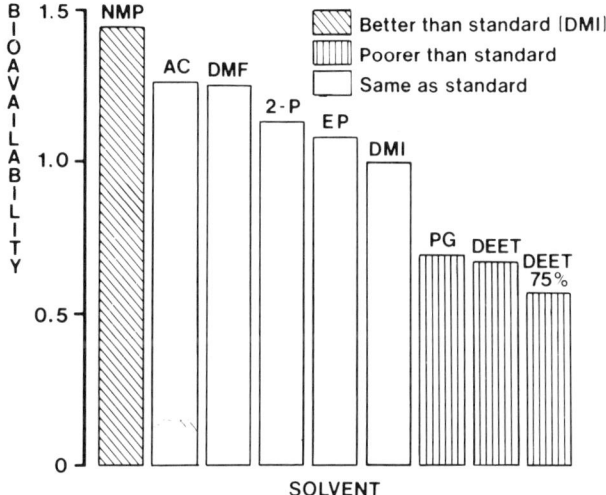

Figure 10 Histogram of the bioavailabilities of steroid solutions; penetration enhancer experiments: NMP, N-methyl-2-pyrrolidone; AC, acetone; DMF, dimethylformamide; 2-P, 2-pyrrolidone; EP, N-ethyl-2-pyrrolidone; DMI, dimethylisosorbide; PG, propylene glycol; DEET, diethyl-m-toluamide; DEET 75%, diethyl-m-toluamide in ethanol.

defined as the area under the blanching curve for the steroid in the test solvent divided by the area for the steroid in DMI.

This experiment has at least two drawbacks: the lack of thermodynamic control and the *occluded* test procedure. This chapter has discussed the importance of correct thermodynamic control; the effect of excessive skin hydration is probably at least as important. Because water is such a good penetration enhancer, it is possible that the marked effect of occlusive hydration obscured the enhancing abilities of the other solvents.

Our second trial therefore maintained the thermodynamic activity of the steroid approximately constant at 10% saturation and tested the formulations using a *nonoccluded* blanching assay, to avoid the swamping effect of hydrating fully the stratum corneum (Bennett et al., 1985). It used aqueous solutions of 2-P, NMP, DMF, PG, and DMI. In some systems we also incorporated 2% Azone (A), 1.5% oleic acid (OA), or 5% OA; these concentrations provided saturated solutions of A or OA, that is, maximum thermodynamic activities of these enhancers.

A histogram (Fig. 11) showed that now 2-P, NMP, PG + OA, PG + A, and DMF increased the bioavailability of the steroid compared with the DMI standard. An

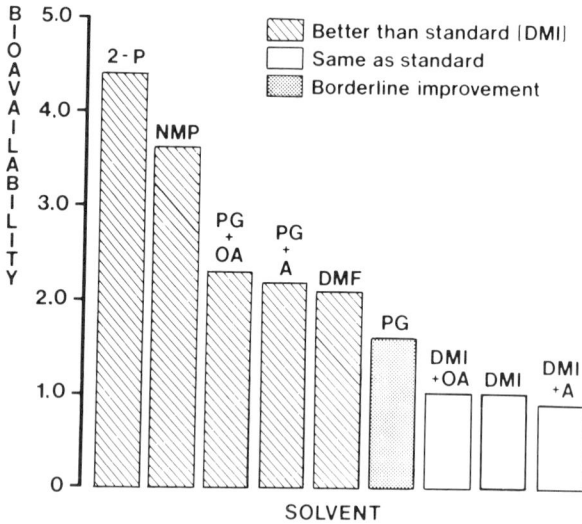

Figure 11 Histogram of bioavailabilities of steroid solutions of controlled thermodynamic activities; penetration enhancer experiments. Key as for Figure 10, plus OA, oleic acid; A, azone.

interesting feature of these results is that OA acted as penetration enhancers only when disolved in PG, and not when incorporated into DMI. For enhancer activity, cis isomers such as oleic acid need to be presented to the skin dissolved in specific polar solvents such as PG (Cooper, 1984). Our results tentatively suggest that the same may be true for Azone.

CORRELATION BETWEEN OPTIMIZATION THEORY AND CLINICAL EFFICACY

The schemes detailed previously for developing topical preparations depend either on in vitro experiments or the cooperation of *healthy* volunteers. It seems appropriate therefore to discuss briefly the many differences between the simple assumptions of laboratory work and what happens in a patient.

During developmental work, investigators often apply model formulations of compounds to membranes they assume to be uniform and homogeneous; pseudo-steady-state designs maintain experimental conditions as near constant as practicable. However, clinical formulations are usually complex, multiphase preparations applied to deranged skin, which is a laminated, specialized, dynamic structure; and interactions lead to many infringements of simple postulates. For example, we usually assume that the stratum corneum provides the rate-limiting step in percutaneous absorption. However, disease and damage, or an occlusive vehicle raising skin hydration and temperature, may all increase permeability and thus reduce the resistance role of the horny layer. After skin application, the dermatological formulation may change in ways that reduce drug diffusion within the vehicle and release from the applied layer. Such variations may cause the base to control transdermal input, not the skin.

The skin is laminated, pierced by appendages, and it is far from a simple, homogeneous membrane. These shunt routes may aid the penetration of large polar molecules, electrolytes and, possibly, many drugs (Scheuplein, 1978a,b; Scheuplein and Blank, 1971). Drugs are often not ideal in a physicochemical sense—in particular, the vehicle pH and how it changes after skin application may affect ionic compounds. Simple diffusion of a single species is rare; other materials may codiffuse, modifying the permeation of the primary agent, while low molecular weight solvents may enter the skin and modify the horny layer.

The colloidal structure of a formulation alters as patients rub it into their skin; components may evaporate or pass into the skin, while body secretions may dilute the base. Drug penetration may well be promoted as solvents evaporate and medicament concentration rises (Coldman et al., 1969). A drug's diffusion coefficient within the skin may alter with time, or with position and concentration in the horny layer, due to vehicle or drug effects. The viable tissues may not function as a perfect sink, and the stratum corneum or dermis may bind the penetrant.

During pseudo-steady-state experiments, we presume that the penetrant concentration in the vehicle remains essentially constant. In practice, finite drug amounts may leave the preparation and the skin may absorb base components or dilute the topical with tissue fluids; the drug may precipitate or supersaturate the vehicle, and emulsions may invert or crack. All such factors can modify the chemical potential of a drug.

Contrary to usual assumptions, few vehicles are inert when interacting with the skin. Glycols may dehydrate the horny layer and occlusive components may hydrate the tissue. Many solvents readily penetrate the stratum corneum, possibly increasing drug solubility within this layer.

A common postulate is that the penetrant remains intact during diffusional processes. However, the drug may degrade chemically by photolytic action, hydrolysis and bacterial mechanisms, or fungal or tissue metabolism. Alternatively, the diffusional state of a drug may change as it complexes with vehicle or skin chemicals.

Finally, many in vitro experimental designs produce pseudo-steady-state estimates. During dermatological treatment, steady-state conditions seldom hold because the patient reapplies the product several times daily and also removes material from the skin (accidentally or by washing). The microenvironment of the body surface also alters throughout the day.

It is apparent that we need to be careful when correlating optimization theory with clinical activity!

PROTOCOL FOR OPTIMIZING A DERMATOLOGICAL FORMULATION

At first sight, skin therapy appears to be a simple type of treatment compared with, for example, oral medication. However, a closer examination suggests that the successful design of a dermatological can involve the most difficult aspects of the science (and art) of formulation, besides often requiring fundamental studies. This is particularly true now that modern formulators must do more than ensure that their products are acceptable simply with respect to cosmetic, compatibility, and stability criteria. Although pharmaceutical elegance in a preparation is still important, the primary concerns are clinical effectiveness and safety, and for these we should control the bioavailability of our modern potent drugs. The final section of this chapter therefore is a concise listing of the necessary steps for consideration in a program aimed at developing a successful topical drug formulation (Fig. 12).

Program for a Topical Drug Formulation

1. Identify precisely the skin disease or condition, or complex of symptoms, to be treated.
2. Determine the anatomical site for drug action. Is this the skin surface (simple drug release from the vehicle required), stratum corneum, viable epidermis, dermis, hair follicles, eccrine sweat glands, apocrine glands, or systemic circulation? Do we need to formulate for a specific body region (e.g., feet, nails, scalp or trunk)?
3. Have we identified the receptor site within the target area? Unfortunately, the subcellular biochemical locus of topical drug action may be unknown.
4. Estimate the skin condition of the "average" patient. Is the tissue broken and inflamed (as in acute eczema) or thickened (e.g., icthyosis, psoriasis), or is the pilosebaceous unit blocked (as for comedones or acne)? A complication for formulation is that successful treatment may soon change the skin's state. Thus, the healing process may rapidly develop a few horny cell layers with a dry surface from a weeping skin with a disrupted stratum corneum.
5. Choose the optimum drug or prodrug for the disorder. Within the pharmaceutical industry, the fundamental molecular structure of a new drug may have been developed elsewhere within the firm, but the formulator should at least be involved early on in respect to decisions about the form to be

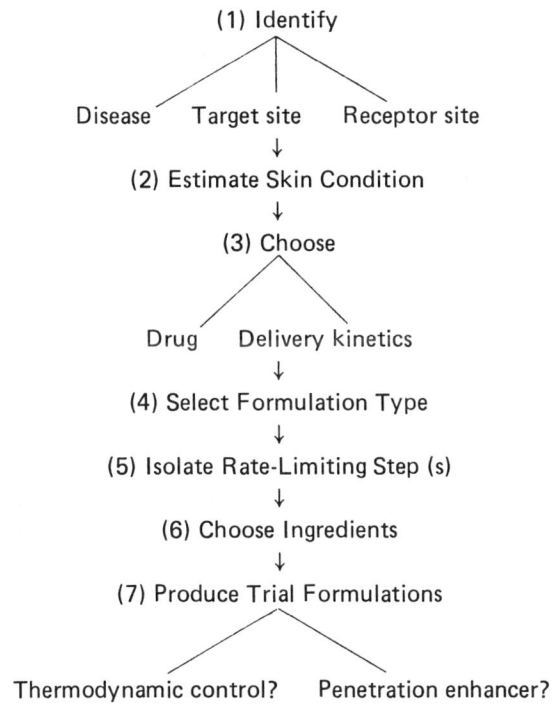
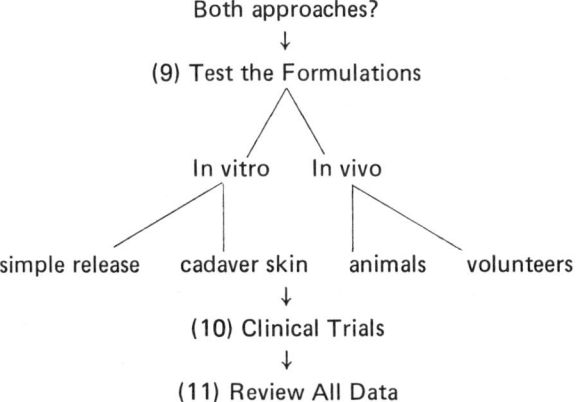

Figure 12 Steps in a program for optimizing a topical drug formulation.

used (ester, salt, etc.). Consider the drug's pharmacological and pharmacokinetic profiles, and its toxicity, sensitizing potential, stability, and susceptibility to degradation and enzyme metabolism. The investigator needs also to generate data on the molecule's physicochemical properties, particularly with respect to the partition coefficient and the diffusion coefficient relevant to the horny layer.

6. Evaluate the optimum kinetics for drug delivery to the receptor site; consider pulsed or pseudo-steady-state treatment, amount and strength of the dosage form, and frequency of application.
7. From a consideration of items 1-6, select the type of preparation. Is this to be a delivery device for systemic therapy or a traditional ointment, cream, gel, lotion, powder, liniment, or aerosol?
8. Decide whether there is a single rate-limiting step in the treatment and its location (within the vehicle, release from the base, partition into the stratum corneum, permeation across the horny layer, partition into the viable tissues, or clearance from these layers). Concentrate on controlling this stage; often this means optimizing the partitioning of the drug from the preparation into the stratum corneum and increasing its subsequent diffusion.
9. Choose stable, compatible, cosmetically and therapeutically acceptable vehicle ingredients. Remember that adjuvants may themselves improve therapy. For example, occlusive components moisturize the skin and thereby help to alleviate many disorders.
10. If the intention is to promote drug penetration, optimize the formulation to its maximum chemical potential (overly potent drugs may require a formulation that retards permeation). Note that a formulation optimized on the basis of in vitro tests may change radically when used clinically. Thus, vehicles often alter after skin application as components evaporate or penetrate the skin and secretions mix with the vehicle.
11. If the drug penetrates skin poorly because of its intrinsic physicochemical properties, consider the value of a suitable penetration enhancer. However, remember that a new enhancer will require a full toxicological screen.
12. For selected trial formulations, perform in vitro release tests using a simple synthetic membrane (or possibly no membrane) and a receptor maintained at sink condition. This procedure ensures that the drug is available for release and is not bound to vehicle components.
13. Perform permeation tests with cadaver skin or other isolated human skin. Such experiments may include a steady-state design together with a program that mimics clinical usage. As far as possible, avoid using animal skin during in vitro tests because for any new compound or formulation good correlations between animal and human data cannot be *guaranteed*.

14. Conduct in vivo studies in animals and human volunteers to determine efficacy, safety, and acceptability. Establish the topical pharmacokinetic profile and bioavailability of the drug from the candidate formulation.
15. Do clinical trials.
16. Throughout the program, review the physicochemical behavior and stability (chemical and microbiological) of the dosage form and package during preformulation studies, scaleup procedures, manufacture, storage, and use.

ACKNOWLEDGMENTS

I thank Dr. R. Woodford of the School of Pharmacy, Portsmouth Polytechnic, for his valued collaboration in vasoconstrictor testing over many years, and present and past graduate students who have worked with me at Bradford University, some of whose data are reviewed here: Dr. D. Southwell, Mr. S. A. Akhter, Miss S. L. Bennett, and Mrs. S. M. Harrison. My appreciation is also due to Mrs. G. Richman for her secretarial skills.

REFERENCES

Akhter, S. A. and Barry, B. W. (1985). Absorption through human skin of ibuprofen and flurbiprofen; effect of dose variation, deposited drug films, occlusion and the penetration enhancer N-methyl-2-pyrrolidone. *J. Pharm. Pharmacol. 37:* 27-37.

Akhter, S. A. and Barry, B. W. (1983). Flurbiprofen penetration and enhancement through cadaver skin; Value of "in vivo mimic" approach with low enhancer concentrations. *J. Pharm. Pharmacol. 34* (Suppl.): 31P.

Akhter, S. A., Barry, B. W., and Meyer, M. C. (1982). Absorption through cadaver skin of Ibuprofen, applied as dry films: Effects of solvents. *J. Pharm. Pharmacol. 34* (Suppl.): 34P.

Allenby, A. C., Creasey, N. H., Edgington, J. A. G., Fletcher, J. A., and Schock, C. (1969). Mechanism of action of accelerants on skin penetration. *Br. J. Dermatol. 81:* 47-55.

Barry, B. W. (1976). Bioavailability of topical steroids. *Dermatologica 152* (Suppl. 1): 47-65.

Barry, B. W. (1983). *Dermatological Formulations: Percutaneous Absorption.* Dekker, New York.

Barry, B. W. and Woodford, R. (1978). Activity and bioavailability of topical steroids. In vivo/in vitro correlations for the vasoconstrictor test. *J. Clin. Pharm. 3:* 43-65.

Barry, B. W., Harrison, S. M., and Dugard, P. H. (1985a). Correlation between thermodynamic activity and vapour diffusion through human skin for the model compound, benzyl alcohol. *J. Pharm. Pharmacol. 37:* 84-90.

Barry, B. W., Harrison, S. M., and Dugard, P. H. (1985b). Vapor and liquid diffusion of model penetrants through human skin; correlation with thermodynamic activity. *J. Pharm. Pharmacol. 37*: 226-235.

Barry, B. W., Southwell, D., and Woodford, R. (1984). Optimization of bioavailability of topical steroids: Penetration enhancers under occlusion. *J. Invest. Dermatol. 82*: 49-52.

Bennett, S. L., Barry, B. W., and Woodford, R. (1985). Optimization of bioavailability of topical steroids: non-occluded penetration enhancers under thermodynamic control. *J. Pharm. Pharmacol. 57*: 570-576.

Coldman, M. F., Poulsen, B. J., and Higuchi, T. (1969). Enhancement of percutaneous absorption by the use of volatile: Nonvolatile systems as vehicles. *J. Pharm. Sci. 58*: 1098-1102.

Cooper, E. R. (1984). Increased skin permeability for lipophilic molecules. In press.

Crank, J. (1975). *The Mathematics of Diffusion,* 2nd ed. Oxford University Press (Clarendon), New York.

Franz, T. J. (1978). The finite dose technique as a valid in vitro model for the study of percutaneous absorption in man. *Curr. Probl. Dermatol. 7*: 58-68.

Harrison, S. M., Barry, B. W., and Dugard, P. H. (1982). Benzyl alcohol vapour diffusion through human skin; dependence on thermodynamic activity in the vehicle. *J. Pharm. Pharmacol. 34* (Suppl.): 36P.

Harrison, S. M., Barry, B. W., and Dugard, P. H. (1983). Factors controlling liquid and vapour diffusion through human skin for the model compound benzyl alcohol. *J. Pharm. Pharmacol. 35* (Suppl.): 32P.

Higuchi, T. (1960). Physical chemical analysis of percutaneous absorption from creams and ointments. *J. Soc. Cosmet. Chem. 11*: 85-97.

Katz, M. and Poulsen, B. J. (1971). Absorption of drugs through the skin. In *Handbook of Experimental Pharmacology*, Vol. 28, Pt. 1. Edited by B. B. Brodie and J. Gillette. Springer-Verlag, New York, pp. 103-174.

Poulsen, B. J. (1972). Diffusion of drugs from topical vehicles: An analysis of vehicle effects. *Adv. Biol. Skin 12*: 495-509.

Resh, W. and Stoughton, R. B. (1976). Topically applied antibiotics in acne vulgaris: Clinical Response and suppression of *Corynebacterium acnes* in open comedones. *Arch. Dermatol. 112*: 182-184.

Ritschel, W. A. (1969). Sorption promoters in biopharmaceutics. *Angew. Chem., Int. Ed. 8*: 699-710.

Scheuplein, R. J. (1978a). The skin as a barrier (Chap. 54). Skin permeation (Chap. 55). Site variations in diffusion and permeability (Chap. 56). In *The Physiology and Pathophysiology of the Skin,* Vol. 5. Edited by A. Jarrett. Academic, New York, pp. 1669-1692, 1693-1730, 1731-1752.

Scheuplein, R. J. (1978b). Permeability of skin: A review of major concepts. *Curr. Probl. Dermatol. 7*: 172-186.

Scheuplein, R. J. and Blank, I. H. (1971). Permeability of the skin. *Physiol. Rev. 51*: 702-747.

Southwell, D. and Barry, B. W. (1983). Penetration enhancers for human skin: Mode of action of 2-pyrrolidone and dimethylformamide on partition and diffusion of model compounds water, *n*-alcohols and caffeine. *J. Invest. Dermatol. 80*: 507-514.

Stoughton, R. B. (1981). Azone (1-dodecylazacycloheptan-2-one) enhances percutaneous penetration. Presented at the Third International Symposium on Psoriasis, Stanford, Calif.

Stoughton, R. B. (1982). Enhanced percutaneous penetration with 1-dodecylazacycloheptan-2-one. *Arch. Dermatol. 118*: 474-477.

Stoughton, R. B. and McClure, W. O. (1983). Azone—A new nontoxic enhancer for cutaneous penetration. *Drug Dev. Ind. 9*: 725-744.

Woodford, R. and Barry, B. W. (1982). Optimization of bioavailability of topical steroids: Thermodynamic control. *J. Invest. Dermatol. 79*: 388-391.

38
Percutaneous Absorption of Corticosteroids
Systemic Effects

Torsten Fredriksson
Central Hospital, Västeras, Sweden

When a corticosteroid is applied to the skin surface, only part of it eventually reaches deeper compartments, possibly producing systemic effects. Some of the applied corticosteroid is rubbed off or shed off by desquamation; some of it becomes bound to receptors; some of it is metabolized in the skin—probably only a fraction, and in most cases into less active compounds (Anjo et al., 1980; Schaefer and Schalla, 1980).

After reaching the bloodstream, the active corticosteroid is metabolized by blood and—mainly—liver enzymes, and it may also be bound to blood proteins. Different steroids are metabolized at different rates and into metabolites of differing activities, and bound to proteins to different degrees. Thus, the systemic effects of a certain corticosteroid may depend not only on its initial or intrinsic activity (including vehicle properties and penetration enhancers such as Azone) but also on its metabolism. This is illustrated by the following example. Budesonide (Fig. 1), a nonhalogenated steroid clinically as effective as most "strong" steroids (Salde and Schröpl, 1982), is metabolized faster in the liver (Andersson et al., 1982) than some clinically comparable steroids, and should thus theoretically produce fewer systemic effects (Fig. 2).

APPROACH TO THE STUDY

The only well-established systemic side effect of topically applied corticosteroids is the influence on the hypothalamic-pituitary-adrenocortical function, that is, adrenal function suppression. In practice, this means determining whether a topically applied corticosteroid depresses cortisol production, since the produc-

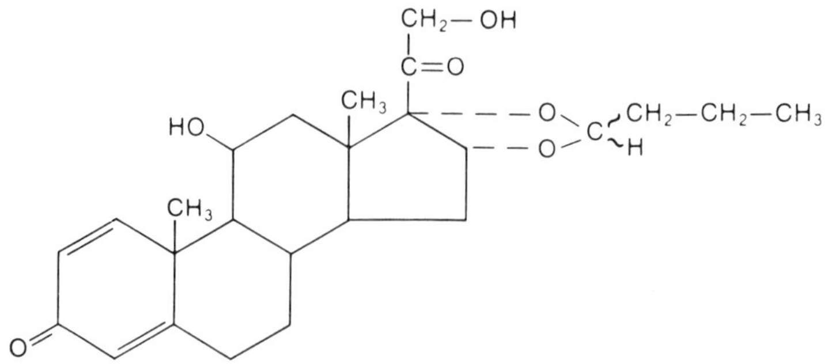

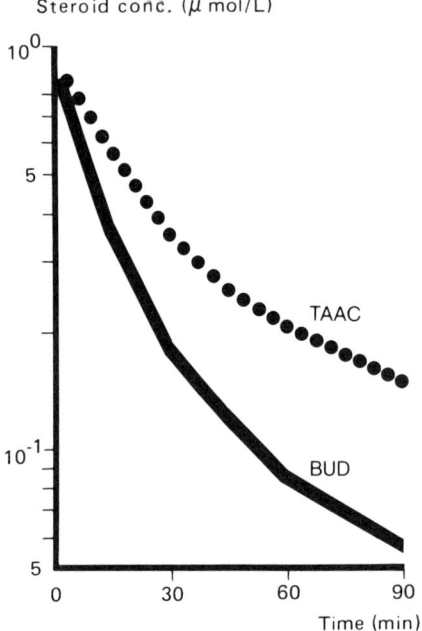

Figure 1 Structural formula for budesonide.

Figure 2 In vitro degradation of budesonide (BUD) and triamcinolone (TAAC) by human liver homogenate. (Modified from Andersson et al., 1982.)

tion of other adrenal hormones does not seem to be influenced to any significant extent. If depressed, the extent is of interest and also how fast adrenal function is restored after treatment has been withdrawn.

Before doing such studies, there are several important points to consider. First, the corticosteroid must be incorporated into the exact vehicle intended for clinical usage, and in the proper concentration, since absorption kinetics are related to vehicle properties and solubility properties in that vehicle. Second, these studies must be done on human volunteers, since there are no suitable animal models allowing extrapolation either to healthy persons or to individuals with diseased skin (the metabolism of corticosteroids is "species specific"). Should healthy volunteers with "normal, nontreated" skin (do such individuals exist?) or patients with steroid-responsive dermatosis such as psoriasis or atopic dermatitis be used? One advantage associated with healthy volunteers is that their skin condition is rather constant during the test period, while patients with diseased skin may improve during treatment, with the absorption barrier gradually being restored. Furthermore, it is more difficult to grade skin condition and barrier function in diseased skin than in the skin of healthy volunteers. Patients with diseased skin are in a stress situation, not only because of their disease but also because treatment is postponed for a few days to obtain basal cortisol values and because they have been asked to take part in a academic study not necessarily aiming to produce relief of their condition. We do not know with certainty whether they have received treatment with other corticosteroids before the test. Their baseline values might be high due to stress, or low due to pretreatment. Most of these problems can be avoided if healthy volunteers are used; but on the other hand, the corticosteroids are intended to be used on diseased skin. Healthy volunteers can be recruited with great accuracy with regard to weight, body surface, area of application, and so on, and the use of them makes crossover studies possible. Area of application is particularly important, since absorption varies, being high in intertriginous areas and the face and on the other extreme low on palms and soles (Anjo et al., 1980).

METHODS AND AMOUNTS

Methods of application are important. Occlusive dressings increase absorption and produce elevated serum concentrations of the steroid and more pronounced adrenal suppression. However, there seems to be a worldwide tendency to use occlusive dressings less than was done a few years ago. Therefore, it is my opinion that occlusive dressings should be used only in comparative studies of healthy volunteers, in search of systemic effects.

Amounts used must also be taken into account. Schlagel and Sandborn (1964) showed that 30 g of an emollient covered the body of an average-sized adult. With an ointment vehicle, more has to be used. However, in clinical practice, how often do we treat the whole body surface, and what patient can afford the cost of such a regimen for an extended period of time? In the United Kingdom Wilson et al. (1981) found that 80% of the outpatients used less than 30 g per week. In Sweden, where medicine is to a high extent subsidized by the government, we have found comparable figures for outpatients (in the Department of Dermatology at Central Hospital in Västeras, 75% of the outpatients use less than 50 g, and 2% more than 100 g, and none more than 150 g per week). Thus, in this group there are few at risk except when very strong steroids are used. Downie et al. (1981) showed that betamethasone dipropionate in a vehicle with high content of propylene glycol produces a slight adrenal depression when 50 g is applied per week (3.5 g twice daily). However, the depression was seen initially, and the adrenal function was in most cases partly restored in these patients during treatment, probably due to barrier function repair. In healthy volunteers there was no significant depression with this regimen. In inpatients we have on occasion treated the whole body surface, but seldom for more than a week, and seldom with "strong" steroids.

FREQUENCY OF APPLICATION

What about frequency of application? Steroids are usually prescribed to be applied two or three times daily. It is my firm belief that few patients are motivated enough to apply any topical remedy three times daily except on small areas such as the hands or the face, and that many with extended lesions do not apply it twice daily when so directed. By "tube-weighing" technique we found that only 60% of randomly selected patients followed the instructions during a 2-week period. On the other hand, Fredriksson et al. (1980) showed that in highly motivated patients one application per day of a halcinonide cream was about as effective as the cream applied three times daily. Since adrenal suppression studies ideally should be done on hospitalized individuals, this is a minor problem, but we cannot always with certainty translate results from such studies to the practical world.

MEASUREMENT OF ADRENAL SUPPRESSION

There are many methods to measure adrenal suppression and its functional integrity (Table 1). From this wide range of diagnostic procedures the U.S. Food and Drug Administration (FDA) made a reasonable selection in their "topical Corticosteroids Testing Guidelines" of August 14, 1980:

> Adrenal suppression studies should be done on new corticoids and usually on optimized formulations of known corticoids as follows:

Table 1 Diagnostic Procedures Employed in the Assessment of the Hypothalamic-Pituitary-Adrenocortical System

Determination or procedure	Control mechanism and/or component assessed
Basal plasma corticosteroid levels	
Basal plasma ACTH levels	
Basal urinary corticosteroid excretion	Basal homeostasis
Cortisol secretion rate	
Urinary free cortisol	
Plasma corticosteroid levels throughout 24 hr	Circadian control mechanism
Response to dexamethasone	Functional integrity of negative feedback control
Response to metypyrone	
Response to pyrogen	Functional integrity of components involved in stress control mechanism
Response to insulin-induced hypoglycemia	
Response to vasopressin	
Adrenocortical response to exogenous corticotrophin, synacthen depot (or ACTH)	Functional integrity of adrenal cortex
Half-life of cortisol	Ability of liver to clear cortisol

Source: Adapted from Landen et al. (1976).

1. Study six adult hospitalized patients with generalized dermatitis, ideally three with psoriasis and three with atopic dermatitis; some with recently acquired disease and some with long-standing chronic disease who have been extensively treated with topical corticoids. Healthy volunteers may be studied but not substituted for patients with dermatitis.
2. Thirty grams of the test drug using the formulation proposed for market (phase III) should be applied daily in divided doses.
3. Take three successive daily baseline levels for plasma cortisol at 8 A.M. and two 24-hr urine samples for 17-hydroxycorticoids.
4. Then apply steroid for 7 days to lesions that cover 30% of the body. Plasma cortisols are then to be done after days 6 and 7 of treatment at 8 AM as well as two 24-hour urine samples for 17-hydroxycorticoids, or urine-free corticoids.

5. If plasma cortisol levels were not pushed below the level of 5 µg in any of the subjects at any time (corroborated by urinary 17-hydroxycorticoid tests; male, below 5 mg/24 hr, female, below 3 mg/24 hr), the steroid should not cause significant adrenal suppression.
6. If there is suppression below 5 micrograms in any of the readings, the sponsor has the obligation to:
   A. Titrate the amount of topical steroid necessary to give suppression of plasma cortisol supported by 24-hr urine samples for 17-hydroxycorticoids.
   B. Perform metypyrone and insulin tolerance tests 2 weeks after the plasma cortisol levels have returned to normal.
   C. Other follow-up tests may be done as medically indicated to fully characterize the pharmacological picture.
7. If 10 g or less per day gives any suppression (5 g over 30% of body to the lesions, twice a day) of plasma cortisol, the drug could be only approved with strong warnings on the label to restrict its use (amount/day and duration).

Note: If the first two patients studied show significant suppression of plasma cortisol and/or urinary 17-hydroxycorticoids, the dose of the test corticoid should be reduced for the next two or three patients. Thus, the "titration" process begins which may require the study of more than six patients. Flexibility in number and type of tests as well as the number of patients studied is required and dependent on the data generated. Other newly developed tests may be included.

AREAS OF UNCERTAINTY

There remain a few question marks. The dosage, 15 g twice daily, is high, since 30–50% of the body surface must be involved. Few of our patients are in this unfortunate situation, but this dosage may be acceptable as a high safety precaution. Five micrograms of cortisol corresponds to 140 nmol/liter (our 8 A.M. range in normal individuals is 280–830 nmol/liter: Fig. 3).

The other question mark involves the "ban" on healthy volunteers, who are necessary to obtain a fair comparison between different corticosteroids and the same corticosteroid in different vehicles. This can be illustrated by a study that compared budesonide with competitive drugs. The systemic effect of the topical glucocorticoid ointments budesonide 0.025%, hydrocortisone-17-butyrate 0.1%, and betamethasone-17,21-dipropionate 0.05% was studied in nine healthy volunteers with crossover design (Scott et al., 1981). Five grams of ointment was applied on about 13% of the total body surface, using occlusive techniques, for three consecutive nights (Fig. 4). The cortisol values in plasma and urine were

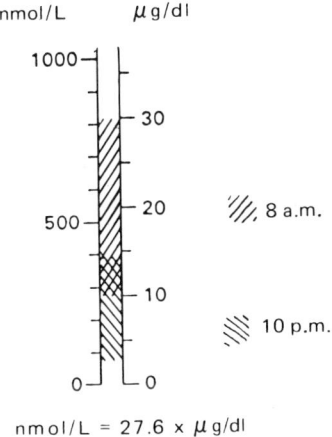

Figure 3 Normal range of plasma cortisol.

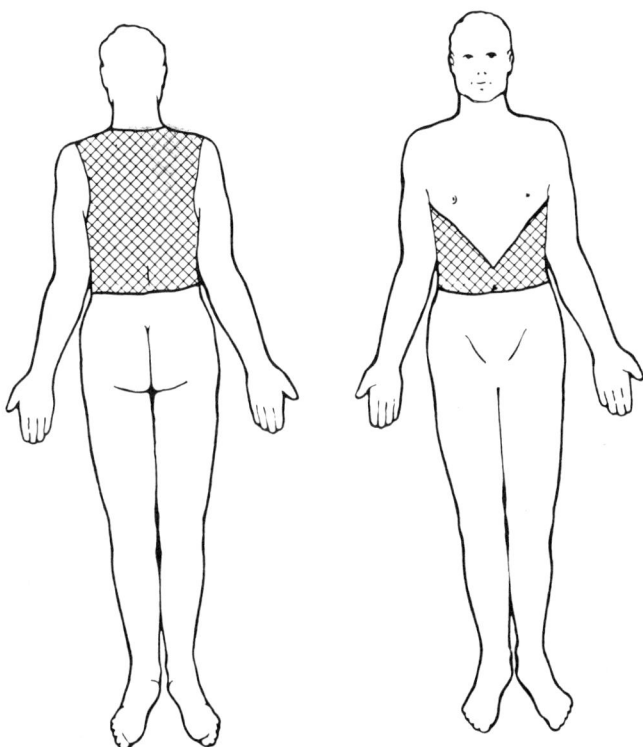

Figure 4 Area occluded.

measured before, during, and 3 days after applications. Although budesonide and betamethasone-17,21-dipropionate are equipotent drugs from a therapeutic point of view (Salde and Schröpl, 1982), the halogenated betamethasone-17,21-dipropionate caused significantly greater decrease in levels of plasma and urinary cortisol. Between the two nonhalogenated glucocorticosteroids, budesonide and hydrocortisone-17-butyrate, no significant difference was found despite the difference in anti-inflammatory effects (Heijer et al., 1981).

SPECIAL CASES

A clinical trial was performed to study adrenal suppression in patients with plaque or discoid psoriasis treated with 7-21 g of topical glucocorticoids (average dose 18 g/24 hr (Salde and Lassus, 1983). Betamethasone-17,21-dipropionate ointment was compared with budesonide 0.025% ointment, using a double-blind group-comparative design. Adrenal suppression was measured via plasma cortisol levels, with and without ACTH stimulation. The suppression of and difference in adrenal suppression were considerably less than in healthy volunteers, as described, but still in the same ranking order (Fig. 6).

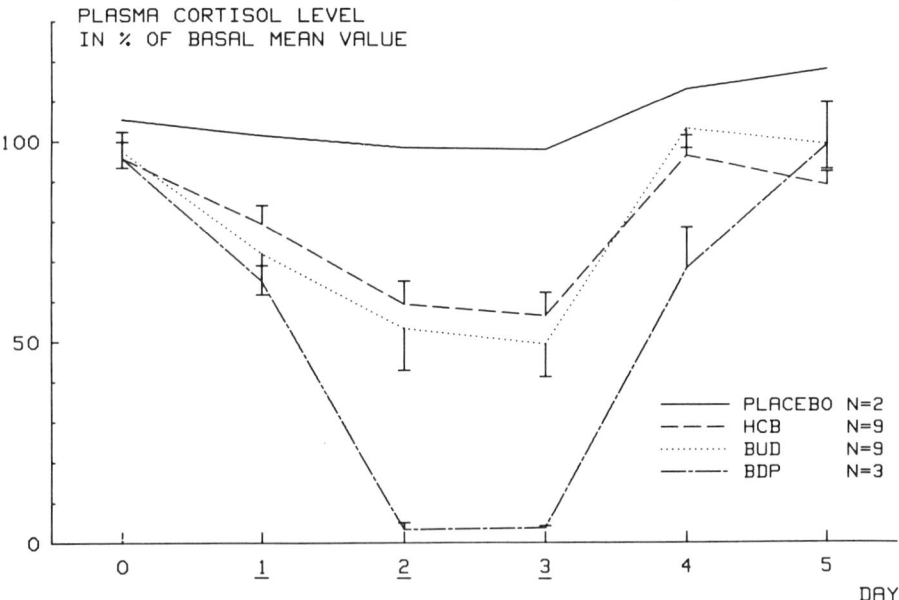

Figure 5 Effect of placebo, hydrocortisone butyrate (HCB), budesonide (BUD), and betamethasone dipropionate (BDP) on plasma cortisol levels. (From Scott et al., 1981.)

Systemic Effects of Corticosteroids

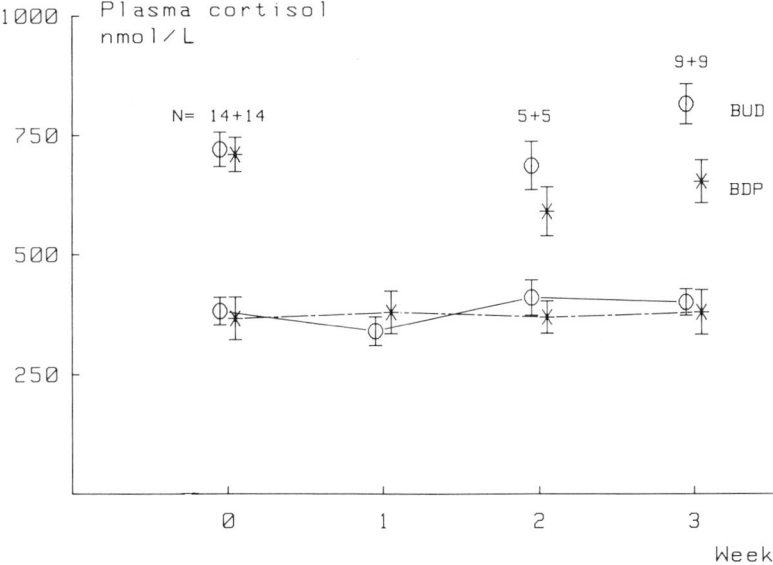

Figure 6 ACTH stimulation test at start and end of treatment. Budesonide (BUD) and betamethasone dipropionate (BDP). (From Salde and Lassus, 1983.)

Munro (1975, 1976) has extensively studied adrenal suppression in patients using essentially the same methods outlined by the FDA, but he has also used occlusive material. From Figure 7 it is evident that occlusion produces almost complete adrenal suppression when 30 g of the "strong" steroid fluocinonid is applied, while the same amount of the same steroid in the same vehicle with stockinette has little effect. It is remarkable how fast adrenal function is restored—usually after a few days, in contrast to systemic administration, where it may take months. This fast recovery to some extent contradicts the exciting theory about the "reservoir effect of human skin" (Vickers, 1980). Of course, in clinical practice topical steroids are not withdrawn as drastically as in these studies, but gradually, to avoid rebound phenomena.

Children constitute a special problem. There are few adrenal suppression studies recorded (Rasmussen, 1978; Weston et al., 1980), and few reports of side effects such as growth impairment (Salde and Lassus, 1983). The situation has been well summarized by Rasmussen (1982):

Children do not absorb drugs differently than adults. Their stratum corneum, which is the rate-limiting membrane in percutaneous absorption, is as thick as that of an adult (Janet Fairley and James E. Rasmussen, unpublished data). However, the ratio of surface area to volume is greater in children than

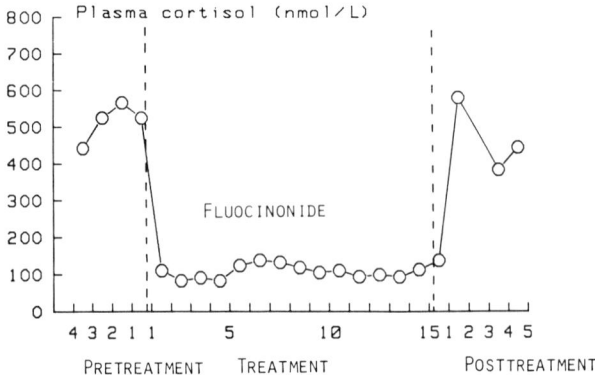
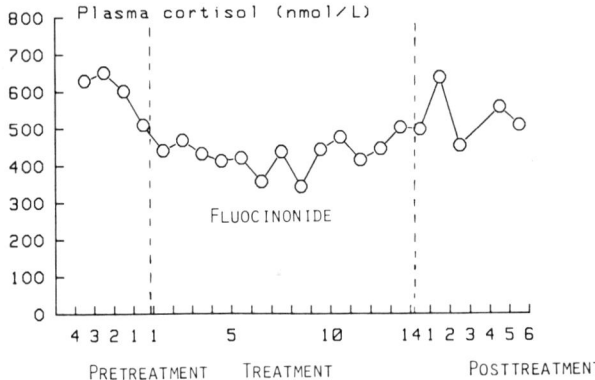

Figure 7 Effect of fluocinonide on plasma cortisol. Occlusion (upper curve) and no occlusion (lower curve). (Modified from Munro, 1976.)

in adults. Young children have nearly twice as much surface area per kilogram of body weight as do adults. Consequently, they absorb more drug per kilogram even though absorption per square centimeter of surface area is the same as an adult. Although not well studied, most high-potency steroids will produce prompt and substantial PHA suppression in children.

Sparkes (1976) stated:

[I]t is probable that the adrenal function of the majority of patients is very little affected by treatment with topical corticosteroids. However, where large quantities of more potent preparations are used adrenal suppression is likely to occur, especially early in the treatment. As long as these large doses are not used for a prolonged period, adrenal atrophy and its attendant complications are unlikely to occur.

That statement is most probably true. Furthermore, there seems to be an international trend to "step down" to weaker steroids, once the condition is under control. In practical dermatology the topical side effects are of much greater concern than the systemic. With regard to both systemic and topical side effects, only the "weak" steroids such as hydrocortisone are really safe in adults as well as in children—provided the indication is correct.

REFERENCES

Andersson, P., Edsbäcker, Å. S., Ryrfeldt, A., and von Bahr, C. (1982). *J. Steroid Biochem. 16*: 787.
Anjo, D. M., Feldmann, R. J., and Maibach, H. I. (1980). In *Percutaneous Absorption of Steroids*. Edited by P. Mauvais-Jarvis, C. F. H. Vickers, and J. Wepierre. Academic, New York, p. 31.
Downie, D. A. W., Swarbrick, P. T., and Salmon, R. M. (1981). *Aust. J. Dermatol. 22*: 113.
Fredriksson, T., Lassus, A., and Bleeker, J. (1980). *Br. J. Dermatol. 102*: 575.
Heijer, A., Hesser, G., Holm, P., and Salde, L. (1981). *J. Int. Med. Res. 9*: 239.
Landon, J., Snitcher, E., and Rees, L. (1976). *Br. J. Dermatol. 94* (Suppl. 12): 61.
Munro, D. D. (1975). Thesis for doctorate in medicine. University of London.
Munro, D. D. (1976). *Br. J. Dermatol. 94* (Suppl. 12): 67.
Rasmussen, J. E. (1978). *Arch. Dermatol. 114*: 1165.
Rasmussen, J. E. (1982). *JAMA 248*: 3030.
Salde, L. and Lassus, A. (1983). Accepted for publication in *Curr. Med. Res Opin*.
Salde, L. and Schröpl, F. (1982). *Z. Hautkr. 57*: 1745.
Schaefer, H. and Schalla, W. (1980). In *Percutaneous Absorption of Steroids*. Edited by P. Mauvais-Jarvis, C. F. H. Vickers, and J. Wepierre. Academic, New York, p. 53.
Schlagel, C. A. and Sandborn, E. C. (1964). *J. Invest. Dermatol. 42*: 253.
Scott, M., Malmsten, L., and Thelin, I. (1981). *Acta Dermatol. Venereol.* (Stockholm) *61*: 543.
Sparkes, C. G. (1976). *Br. J. Dermatol. 94* (Suppl. 12): 77.
Vickers, C. F. H. (1980). In *Percutaneous Absorption of Steroids*. Edited by P. Mauvais-Jarvis, C. F. H. Vickers, and J. Wepierre. Academic, New York, p. 19.
Weston, W. L., Sams, W. M. Morris, H. G., et al. (1980). *Pediatrics 65*: 103.

39
Vehicle Effects on Skin Penetration

Eugene Cooper*
Miami Valley Laboratories, Procter and Gamble Company, Cincinnati, Ohio

The remarkable barrier properties of skin have been the subject of several reviews (Barry, 1983; Katz and Poulsen, 1971; Scheuplein and Blank, 1971). The key to topical delivery of drugs is in large part the ability to alter this barrier function of skin. Dimethyl sulfoxide (DMSO) (Scheuplein and Blank, 1971) and soaps (Bettley, 1961; Betteley and Donoghue, 1960) can increase the cutaneous penetration of chemical agents. Except for the recent introduction of 1-dodecylazacycloheptan-2-one (Azone) (Stoughton, 1982), there have been few new developments in the field of penetration enhancers. The recognition of the advantages of using skin as the port of entry for drugs is becoming a major impetus for discovering materials that increase skin penetration, and it is expected that new technologies will be developed in the near future.

This chapter examines the existing data on skin penetration enhancers in light of the composition and structure of the skin and proposes simple guidelines for altering the barrier properties of skin. Skin is a complex and heterogeneous membrane; simple models will not account for all the observed effects. Such models, however, can account for the general observations and can provide a sensible framework from which to build new agents to alter the barrier properties. This chapter discusses the basic factors affecting diffusion and their implications with respect to the stratum corneum composition. The action of known penetration enhancers is interpreted in light of the model, and future possibilities are explored.

**Present affiliation*: Alcon Laboratories, Inc., Fort Worth, Texas

DIFFUSION FACTORS

The rate of movement at which a molecule will diffuse through a given medium depends on the size and shape of the molecule and on the energy required to make a hole in the barrier medium. Elegant theories (Kumins and Kwei, 1968) are available to describe this process, but in qualitative terms one knows the diffusion in liquids is much more rapid than in solids, and that for fluids the rate of diffusion is inversely proportional to the fluid viscosity. For diffusion in polymers (e.g., proteins), the structural and chemical properties of the polymer control diffusion and the degree of solvent swelling can greatly alter the diffusional process. Thus, alterations in the viscosity and crystallinity (or structural properties) of a medium can greatly affect the rate of diffusion in the medium.

COMPOSITIONAL AND STRUCTURAL FACTORS

Although the skin has a complex structure and composition, for qualitative thinking one can focus on its gross composition. The skin's main barrier, the stratum corneum, consists mostly of keratinized protein, some lipid, and varying amounts of water (Anderson and Cassidy, 1973). The arrangement of these materials is important to the extent that parallel or series pathways exist. That is, if the lipid and aqueous (hydrated protein) pathways are parallel, one does not have to alter both pathways to significantly alter transport. If the pathways are in series, then both pathways must be altered unless one barrier is dominant. The existence of parallel pathways is supported by the lack of dependence of flux on oil/water partition coefficient as the partition coefficient decreases beyond the value for glycerol (Cooper, 1984; Scheuplein and Blank, 1971), and the fact that surfactants alter the permeability of polar molecules much more than nonpolar molecules (Cooper, 1982). The key to altering the polar pathway will be to swell the protein matrix or change its structure, and the key to altering the lipid pathway will be to alter its crystallinity or its viscosity.

PENETRATION ENHANCERS

Surfactants

Decylmethyl sulfoxide ($C_{10}MSO$) greatly increases the penetration of salicylic acid at pH 9.9 but only slightly increases salicylic acid penetration at pH 2.65 (Cooper, 1982). This finding is consistent with the observation that $C_{10}MSO$ alters the polar pathway but not the lipid pathway. Similar results were obtained for the effect of sodium dodecyl sulfate on the penetration of urea (polar) and 1-pentanol (nonpolar). Scheuplein and Ross (1970) and Oertel (1977) have shown that surfactants alter the protein conformations and essentially "open up" the protein-controlled polar pathway. Further confirmation of this mechanism can be found in the effect of thermal denaturation (Cooper, 1982) on the transport of polar and nonpolar molecules. As predicted, the transport of polar molecules is affected by thermal denaturation to a much greater extent than that of nonpolar molecules.

The ability of a surfactant to alter transport is a function of the hydrophilicity (Laughlin, 1978) of the polar head group and to a lesser degree a function of the hydrocarbon chain. The optimum chain length often occurs at 12 carbons (Cooper and Berner, 1985), but unsaturated, long chains are effective as well. The ranking of the polar head groups is given in Table 1, where the ethoxylates and alcohols have virtually no effect on transport through the polar pathway.

Binary Systems

Surface-active agents, even those that do not alter the skin protein, can be used in combination with a polar solvent like propylene glycol to greatly enhance the penetration of nonpolar species. For example, penetration of salicylic acid from saturated solutions of propylene glycol or oleic acid is much less than from the mixture of the two solvents (Table 2). If it is assumed that salicylic acid penetrates predominantly through the lipid pathway, it is reasonable to assume that the binary vehicle is altering the stratum corneum lipids. The incorporation of unsaturated fatty acids into *Escherichia coli* (Davis and Silbert, 1974) or liposomes (De Gier et al., 1968) greatly reduces the membrane barrier properties, which is consistent with a change in the membrane fluidity (viscosity) as a result of the incorporation of unsaturated lipids.

For the enhancement of the penetration of lipophilic molecules, the hydrocarbon chain appears to be the dominant factor rather than the polar head group (Cooper, 1984). The cis isomer is preferred when only one double bond is present. The results appear to be consistent with the interpretation that the introduction of molecules to reduce crystallinity will result in increased transport.

Table 1 Hydrophilicity of Surfactant Head Groups in Order of Decreasing Hydrophilicity/Protein Interaction

Head group	Example
Ionic	Sodium dodecyl sulfate
Zwitterionic	Dodecyl dimethylammoniopropane sulfonate
Sulfoxide	Dodecyl methyl sulfoxide
Ethoxylate	Dodecanol hexaethoxylate
Alcohol	Dodecyl alcohol

Table 2 Penetration of Salicylic Acid Across Human Epidermis in Vitro from Saturated Solutions

Vehicle	Relative penetration
Propylene glycol	1
Oleic acid	1
Propylene glycol/oleic acid (50/50)	20

Source: Cooper, 1984.

Solvents

Solvents such as DMSO, 2-pyrrolidone, and dimethylformamide can swell the stratum corneum and should be able to solubilize the lipids. Thus their effects can be all encompassing and somewhat complex. One would expect in general that these solvents would increase penetration by creating a "solvent" pathway or by fluidizing the lipids.

The effect of these solvents on penetration is dependent on solvent concentration (Scheuplein and Blank, 1971); little effect is observed for DMSO unless high concentrations are employed. In our laboratory the flux of salicylic acid from DMSO was measured as a function of salicylic acid concentration. The flux increased with concentration up to about 20% salicylic acid and then decreased beyond this concentration. The peak flux results from an increasing driving force competing with a decreasing DMSO effect.

SUMMARY

The specific interactions of penetration enhancers with the stratum corneum may vary considerably, but for qualitative discussion their basic effects can be separated into two categories:

Protein structural changes
Lipid fluidization

Strong detergents such as ionic surfactants fall into the first category and lipid solvents or unsaturated lipids appear to be in the second. New penetration enhancers will most likely be found among agents that can alter the crystallinity of the stratum corneum lipids and/or open up the protein structures.

REFERENCES

Anderson, R. L. and Cassidy, J. M. (1973). *J. Invest. Dermatol. 61*: 30.
Barry, B. W. (1983). In *Dermatological Formulations.* Dekker, New York.
Bettley, F. R. (1961). *Br. J. Dermatol. 73*: 448.
Bettley, F. R. and Donoghue, E. (1960). *Nature 17*: 185.
Cooper, E. R. (1982). In *Solution Behavior of Surfactants.* Edited by K. L. Mittal and E. J. Fendler. Plenum, New York, p. 1505.
Cooper, E. R. (1984). *J. Pharm. Sci. 73*: 1153.
Cooper, E. R. and Berner, B. (1985). In *Surfactants in Cosmetics.* Edited by M. M. Rieger. Dekker, New York, p. 1950.
Davis, M. B. and Silbert, D. F. (1974). *Biochim. Biophys. Acta 373*: 224.
DeGier, J., Mandersloot, J. G., and Van Deenan, L. L. M. (1968). *Biochim. Biophys. Acta 150*: 666.
Katz, M. and Poulsen, B. J. (1971). In *Handbook of Experimental Pharmacology.* Edited by B. B. Brodie and J. Gillette. Springer-Verlag, New York, p. 103.
Kumins, C. A. and Kwei, T. K. (1968). In *Diffusion in Polymers.* Edited by J. Cronl and G. S. Park. Academic Press, New York, p. 107.
Laughlin, R. G. (1978). In *Advances in Liquid Crystals.* Academic, New York, p. 41.
Oertel, R. P. (1977). *Biopolymers 16*: 2329.
Scheuplein, R. J. and Blank, I. H. (1971). *Physiol. Rev. 51*: 702.
Scheuplein, R. J. and Ross, L. (1970). *J. Soc. Cosmet. Chem. 21*: 853.
Stoughton, R. B. (1982). *Arch. Dermatol. 118*: 474.

40
Absorption of Triethanolamine 7-[^{14}C] Salicylate in Human and Animal Joints

Joseph L. Rabinowitz and Martin D. Rabinowitz
Veterans Administration Medical Center, University of Pennsylvania, Philadelphia, Pennsylvania

Interest in alternatives to peroral delivery of medications, particularly transdermal delivery (the introduction of medication through the skin, rather than by oral ingestion or injection) has existed for years. Salicylates were one of the first groups of medications to be prepared in ointment form for topical absorption. Salicylates have been of great interest because oral aspirin shows a significant incidence of gastrointestinal symptoms, increased risk of gastric ulcer, and so on (Arthritis Foundation, 1976; McCarthy, 1979; Silvoso et al., 1979). In 1952 triethanolamine was found to be a good base for the cutaneous penetration of many materials, including salicylates (Flesch et al., 1955; Gaudin, 1952; Nothman and Wolff, 1933; Rujahn and With, 1937; Strakosch, 1943). This chapter discusses the methods used and results obtained in our investigations of the knee joints of humans and various species of animals after local massage with an ointment containing 10% triethanolamine salicylate (TEA/S), also known as trolamine salicylate.

HISTORICAL DEVELOPMENT

Interest in alternative routes of salicylate administration began in the 1930s when the properties of topical salicylate preparations were first explored. In 1952 an ointment of 10% triethanolamine salicylate was found to achieve good subcutaneous penetration (Gaudin, 1952). After penetration through the skin, the triethanoloamine salicylate compound released the salicylate moiety, permitting it to exert its analgesic and anti-inflammatory properties locally. The penetration of topically applied salicylate into joints, however, has not been fully investigated.

Previous animal studies have shown that TEA/S is rapidly absorbed through the skin (Gaudin, 1952; Rujahn and With, 1937). Several clinical studies of the effectiveness of TEA/S cream in humans have demonstrated favorable results in a variety of localized rheumatic disorders (Strakosch, 1943; Stahl, 1969) and have reported that active treatment is more effective than placebo (C. W. Waggoner, personal communication, 1983). In a double-blind study of patients with rheumatic pain (Golden, 1978), topical salicylate was found to provide prompt subjective relief with fewer adverse effects than oral aspirin.

TEA/S is the active ingredient in various topical analgesic creams used for sore muscles, joint stiffness, strains, and so on. The percutaneous absorption of salicylate is well known (Rabinowitz et al., 1982). While dermatologists have been aware of the need for improving penetration of drugs used to treat the skin, the availability of suitable agents has been limited.

We performed several radioisotope studies to compare the local, articular, and systemic absorption of oral and topical salicylate preparations. The levels of [^{14}C] salicylate in periarticular tissues, synovial fluid, blood, and urine were compared in both dogs and humans after topical administration of triethanolamine 7-[^{14}C] salicylate and oral administration of 7-[^{14}C] acetylsalicylic acid (Rabinowitz et al., 1982, 1984).

METHODOLOGY

The preparation of ^{14}C-labeled salicylates and aspirin has been described (Rabinowitz et al., 1982). The chemical and radioactive purity of all materials was predetermined by thin-layer chromatography, radioassay, and nuclear magnetic resonance (NMR) (Rabinowitz et al., 1982). Molecular and radioactive equivalent doses of salicylate and aspirin were present in each preparation; calculation and techniques have been presented previously (Rabinowitz et al., 1982).

The ^{14}C content was determined by radioassay. The chemical content of salicylate was determined by the ACA method (Natelson, 1957). TEA/S was also assayed by NMR for qualitative and quantitative identification (Jackman and Sternhell, 1969). When TEA/S was prepared from authentic materials, its NMR spectrum was found to be identical to that of TEA/S in commercial preparations (Rabinowitz et al., 1982). The triethanolamine [^{14}C] salicylate was also assayed and found to have the same NMR spectrum.

Canine Study

Each of five male 8-month-old beagle dogs received by mouth a 500-mg capsule of 7-[^{14}C] aspirin: specific activity 140 dpm/μg of [^{14}C] salicylate, 2.77 mM = 24.3 μCi, specific activity 8.77 μCi/mM (Blahd, 1971; Chase and Rabinowitz, 1967; Medical International Radiation Dose Committee of the Society of

Nuclear Medicine, 1969; Quimby and Feitelberg, 1963; Rabinowitz et al., 1982, 1984).

Each of a second group of five male 8-month-old beagle dogs received 10 g of labeled TEA/S cream containing 7-[^{14}C]salicylate of the same total equimolar amount and radioactivity. The right knee of each dog was shaved and the cream was rubbed in thoroughly until completely absorbed into the skin (Rabinowitz et al., 1982).

After 30 and 60 min, samples of blood and urine were obtained from the anesthetized dogs. In the TEA/S group, tissue samples were taken at the point of cream application. At the conclusion of the surgery, the dogs were disposed of according to humanitarian rules and the Nuclear Regulatory Commission regulations for ^{14}C-labeled animal remains.

Human Study

Six male subjects (55 to 62 years of age) with seropositive, adult-onset rheumatoid arthritis were studied. All patients met American Rheumatism Association criteria for classical or definite rheumatoid arthritis (Arthritis Foundation, 1976; Ropes et al., 1958).

Each subject had active knee synovitis with recurrent effusions that required synovial fluid aspiration at frequent intervals. Synovial fluid leukocyte counts ranged from 7500 to 12,000 WBC/mm^3. All patients had been on a stable dose of oral aspirin for at least 6 months. One patient was also taking Ibuprofen, and two were on chronic myochrysine therapy.

Informed written consent was obtained from each patient before his participation. All studies conformed to the standards set forth by the Declaration of Helsinki and the regulations of the Human Research and Nuclear Medicine Committee of the USVAMC (Wagner, 1968).

Early observations indicated great individual variability in the absorption of the topical and the oral preparations. For this reason, we decided to test each patient for both preparations, comparing the results only to those of the same patient. We waited approximately 6 weeks from one study to the next.

Patients abstained from salicylates for at least 6 hr before each study period. In the first part of the experiment, each patient received a 500-mg capsule of [^{14}C]aspirin. In the second part of the experiment, each patient was given 10 g of the triethanolamine [^{14}C]salicylate cream, which was gently massaged into the skin over one knee. Care was taken to continue application of the cream until all the material was absorbed. The skin surface area to which the topical salicylate was applied was approximately 25-30 cm square.

Blood and urine samples were obtained just before the administration of the oral or topical medication, and again at 60 and 120 min, at which time a synovial fluid aspiration was performed under sterile conditions. The synovial aspirations were performed after careful removal of the topical preparation from the skin (by washing with alcohol and Phisohex). The zero-time samples of blood were used to determine salicylate and ^{14}C background content; if either was above background, the patient was not given the medication, and the experiment was delayed until appropriate readings were obtained (Rabinowitz et al., 1982).

Measurement of Salicylate

All tissue samples were weighed. Aliquots of the tissue material were then homogenized with 20 volumes of 0.1 M sulfuric acid. Aliquots of the acidified homogenates of each of the tissues (20-40 ml) were then extracted three times each with 10 volumes of absolute ether. The ether extracts were combined and mixed with 10-15 g of anhydrous magnesium sulfate by shaking. After 3 hr, the magnesium sulfate was filtered and the anhydrous ether solution concentrated to a small volume. The salicylates from the ether extracts were isolated by thin-layer chromatography. Thin-layer plates (Silica Gel HF, Analabs, North Haven, Conn.) were spotted with the concentrated ether solution containing the salicylates. The plates were developed in methanol/acetic acid/ether/benzene (Rabinowitz et al., 1982). For acetylsalicylic acid, the Rf was determined to be 0.76, and for salicylic acid, the Rf was 0.85 (Stahl, 1969). The radioactive spots containing salicylates were scraped from the plate and reextracted in ether. This ether solution was evaporated, and the residue mixed with liquid scintillation phosphor solution and assayed for radioactivity.

RESULTS

Canine Study

The blood level of [^{14}C] salicylate at 30 and 60 min was 10-100 times lower after administration of topical TEA/S than after administration of an equimolar quantity of oral aspirin. Despite this, TEA/S application resulted in higher local tissue salicylate concentrations than those obtained from oral aspirin. These results suggest that topically applied TEA/S ointment was primarily absorbed locally by direct penetration. As expected, the skin showed the highest salicylate level after application. In addition, good salicylate concentrations were seen in a number of other tissues, including the ligament, tendon, cartilage, fascia, and fat pad. The adjacent muscle showed greater salicylate concentrations from topical TEA/S application than from oral aspirin. Approximately equal salicylate concentrations were noted in bone, synovial fluid, and synovium.

At distances greater than 10 cm from the point of cream application, tissue samples showed only trace salicylate levels.

Human Study

Oral [^{14}C]aspirin was absorbed into blood and synovial fluid and was excreted in the urine. After topical application of triethanolamine [^{14}C]salicylate, [^{14}C]-salicylate was found in the synovial fluid, indicating that it had been absorbed into the joint (through the skin through the blood system or directly). Concentrations after 2 hr were greater than those found after 1 hr.

The [^{14}C]salicylate concentrations in synovial fluid after the topical application of the triethanolamine [^{14}C]salicylate were found to be about half the concentrations found after the oral ingestion of [^{14}C]aspirin after both 1 and 2 hr. Blood [^{14}C]salicylate levels remained low after topical TEA/S application at both time intervals. The [^{14}C]salicylate blood levels at all time intervals were hundreds of times less from topical application than after peroral aspirin administration.

Our clinicians found that four of six patients reported equal subjective improvement after 1 and 2 hr from both topical salicylate and oral aspirin. There were no cases of gastrointestinal symptoms, skin irritation, or other adverse effects (Rabinowitz et al., 1982, 1984).

CONCLUSIONS

This study was designed to obtain accurate quantitative bioavailability data on the comparative absorption of oral and topical salicylates in specific tissues. For this purpose, ^{14}C-radioactive tracer methods were used. The use of trace amounts of radioactive materials facilitated the accurate measurement of salicylate levels in the tissues assayed, without producing significant human exposure (Chase and Rabinowitz, 1967; Quimby and Feitelberg, 1963; Wagner, 1968). Information on the ability of salicylates to penetrate the joint space and periarticular tissues was obtained. Our results demonstrated that topical salicylate can be absorbed through the skin, achieving significant salicylate levels directly or indirectly in the knee joint and surrounding tissues (Rabinowitz et al., 1982, 1984).

In canines, topical salicylate was clearly superior to oral aspirin in terms of local tissue concentrations achieved, despite lower blood levels. The highest salicylate concentrations were found in the areas where the ointment was directly applied. Measurable intra-articular concentrations of salicylate after topical application were observed. All the data support direct penetration as the initial route of absorption, with subsequent blood absorption and circulatory travel. Data obtained after 2 hr suggested that absorption may be increased through longer duration of the massage of the topical material. (See Figs. 1, 2, and 3.)

Our nuclear magnetic resonance spectra data demonstrated that the TEA/S preparation is a salt. This salt is lipid soluble, and as such could be transported intact through the lipid layers of the skin. This property may explain the high local tissue levels observed despite low circulatory levels.

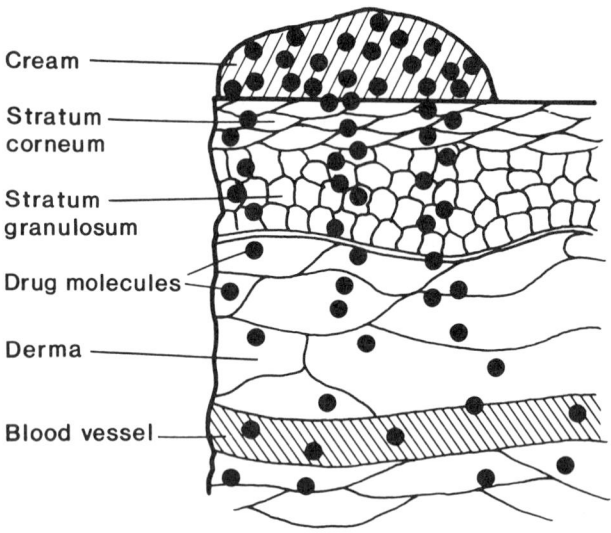

Figure 1 Schematic representation of the penetration of a pharmacologically active compound through the skin. The cream on the surface of the skin contains TEA/S and a vehicle (usually cold cream, a fatty material). TEA/S contains a pharmacologically beneficial compound (i.e., salicylic acid) and a compound that facilitates the penetration of the active ingredient (i.e., triethanolamine). After rubbing with the cream, the skin's stratum corneum may be disrupted by the triethanolamine in a way that permits the penetration of TEA/S; this penetration continues to the stratum granulosum and then through the fatty and muscular regions of the derma. As illustrated, the concentration of TEA/S per unit weight should be highest on the stratum corneum, and should slowly diminish when further from the surface. Finally, the TEA/S molecule, intact or broken into its components, passes through the capillary membranes of the blood vessels and enters the circulatory system. The TEA/S and/or its constituents then travel with the blood, lowering concentrations in the derma; this permits further movement of additional fresh TEA/S down from the skin.

Obviously, blood salicylate levels at the beginning of the rubbing will be smaller than tissue salicylate levels near the area of penetration (rubbing). After some time, however, tissues distant from the area of application will receive the salicylate through the blood supply. Many hours later the circulatory system will be instrumental in removing the metabolically detoxified materials from all the tissues and transporting them to the kidneys for eventual excretion by the urine. In peroral absorption, aspirin is transported almost totally through the actions of the circulatory system, so regions of poor blood supply will necessarily receive smaller salicylate concentrations than areas with good perfusion.

Absorption of Trolamine Salicylate in Joints 537

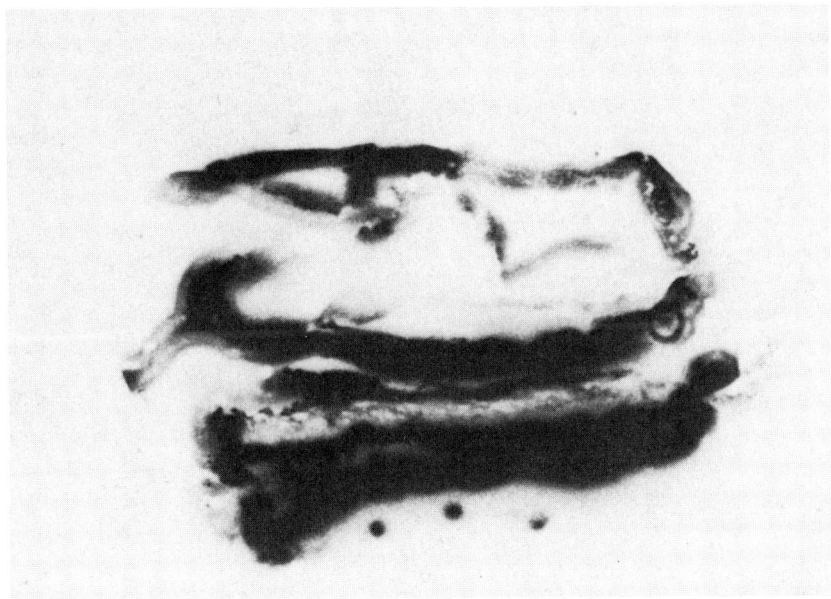

Figure 2 Negative print of an autoradiograph of the skin and adjacent tissues from a shaved dog's knee after 1 hr of gentle massaging with triethanolamine 7-[^{14}C]salicylic acid. The skin and adjacent tissue of the knee were then thoroughly washed to remove excess cream (soap and alcohol). To prepare this autoradiograph, 1 cm^2 of washed knee skin and adjacent tissue was removed from the animal, immediately frozen with powdered dry ice, and sectioned with a frozen (-20°C) microtome and 200-µm-thick serial sections made. The serial frozen sections were placed on thin glass cover slides and placed on Kodak autoradiographic film, with the tissues next to the film. A 25-g weight was placed on top of each cover slide, and the sections were put in a lead-shielded box. All these operations were performed in a cold room (0°C). The lead-shielded box was stored at -20°C. After 5 weeks the film was separated from the sections and thawed in a dark room, and the autoradiographic film was then developed.

The TEA/S may penetrate through the oily hair follicles on the skin, pass through the stratum corneum, and then through the stratum granulosum. In this photo, the dark areas represent radioactivity due to ^{14}C from the 7-[^{14}C]salicylic acid. Notice that the penetration of the salicylate is not regular; it appears to follow certain tissue compositions (possibly lipophilic areas). The muscular tissues show less darkness, thus indicating less content of salicylate than the fatty areas. Remnants of a capillary later on the slide also show radioactivity. Autoradiographs of tissues handled identically, but rubbed with TEA/S not containing 7-[^{14}C]salicylate, failed to show radioactive spots in any specific area. Scale = 1 in. of photograph = 1.5 mm in this section.

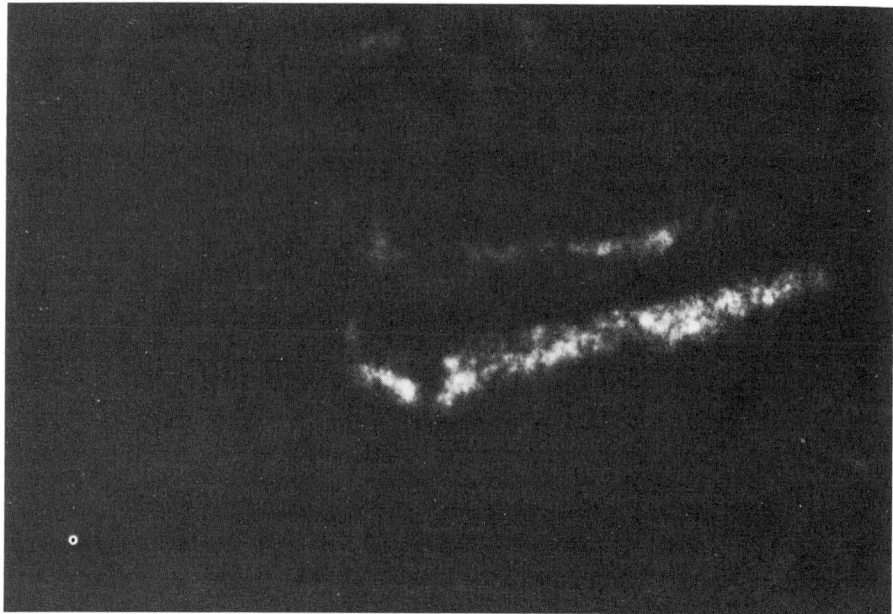

Figure 3 Positive print of an autoradiograph of a slice of a dog knee skin (same type as in Fig. 2). Radioactivity is shown by white dots, which represent the position of the ^{14}C of 7-[^{14}C]salicylic acid in the tissue. The highest concentrations were found on the surface, with diminishing concentrations further away from the skin. Penetration of salicylate is irregular, following tissues that may be richer in lipophilic materials. Scale: 1 in. photograph = 1.5 mm in this section.

We have shown that significant tissue and intra-articular salicylate levels can be achieved with topical application of TEA/S. The lipid solubility of this material permits it to remain near the site of application, from which it appears to be slowly absorbed into the bloodstream and eventually excreted. This very slow absorption is a highly desirable feature, since it permits longer relief of local discomfort without systemic side effects.

Recent work (Baldwin et al., 1984) on the penetration of trolamine salicylate into the skeletal muscle of the pig utilizing trolamine 7-[^{14}C]salicylate has also shown a high [^{14}C]salicylate penetration. About 13 times higher levels in muscle than that of blood and 49 times than those of muscle taken from untreated areas were measured in the pig. Results observed in this study were similar to those reported by us (Rabinowitz et al., 1982). Although different ^{14}C counting and separation techniques were used in this study and a different mode of application was employed, the observed penetration results for the pigs were similar to those observed in canines and in humans.

SUMMARY

We believe that topical application of TEA/S permits steady low-level absorption, and that this material remains in the adjacent areas while it is slowly being utilized; then it is steadily, slowly absorbed into the bloodstream, eventually passing through the kidney and being excreted in the urine. Autoradiography performed on sections of dog knees and early experiments with mice and rats indicated also a slow penetration throughout the tissues from the skin toward the muscles and fascia.

This specific work demonstrated that there is a very slow local absorption of the topically applied ointment, and that no significant amounts of salicylate are to be found at distances greater than 10 cm from the applied area. We believe that direct lipid penetration for a short distance (about 1 cm) is likely to be the first step in the mechanisms involved in the absorption of the lipid-soluble TEA/S preparations; these absorptions probably are highest if they occur through the lipid-rich areas of the skin. The capillaries may then very slowly pick up the salicylate from these areas. This slow penetration is advantageous, for it permits a high concentration of the active ingredient to remain in the area of application. The adjacent areas (of fat, fascia, muscle, synovium, etc.) below the massaged skin showed the highest levels of salicylate. This may explain why blood levels of salicylate are so very low after topical application, contrary to peroral administration, which yields immediately very high blood salicylate levels.

REFERENCES

Arthritis Foundation. (1976). *Arthritis Foundation Annual Report*. Arthritis Foundation Books, New York.

Baldwin, J. R., Carrano, R. A., and Imondi, A. R. (1984). Penetration of trolamine salicylate into the skeletal muscle of the pig. *J. Pharm. Sci. 93*: 1002–1004.

Blahd, W. M. (1971). *Nuclear Medicine*. McGraw-Hill, New York.

Chase, G. D. and Rabinowitz, J. L. (1967). *Principles of Radioisotope Methodology*, 3rd ed. Burgess, Minneapolis.

Flesch, P., Sabanove, A., and Brown, C. S. (1955). Laboratory methods for studying percutaneous absorption and the chemical effects of topical agents upon human skin. *J. Invest. Dermatol. 24*: 289–300.

Gaudin, O. (1952). U.S. Patent 2,596,674.

Golden, E. (1978). A double-blind comparison of orally ingested aspirin and a topically applied salicylate cream in the relief of rheumatic pain. *Curr. Ther. Res. 24*: 524–529.

Jackman, L. M. and Sternhell, S. (1969). *Application of Nuclear Magnetic Resonance Spectroscopy in Organic Chemistry*, 2nd ed. Pergamon, New York.

McCarthy, D. J., Editor. (1979). *Arthritis and Allied Conditions*, 9th ed. Lea & Febiger, Philadelphia.

Medical International Radiation Dose Committee of the Society of Nuclear Medicine (1969). *J. Nucl. Med. 10* (Suppl. 3 and 10).

Natelson, S. (1957). *Microtechniques of Clinical Chemistry for the Routine Laboratory*. Thomas, Springfield, Ill.

Nothman, M. and Wolff, M. (1933). The absorption of salicylic acid by human skin. *Klin. Wochenschr. 12*: 345-346.

Quimby, E. and Feitelberg, S. (1963). *Radioactive Isotopes in Medicine and Biology*. Lea & Febiger, Philadelphia.

Rabinowitz, J. L., Feldman, E. S., Weinberger, A., and Schumacher, H. R. (1982). Comparative tissue absorption of oral [^{14}C] aspirin and topical triethanolamine [^{14}C] salicylate in human and canine knee joints. *J. Clin. Pharmacol. 22*: 42-48.

Rabinowitz, J. L. and Baker, D. (1984). Absorption of labeled triethanolamine salicylate in human and canine knee joints. II. *J. Clin. Pharmacol. 24*: 532-539.

Ropes, M. W., Bennett, G. A., Cobb, S., Jacox, R., and Jessar, R. A. (1958). Revision of diagnostic criteria for rheumatoid arthritis. *Bull. Rheum. Dis. 9*: 175-176.

Rujahn, C. A. and With, E. (1937). The degree of percutaneous absorption of salicylic acid and esters from preparations sold for the treatment of arthritis. *Arch. Exp. Pathol. Pharmacol. 175*: 26-37.

Silvoso, G. R., Ivey, K. J., Butt, J. H., Lockhard, O. O., Holt, S. D., Sick, C., Baskin, W. N., MacKercher, P. A., and Hewett, J. (1979). Incidence of gastric lesions in patients with rheumatic disease on chronic aspirin therapy. *Ann. Intern. Med. 91*: 517-520.

Stahl, E. (1969). *Thin Layer Chromatography*. Springer-Verlag, New York.

Strakosch, E. A. (1943). Studies on ointments. IV. Local action of salicylic acid. *Arch. Dermatol. Syphilol. 48*: 348-392.

Wagner, H. (1968). *Principles of Nuclear Medicine*. Saunders, Philadelphia.

41
In Vivo Skin and Nitroglycerin Transdermal Delivery

Ronald C. Wester
University of California School of Medicine, San Francisco, California

Nitroglycerin (glyceryl trinitrate: GTN) is a potent vasodilator used in the treatment of angina pectoris, congestive heart failure, and acute myocardial infarction (Elkayam and Aronow, 1982). Part of the expanding use of nitroglycerin has come from the introduction of transdermal systems that offer sustained nitroglycerin delivery over longer periods of time. Administration of nitroglycerin ointment increases exercise capacity in patients with angina (Awan et al., 1978; Davidov and Mroczek, 1976; Reichek et al., 1974). Several new solid-state transdermal delivery systems (patches) are used for treatment of angina (Dasta and Geraets, 1982). These delivery systems yield sustained GTN concentrations in plasma (Gonzales et al., 1982; Karin et al., 1981; Muller et al., 1982). The sustained delivery is attributed to engineering in the device and little credit is given to the role of the skin. This chapter discusses the skin's attributes for nitroglycerin percutaneous absorption/transdermal delivery.

FACTORS INFLUENCING PERCUTANEOUS ABSORPTION

Table 1 lists the 10 steps to percutaneous absorption. Each step has an influence on the percutaneous absorption of chemicals. The first step is vehicle release, and this is where the controlling elements of transdermal delivery are located. Step 2 is absorption kinetics, and this is where the skin's role supposedly begins.

Table 1 Ten Steps to Percutaneous Absorption

1. Vehicle release
2. Absorption kinetics
    A. Skin site of application
    B. Individual variation
    C. Skin condition
    D. Occlusion
    E. Drug concentration and surface area
    F. Multiple dose application
3. Excretion kinetics
4. Effective cellular and tissue distribution
5. Substantivity
6. Wash and rub resistance
7. Volatility
8. Binding
9. Anatomic pathways
10. Cutaneous metabolism

Source: Wester and Maibach (1983).

Concentration of Dermally Applied Dose

Table 2 gives the percutaneous absorption in the rhesus monkey for increasing concentrations of nitroglycerin applied as ethanolic solutions to a constant skin surface area for 24 hr. The percentage dose absorbed was fairly constant over the range of 0.01-1.0 mg/cm^2. However, for 7 and 10 mg/cm^2 the efficiency of absorption decreased, suggesting a saturation of the skin's absorption process. Thus, concentration can limit absorption.

Surface Area

When concentration becomes limiting, the systemic availability of a transdermal drug can be increased with a larger surface area. However, consumer acceptance will limit the size of the transdermal systems. Table 3 shows the interaction of surface area and concentrations on the ability of the skin to efficiently absorb nitroglycerin. For a constant dose (40 mg), the surface area will determine concentration per unit of skin area, and this will determine the efficiency of skin absorption. The 20-mg/cm^2 dose on the smaller surface area in Table 3 is in the skin saturation range shown in Table 2 (Noonan and Wester, 1980).

Table 2 Effect of Dermal Concentration on Percutaneous Absorption of Nitroglycerin

Nitroglycerin concentration (mg/cm^2)	Percentage of dose absorbed	Total absorbed (mg)
0.01	41.8	0.004
0.1	43.5	0.04
1.0	36.6	0.4
7.0	26.6	1.9
10.0	7.8	0.8

Source: Wester (1983).

Transdermal Device Thickness and Nitroglycerin Absorption

Table 4 shows the influence of transdermal device thickness and nitroglycerin transdermal delivery. Devices were made with a surface area of 5 cm^2 and thickness of 0.6 cm. The total nitroglycerin content in each device was 40 mg and of this, 6.5 ±0.08% was absorbed by rhesus monkeys for a 24-hr application period. Some of these original devices were then sliced horizontally into four pieces, each with combined dimensions of 20 cm^2 × 0.15 cm. As an analogy, consider the original device to be four stacked coins of dimensions 5 cm^2 × 0.6 cm and then place the coins on a surface side by side, giving dimensions of 20 cm^2 × 0.15 cm. Thus, the total nitroglycerin dose remains at 40 mg and the device formulation was identical. The thickness of the device was decreased by one-fourth, and concomitantly the surface area was increased by 4 (which in turn decreased concentration per unit skin area). The percentage dose absorbed then increased fourfold. Thus, the efficiency of absorption (and transdermal delivery) was greatly increased by altering some of the factors that influence percutaneous absorption.

Table 3 Skin Surface Area and Percutaneous Absorption of Nitroglycerin

Total dose (mg)	Surface area (cm^2)	Concentration (mg/cm^2)	Percentage of dose absorbed
40	2	20	13.4±1.2
40	50	0.8	36.4±4.3

Source: Wester (1983).

Table 4 Transdermal Device Thickness and Nitroglycerin Absorption

Total dose (mg)	Device dimensions	Percentage of dose absorbed
40	5 cm^2 × 0.6 cm	6.5±0.08
40	20 cm^2 × 0.15 cm	22.4±1.3

Source: Wester (1983).

Transdermal Device Formulation

Concentration, surface area, and device thickness can determine, and also limit, efficiency of transdermal delivery. Formulation also interacts with these factors and can be used to enhance absorption. Table 5 gives the percentage of nitroglycerin dose delivered in rhesus monkeys for several transdermal formulations. With all variables but vehicle controlled, formulation D obviously showed enhanced transdermal absorption. The efficiency of absorption for formulation D could be further enhanced by reducing the concentration of nitroglycerin per unit skin area from 10 (saturating dose) to 2.5 mg/cm^2 (see Table 2).

Skin Stripping and Transdermal Delivery

Skin contains the sink conditions for which a transdermal device must deliver its drug. If a transdermal device is the rate-limiting step, alteration of the skin should not affect drug delivery. Skin stripping with cellophane tape removes the outer layers of the stratum corneum and thus removes some of the skin's barrier properties. An ethanolic solution of nitroglycerin was applied to intact and stripped skin (Table 6). Stripped skin gave enhanced absorption. The same results were obtained with nitroglycerin in a transdermal device. Thus, the skin was the rate-limiting step in transdermal delivery, not the device.

Table 5 Formulation and Transdermal Delivery of Nitroglycerin

Device formulation	Nitroglycerin concentration (mg/cm^2)	Percentage of dose delivered
A	10	4.9±2.1
B	10	9.4±1.7
C	10	4.6±1.2
D	10	28.1±1.9
D	2.5	37.4±3.6

Source: Wester (1983).

Table 6 Skin Stripping and Transdermal Delivery of Nitroglycerin

Nitroglycerin dosage form	Percentage of dose absorbed	
	Intact skin	Stripped skin
Ethanolic solution	30.8±5.4	55.1±4.1
Device	28.2±6.1	63.3±6.3

Source: Wester (1983).

Table 7 Apparent Transdermal Absorption Rates and Transdermal Dosage Forms of Nitroglycerin Administered to Healthy Volunteers

Parameter	Absorption rate ($\mu g/hr \cdot cm^2$)		
	Nitro-BID ointment	Nitro-DUR system	Nitrodisc system
Mean	5.15	8.09	5.55
± SD	1.07	6.35	3.04
n	5	4	4

Source: Noonan et al. (1983).

APPARENT TRANSDERMAL ABSORPTION RATES (HUMANS)

Noonan and co-workers determined the absolute bioavailabilities of nitroglycerin for an ointment dosage form (Nitro-BID) and for two transdermal delivery systems (Nitro-DUR, Nitrodisc). The amounts of nitroglycerin absorbed were 4.7±2.0, 3.9±3.0, and 1.6±0.4 mg, respectively. The apparent absorption rates were determined after normalizing for surface area differences. Table 7 shows that the mean absorption rates were not significantly different from each other. They concluded that absorption of nitroglycerin through the skin was the rate-limiting step of the transdermal delivery process.

SUMMARY

The skin plays an active role in nitroglycerin transdermal delivery and probably is the rate-limiting step. Thus factors that affect percutaneous absorption (concentration, surface area, vehicles, etc.) must be considered in the study design for bioavailability from transdermal systems. These percutaneous absorption factors must be controlled variables when a transdermal system is evaluated.

REFERENCES

Awan, N. A., Miller, R. R., Maxwell, K. S., and Mason, D. T. (1978). Cardiocirculatory and antianginal actions of nitroglycerin ointment—Evaluation by cardiac catheterization, forearm plethysmography and treadmill stress testing. *Chest 73*: 14–18.

Dasta, J. F. and Geraets, D. R. (1982). Topical nitroglycerin: A new twist to an old standby. *Am. Pharm. NS22*: 85–88.

Davidov, M. E. and Mroczek, W. J. (1976). The effect of nitroglycerin ointment on the exercise capacity in patients with angina pectoris. *Angiology 27*: 205–211.

Elkayam, U. and Aronow, W. S. (1982). Glyceryl trinitrate (nitroglycerin) ointment and isosorbide dinitrate: A review of their pharmacological properties and therapeutic use. *Drugs 23*: 165–194.

Gonzales, M. A., Hsiao, J., Blanford, M. F., and Golub, A. L. (1982). Determination of nitroglycerin (GTN) in plasma by gas-liquid chromatography. Abstracts, 1982 Midwest Regional Meeting of the American Pharmaceutical Association and the American Physical Society, May.

Karin, A., Schubert, E., Schoenhard, G., Arnold, J., Berzer, A., and Boyer, S. (1981). Transdermal absorption of nitroglycerin in man. Abstracts, Eighth International Congress of Pharmacology, Tokyo, p. 556.

Muller, P., Imhof, P. R., Burkart, F., Chu, L.-C., and Gerardin, A. (1982). Human pharmacological studies of a new transdermal system containing nitroglycerin. *Eur. J. Clin. Pharmacol. 22*: 473–480.

Noonan, P. K. and Wester, R. C. (1980). Percutaneous absorption of nitroglycerin. *J. Pharm. Sci. 69*: 365.

Noonan, P. K., Rigod, J. F., Williams, R. F., and Benet, L. Z. (1983). Transdermal absorption rates of nitroglycerin in healthy volunteers. Presented at the Tenth International Symposium on the Controlled Release of Bioactive Materials, pp. 332–335.

Reichek, N., Goldstein, R. E., Redwood, D. R., and Epstein, S. E. (1974). Sustained effects of nitroglycerin ointment in patients with angina pectoris. *Circulation 50*: 348–352.

Wester, R. C. (1983). Role of skin in nitroglycerin transdermal delivery. Presented at the Tenth International Symposium on the Controlled Release of Bioactive Materials, pp. 329–331.

Wester, R. C. and Maibach, H. I. (1983). Cutaneous pharmacokinetics: 10 steps to percutaneous absorption. *Drug Metab. Rev. 14*: 169–205.

42
Pharmacodynamics and Percutaneous Absorption
Minoxidil Stimulates Cutaneous Blood Flow in Balding Humans

Ronald C. Wester and Howard I. Maibach
University of California School of Medicine, San Francisco, California

Richard H. Guy
University of California School of Pharmacy, San Francisco, California

Ervin Novak
The Upjohn Company, Kalamazoo, Michigan

Minoxidil, an orally effective, direct-acting peripheral vasodilator prescribed for hypertension, occasionally produces hypertrichosis. It has been hypothesized that the mechanism for minoxidil stimulation of hair growth is its potent vasodilation. The microcirculation surrounding the hair follicle is decreased, leading to hypertrichosis. A minoxidil topical preparation would stimulate the microcirculation surrounding the hair follicle. This was tested in a double-blind study for 0, 1, 3, and 5% minoxidil solutions using laser Doppler velocimetry (LDV) and photopulse plethysmography (PPG) to noninvasively measure cutaneous blood flow and blood perfusion in balding scalps of 16 human volunteers. A 0.25-ml volume of the formulations was uniformly spread over 100 cm^2 of the bald scalp and cutaneous blood flow recorded for 4 hr on two consecutive days.

Blood flow data were analyzed using analysis of variance, and vital signs were analyzed using paired t-test and analysis of variance. When the data were summarized over time, the 5% minoxidil solution had increased blood flow when compared to other treatments. LDV response on day 1 ($p < 0.0001$) increased within 15 min of application, and maintained increased blood flow at least through hour 1. Day 2 blood flow stimulation ($p < 0.0001$) was threefold within 15 min of application and lasted for about 1 hr. PPG response was significant ($p < 0.01$) only for day 2 application of the 5% minoxidil solution.

Reproduced from *J. Invest. Dermatol. 85*: 515, 1984 with permission of the publisher.

LDV measures a single microcirculatory flow parameter and PPG measures changes in microcirculatory blood volume. Both optical techniques showed that the 5% minoxidil solution stimulated the microcirculation of the bald scalp. Analysis of vital signs for days 1 and 2 gave no indication of minoxidil systemic effect, suggesting that the blood flow stimulation was direct following topical application.

INTRODUCTION

The antihypertensive agent minoxidil may be useful in the development of a model for studying hypertrichosis, male pattern baldness, and other alopecias. Some patients using minoxidil for control of their hypertension have experienced a general and unpredictable hypertrichosis of their facial and body vellus hairs. Changes in the hair growth patterns of these patients have been observed in the area between the eyebrows and existing hairline, in the malar and temporal areas, between the eyebrows, and on the back, arms, shoulders, and legs. The incidence of the hypertrichosis has been between 30 and 50% for males and 50 and 85% for females.

Minoxidil is an orally effective, direct-acting peripheral vasodilator that reduces elevated systolic and diastolic blood pressure by decreasing peripheral vascular resistance. Microcirculatory blood flow in animals is enhanced or maintained in all systemic vascular beds. In man, forearm and renal vascular resistance decline, forearm blood flow increases, and renal blood flow and glomular filtration rate are preserved (Gottlieb et al., 1972; *Physicians Desk Reference*, 1981; Weiss et al., 1982).

It has been hypothesized that the mechanism for minoxidil stimulation of hair growth is its potent vasodilation. The microcirculation surrounding the hair follicle is stimulated, thus leading to hypertrichosis. If this is true, then a minoxidil topical preparation applied to the scalp could lead to direct stimulation of the microcirculation surrounding the hair follicle, and perhaps a reversal of the alopecia process. New methods, laser Doppler velocimetry and photopulse plethysmography, were used to measure noninvasively the cutaneous blood flow in bald but otherwise healthy volunteers following topical application of minoxidil solutions or vehicle only, to balding scalp areas.

METHODS

The double-blind study involved 16 male volunteers, aged 24 to 76 years, from whom informed consent was obtained. All volunteers had balding scalps, but were otherwise healthy. A complete physical exam, including subject's medical history and a recording of vital signs (pulse, respiration, body weight, and blood pressure) was conducted at the time of selection. Volunteers were not to be on any form of medication for 14 days before the study and were not to receive medication other than the test drug during the study.

The laser Doppler velocimetry (LDV) method operates on the Doppler principle. Light from a 5-mW helium-neon laser is transmitted to the skin through a quartz optical fiber. The light is backscattered from stationary skin components and by red blood cells moving in the dermal capillaries, which are encountered as the radiation penetrates to a depth of 1–1.5 mm (approximately 0.05 in.). A second optical fiber collects the reflected light and the frequency-shifted component is converted to a single flow parameter. Photopulse plethysmography (PPG) utilizes a diode-emitting infrared light and determines changes in blood volume passing through the microcirculation by the percentage of incident radiation absorbed. Both techniques are noninvasive (Guy et al., 1981a,b, 1983; Holloway and Watkins, 1977; Watkins and Holloway, 1978).

On day 1 before drug was applied, blood pressure and pulse rates were obtained. Baseline measurement of blood flow in the scalp skin at the intended site of drug application was made with both techniques, LDV on one half of the scalp and PPG on the other half.

The topical formulations used were vehicle only, and minoxidil in 1, 3, and 5% concentrations in a vehicle of varying proportions of propylene glycol/ethanol/water. Volunteers were randomly assigned to one formulation. A volume of 0.25 ml of formulation was distributed uniformly over 100 cm^2 of the bald scalp area. A 15-min "drying period" after drug application was allowed before recording was started. The LDV and PPG probes were positioned on the scalp at the site drug application. Cutaneous blood flow was recorded continuously for 40–60 min, and then intermittently for 4 hr. Blood pressure and pulse rates were taken after the 4-hr recording. Volunteers were asked to not wash the scalp before day 2.

On study day 2 (following day), vital signs were obtained and a baseline blood flow measurement obtained. This measurement was both the 24-hr measurement for day 1 and the predrug measurement for day 2. The same randomly assigned formulation from day 1 was reapplied to the same scalp site and cutaneous blood flow recorded as on day 1. Vital signs were again obtained after the 4-hr session.

The blood flow data were analyzed using analysis of variance techniques and the paired t-test. Change from baseline (difference scores) were analyzed using the paired t-test within treatment groups. Differences between treatment groups were evaluated using analysis of variance. A summary result was obtained by averaging the scores across the periods (excluding the predrug score). An analysis of variance model with factors, time period at treatment (minoxidil solution), was used to obtain the significance levels for the summary results. Vital signs were analyzed using the paired t-test within treatment groups and analysis of variance across treatment groups.

RESULTS

Table 1 gives the LDV blood flow measurements for day 1 application of 0, 1, 3, and 5% minoxidil solution. When the data were summarized over time periods, the 5% solution had increased blood flow ($p < 0.0001$) when compared to other treatments. Figure 1 shows that the 0% solution showed a slight increase in blood flow through the first 40 min of recording. This is the time period of continuous recording, suggesting that the presence of the probe or the vehicle itself had some small vasodilation effect. The 1, 3, and 5% solutions produced increases in blood flow, suggestive of a dose response.

Table 2 gives the LDV blood flow measurements for day 2. When the data were summarized over time periods, the 5% solution had increased blood flow ($p < 0.0001$). Figure 2 shows no differences with the 24-hr measurement, nor with the time curves for the 0, 1, or 3% solutions. The 5% solution shows a threefold increase in blood flow, which was maintained for the first hour following drug application. After 1 hr blood flow was the same for all applications.

Table 3 gives the PPG blood flow measurements for day 1. There were no significant treatment differences. Figure 3 shows the time curves for the applications.

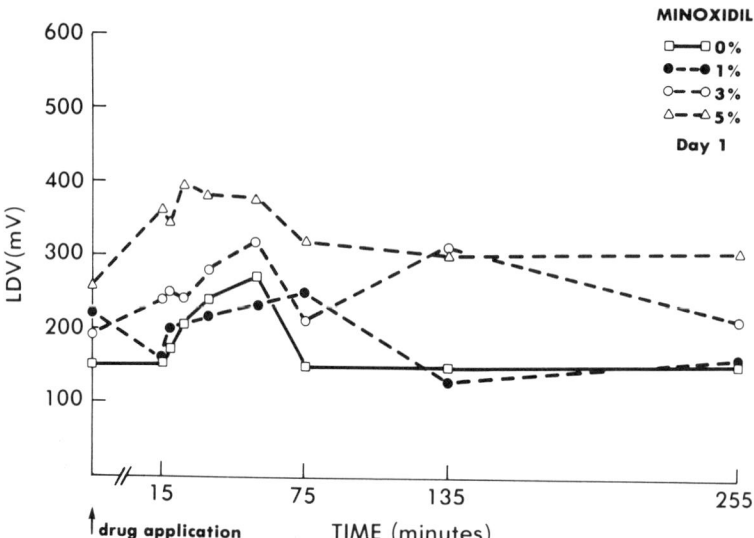

Figure 1 Laser Doppler velocimetry (LDV) blood flow versus time curve following day 1 application of 0, 1, 3, and 5% topical minoxidil to bald human scalps. LDV response is in millivolts (mV).

Table 1 Measurement of Blood Flow by Laser Doppler Velocimetry: Day 1

| | Minoxidil solution ||||||||| Significance level ||
| Time (min) | 0% (n = 3) || 1% (n = 4) || 3% (n = 4) || 5% (n = 5) || | |
	Mean	Difference	Mean	Difference	Mean	Difference	Mean	Difference	Mean	Difference
Predrug	149.3		221.0		190.0		261.6		0.7568	
15	156.0	6.7	163.0	−58.0	242.0	52.0	365.0[a]	50.0[a]	0.2778	0.7556
20	176.0	26.7	201.0	−20.0	254.0	64.0	337.6	76.0	0.6113	0.8405
25	209.3	60.0	208.0	−13.0	243.0	53.0	369.6	108.0	0.5737	0.7547
35	242.7	93.3	217.0	−4.0	288.0	98.0	383.2	121.6	0.5801	0.5838
55	273.3	124.0	234.0	13.0	320.0	130.0	374.4	112.8	0.7082	0.6789
75	150.7	1.3	251.0	30.0	210.0	20.0	308.0	46.4	0.3520	0.9165
135	148.0	−1.3	130.0	−91.0	314.0	124.0	299.2	37.6	0.1421	0.4088
255	156.0	6.7	162.0	−59.0	215.0	25.0	308.8	47.2	0.2425	0.7583
Summary (excluding predrug)	(n = 24) 189.0	(n = 24) 39.7	(n = 32) 195.8	(n = 32) −25.3	(n = 32) 260.8	(n = 32) 70.8[b]	(n = 39) 342.7	(n = 39) 75.6[b]	0.0001[c]	0.0151[d]

[a] n = 4.
[b] Statistically significant change from baseline ($\alpha \leq 0.01$).
[c] Statistically significant ($\alpha \leq 0.01$): 5% > others.
[d] Statistically significant ($\alpha \leq 0.05$): 3% and 5% > 1%.

Table 2 Measurement of Blood Flow by Laser Doppler Velocimetry: Day 2

| | \multicolumn{8}{c}{Minoxidil solution} | | |

Time (min)	0% (n = 3) Mean	Difference	1% (n = 4) Mean	Difference	3% (n = 4) Mean	Difference	5% (n = 5) Mean	Difference	Significance level Mean	Difference
Predrug	150.7		156.5		164.0		138.4		0.9793	
15	218.7	68.0	167.0	10.5	222.0	58.0	515.8	377.4	0.1869	0.1405
20	192.0	41.3	160.0	3.5	242.0	78.0	499.0	360.6	0.1341	0.0818
25	198.7	48.0	192.5	36.0	264.0	100.0	483.8	345.4	0.1931	0.0993
35	234.7	84.0	229.0	72.5	224.0	60.0	504.6	366.2[a]	0.2067	0.0832
55	205.3	54.7[a]	230.0	73.5	221.0	57.0	480.6	342.2	0.2070	0.0961
75	158.7	8.0	226.0	69.5	193.0	29.0	219.2	80.8	0.8737	0.8571
135	189.3	38.7	251.0	94.5	210.0	46.0	220.0	81.6[b]	0.9588	0.9568
255	218.7	68.0	160.0	3.5	309.0	145.0	304.0	165.6[b]	0.3526	0.3484
Summary (excluding predrug)	(n = 24) 202.0	(n = 24) 51.3[b]	(n = 32) 201.9	(n = 32) 45.4	(n = 32) 235.6	(n = 32) 71.6[b]	(n = 39) 403.4	(n = 39) 265.0[b]	0.0001[c]	0.0001[c]

[a] Statistically significant change from baseline ($\alpha \leq 0.05$).
[b] Statistically significant change from baseline ($\alpha \leq 0.01$).
[c] Statistically significant ($\alpha \leq 0.01$): 5% > others.

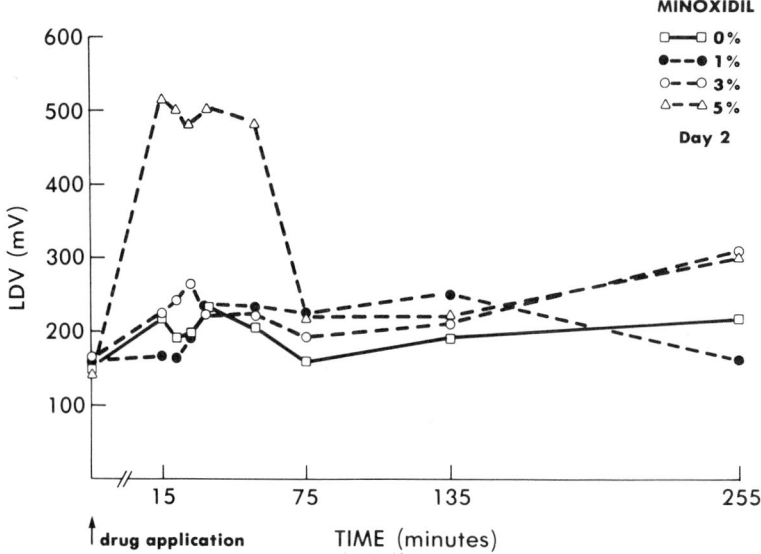

Figure 2 LDV blood flow versus time curve following day 2 application of 0, 1, 3, and 5% topical minoxidil to bald human scalps. LDV response is in millivolts (mV).

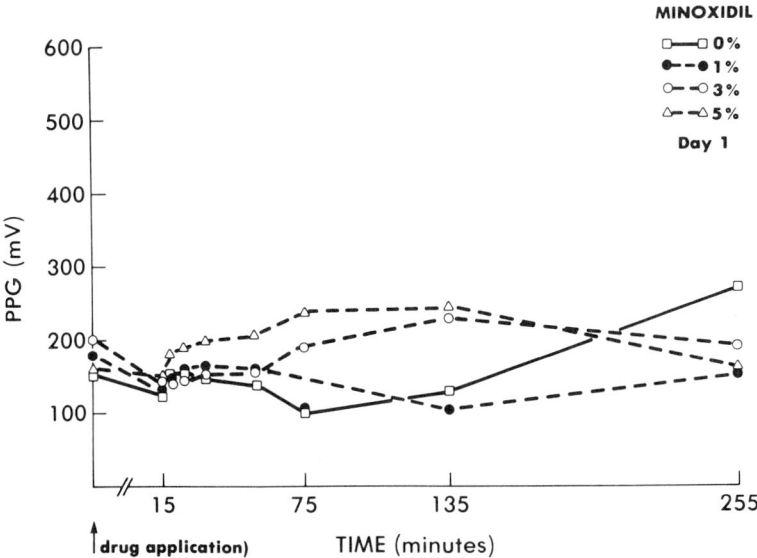

Figure 3 Photopulse plethysmography (PPG) blood perfusion versus time curve following day 1 application of 0, 1, 3, and 5% topical minoxidil to bald human scalps. PPG response is in millivolts (mV).

Table 3 Measurement of Blood Flow by Photopulse Plethysmography: Day 1

Time (min)	0% (n = 3)		(1% (n = 4)		Minoxidil solution 3% (n = 4)		5% (n = 5)		Significance level	
	Mean	Difference	Mean	Difference	Mean	Difference	Mean	Difference	Mean	Difference
Predrug	148.3				202.5		160.0		0.8970	
15	121.7	-26.7	127.5	-51.3	141.3	-61.3	135.0[a]	-21.3[a,b]	0.9869	0.9099
20	155.0	6.7	151.3	-27.5	145.0	-57.5	179.4	19.4	0.9230	0.3779
25	156.7	8.3	158.8	-20.0	146.3	-56.3	191.0	31.0	0.8500	0.2331
35	146.7	-1.7	165.0	-13.8	148.8	-53.8	200.0	40.0	0.6914	0.1943
55	135.0	-13.3	157.5	-21.3	158.8	-43.8	205.0	45.0	0.5901	0.3325
75	98.3	-50.0	102.5	-76.3	192.5	-10.0	235.0	75.0	0.2011	0.2526
135	130.0	-18.3	102.5	-76.3	231.3	28.8	242.0	82.0	0.2444	0.1869
255	273.3	125.0	147.5	-31.3	190.0	-12.5	152.0	-8.0	0.6625	0.1869
Summary (excluding predrug)	(n = 24) 152.1	(n = 24) 3.8	(n = 32) 139.1	(n = 32) -39.7[c]	(n = 32) 169.2	(n = 32) -33.3	(n = 39) 193.9	(n = 39) 34.3[c]	0.0937	0.0009[d]

[a] n = 4.
[b] Statistically significant change from baseline (α ≤ 0.05).
[c] Statistically significant change from baseline (α ≤ 0.01).
[d] Statistically significant (α ≤ 0.01): 5% > 1% and 3%.

Table 4 gives the PPG blood flow measurements for day 2. When the data were summarized over time periods, the 5% solution had increased blood flow ($p < 0.0016$) when compared to other treatments. Figure 4 shows an elevated blood flow at 24 hr following day 1 application. This was maintained by day 2 drug application through hour 2.

Tables 5 and 6 summarize the vital signs for days 1 and 2. There is no indication of a systemic effect for minoxidil as monitored by pulse rate and blood pressure.

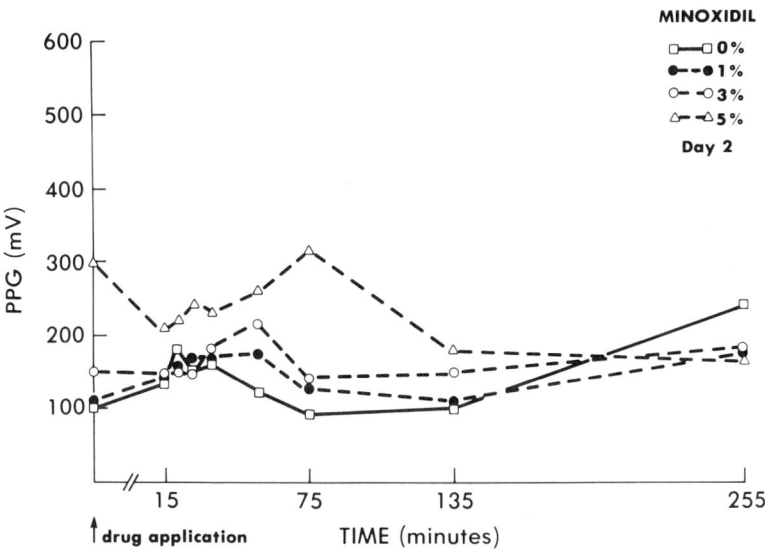

Figure 4 PPG blood perfusion versus time curve following day 2 application of 0, 1, 3, and 5% topical minoxidil to bald human scalps. PPG response is in millivolts (mV).

Table 4 Measurement of Blood Flow by Photopulse Plethysmography: Day 2

	Minoxidil solution									
	0% (n = 3)		1% (n = 4)		3% (n = 4)		5% (n = 5)		Significance level	
Time (min)	Mean	Difference	Mean	Difference	Mean	Difference	Mean	Difference	Mean	Difference
Predrug	100.0		112.5		150.0		303.0		0.0524	
15	136.7	36.7	142.5	30.0	135.0	-15.0	210.0	-93.0	0.7237	0.4616
20	181.7	81.7	162.5	50.0	148.8	-1.3	223.0	-80.0	0.8189	0.4297
25	153.3	53.3	168.8	56.3	148.8	-1.3	236.0	-67.0	0.6218	0.5734
35	161.7	61.7	167.5	55.0	183.8	33.8	233.0	-70.0	0.7964	0.5131
55	121.7	21.7	176.3	63.8	217.5	67.5	262.0	-41.0	0.4606	0.6928
75	91.7	-8.3	125.0	12.5	140.0	-10.0	315.0	12.0	0.1074	0.9913
135	101.7	1.7	110.0	-2.5	148.8	-1.3	177.0	-126.0	0.4023	0.2111
255	243.3	143.3	175.0	62.5	175.0	25.0	166.0	-137.0	0.8847	0.0901
Summary	(n = 24)	(n = 24)	(n = 32)	(n = 32)	(n = 32)	(n = 32)	(n = 39)	(n = 39)		
(excluding predrug)	149.0	49.0[a]	153.4	40.9[b]	162.2	12.2	227.8	-75.3[a]	0.0107[c]	0.0003[d]

[a]Statistically significant change from baseline ($\alpha \leq 0.05$).
[b]Statistically significant change from baseline ($\alpha \leq 0.01$).
[c]Statistically significant ($\alpha \leq 0.05$): 5% > others.
[d]Statistically significant ($\alpha \leq 0.01$): 5% < others.

Table 5 Summary of Vital Signs: Day 1

	Minoxidil solution															
	0% (n = 3)			1% (n = 4)			3% (n = 4)			5% (n = 5)			Significance levels		
Vital signs	Sys-tolic	Dia-stolic	Pulse	Sys-tolic	Dia-stolic	Pulse	Sys-tolic	Dia-stolic	Pulse	Sys-tolic	Dia-stolic	Pulse	Sys-tolic	Dia-stolic	Pulse
Before	115.7	79.0	80.7	113.0	79.0	78.0	115.5	77.8	78.5	120.4	83.2	83.0	0.8395	0.7141	0.9303
After	116.0	85.3	74.0	118.0	82.0	76.3	115.3	77.0	69.0	115.2	81.2	82.8	0.9881	0.5934	0.6396
Difference	−0.3	−6.3[a]	6.7	−5.0	−3.0	1.8	0.3	0.8	9.5[a]	5.2	2.0	0.2	0.3324	0.5312	0.7092

[a]Statistically significant ($\alpha \leq 0.05$).

Table 6 Summary of Vital Signs: Day 2

Vital signs	Minoxidil solution												Significance levels		
	0% (n = 3)			1% (n = 4)			3% (n = 4)			5% (n = 5)					
	Sys-tolic	Dia-stolic	Pulse	Sys-tolic	Dia-stolic	Pulse	Sys-tolic	Dia-stolic	Pulse	Sys-tolic	Dia-stolic	Pulse	Sys-tolic	Dia-stolic	Pulse
Before	116.0	76.7	81.0	119.5	80.3	67.8	107.0	76.5	69.0	116.2	79.6	80.4	0.5431	0.9122	0.2880
After	115.7	75.3	70.3	111.8	78.0	73.5	109.0	74.5	71.2	111.6	80.0	74.0	0.9422	0.7868	0.9476
Difference	0.3	1.3	10.7	7.8	2.3	-5.8[a]	-2.0	2.0	-2.3	4.6	-0.4	6.4	0.3721	0.9763	0.0283[b]

[a] Statistically significant ($\alpha \leq 0.05$).
[b] Statistically significant ($\alpha \leq 0.05$); 0% different from 1%.

DISCUSSION

The two optical procedures (LDV and PPG) use different approaches to generate a voltage related to perfusion of the cutaneous microcirculation. The LDV method operates using the Doppler principle. Light is backscattered from the stationary skin components and by erythrocytes moving in the dermal capillaries. The instrument separates out the frequency-shifted (i.e., Doppler-shifted) component and converts it to a single "flow parameter," which is registered as a voltage output. This output correlates with peripheral cutaneous circulation. The PPG emits infrared radiation, the frequency of which covers wavelengths strongly absorbed by hemoglobin. It follows that changes in blood volume in the region of skin under the probe cause the PPG output to change because the percentage of incident radiation absorbed is altered. Minoxidil enhances microcirculatory blood flow, and this was detected by both LDV and PPG procedures following topical application. The lack of any systemic effects on pulse rate and blood pressure suggests that the activity of minoxidil is local through percutaneous absorption following topical application.

The most significant point of this study is that the pharmacodynamics of topical minoxidil can now be studied in the bald scalp, the site of action. These pharmacodynamic data are most relevant in designing and interpreting clinical efficacy studies. For example, the data show the time course of topical minoxidil activity to be much less than would be anticipated for a topical preparation. Usually percutaneous absorption is a slow process. The major activity for minoxidil lasts for only an hour following application. This suggests that multiple daily applications may improve response and subsequent efficacy. Second, the response on day 2 was greater than day 1. This suggests an increase in topical bioavailability (rate and/or amount of absorption), or perhaps some activation of minoxidil from day 1 application. Skin exhibits a reservoir effect where some chemicals can be retained following topical application. This chemical is normally lost during skin exfoliation. However, subsequent treatments such as occlusion can inhibit this loss process and the reservoir chemical is subsequently absorbed. Pharmacodynamic studies following chronic application could indicate when (or indeed if) steady-state conditions are established.

Positive pharmacodynamic results such as this are exciting; however, clinical relevance to hair growth requires appropriate controlled efficacy studies. The effect of vasodilation on hair growth has not been shown. Also, the correlations of pharmacodynamics and percutaneous absorption have not been established. It would seem unusual for percutaneous absorption to be completed in an hour (the time of pharmacodynamic response). Perhaps a threshold concentration is needed in the scalp to maintain vasodilation. The suggestion of a dose response might indicate this.

Comparison of responses by LDV and PPG seems to indicate that LDV is the more sensitive technique to monitor vasodilation. Subsequent studies with minoxidil probably could be done with this technique only, unless there is a special necessity to look at PPG measurement of blood perfusion.

In summary, both laser Doppler velocimetry and photopulse plethysmography are able to show pharmacodynamic responses for topical minoxidil applied to bald human scalps.

REFERENCES

Gottlieb, T. B., Katz, F. H., and Chidsey, C. A. (1972). Combined therapy with vasodilator drugs and β-adrenergic blockade in hypertension: A comparative study of minoxidil and hydralazine. *Circulation 43*: 571–582.

Guy, R. H., Maibach, H. I., and Wester, R. C. (1981a). Percutaneous penetration monitored by laser Doppler velocimetry. American Pharmaceutical Association abstract 27, Orlando, Fla.

Guy, R. H., Maibach, H. I., and Wester, R. C. (1981b). Non-invasive monitoring of percutaneous absorption in vivo. *Clin. Res. 30*: 157A.

Guy, R. H., Wester, R. C., Tur, E., and Maibach, H. I. (1983). Non-invasive assessments of the percutaneous absorption of methyl nicotinate in man. *J. Pharm. Sci. 72*: 1077–1079.

Holloway, G. A., Jr. and Watkins, D. W. (1977). Laser Doppler measurement of cutaneous blood flow. *J. Invest. Dermatol. 69*: 306–309.

Physicians' Desk Reference, 35th ed. (1981). Loniten®, Medical Economics Co., Oradell, N.J., p. 1826.

Watkins, D. W. and Holloway, G. A., Jr. (1978). An instrument to measure cutaneous blood flow using the Dopple shift of laser light. *IEEE Trans. Biomed. Eng. BME-25*: 28–33.

Weiss, V. C., West, D. P., Robinson, L. A., and Mueller, C. E. (1982). Topical minoxidil in alopecia areata. Presented at the Third Annual Meeting of the American College of Clinical Pharmacologists, June, Kansas City, Mo. Abstr. 78.

43
Vehicles as Penetration Enhancers

Christopher L. Gummer
University of California School of Medicine, San Francisco, California

It is generally believed that the vehicle component of a dermatological formulation can appreciably affect the penetration of compounds through the skin (Christie and Moore Robinson, 1970; Jimbo et al., 1983; Tissot and Osmundson 1966). Most publications regarding the variable activity of vehicles are comparisons of existing formulations or of single solvents that do not reflect the actions of a completed formulation. However, since no concise definition of a "vehicle" exists, one must be cautious in the interpretation of experimental data that reports the increased percutaneous penetration of drugs from a variety of formulations. For a compound to act as a vehicle/penetration enhancer it should:

1. Confer stability on the drug, presenting it in an active form at therapeutic levels.
2. Be suitable for use in certain dermatoses and/or be cosmetically acceptable.
3. Produce either no change or a controlled, reversible change in the epidermis.
4. Enhance penetration of another, presumably "active" agent.
5. Offer subjective or "cosmetic" qualities.

A vehicle may therefore be a means of applying a drug to the skin surface, releasing the drug at a therapeutic level, and increasing or decreasing the penetration of the drug through the skin without permanently altering the structural integrity of the epidermis.

COSMETIC AND THERAPEUTIC EFFECTS

Prolonged treatment, particularly to the exposed areas, dictates that the vehicle be cosmetically acceptable for everyday use. Such vehicles are usually of an aqueous or emulsion type and often pigmented, allowing the application of a thin, often invisible film. Other vehicles are chosen for their therapeutic effects (e.g., to give relief from itching or pain, to act as emolients and moisturizers for dry skin, or to remove dirt and exudate). Similarly the vehicle should be inert and should not cause contact irritation or promote bacterial growth. Dermatologic vehicle formulation is often dictated by patient compliance or by the request of the dermatologist before the formulator can begin to consider increasing the effect of the vehicle on penetration.

VEHICLES AS PENETRATION ENHANCERS

If one assumes that the skin is a perfect sink, the rate-limiting step for the penetration of a drug will be the presentation of the drug to the skin surface, that is, its release from the vehicle to the skin. A number of factors will influence this step:

1. The solubility of the drug.
2. The concentration of the drug.
3. Replenishment of the skin/vehicle interface.
4. Partitioning of the drug from the vehicle.

DRUG SOLUBILITY

Dempski et al. (1969) sum up the problems of drug solubility by saying that the drug should be "sufficiently soluble ... but not so soluble." Ostrenga et al. (1971) suggest that the concentration of the diffusable drug in the vehicle should be optimized by ensuring that all the drug is in solution. Similarly Iyer and Vasavada (1979) state that drug release is maximum for vehicle systems at near saturation. Busse et al. (1969), using betamethasone derivatives in various ointments, concluded that drug release is greatest from the vehicle in which it is least soluble. Katz and Poulsen (1972) found that the penetration of corticoid was increased by first solubilizing all the corticoid. It appears therefore that the penetration of a drug from a given vehicle can be increased by presenting the drug in a molecular form (i.e., in solution). However it is difficult to elucidate whether solubilizing the drug aids penetration through the skin or simply aids diffusion through the vehicle to replenish the vehicle/skin interface.

Coldman et al. (1969), working in vitro, found that the penetration of fluocinolone acetonide could be increased eightfold by increasing the ratio of volatile to nonvolatile component in the vehicle. On application, the volatile component evaporated, thereby supersaturating the nonvolatile vehicle and providing a greater steroid/skin interface. It is not clear, however, whether the volatile component directly affects the skin lipids and this in turn affects penetration. One wonders whether a layer analogous to the epicutile on the outer aspect of hair shaft cuticle cells is also present on the outer cell layers of the stratum corneum. Solubilizing, or denaturing such a layer may have a marked effect on penetration.

For multiphase vehicle systems (e.g., emulsions), it is important to consider the relative volumes and solubilizing powers of the component phases, since these will affect both the distribution of the drug in and its partitioning from the vehicle. Drug solubility (in a nonvolatile vehicle) should therefore be optimized by using the minimum volume of solvent to completely solubilize the drug, thereby both aiding diffusion through the vehicle and presenting the drug to the skin in a molecular form.

DRUG CONCENTRATION

Obviously the more drug included in the vehicle, the more is available for penetration (Coldman et al. 1969). Higuchi (1960), working in vitro, showed that doubling the drug concentration produced only a 40% increase in penetration. Also the penetration of hydrocortisone butyrate in vitro increases with concentration, though the increase is less than linear (Ponec and Polano, 1972). Similarly the penetration of aliphatic alcohols is not necessarily proportional to an increase in concentration (Drill and Lazar, 1983). Akerman et al. (1979) showed that the anesthetic effects of topical lidocaine on guinea pigs could be increased by increasing its concentration in a dimethylacetamide vehicle. Wurster (1965) points out that it is important to consider the relative concentration of a drug in a multiphase vehicle and indicates that the drug concentration should be optimized in the phase that is in contact with the skin (e.g., oil in the case of a water-in-oil emulsion).

The concentration of the drug in the vehicle directly affects the thermodynamic activity, a product of the concentration and the activity coefficient. Rapid release of the drug depends on a high thermodynamic activity in the vehicle (Higuchi, 1960). For specific drug concentrations the thermodynamic activity may be 1000-fold different from one vehicle to another, making comparison extremely difficult (Drill and Lazar, 1983). Interactions of acidic drugs in basic vehicles and vice versa, and the inclusion of skin secretions to the vehicle after application, would be expected to alter the pH of the system, hence the thermodynamic activity of the drug. One must consider therefore the nature of the dermatoses to be treated when attempting to optimize drug release from a vehicle formulation.

SKIN/VEHICLE INTERFACE

More drug will be absorbed per unit time at a given drug concentration if the treatment is applied to a larger surface area (Guy and Hadgraft, 1980). This may be optimized by ensuring that the maximum concentration of drug per unit area is maintained. One of the major problems of patient compliance with topical preparations is simply a question of "How much do I put on?" This is probably of little importance with aqueous and volatile vehicles, which are easily spread into thin layers. However as the viscosity of the vehicle increases there is a concomitant increase in the thickness of the application, and therefore diffusion through the vehicle to the skin interface may limit drug supply. From the Stokes-Einstein equation (Eq. 1) it can be seen that as the viscosity decreases, the diffusion coefficient increases (Wurster, 1965):

$$D = \frac{Kt}{6\pi r \eta} \tag{1}$$

where D is the diffusion coefficient, K is the Boltzmann constant; η is the viscosity, and r is the radius. It can be assumed that a decrease in the viscosity of the vehicle will favor diffusion through the vehicle and thereby reduce the problem of the thickness of application. One may also assume that both diffusion through the vehicle and diffusion through the skin depend on molecular size. Wurster (1965) has shown that a relatively large increase in molecular size is required before diffusion is significantly reduced. One may assume then, that in contrast to changes in vehicle viscosity, increasing the molecular size of a drug is unlikely to adversely affect percutaneous penetration.

SKIN HYDRATION

Penetration is enhanced by increasing the water content of the skin (Scheuplein, 1978). One possible reason for the discrepancies between in vitro and in vivo experiments is that almost all in vitro work is carried out on skin under maximum conditions of hydration. Fritsch and Stoughton (1963) showed that both increased temperature and increased relative humidity caused an increase in penetration of salicyclic acid through excised human skin. Dutkiewicz (1957) also showed that the cutaneous absorption of aniline was increased by 50% by raising the humidity of the air by 40%. By using two cell systems, one hydrated and one containing a desiccant, Wurster and Kramer (1961) showed that the penetration of salicylate esters through human skin in vivo was significantly enhanced by conditions of increased hydration. There is also a wealth of information regarding increased cutaneous penetration of steroids using occlusive plastic films (McKenzie and Stoughton, 1962; Sulzberger and Witten, 1961), indicating the beneficial effects of increased hydration.

Given the very viscous nature of many dermatological preparations (e.g., petrolatum, white soft paraffin, isopropyl myristate, lanolin) and preparations containing an aqueous phase (e.g., emulsions), we would expect different vehicles to increase the level of hydration of the skin, thereby favoring the release of water-soluble drugs from the vehicle (Wurster and Dempski, 1961) and increasing absorption. Wahlberg (1971), working in vivo with the guinea pig, showed that petrolatum was a preferable vehicle to water for sodium chromate because it provided both stability and reduced transepidermal water loss by virtue of its occlusive properties. It appears that increased occlusivity is a preferable method of hydrating the skin in comparison to applying an aqueous phase to promote penetration (Baker, 1969).

The effect of the vehicle on the degree of hydration of the epidermis is therefore another parameter to be considered in the formulation of a topical preparation.

PARTITION COEFFICIENT

Washitake et al. (1975), studying the absorption of salicylic acid and carboxamine from various oily vehicles, concluded that vehicles with a strong drug affinity showed poor release rates and reduced skin absorption. Zatz and Dalvi (1983), using mouse skin in vitro, also found that by using a water solvent for n-alkanols, an increase in carbon chain length was accompanied by an increase in partition coefficient. Using isopropyl palmitate as the solvent produced an opposite trend. In each case, however, the increase in affinity for the vehicle (i.e., reduced partition coefficient) resulted in a reduction in the degree of penetration. Bronaugh et al. (1981) working in vitro, showed that the penetration of N-nitrosodiethanolamine (NDELA), a normal cosmetic impurity, was 250 times greater through human skin using isopropyl myristate as the solvent than with either propylene glycol or water. The investigators relate this increase to a partition coefficient of NDELA in isopropyl myristate of 230 compared with partition coefficients from propylene glycol and water of approximately 1.8 and 1.0, respectively.

Due to the complex nature of vehicles, partitioning may occur between independent vehicle phases and may be considered to be a rate-limiting step. Little work has been done on phase changes within vehicles, such as phase inversion in emulsions, after application to the skin, and the effect of such changes on the partitioning of the drug from the vehicle (Barry, 1983).

One must also consider that the partition coefficient of the drug from the vehicle to the skin as established for normal skin may not be applicable to diseased skin, where the stratum corneum may be absent. Partitioning is therefore from the vehicle to a more aqueous phase and must be considered in vehicle design.

VEHICLE ADDITIVES

Numerous compounds may be added to dermatologic preparations to enhance the penetration of the effective compound. Many are however limited in their function as vehicles per se by their deleterious effect on the skin, a consideration of paramount importance when dealing with dermatoses in which the skin barrier may already be disrupted. Such compounds may be added to existing formulations in finite amounts to improve the availability of the drug. Numerous compounds have been studied for their effects as penetration enhancers. Among the most popular and regularly used are dimethyl sulfoxide (DMSO) and propylene glycol (PG).

Dimethyl Sulfoxide

After initial fears that DMSO caused changes in the refractive index of the lens of the eye in rabbits, pigs, and dogs, an extensive study by Brobyn (1975) concluded that DMSO was safe to use in humans, causing no such changes to the eye. However, DMSO is a potent irritant, causing a burning sensation on application followed by erythema and prolonged itching (i.e., nonimmunologic contact urticaria). After continued use the skin is often dry and scaly (Goldman et al., 1967), Forster and Stoklaska (1969) also noted that irritation and edema occurred in rat and guinea pig paws after a 1-hr application of 89% DMSO.

Even a brief scan of the literature shows that there is little doubt that DMSO and its associated compounds dimethylformamide and dimethylacetamide can significantly enhance the percutaneous penetration of a number of drugs (Maibach and Feldmann, 1967). Stüttgen and Bauer (1982) showed that both 49 and 99% DMSO increases the uptake of antimycotics into the nail plate. Hwang and Danti (1983), using in vivo studies on the rabbit, concluded that the penetration of flufenamic acid was greatly enhanced by the addition of 5% DMSO. The concentration of DMSO does appear, however, to be vehicle dependent. Sweeney et al. (1966) reported that for a number of compounds dissolved in water and DMSO, below 50% DMSO produced virtually no change in penetration rates, whereas above 60-70% the increase was apparently exponential. However DMSO is not a universal penetration enhancer, as shown by Stelzer et al. (1968), also using the rabbit in vivo. The addition of DMSO did not increase the penetration of sodium salicylate from a polyethylene glycol vehicle. Similarly Cramer and Cates (1974) showed that DMSO would increase the penetration of a polar steroid (hydrocortisone sodium succinate) through rat skin but did not increase the penetration of the highly lipid-soluble cortisone acetate.

The mode of action of DMSO remains speculative. It is a powerful solvent and as has been discussed, solubilizing the drug in the vehicle would be expected to increase skin penetration. DMSO and its acetamide and formamide analogs increase transepidermal water loss (Baker, 1968). Scheuplein (1970) suggests that the intense hygroscopicity causes the displacement of normally bound water to a more structured and loosely bound form. This would enhance the passage of water and other molecules. It is possible that the epidermis holds a large concentration of DMSO and instead of requiring the drug to partition from the vehicle to the skin, may act as a continuous phase through the epidermis. Elfbaum and Laden (1967) showed that the rate constant for DMSO was approximately 100 times greater than for picrate ions, indicating a more rapid and independent transfer through the skin. They also noted that the skin samples after in vitro application of high concentrations of DMSO were more wrinkled and less pliable than the control, buffer-treated sample. DMSO appears then to enhance penetration by either solubilizing the drug in the vehicle or by preceding the compound in penetration and altering the biochemical and structural integrity of the skin.

Propylene Glycol

The addition of propylene glycol will enhance the penetration of a number of compounds, though to a much lesser degree than DMSO. It is however much less irritant.

The literature to date implies that although PG readily penetrates the skin (Poulsen and Ponec, 1976), it does not carry the drug molecule through. It would seem to be more important in the role of a solubilizer. Poulsen and Ponec (1976) found that increasing the concentration of PG increased the penetration of hydrocortisone only up to the point where all the hydrocortisone had been dissolved. Further addition of PG reduced the degree of penetration. The penetration of fluocinilone acetamide in white soft paraffin can be increased by first dissolving in propylene glycol and then dispersing in the vehicle. Portnoy (1965) found that by using this method solubilized fluocinilone acetamide showed greater penetration than when presented as a microcrystalline form. Propylene glycol therefore appears to enhance the penetration of various drugs by presenting them in a molecular form. Its ability to adversely affect partitioning of the drug from the vehicle, at high concentrations, requires that its inclusion to the vehicle be tailored to the drug in question.

The vehicle literature contains many references to penetration enhancers that produce minimal irritation and are of low toxicity. Two recent compounds are:

1. N,N-dimethyl-m-toluamide: Windheuser et al. (1982) found an increased penetration of hydrocortisone in both hairless mouse skin in vitro and human skin in vivo.
2. Azone (1-dodecylazacycloheptan-2-one): Stoughton (1982) found enhanced penetration of a number of germicides and antibiotics. He showed that the penetration of fluoruracil could be increased by 80 times following the addition of 1.8% Azone to the vehicle. Further increases in the concentration of Azone did not increase penetration.

IDEAL VEHICLES

It is obvious that no one universal vehicle will accomplish all the tasks required by the dermatologist. There are however a number of reasonably predictable considerations regarding the formulation of efficient vehicles that will produce more effective topical preparations:

1. The vehicle should be suitable for use in specific dermatoses and preferably should be cosmetically acceptable.
2. Possibly it should be therapeutic in its own right.
3. It should have no or minimum dermal or systemic side effects (e.g., irritant or allergen).
4. It should contain a solubilizer to ensure that all the active compound is in solution.
5. It should be of sufficiently low viscosity to allow diffusion of the drug through it and to allow ease of application.
6. The drug should have a high thermodynamic activity when dissolved in the completed vehicle formulation.
7. The drug/vehicle partition coefficient must favor release of the drug from the vehicle to the skin membrane.

The development of vehicle penetration enhancers allows many technological approaches. The two techniques receiving the greatest attention to date are vasoconstriction assays (largely with corticoids) and in vitro assays. Both allow some degree of extrapolation for in vivo human skin; exact correlations, however, may not be possible at present. Until more is known about the quantitative relationships, we believe that the most exact correlations to the clinical situation will be obtained with in vivo dermatopharmacokinetic studies in appropriate animal models and man.

REFERENCES

Akerman, B., Haegerstorm, G., Pring, R. G., and Sandberg, R. (1979). Penetration enhancers and other factors governing percutaneous local anaethesia with lidocaine. *Acta Pharmacol. Toxicol. 45*: 58–65.

Baker, H. (1968). The effects of dimethyl sulphoxide, dimethyl formamide and dimethyl acetamide on the cutaneous barrier to water in the skin. *J. Invest. Dermatol. 50*: 283.

Baker, H. (1969). Experimental studies on the influence of vehicles on percutaneous absorption. *J. Soc. Cosmet. Chem. 20*: 239.

Barry, B. W. (1983). Dermatological formulations. Percutaneous absorption. In *Drugs and Pharmaceutical Sciences*, Vol. 18. Dekker, New York.

Brobyn, R. D. (1975). In *Biological Actions of Dimethyl Sulphoxide*. Edited by S. W. Jacob and R. Herschler. *Ann. N.Y. Acad. Sci. 243*: 497.

Bronaugh, R. L., Congolon, E. R., and Scheuplein, R. J. (1981). The effect of cosmetic vehicles on the penetration of *N*-nitrodiethanolamine through excised human skin. *J. Invest. Dermatol. 76*: 94-96.

Busse, M. J., Hunt, P., Lees, K. A., Maggs, P. N. D., and McCarthy, T. M. (1969). Release of betamethasone derivatives from ointments—In vivo and in vitro studies. *Br. J. Dermatol. 81*: 103.

Christie, G. A. and Moore-Robinson, M. (1970). Vehicle assessment—Methodology and results. *Br. J. Dermatol. 82*: 93.

Coldman, M. F., Poulsen, B. J., and Higuchi, T. (1969). Enhancement of percutaneous absorption by the use of volatile:nonvolatile systems as vehicles. *J. Pharm. Sci. 58*: 1098.

Cramer, M. B. and Cates, L. A. (1974). Effects of DMSO and trimethylphosphine oxide on the percutaneous absorption of corticosteroids in the rat. *J. Pharm. Sci. 63*: 793.

Dempski, R. E., Portnoff, J. B., and Lase, A. W. (1969). In vitro release and in vivo penetration studies of a topical steroid from non-aqueous vehicles. *J. Pharm. Sci. 58*: 579.

Drill, V. A. and Lazar, P., Editors. (1983). *Cutaneous Toxicology*. Target Organ Toxicology Series. Raven, New York.

Dutkiewicz, T. (1957). *Med. Pracy. 8*: 25.

Elfbaum, S. G. and Laden, K. (1967). The effect of DMSO on percutaneous absorption. A mechanistic study. *J. Soc. Cosmet. Chem. 19*: 119-127.

Feldmann, R. J. and Maibach, H. I. (1966). Percutaneous penetration of [^{14}C]-hydrocortisone in man. II. Effect of certain bases and pretreatments. *Arch. Dermatol. 94*: 649-651.

Forster, O. and Stoklaska, E. (1969). The effect of repeated application of dimethyl sulphoxide to paws of rats and guinea pigs. *Pharmacology 2*: 9-13.

Fritsch, W. C. and Stoughton, R. B. (1963). The effect of temperature and humidity on the penetration of [^{14}C] acetylsalicylic acid in excised human skin. *J. Invest. Dermatol. 41*: 307.

Goldman, L., Ingleman, J. M., and Kitzmiller, K. (1967). Investigative studies with DMSO in dermatology. *Ann. N.Y. Acad. Sci. 141*: 428.

Guy, R. H. and Hadgraft, J. (1980). A theoretical description relating skin penetration to the thickness of the applied medicament. *Int. J. Pharm. 6*: 321-332.

Higuchi, T. (1960). Physical chemical analysis of percutaneous absorption process from creams and ointments. *J. Soc. Cosmet. Chem. 11*: 85.

Hwang, C. C. and Danti, A. C. (1983). The percutaneous absorption of flufenamic acid in rabbits. Effect of various nonionic surface active agents. *J. Pharm. Sci. 72*: 857.

Iyer, B. V. and Vasavada, R. C. (1979). Evaluation of lanolin alcohol films and kinetics of triamcinolone acetonide release. *J. Pharm. Sci. 68*: 782-787.

Jimbo, Y., Ishihara, M., Osamura, H., Takano, M., and Ohara, M. (1983). Influence of vehicles on penetration through human epidermis of benzyl alcohol, isoeugenol and methyl isoeugenol. *J. Dermatol. (Japan) 10*: 241.

Katz, M. and Poulsen, B. J. (1972). Corticoid, vehicle, and skin interaction in percutaneous absorption. *J. Soc. Cosmet. Chem. 23*: 565-590.

McKenzie, A. W. and Stoughton, R. D. (1962). Method for comparing the percutaneous absorption of steroids. *Arch. Dermatol. 86*: 608-610.

Ostrenga, J., Steinmetz, C., and Poulsen, B. (1971). Significance of vehicle composition. I. Relationship between topical vehicle composition, skin permeability and clinical efficacy. *J. Pharm. Sci. 60*: 1175.

Polano, M. K. and Ponec, M. (1976). Dependance of corticosteroid penetration on the vehicle. *Arch. Dermatol. 112*: 675-680.

Ponec, M. and Polano, M. K. (1972). Hydrocortisone butyrate penetration through the epidermis in vitro. *Arch. Dermatol. Forsch. 245*: 381-389.

Portnoy, B. (1965). The effect of formulation on the clinical response of topical fluocinolone acetonide. *Br. J. Dermatol. 77*: 579-581.

Scheuplein, R. J. (1978). Permeability of skin: A review of major concepts. *Curr. Probl. Dermatol. 7*: 58-68.

Scheuplein, R. J. and Ross, A. B. (1968). Effects of surfactants.

Stelzer, J. M., Colaizzi, J. L., and Wurdack, P. J. (1968). Influence of DMSO on the percutaneous absorption of salicylic acid and sodium salicylate from ointments. *J. Pharm. Sci. 57*: 1732-1737.

Stoughton, R. B. (1982). Enhanced percutaneous penetration with 1-dodecylazacycloheptan-2-one (Azone). *Arch. Dermatol. 118*: 474-477.

Stüttgen, G. and Bauer, E. (1982). Bioavailability, skin and nail penetration of topically applied antimycotics. *Mykosen 25*: 74-80.

Sulzberger, M. B. and Witten, V. H. (1961). Thin pliable plastic films in topical dermatological therapy. *Arch. Dermatol. 84*: 1027.

Sweeney, (1966). The effects of DMSO on the epidermal water barrier. *J. Invest. Dermatol. 46*: 300.

Tissot, J. and Osmundson, P. E. (1966). Influence of vehicles on the topical activity of fluorometholone. *Acta Dermatovenereol.* (Stockholm) *46*: 447-452.

Wahlberg, J. E. (1971). The vehicle role of petrolatum. *Acta Dermatovenereol.* (Stockholm) *51*: 129-134.

Washitake, M., Anma, T., Tanaka, I., Arita, T., and Nakano, M. (1975). Percutaneous absorption of drugs. IV. Percutaneous absorption of drugs from oily vehicles. *J. Pharm. Sci. 64*: 397-401.

Windheuser, J. J., Haslam, J. L., Caldwell, L., and Shaffer, R. (1982). The use of *N,N*-diethyl-*m*-toluamide to enhance the transdermal delivery of drugs. *J. Pharm. Sci. 71*: 1211.

Wurster, D. E. (1965). Some factors related to the formulation of preparations for percutaneous absorption. *Am. Perf. Cosmet. 80*: 21-28.

Wurster, D. E. and Dempski, R. E. (1960). Adsorption of lipid-soluble substances by human keratin. *J. Am. Pharm. Assoc. 49*.

Wurster, D. E. and Kramer, S. F. (1961). Investigation of some factors influencing percutaneous absorption. *J. Pharm. Sci. 50*: 288-293.

Zatz, J. L. and Dalvi, E. R. (1983). Evaluation of solvent-skin interaction in percutaneous absorption. *J. Soc. Cosmet. Chem. 34*: 327-334.

44
Effect of a Water Vapor-Permeable Film on the Percutaneous Penetration of Hydrocortisone

Dennis M. Anjo* and Howard I. Maibach
University of California School of Medicine, San Francisco, California

Although considerable enhancement of corticoid efficacy is made possible by the use of appropriate vehicles, no presently available vehicle system promotes penetration to that obtained with occlusion (Feldmann and Maibach, 1965; Maibach and Feldmann, 1967). The mechanism of penetration enhancement with occlusion is incompletely understood. This chapter utilizes a water vapor permeable film to inspect one possible mechanism, namely, that related to the prevention of loss of chemical from the skin.

MATERIALS AND METHODS

Absorption was quantified on the basis of the percentage of radioactivity excreted in urine for 6 days following application of a known amount of the labeled compound to the skin. This method, used for measuring in vivo percutaneous penetration, is the procedure of Feldmann and Maibach adapted to the rhesus monkey. Methodology is detailed elsewhere (Maibach and Feldmann, 1967).

Rhesus monkeys (4-8 kg) trained for metabolic studies were randomly selected from the colony. To be selected, the monkeys had to be clear of any previously administered ^{14}C-labeled compound. Hydrocortisone labeled with radioactive carbon, 0.35 μCi, was applied to lightly clipper-shaved skin of the ventral forearm with a dose of 4 μg/cm^2. Previous experience with testosterone absorption suggests that clipper shaving does not alter penetration in this animal (Wester and Maibach, 1975). The area was not occluded in the control experiment.

---

*Present affiliation: California State University, Long Beach, California

For the covered experiment the same monkeys were prepared in like manner but the applied hydrocortisone was covered with Gortex laminate cloth, held at the edges with adhesive tape. The cloth was large enough that no tape was near the applied compound. The monkeys were placed in metabolism chairs; their hands were secured to avoid wiping off the applied compound.

Hydrocortisone labeled with ^{14}C was applied to the skin in acetone; the solvent was quickly evaporated by gentle blowing, leaving pure compound in situ.

The concentration of hydrocortisone applied to the skin was 4 $\mu g/cm^2$. An application of 4 $\mu g/cm^2$ is the amount deposited by a thin film of 0.25% solution. The applied concentrations were relevant to the clinical situation. The application site was washed with soap and water at 24 hr and the monkey returned to the metabolic chair to continue the urine collection. In the metabolic chair, a barrier totally separates the site of applications from the area of urine collection. This ensures against any possibility of chemical falling off the skin and contaminating the urine.

Urinary excretion values were corrected for excretion of radioactivity by other routes and for retention of radioactivity in the body by using data obtained from administration of an intravenous dose of ^{14}C-labeled hydrocortisone (Feldmann and Maibach, 1965).

Urine was wet washed and the [^{14}C]CO$_2$ trapped and prepared for liquid scintillation counting (Maibach and Feldmann, 1967). A microcomputer was utilized for calculation.

The Gortex laminate film, fabricated of expanded polytetrafluoroethylene, has 9 billion pores/in. Each pore is 20,000 times smaller than a water drop yet 700 times larger than a vapor molecule. This film prevents penetration by liquid water while allowing the diffusion of moisture vapor—as if the film was not there.

RESULTS

The excretion from control animals at 144 hr was 8.008, 5.965, and 2.041% (average of 5.34 ±3.3%) of the applied dose. With the laminate cloth covered animals, the excretion was 3.308, 2.906, and 5.359% (average of 3.860 ±1.311%) (Table 1). Because the same animals were used for both experiments, a paired comparison was done. Using Student's t comparison, two experiments were not significantly different (p = 0.548).

DISCUSSION

Previous studies with occlusion such as in biological assays (vasoconstriction) or in direct permeability measurements (urinary and fecal excretion) demonstrate that occlusion enhances penetration greatly (Feldmann and Maibach, 1965;

Table 1 Penetration (% of applied dose)

Monkey	Time (hr)									
	0–4	4–8	8–12	12–24	24–48	48–72	72–96	96–120	120–144	0–144
	Hydrocortisone under water vapor-permeable film									
1	0.0345	0.0655	0.00238	0.136	0.298	0.563	1.803	0.061	0.324	3.308
2	0.0262	0.0750	0.0357	0.2001	0.539	0.689	0.594	0.347	0.404	2.906
3	0.0298	0.476	a	0.281	0.667	1.308	1.540	0.782	0.704	5.359
							Average		3.860	
							S.D.		1.314	
	Hydrocortisone control (without a film cover)									
1	0.0607	0.101	0.133	0.745	1.821	2.178	0.966	0.981	1.021	8.008
2	0.0143	0.0584	a	0.354	1.159	1.409	1.278	1.730	1.100	5.965
3	0.0155	a	a	0.431	0.441	0.467	0.362	0.311	0.637	2.041
							Average		5.34	
							S.D.		3.3	

aNo urine voided.

McKenzie, 1962). With hydrocortisone on human skin, the enhancement factor is approximately 10-fold (Feldmann and Maibach, 1965).

Studies of the effect of certain chemicals on mitotic rate in human skin showed a distinct enhancement of activity with topical administration from nonocclusive adhesive tape systems (Fisher et al., 1978). Presumably, either this tape system has a penetration-enhancing effect different from that of this film or a different mechanism of antimitotic action is involved. The latter is a distinct possibility, since nonocclusive adhesive tape is antimitotic by itself (Fisher et al., 1978).

The data from the present experiment suggest that keeping hydrocortisone on skin by preventing its loss through rubbing, movement, and sweating does not—in the system evaluated—enhance penetration. We doubt that increased temperatures under occlusion play a significant part in enhancing penetration, for actual temperature measurements show that several plastic films allow for heat release, so that elevated temperature does not occur. The water content of skin, not affected by the film in this experiment, is a likely candidate for further study in terms of the penetration enhancing factor.

The data suggest that the more comfortable laminate cloth will probably not offer the dermatologic patient the efficacy found with water-impermeable occlusive fabric. This hypothesis must still be verified in a clinical trial. Furthermore, we would not extend this lack of effect of water-permeable laminate cloth or penetration to other chemicals until such are specifically studied. Certain easily washed or rubbed off chemicals might offer more promise for increased efficacy with this approach. In this model the sparingly soluble hydrocortisone alcohol might be handled differently from more water-soluble compounds.

As an incidental comment, if this laminate does not enhance penetration, it may be a useful cover over skin-drug application sites to prevent contamination of metabolic cases.

REFERENCES

Feldmann, R. J. and Maibach, H. I. (1965). Penetration of [^{14}C] hydrocortisone through normal skin. *Arch. Dermatol. 91*: 661-666.

Fisher, L. B., Maibach, H. I., and Trancik, R. J. (1978). Effects of occlusive tape systems on the mitotic activity of epidermis. *Arch. Dermatol. 114*: 384-386.

Maibach, H. I. and Feldmann, R. J. (1967). The effect of DMSO on percutaneous penetration of hydrocortisone and testosterone in man. *Ann. N.Y. Acad. Sci. 141*: 423-427.

McKenzie, A. W. (1962). Percutaneous absorption of steroids. *Arch. Dermatol. 86*: 611.

Wester, R. C. and Maibach, H. I. (1975). Rhesus monkey as an animal model for percutaneous penetration. In *Animal Models in Dermatology*. Edited by H. I. Maibach. Churchill-Livingstone, New York, pp. 133-137.

Index

Acetylsalicylic acid (*see also* Aspirin), 270, 530
Activation energy, 98
Aflatoxin (*see also* Mycotoxin), 388, 423
Air flow, 314
Air temperature, 315
Albumin, 47
Alcohols, 219
Alopecia, 546
Animal model, 192, 251-266, 269, 273, 309
Anthralin, 296
Apocrine glands, 290
Artificial membranes (*see also* Synthetic membranes), 373-386, 443
Aspirin, 480
Azone, 493, 523, 565

Benzo(a)pyrene, 69
Benzoic acid, 270, 309
Benzyl alcohol, 491
Binding, 43-56, 284
  drug, 11
  protein, 43

Bioavailability, 87, 248, 489, 543
Biological response, 247
Blanching, 337
Blood flow (*see also* Capillaries), 393-407, 545
Body surface area, 463
Butanol, 491
Butyl acetate, 491
Butylated hydroxytoluene, 153-163

Caffeine, 309
Capillaries, 335
Cat, 260
Cinnamyl anthranilate, 271
Chimpanzee, 260
Compartments
  pharmacokinetic model, 291
  skin, 165
  stratum corneum, 165
Concentration profile, 282
Cortisol, 44, 45
Cortisone, 272, 359
Corticosteroids, systemic effects, 511-521
Corticosterone, 44, 45
Cyproterone acetate, 291

DDT, 316
Decontamination, 327–333, 363
Decylmethyl sulfoxide, 524
Depilatory, 145
Deposition, 141–152
Dermatome, 268
Dermis, 335–346
Desoxymethasone, 290
Dexamethasone, 44, 469
Diethyl malonate, 316
N,N-Diethy-m-toluimide, 309
Diffusion, 3–15, 523
  cell, 99, 261, 268, 307, 448
  coefficient, 62, 340, 375, 490
  through stratum corneum, 10, 282
  through viable epidermis, 16, 282
Diisopropyl fluorophosphate, 316
Dimethyl acetamide, 493
Dimethylformamide, 493, 526
Diseased skin, 129, 292–295
  acne, 506
  eczema, 292, 506
  icthyosis, 506
  models, 294–295
  mycosis fungoides, 131
  psoriasis, 130, 292, 506
DMSO, 453, 482, 493, 526, 564
Dog, 260, 530
Dose, 347–357, 398, 548
  concentration, 125, 317, 540, 561
  finite, 175, 444
  infinite, 6, 168
  multiple, 11, 237, 352
  regimen, 125, 297
  surface area, 125, 354, 540
  time of exposure, 125
  washing, 237, 363
Drug delivery
  blood, 537
  muscle, 469–487, 537
  nitroglycerin, 539–544
  periarticular tissue
  subcutaneous, 485
Drug metabolism, 284
Drug release, thermodynamic control, 437

Epidermal tumors, 127
Erythema, 336
Escin, 336, 482
Essential fatty acid deficiency, 294
Estradiol, 472
Evaporation, 305–325

Facilitated transport, 87–95
Fatty acids, 219, 288
Forearm, 227
Fick's law, 3, 58, 340
Flufenamic acid, 472
Fluocinolone acetonide, 309, 435
Foreskin
  adult, 225, 261
  newborn, 225, 261
Fragrances, 276
Fuzzy rat, 188

Goat, 260
Griseofulvin, 493
Guinea pig, 153, 256, 359, 363

Hair dye, 409–422
Hairless mouse, 142–147, 150, 259
Hairless rat, 259
Hand, 227
Heptane, 491
Histoautoradiography, 283
Horse, 260
Human, 133, 144–147, 150, 213, 252, 409, 423, 529, 545
Humidity, 234, 315
Hydration, 231, 562
Hydrocortisone, 8, 45, 66, 137, 327, 462, 569
Hydrophilic ointment, 360
Hydrophobic compounds, 270, 387
Hydrophobic membranes, 442

Ibuprofen, 495
In vitro techniques, 267–279

Index

In vivo methods, 245-249
Indomethacin, 10, 479
Infant, 213-222, 261
Isopropyl fluorophosphate, 472
Isopropyl myristate, 491

Knee synovitis, 531

Lag-time, 8
Laser Doppler velocimetry, 393, 545
Leg, 227
Lidocaine hydrochloride, 45
Lindane, 45, 309
Lipids, 133

Malathion, 45, 52, 309, 329, 462, 472
Mercuric chloride, 45
Metabolism, 57-64, 65-85, 426
    conjugation, 68
    enzyme induction, 76
    hydrolytic reaction
Methotrexate, 10
8-Methoxypsoralen, 44, 289
Methyl nicotinate, 336
3-Methylcholanthrene, 73
Minoxidil, 396, 545
Model
    capillary diffusion, 343
    computer simulation, 165-180
    mathmatical, 3-15
    multicompartmented membrane, 165-180
    pharmacokinetic, 3, 401
    skin barrier, 35
Monkey, 254, 359, 363, 409, 569
Mosquito repellents, 305-325
Mouse, 259
Mycotoxin, 423-429
    aflatoxin, 423
    T-2 toxin, 423

Newborn, 213, 225, 261, 351, 463

Nitroaromatic compounds, 275
Nitro-BID, 543
Nitrodisc, 541
Nitro-DUR, 543
Nitroglycerin, 396, 539-544
Nonionic surfactant
    octoxynol 9 (Triton X-100), 271, 388
    oleth 20 (Volpo 20), 271
Norepinephrine, 10
Nude rat, 259

Occlusion, 97, 131, 513, 569
Oleic acid, 494, 526
Organic solvents, 137

Paraquat, 227-230
Parathion, 45, 309, 329, 388, 462, 472
Partition, 46
Partition coefficient, 98, 107, 276, 490, 563
    skin-vehicle, 5
    stratum corneum-epidermis, 8
Penetration
    amphiphilic molecule, 119
    delipidization, 133-139
    dipole moment, 119
    enhancers, 33, 489, 523, 559
    hair follicles, 535
    ionization, 119
    kinetics, 396
    lipid pathways, 35
    molecular weight, 118
    parallel pathways, 20
    physicochemical effects, 21, 25
    polar pathways, 37
    shunt routes, 505
Permeability constant, 98, 198, 446
Permeation
    and partitioning, 21, 25
    age, effect of, 183-212, 213, 223, 463

[Permeation]
  chemical and thermal action, effect of, 32
  hydration, effect of, 231
  mechanism, 191
  non steady-state, 58, 168, 295
  pH, 29, 120
  phenol, effect of, 34
  sex, effect of, 201, 273, 274
  steady-state, 58, 188
  of stripped skin, 30
  of viable epidermis and dermis, 31
  of weak electrolytes, 28
Pharmacodynamics, 545–558
Pharmacokinetics, 153–163, 281, 338
Photopulse plethysmography, 393, 545
Pig, 309
Polychlorinated biphenyls (PCBs), 328, 363–372
Prodrugs, 58, 61, 64, 506
Progesterone, 309, 472
Propylene glycol, 494, 526, 565
Pyrolidones, 493

Rabbit, 252
Radial transport, 335–356
Radioactivity
  blood, 246
  excreta, 246
Rat, 142–150, 252
Receptor fluid, 271, 387
Reservoir, 8, 11, 44, 493, 557
Resorption, 281–303
Rubbing, 359–361

Safrole, 276
Salicylate, 90, 480, 530
Scalp, 545
Scopolamine, 10
Serum, 388
Sink, 335

Skin
  appendages, 284
  layer localization, 281–303
  sections, 283, 284
  storage, 312
  surface biopsy, 282
  thickness, 194
Soap, 141–151
Sodium lauryl sulfate, 388
Soman, 322
Stratum corneum, 412
  diffusion, 97, 98
  hydration, 97
  stratum compactum, 287
  thickness, 97, 98, 101, 273
Structure-activity correlations, 107–123
Substantivity, 3, 150, 332
Suction blister technique, 282
Surface disappearance, 247
Surface recovery, 247
Synthetic membranes (*see also* Artificial membranes), 373–386, 439

Tape stripping, 282, 283, 285, 542
Temperature, 97, 234, 352
Testosterone, 11, 44, 45, 51, 66, 272, 309
Thermodynamic activity, 454, 489, 561
Thyropyronine, 44, 48
Toluene, 491
Total body exposure, 461–466
Transdermal delivery, 8, 10, 529
Transdermal device
  formulation, 542
  thickness, 541
Transepidermal pathway, 205
Transepidermal water loss, 98–104, 185
Transfollicular pathway, 201
Transport coefficient, 339
Triamcinolone acetonide, 45

Index

3,4,4'-Trichlorocarbanilide (Triclocarban), 141–151, 223–226
Triethanolamine, 529
Triethanolamine salicylate, 480, 529
Triphenylstibine sulfide, 286

Ultraviolet (UV) irradiation, 289
Urea, 270, 494, 524

Vapor pressure, 120, 315
Variability
  individual, 128, 223

[Variability]
  site, 128, 183, 273, 274, 461
Vasoconstriction, 337
  assay, 490
Vasodilation, 402, 545
Vehicle, 317, 523–527, 559–568
  dynamics, 451
  thickness, 8
Volatility (*see also* Evaporation), 3, 305

Wash, 363
Water, 99, 134